Clinical Practice in Sexually Transmissible Diseases

Clinical Practice in Sexually Transmissible Diseases

D. H. H. Robertson
MB ChB FRCP(Ed) DTM&H(Liverpool)
Consultant Physician, Department of Genito-Urinary Medicine, Royal Infirmary of Edinburgh; Senior Lecturer, Genito-Urinary Medicine Unit, Department of Medicine, University of Edinburgh

A. McMillan
BSc MD FRCP(Ed)
Consultant Physician, Department of Genito-Urinary Medicine, Royal Infirmary of Edinburgh; Senior Lecturer, Genito-Urinary Medicine Unit, Department of Medicine, University of Edinburgh

H. Young
BSc PhD MRCPath
Senior Lecturer, Department of Bacteriology, University of Edinburgh, and Royal Infirmary of Edinburgh

SECOND EDITION

CHURCHILL LIVINGSTONE
EDINBURGH LONDON MELBOURNE AND NEW YORK 1989

CHURCHILL LIVINGSTONE
Medical Division of Longman Group UK Limited

Distributed in the United States of America by Churchill
Livingstone Inc., 1560 Broadway, New York, N.Y. 10036,
and by associated companies, branches and representatives
throughout the world.

First Edition (Published by Pitman Medical Limited) 1980
Second edition 1989

ISBN 0-443-03260-2

British Library Cataloguing in Publication Data
Robertson, D. H. H. (David Hunter
    Henderson), *1924–*
    Clinical practice in sexually transmissible
    diseases — 2nd ed.
    1. Man. Sexually transmitted diseases
    I. Title   II. McMillan, A. (Alexander)
    1947–   III. Young, H. (Hugh), *1945–*
    616.95'1

Library of Congress Cataloging in Publication Data
Robertson, D. H. H. (David Hunter Henderson)
    Clinical practice in sexually transmissible diseases /
    D. H. H. Robertson, A. McMillan, H. Young. — 2nd ed.
        p.   cm.
    Includes index.
    1. Sexually transmitted diseases. I. McMillan, Alexander.
    II. Young, Hugh, 1945–   III. Title.
    [DNLM: 1. Sexually Transmitted Diseases. WC.140 R649c]
    RC200.R63 1989
    616.95'1 — dc19

Printed in Great Britain at The Bath Press, Avon

Preface to the Second Edition

The objectives of this second edition continue to be those outlined in the preface to the first. The nine years that have passed have brought many scientific advances and it has been our fascinating task to incorporate these and develop the text, which has been rewritten virtually in its entirety.

In Chapter 1 we have described the pattern of human sexual behaviour as the background to infection and assembled information which sheds light on its nature and evolution. In Chapter 2 we have given attention to the taxonomy and classification of the infective organisms or agents referred to in the book. We hope these chapters will help clinicians to develop or renew their understanding of these subjects. A new chapter has been devoted to the problems arising from infection with the human immunodeficiency viruses (HIV), and other persistent virus infections have been given fuller attention. The opportunistic pathogens which are such an important feature of HIV infection are considered in Chapter 2 and again from the clinical point of view in Chapter 31. Much new and important information has been assembled relating to the classical sexually transmitted pathogens and in particular to *Neisseria gonorrhoeae* and *Treponema pallidum*. Epidemiological, psychosocial and educational matters are touched upon in Chapters 3–5 and an approach to the clinical investigation of the patient is outlined in Chapter 6. The book covers those sexually transmissible diseases in which the traditional clinical services have been very effective in specific diagnosis, effective specific treatment and contact tracing, activities where secondary prevention is of prime importance as a method of control. Much of the book, however, is devoted to persistent virus infections in which primary prevention provides only a weak and uncertain means of control. In this connection the impact of the human immunodeficiency viruses has set in train extremes of suffering for the patient and testing questions for society. Far-reaching complexities also surround papillomavirus infection, not least in the organization of life-long follow-up of women.

Sound knowledge of the sexually transmissible diseases and firm application of principles developed in this subject remain among the indispensible essentials of medical practice.

Edinburgh, 1989   D.H.H.R.
                                   A.M.
                                   H.Y.

Preface to the First Edition

This book has been written primarily for those who are actively engaged in the increasingly demanding clinical practice of venereology and who, by so doing in the United Kingdom at least, now tend to undertake so large a part of the primary care of adolescents and young adults. We have attempted to bring together information which is widely scattered in the literature and to present an appreciation of clinical and laboratory aspects of the various subjects in a way which we believe will be useful to our colleagues. It is our hope that the book will be of value, as a reference in teaching and also to the wider range of clinicians, for instance gynaecologists and urologists, who participate as we do in the practice of sexual and reproductive medicine and will therefore often require to consider the full range of sexually transmitted diseases. General practitioners and other clinicians, who are involved in clinics set up for counselling and for giving contraceptive and kindred advice, will find some answers to their questions, and physicians, who may not ordinarily look after adolescents and youngs adults, may find the inclusion of sexually transmissible infections in their differential diagnosis a rewarding exercise. It is clear that when precise information about the organisms involved is regarded as an essential discipline in the diagnosis of genito-urinary and pelvic inflammatory disease, the importance of transmission by sexual intercourse will become better appreciated and the application of isolation methods, more searching than conventional bacteriological investigations, will help in developing more rational care of patients.

Although this book is primarily for medical readers it is hoped that those involved in nursing or counselling patients, tracing contacts or in health education will be able to obtain some of the factual information which they require. Barriers between disciplines are tending to become inappropriate and those who share objectives in patient care will require to pool their knowledge to obtain the best results possible.

There is more to be achieved by those concerned than a technical understanding of one aspect of clinical medicine and microbiology because psychological and social barriers intrude and hamper at every level. Some aims of this text are primarily intellectual and are fundamental to practice in a subject which involves deep personal feelings to such an extent that patient, doctor and society may appear not infrequently to be bewitched. The reader will be encouraged to adopt a logical attitude essential in clinical practice and an approach to the subject based on an acceptance of human diversity.

Edinburgh, 1980

D.H.H.R.
A.M.
H.Y.

Acknowledgements

We wish to acknowledge the advice, help and discussion given by many friends and colleagues in the Royal Infirmary of Edinburgh and University of Edinburgh. We wish to give our appreciation and thanks also to: Professor R. V. Short, Professor of Reproductive Biology, Monash University, Melbourne, Australia, and the publishers, Australian Academy of Science, for permission to use Figs. 1.1 and 1.2; Professor J. M. Tanner, Professor of Child Health and Growth at the Institute of Child Health, University of London, and Honorary Consultant Physician at the Hospital for Sick Children, Great Ormond Street, London, and the publishers, Open Books Publishing Ltd., London, for permission to use Figs. 1.3 and 1.4; Professor D. C. G. Skegg, Professor of Preventive and Social Medicine, University of Otago, Dunedin, New Zealand, and the *Lancet*, 7 Adam Street, London, for permission to use Fig. 1.6. Fig. 1.7 is derived from data which is Crown copyright and is reproduced with permission of the Controller of Her Majesty's Stationery Office. The authors also wish to give their appreciation and thanks to: Ms Kathleen E. Kiernan for permission to use data from which Fig. 1.8 is derived; Ms Audrey C. Brown of the Office of Population Censuses and Survey and Ms Kathleen E. Kiernan, Centre for Population Studies, London School of Hygiene and Tropical Medicine, for permission to use data from which Fig. 1.9 is derived; Dr Philip Blumstein and Dr Pepper Schwartz of the University of Washington, USA, for permission to use data from their book *American Couples*, William Morrow and Co., New York (1983), from which Figs. 1.10, 1.11 and 1.13 have been constructed; Professor A. P. Bell and Professor M. S. Weinberg of Indiana University, USA, for permission to use data from their book *Homosexualities: A Study of Diversity among Men and Women*, Simon and Schuster, New York (1978), from which Figs. 1.12 and 1.14 and Table 1.5 have been constructed; Dr H. Alzate of the University of Caldas, Manizales, Colombia, and the publisher of *Archives of Sexual Behaviour*, Plenum Publishing Corporation, New York, for permission to include the data shown in Table 1.3; Professor Harold T. Christensen, Professor Emeritus of Sociology, Purdue University, Lafayette, Indiana, for permission to include data in Table 1.1; Professor B. Roizman, Joseph Regenstein Distinguished Service Professor and Chairman, Department of Molecular Genetics and Cell Biology, The University of Chicago, for his courtesy and help in connection with matters relating to the taxonomy of human herpes viruses; Dr Mary P. English, formerly Consultant Mycologist, Bristol Royal Infirmary and Research Fellow, University of Bristol and Dr P. M. Stockdale, Commonwealth Mycological Institute, Ferry Lane, Kew, Surrey, for their help with taxonomy; The World Health Organization, Geneva, for permission to include Figures 3.1 and 3.8; The Office of Health Economics, 195 Knightsbridge, London SW7, for permission to use Figs. 3.2, 3.3 and 3.4; Dr D. B. L. McClelland, Regional Director, Edinburgh, and South East Scotland Regional Blood Transfusion Centre, Royal Infirmary of Edinburgh, for helpful discussion and information in connection with the precautions used against HIV infection; The Health Education Council, 78 New Oxford Street, London, and Mr Colin Forbes, Marketing Director of Forbes Publications Limited, 120 Bayswater Road, London W2 3JH, for permission to include material from *The Schools Council's Project* on Health Education as detailed in Chapter 4; Dr M. S. R. Hutt, Geographical Pathology Unit, Department of Histopathology, St Thomas's Hospital Medical School, London, and the *British Medical Bulletin* (Churchill Livingstone, Publishers) for permission to use data on the proportional frequencies of endemic (African) Kaposi's sarcoma given in Chapter 5; Mrs Catherine Harrison, Research Associate, Department of Genito-Urinary Medicine and Mr Ray Harris of the Drummond Street Reprographics Unit, University of Edinburgh, for their help in the preparation of the world map in Figures 5.1, 13.1, 13.2 and 31.3; The Organizer of National External

Quality Assessment Scheme, Dr. J. J. S. Snell of the Division of Microbiological Reagents and Quality Control, Public Health Laboratory Service, 61 Colindale Avenue, London NW9 5HT, for permission to publish the data in Table 8.3; Ms Anne B. Prasad, Executive Editor, British National Formulary, for her patient help and correspondence which encouraged the present authors to try to bring reason into statements of penicillin dosage in Chapter 10 particularly; Dr Clive Osmond and other members of the MRC Environmental Epidemiology Unit, University of Southampton, for their permission to use diagrams on cervical cancer in Chapter 25, namely Figs. 25.1 and 25.2 (these figures are Crown copyright, reproduced with permission of the Controller of Her Majesty's Stationery Office); Wellcome Foundation Ltd. for permission to use information from recent data sheets on Zovirax (acyclovir) and Retrovir (zidovudine) respectively in Chapters 26 and 31; Professor L. G. Whitby, Professor I. W. Percy-Robb, Dr A. F. Smith and Blackwell Scientific Publications, who have kindly agreed to allow us to use extracts from their book *Lecture Notes on Clinical Chemistry*, 3rd edition, 1984, as a note to our chapter on Viral Hepatitis (Note 30.1); Dr B. G. Gazzard, Dr D. C. Shanson and the *Lancet* for permission to include Fig. 31.2; Mr Paul E. Bishop, Research Associate, Department of Genito-Urinary Medicine, University of Edinburgh, for his kindness in preparing Note 31.4; Professor Kenneth Mellanby, Monks Wood Experimental Station, Abbots Ripton, Huntingdon, for permission to include Fig. 36.1; Dr J. F. Peutherer and Dr I. W. Smith, Senior Lecturers, Department of Bacteriology, University of Edinburgh, for much help and advice on virus disease; Dr R. Heyworth, Senior Biochemist, Department of Clinical Chemistry, Royal Infirmary of Edinburgh, for his help and advice.

The contribution of members of the Department of Medical Illustration of the University of Edinburgh is gratefully acknowledged. The authors wish to thank Mrs J. M. Gilbertson for her skill in applying modern technology in the preparation of the manuscript and for her patience and help.

The authors are also indebted to the staff of Churchill Livingstone, Edinburgh, our publishers, for their encouragement and help.

Edinburgh, 1989   D.H.H.R.
A.M.
H.Y.

Contents

1

Human sexuality: the background to infection

In their classic comparative study of sexual behaviour patterns in contemporary societies, ranging from the isolated primitive to the industrialized and urban, Ford & Beach (1952) identify two main themes. The first relates to activities which are a direct expression of the biological nature of man whereas the other relates to activities derived from social customs and pressures, which differ widely from one society to another. Human sexual responses are not instinctive in the sense of being determined exclusively by the action of genes but are to a large extent taught and indeed in some societies children may learn that sex is a subject to be avoided. Adult members of different societies have very different ideas as to what is proper or normal in sexual relations and what is immoral. In the scientific appraisal of human sexuality avoidance of value judgements by students is an essential and insight is to be gained from cross-cultural and cross-species studies. With the extreme privacy that human societies insist upon in matters of sex and the difficulties in making direct observations, an appreciation of the patterns of sexual behaviour in other mammals, and in primates in particular, provides a significant starting point for such an analysis in mankind.

In this chapter the term sexual behaviour is used to refer exclusively to behaviour which involves stimulation and excitation of the sexual organs and which may bring risks of acquiring infection. For those who wish to understand sexual tendencies and habits of humans, whether hetero-, homo- or bisexual, this goal cannot be reached merely by introspection but only by very much wider study and research (Ford & Beach 1952).

EVOLUTION AND COMPARATIVE ANATOMY IN HUMAN SEXUALITY

In all living species of primate which exhibit habitual monogamy the sexes are similar in size i.e., sexual dimorphism is absent. Where males have access sexually to more than one female it follows, since the sexes are about equal in number, that competition will lead to aggressive encounters between males and larger size will confer a reproductive advantage. Sexual dimorphism in body size, with men being about 20% heavier than women at any given age, would lead a stranger to our species to conclude that mankind was more likely to be polygynous than monogamous (Short 1976a).

Human sexual behaviour is infinitely variable within the range of cultural constraints imposed upon it; either polyandry, polygamy, monogamy, serial monogamy, promiscuity, homosexuality or even celibacy may be regarded as a norm for a particular community. Short (1976a, b, 1979, 1981) provides helpful insight into this elusive subject by considering possible relationships between morphology and behaviour in man and the closely related primates, the great apes.

Assumption of a close relationship between man and the great apes depends mainly on a subjective evaluation of similarities in anatomical structure and physiological function (Le Gros Clark 1971). More recently it has been considered that the times of divergence during evolution would be a more secure basis for classification. Sarich & Wilson's measurements (1967) of the small differences in amino-acid sequences between albumins and later the analysis of the individual DNA in each species by hybridization techniques have provided a valuable basis for estimates of relationship between living creatures (Gribben & Cherfas 1982, Notes and News (Lancet) 1982). Refinements in DNA-DNA hybrid technology now show that man and chimpanzee are extremely closely related to each other, more so than either is to the gorilla, indicating that of these species the gorilla was the first to diverge (Diamond 1984, Sibley & Alquist 1984).

The somatic features illustrated in Figures 1.1 and 1.2 correlate well for the breeding system in the wild for the orang-utan, gorilla and chimpanzee. For the orang-utan the frequency of copulation is extremely low and the testes are very small — there is no need for a high spermatogenic capacity — but competition between males is fierce and the adult male is twice the size of the female. The gorilla, with a mating system different from the orang-utan, is typically polygynous

1

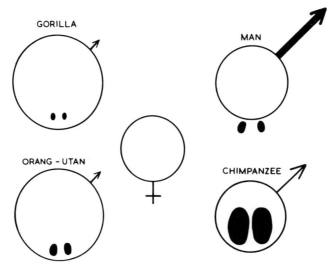

Fig. 1.1 The size of the circles represents the body size of a breeding male, relative to the size of a typical female (central circle) for each of the four species; also represented are the size and location of the testes and relative size of the erect penis (Short 1979).

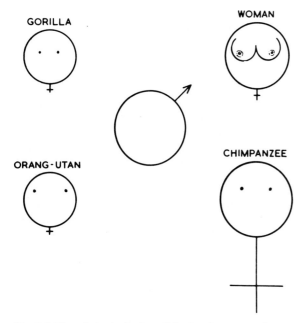

Fig. 1.2 The relative body sizes of the females compared to a typical male, with schematic depiction of the relative development of the mammary glands and of perineum before the first pregnancy (Short 1979).

with the male massively larger than the female. Intercourse, however, is at most an annual event and, in keeping with this state of affairs, the testes to body weight ratio is the lowest for any primate. For the chimpanzee the reduced extent of sexual dimorphism is presumably a consequence of the promiscuous mating system as inter-male competition is less intense. Testicular size, both relative and absolute, is, however, by far the largest and explained by the extremely high copulating frequencies. In man a polygynous mating system is suggested by sexual dimorphism in body size. Regarding sexual function, Caucasian men can maintain a normal sperm output at an ejaculatory frequency of 3.5 times per week; copulating frequency in younger western men is of the order of 2–3 times per week and declines with age. The fact that the human testis (Note 1.1) is considerably larger than that of the gorilla or orang-utan does seem to be related to man's copulatory frequency, which is much less than that of the chimpanzee which has a testicle size large enough to produce sufficient spermatozoa for at least four ejaculations a day (Short 1981).

BEHAVIOUR PATTERNS AND INFECTION IN PRIMATES; IMPORTANCE OF TERRITORY AND SEXUAL FIDELITY AS PROTECTION TO MEMBERS OF THE GROUP

Disease has played an important part in the evolution of behaviour. It is Freeland's (1976) hypothesis that in primates numerous behaviour patterns help the individual avoid new diseases and aid in the control of a disease the animal may harbour. Among other mechanisms, sexual fidelity by individuals to other members of their social group is the result of selection for the avoidance of new diseases. The maintenance of a home range or territory, also, is itself an effective disease-avoidance mechanism. Those mating within their own group have a higher probability of mating with those with the same pathogens as themselves and a lower probability of acquiring new pathogens. Individuals having promiscuous sexual contacts with those outside the social group lower both the probability of surviving or of leaving offspring. In nature friendly or inter-group interactions are rare although they do occur in particular situations. Admission of new 'blood' on occasions is selectively favoured to avoid overmuch in-breeding but the introduction of such an individual is generally gradual to allow time for both the group or a new member to become immune to lethal or pathogenic doses of strange disease-producing organisms.

PATTERNS OF HUMAN SEXUAL BEHAVIOUR IN THE HUNTER-GATHERERS

In the search for the answer to the question 'What is the normal pattern of human social and sexual behaviour?' Short (1981) considers that it cannot be answered by studying contemporary human society, since the extensive modifications of human behaviour by civilization have taken place only in the last few thousand years whereas man has been in existence for several million. Some 99% of this existence is likely to have been that of a hunter-gatherer. Morphology has suggested a polygynous or possibly promiscuous but not a monogamous existence. In 185 contemporary human societies, uncontaminated by western culture, Ford & Beach (1952) found that 74% were basically polygynous although for economic reasons and the shortage of women about half had to adopt a monogamous life style. The human species shows strong male-female pair-bonding and long-term consortships, reinforced by love and by a relatively high copulating frequency. The latter is consequent upon the suppression of cyclical oestrus in the female, who is therefore made constantly attractive to the male, and potentially receptive to him at any time from puberty onwards. How then should this pair-bonded monogamy be equated with evidence from body size that man is likely to have been polygynous?

One possible explanation is that we have indulged in serial monogamy, and that because of the differences in the fertile lifespan of men and women, this would have resulted in a degree of sexual selection. In contemporary societies men tend to choose female partners who are younger than themselves. Female fertility declines markedly after the age of about 40 and ceases entirely at the menopause, whereas male fertility persists throughout life. If males practised serial monogamy and always sought younger women, for whom there would be much competition, the successful would contribute a disproportionately large share of his genes to the succeeding generation, and sexual selection would operate.

There are objections to the sociobiological approach to seeking answers for behaviour in mankind (Harré 1979); the biological basis of life is seen always as a source of problems, never of solutions. The rapidity with which change in behaviour can occur seems to require explanation in terms of matters other than biological, and the elaboration of human social life and the complexities of it go far beyond necessities of survival. The most striking thing about the human nervous system is its redundancy with respect to biological needs and the most fundamental principle around which human life is organized is a craving for recognition as being worthy in the opinion of others.

PATTERNS OF HUMAN SEXUAL BEHAVIOUR AND THE EFFECTS OF NUTRITION

In developed countries there has been a spectacular decline in the age of menarche (Fig. 1.3) although more recent evidence suggests that this downward trend has come to a halt (Dann & Roberts 1973, Marshall & Tanner 1974) to give a mean menarchal age of 12.6–13.5 years. During the period 1830–1960 secular diminution in age of menarche (pronounced menarkee from the Greek *arche* meaning beginning) was calculated to be about 3–4 months per decade. The highest menarchal ages are now to be found among the poorest countries and the trend towards earlier maturation is occurring in many others where improved nutrition, particularly an increase in the protein content of a child's diet, has been shown convincingly to be the cause of this change. In Britain the rich and poor are now beginning to reach the limit of their genetic potential as the latest data show no differences which reflect discrepancies in their family income. In Hong Kong, however, the data show a difference of 9 months between rich and poor, presumably because the poor are much worse off than the poor in Britain. A most convincing argument for nutritional causes is the example of the Lapps who had practically the same age of menarche, $16\frac{1}{2}$ years, from 1780 to 1930, while maintaining their pastoral nomadic way of life. During the same period the neighbouring Norwegians, being settled farmers, became two years earlier in their age at menarche (Marshall & Tanner 1974).

In the sequence of events at puberty (Fig. 1.4) amongst any group of boys or girls there is an enormous

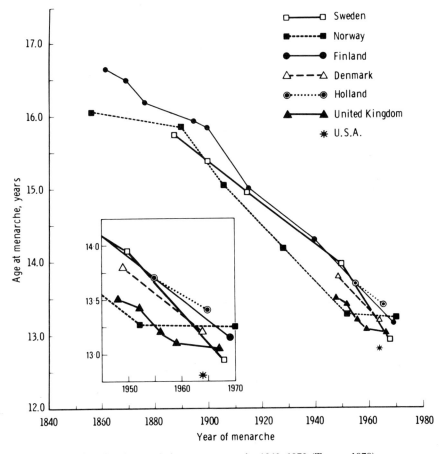

Fig. 1.3 Secular trends in age at menarche 1860–1970 (Tanner 1978).

variability. This situation, described by Tanner (1978) as 'an ineluctable fact of biology' raises difficult social and educational problems. Although boys become fertile before girls they are at a very early stage in their pubertal development and are still physically immature. There is little information about the secular changes in the time of onset of male puberty but evidence for both sexes suggests that psychosexual development is determined by nutritional events which control the time of onset of puberty.

After the menarche a two-year period of adolescent infertility — about 60% of menstrual cycles are anovular (Doring 1969) — will give this degree of protection against unplanned pregnancy. In developed countries sexual maturity occurs in girls at an early age as a result of good nutrition. Intellectual maturity, however, upon which her capacity to cope with her sexuality depends, is, however, more dependent upon chronological age and comes much later. The social consequences of the lowering of the age of puberty can be profound: earlier sexual activity requires earlier access to sex education (see Ch. 4).

Reproductive patterns in three settings are shown diagrammatically in Figure 1.5; the hunter/gatherers (Kung) of the Kalahari are contrasted with the Hutterites and a view of western society.

NORMS OF HUMAN SEXUAL BEHAVIOUR IN CONTEMPORARY SOCIETY

Within the varied pattern of human sexual behaviour it is useful to examine a number of its facets as these may determine not only the identity but also the incidence of the specific disease or diseases acquired.

In the BBC Reith lectures for 1962, entitled 'This Island Now', Professor Carstairs, Professor of Psychological Medicine of the University of Edinburgh, outlined many of the points of change which were occurring at that time in the United Kingdom (Carstairs 1963). He touched on the changing role of women and the abandonment of chastity as a supreme moral value. He recognized that sexual experience before marriage with precautions against pregnancy would become a

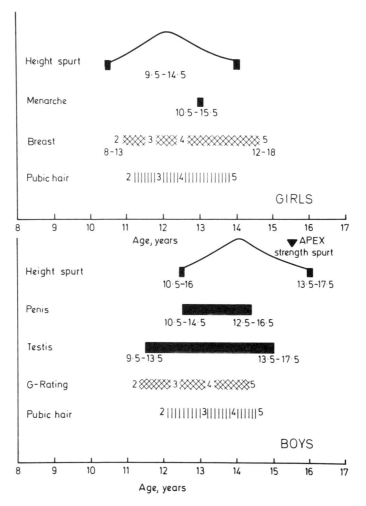

Fig. 1.4 Sequence of events at puberty in girls and boys.

The solid areas, marked 'Testis' and 'Penis', represent the period of accelerated growth of these organs and the vertical lines and rating numbers marked 'Pubic hair' stand for its advent and development. The range of ages at which spurts for height, testis growth and penis growth begin and end are inserted underneath the first and last points of the curves and bars.

The upper part of the figure shows the average age at which each event takes place in girls at puberty. The first event to be noticed is the advent of breast-stage 2, called the breast bud. The average age at which this occurs is about 11.0 years but the range extends from 9–13. The menarche occurs relatively late in puberty (12.8–13.2 years) in various present-day populations. The period of adolescent (relative) infertility lasts for 1–1½ years after the menarche. Ratings for stages of breast development, pubic hair and genitalia (G.rating) are given in Tanner (1962) and also discussed in Tanner (1978).

recognized preliminary to marriage. Changes in attitudes to sex have been profound and it is now commonplace to discuss openly subjects once taboo outside limited circles. In the United Kingdom, male homosexuals have been freed from prosecution for sexual acts in private between adults; abortion has been legalized; contraceptives have been made very readily available and divorce is easier to obtain. The distinguished judge, Sir Leslie Scarman, pointed out (1974) that with concepts derived from the human rights movement, men and women now expect to have opportunities of achieving personal happiness, unfettered by the views of others.

This 'sexual revolution' has been studied in many countries, particularly in the United States, although, in this difficult and costly subject to study, the non-random nature and small sizes of the population samples studied (Farkas et al 1978) often make it uncertain to what extent the changes reported applied to society in general. Many of these reports, however, showed trends that were similar although they varied geographically according to the predominant mores.

A number of reports on students supported the conclusion that, during the decade 1958–1968, change had been occurring in the sexual experience of females

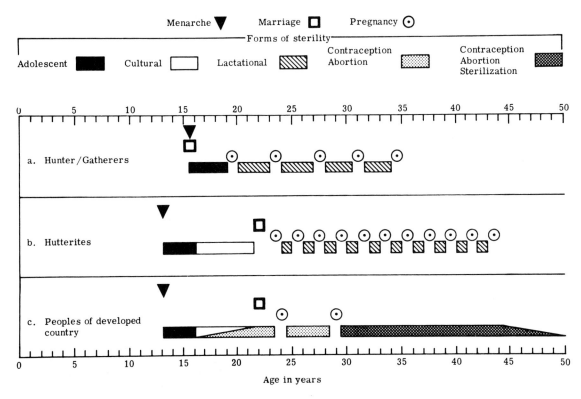

Fig. 1.5 Differing patterns of human fertility in hunter/gatherers of the Kalahari, Hutterites of North America and peoples of developed countries (adapted from Short 1976a). **a.** The menarche is relatively late (15½ years) and coincident with marriage. Adolescent sterility defers birth of first child to 19½. Lactational sterility keeps births 4 years apart. Maternal mortality results in family of 5, 3 of whom would survive into reproductive life. **b.** North American Hutterites, an anabaptist sect, practise no form of contraception. Menarche is at 13 and taboo prevents premarital intercourse. Marriage occurs at the age of 22. Supplemental food is given a few months after birth and weaning takes place within a year. Lactational amenorrhoea is therefore short and births occur every 2 years to give a family size of 11. **c.** Menarche is at 13; taboo against premarital intercourse breaks down in late teens and this requires the use of contraception and abortion. Lactation is so short in duration that it does not induce amenorrhoea and if the desired family size is 2, contraception, abortion or sterilization is necessary for 20 years. As a result there is an enormous increase in number of menstrual cycles in comparison with (a) and (b).

Table 1.1 Trends in three liberal attitudes found in three groups of students of various origins. (Adapted from Christensen & Gregg 1970).

Attitudes	Year	Highly restrictive culture (USA)		Moderately restrictive culture (USA)		Very liberal culture (Denmark)	
		Males %	Females %	Males %	Females %	Males %	Females %
Opposition to censorship of pornography:	1958	42	54	47	51	77	81
	1968	61	58	71	59	99	97
Acceptance of non-virginity in marital partner:	1958	5	11	18	23	61	74
	1968	20	26	25	44	92	92
Approval of premarital coitus:	1958	23	3	47	17	94	81
	1968	38	24	55	38	100	100
Total numbers in sample:	1958	94	74	213	142	149	86
	1968	115	105	245	238	134	61

to a significantly greater extent than in males. Sexual intercourse took place increasingly during a 'going steady' relationship and the commitment of 'engagement' had become less important as a preliminary. Feelings of guilt connected with intercourse lessened. In a study, for example, of a highly restrictive Mormon culture in the intermountain region of western United States (USA); a moderately restrictive midwestern culture in central USA; and a highly permissive Danish–Scandinavian–culture, Christensen & Gregg (1970) identified often marked changes in attitudes in students, particularly in the female. Values for three items, selected to show trends in liberal attitudes, are given in Table 1.1. It was found that there was also a relationship between attitudes and behaviour and, in particular, approval of coitus was a better predictor of coital behaviour for both males and females at the end of the decade than at the beginning. Attitudes towards sex had become more liberal; sexual intercourse was justified when there was commitment or affection between partners, a traditional Scandinavian pattern. There was also a suggestion in the Scandinavian sample that there was a trend for sexual intercourse not to be confined to one partner. Two negative accompaniments of premarital coitus were identified — the first, the feeling of yielding to force or pressures other than personal desire, and the second, coitus followed by guilt or remorse; both tended to be higher in restrictive than permissive cultures, higher in females than in males and higher in 1985 than in 1968 (Christensen & Gregg 1970).

RESTRICTIVE, DOUBLE-STANDARD AND NON-RESTRICTIVE PATTERNS IN PRESENT-DAY SOCIETY

In populations with Judaeo-Christian origins and in plural westernized communities in particular it is possible to distinguish three main types of society in a more generalized way (Fig. 1.6) (Skegg et al 1982). In Type A both men and women are strongly discouraged from having sexual relationships outside marriage; such a restrictive pattern is seen among active members of religious groups. In Type B, women are expected to have only one partner, whereas men are expected to have many. This pattern of disparity between men and women, where there is a double standard of behaviour, is characteristic of some Latin American societies and in the last century was characteristic of many European and other societies. Men tend to seek their extramarital sexual contacts with female prostitutes, who form a reservoir of sexually transmissible infection. In Type C both men and women tend to have several sexual partners during their lives, a pattern which has emerged in

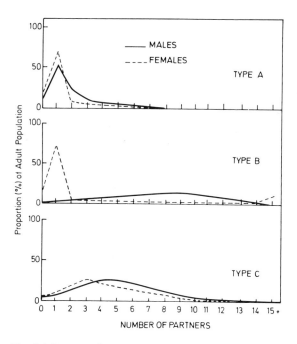

Fig. 1.6 Patterns of sexual behaviour in society (Skegg et al 1982). Type A: Endogamous marriage and monogamy prevail. Both men and women are strongly discouraged from having more than one sexual partner. Type B: Women are expected to have only one partner but men are expected to have many. Sexual contact for men outside marriage is provided by female prostitutes. Type C: Women and men have several partners during their lifetime.

many western countries. The incidence of sexually transmitted disease is expected to be low in Type A communities and high in Types B and C.

TRENDS IN SEXUAL BEHAVIOUR

Canada

Trends in the changes in sexual behaviour, shown in US studies of the late 1960s and early 1970s, are similar to those recorded more recently in Canadian students (Barrett 1980). In Toronto the percentage of unmarried students claiming to have had sexual intercourse increased statistically significantly between 1968 (M 40%; F 32%) and 1978 (M 62%; F 58%). The major change for males took place between 1968 and 1971 and for females between 1971 and 1974. About 12–13% of unmarried students reported no sexual contact of any kind with another person between high-school and the time of the survey. About 16% of males and 7% of females reported some sexual acts which they would classify as homosexual but mostly this appears to have been post-pubertal experimentation and the survey did not define sexual orientation. In both the 1974 and 1978 surveys the majority of students claimed to have had either one or two sexual partners in their lifetime, about 23% had 3–5 partners and about 17% reported more than 6 partners. The results showed a high degree of risk-taking at first intercourse; in 1974, 57% of both sexes reported either using no contraception, coitus interruptus or rhythm the first time they had intercourse. The decline in this percentage in 1978 to 40% for males was not statistically significant but to 46% for females highly so. About one in ten of sexually experienced unmarried students (male and female) had participated in an unplanned pregnancy terminated by induced abortion.

In Alberta in a study of 2062 Canadian students between the ages of 18 and 25, Hobart (1979) records that one consequence of the cultural sexual revolution over the last two decades was an increase in premarital sexual intercourse among women students but not men. Men showed a comparable increase in premarital intercourse earlier — during and after World War II — although it seemed that the revolution was still far from completed by the middle and late 1960s. There is evidence of convergence of male and female patterns, both in the profession and practice relating to sex (Table 1.2).

Table 1.2 Study of premarital sexual experience in students (1848 Anglophone and 414 Francophone) in Alberta, Canada (data from Hobart 1979).

Canadian students	Sex	Percentage with premarital sexual experience	
		1968	1977
Anglophone	M	56	73
	F	44	63
Francophone	M	63	59
	F	30	65

Latin America

Information on sexual behaviour in Latin America is scanty. In a small survey (113 subjects) of female students in Manizales, Colombia (Alzate 1978), the incidence of premarital coitus was 34%. Of the coitally-experienced, 56% professed to have had oral–genital contact and 28% said they had experienced anal intercourse. Many never used any contraceptive method and 11% had had an induced abortion. In a follow-up study Alzate (1984) noted that in the case of men 92% had had sexual intercourse with prostitutes. 65% of them had their first coitus with prostitutes and 41% had patronized prostitutes during the previous 12 months. Concerning heterosexual activities other than vaginal intercourse, 62% admitted oral–genital contact and 24% of them had practised anal coitus. Alzate's description of the social setting fits that given for Type B society

Table 1.3 Sexual experiences of Colombian male university students. Comparisons between 1975 and 1980 (from Alzate 1984).

Experience	1975 Percentage	(No.)	1980 Percentage	(No.)
Ever had coitus with prostitute	92	(49)	74	(155)
Coitus with prostitute as partner at first coitus	65	(99)	39	(155)
Coitus with prostitute in the 12 months preceding survey	41	(99)	20	(153)
Had a venereal disease	49	(49)	25	(150)

(Skegg et al 1982) but, on comparing the 1975 results with those for 1980 (Alzate 1984), he noted that, although rates of sexual activities with prostitutes among males remained high by US standards, there had been a remarkable change (Table 1.3).

Britain

In the United Kingdom major changes have taken place during the last 50 years or more. Among the oldest women in Dunnell's survey (1976) viz., those born between 1926 and 1930, it was estimated that fewer than one-fifth had had intercourse by the age of 20; for women born 20 years later, between 1946 and 1950, this proportion had doubled to more than two-fifths. For the next cohort of women, those aged 20–24 at the time of this interview (1976) half had become sexually active by the age of 20 (Fig. 1.7). Premarital sexual intercourse also appears now to be the norm (Kiernan 1980) (Fig. 1.8) although cohabitation remains a minority practice, as in France near here also, and contrasts with Scandinavian practice (Fig. 1.9) (Brown & Kiernan 1981).

Enquiries in 1977 (Anderson et al 1978) about the sexual behaviour of male and female undergraduates at Oxford University showed that 59% of the women and 52% of the men had experienced sexual intercourse. No contraception had been used by 27% of the women on the first occasion that they had had intercourse: during the four week period preceding receipt of the questionnaire 10% of the sexually active women had had intercourse on one or more occasions without using a contraceptive. The use of contraception increased with the frequency of intercourse and the stability of the relationship. 21% of the experienced women and 18% of the experienced men first had intercourse when they

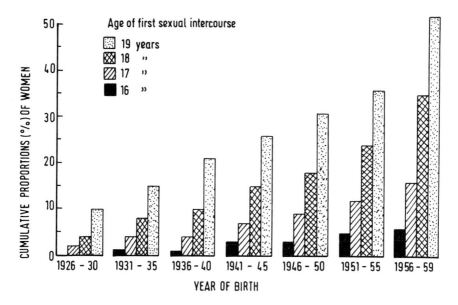

Fig. 1.7 Cumulative proportions (percentage) of UK women who first had sexual intercourse by the ages of 16, 17, 18 and 19 (derived from data in Dunnell 1976).

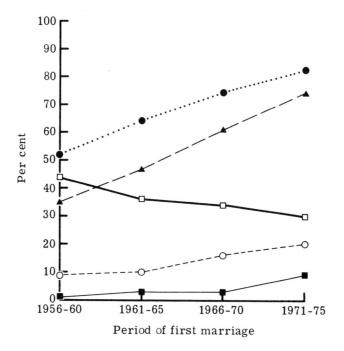

Women in their first marriage reporting pre-marital intercourse with husband ;

●······● when age of marriage was under 20 years

▲— —▲ at all ages of marriage

□———□ for less than 6 months

○-----○ for 2 years or more

Fig. 1.8 Premarital sexual experience in England and Wales (derived from data in Kiernan 1980).

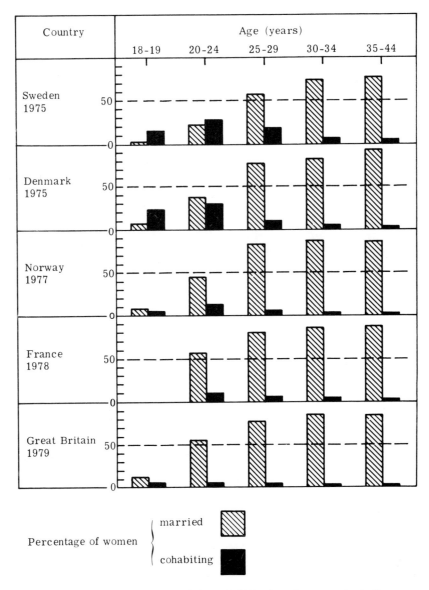

Fig. 1.9 Percentage of women married or cohabiting in various countries in Europe (derived from data in Brown & Kiernan 1981).

were 16 or less, 47 and 49% respectively when aged 17–18 years of age. For 39% of the women and 37% of the men sexual intercourse had been with one partner only, for 27 and 32% respectively with two or three partners, and for 34 and 31% respectively with more than three partners. The proportion of women who had had more than three partners rose from 23% of those who had been having intercourse for less than 4 years to 75% of those who had been having intercourse for more than 4 years. Corresponding figures for the men were almost identical (22 and 79% respectively). Most relationships were described as 'steady' but about 9%

of the women and 8% of the men had had intercourse with more than one partner during the previous 4-week period.

United States

Extensive studies in the United States by Philip Blumstein and Pepper Schwartz (1983) provide insight and contrasts in American couples. Heterosexual men are less monogamous than heterosexual women, a component of their traditional gender role (Fig. 1.10) already discussed in its more striking form in relation to Colombian couples. Within the early years of their relationship

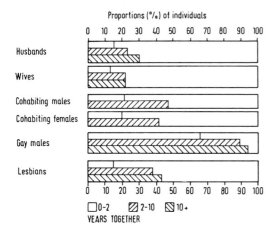

Fig. 1.10 Proportion (percentage) respectively of husbands, wives, cohabiting males, cohabiting females, gay men and lesbians reporting instances of sex outside relationship. Very few of those cohabiting had been together more than 10 years. (Adapted from Blumstein & Schwartz 1983, p. 274.)

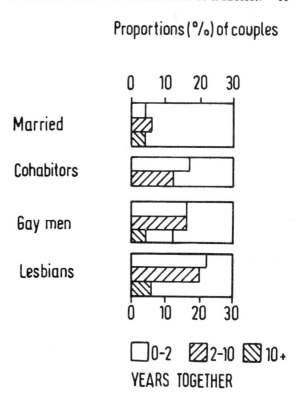

Fig. 1.11 Proportion (percentage) of couples who had broken up 18 months after original survey (adapted from Blumstein & Schwartz 1983, p. 308).

cohabiting couples are no less monogamous than the married but the difference is much more dramatic in established relationships (Fig. 1.10) where, for both sexes cohabiting for a period of 2–10 years, over 40% had sex with someone else. After a couple of years some couples, who had lived together, marry and the ones who do not are more likely to favour an open relationship. Virtually all gay men have other sexual relationships whether they cohabit or not. Lesbians in contrast often have tight-knit friendship groups formed on relationships of a loyal nature and such relationships become actively sexual or erotic. American couples, like those elsewhere sometimes break up but cohabiting individuals, gay men and lesbians are all and approximately equally more likely to do so. Lesbians have the highest break-up rate of all couples (Fig. 1.11) (Blumstein & Schwartz 1983).

PROSTITUTION

Prostitution in women is defined most precisely by Paul Gebhard (1982) who emphasizes its two essential elements: (1) the exchange of money or valuable materials in return for sexual activity with physical contact and (2) the relatively indiscriminate availability of such a transaction to individuals other than spouses or friends. Sexual activity with strangers or with persons for whom there is no affectionate feeling does not itself constitute prostitution if the economic element is absent. His definition represents one end of a continuum ranging from the socially accepted arrangement of marriage, where one male is morally and legally entitled to sexual gratification in exchange for support,

to the other extreme where the arrangement is of a very brief duration and involves numerous males.

The complexity of modern life, with accelerated cross cultural diffusion and rapid transportation, makes a brief description of the exact character of prostitution in any given nation quite impossible. With reference to the nature of the sexual interaction itself Gebhard (1982) comments that in female prostitution the prostitute rarely or never reaches orgasm whereas the client almost invariably does; in contrast, in male homosexual prostitution the prostitute almost invariably reaches orgasm but the client frequently does not.

HOMOSEXUALITY IN MEN AND WOMEN

The basic reflexes leading to consummation of the sexual act in individuals are identical whether stimulation is provided by a heterosexual or a homosexual partner. It is a misconception that male homosexuals invariably prefer effeminate male partners and that homosexual women are attracted predominantly to women with masculine traits. The view that a male/female polarity is present in homosexual relationships reflects a strong culturally induced conviction that such a polarity is essential or innate. Male homosexuals, however, are more attracted by masculine partners than by effeminate ones; among lesbians attraction is not solely a matter of gender-role designation but more an emotional and sexual involvement with women (Beach 1979).

Although gonadal hormones secreted in adulthood may influence potency they almost certainly do not control preference for male or female sex partners. The hypothesis, derived from work on experimental animals, that brain differentiation in the human fetus may be influenced by steroids may be correct and also that such differentiation may also permanently affect the neuro-endocrine functions of the hypothalamus. It is however far from settled that such changes have anything to do with the choice of sexual partners by adult men and women (Beach 1979).

Data on the incidence of homosexuality in the general population are largely those obtained in the United States by Kinsey et al (1948). In the population sampled, individuals varied from those whose sexual acts were wholly with the opposite sex to those whose sexual acts were exclusively with the same sex: men and women could be rated according to Table 1.4 the scale shown in Table 1.4. Much attention was given to the observation near here that 37% of the males interviewed had shared in at least one homosexual experience to the point of orgasm between adolescence and old age, but Bancroft (1983) reminds us of the suggestion of Gagnon & Simon (1973) that this figure exceeded the actual rates because Kinsey's sample included a disproportionate number of criminal and delinquent males. Gagnon & Simon (1973), in their re-analysis of Kinsey's data, found that, in the cases of 2900 young college men, largely between 18 and 25, 30% had experienced at least one homosexual experience in which *either* the interviewee or his male partner was stimulated to the point of orgasm. Of these 30% slightly more than one-half (16% of the total) had shared no such experience since the age of 15 and an additional third (9% of the total) had experienced all their homosexual acts during adolescence or only incidentally in their late teens. The remainder, some 3% of the 2900, were exclusively

homosexual and 3% had substantial homosexual histories as well as heterosexual. In the case of women college students in a comparable re-analysis there is a striking sex difference. Only 6% had had at least one homosexual experience and less than 1% were exclusively homosexual.

Gagnon & Simon (1973) describe Kinsey's studies as portraying sexual man in the 'decorticated state', indifferent to the dimension of sexuality in social life, and in contrast to Freud's writings where sex itself seems 'disembodied'. Bell & Weinberg (1978) criticize the preoccupation that clinicians have with the sexual aspects of homosexual individuals' lives, excluding consideration of their social circumstances, and show that homosexual adults are a remarkably diverse group. From analysis of data based on what their respondents, both men and women, reported to be true of themselves in a face-to-face interview Bell & Weinberg (1978) derived a 'typology of homosexuality'.

1. Close-coupleds. The two partners live together and have a close relationship; they tend to look to each other rather than to outsiders for sexual and interpersonal satisfactions.

2. Open-coupleds. The two partners live together and have a special sexual relationship with each other but in addition they tend to seek satisfactions with individuals outside their partnership.

3. Functionals. These individuals come closest to the notion of 'swinging singles'. They enjoy a wide variety of sexual partners and seem to organize their lives around their sexual experiences.

4. Dysfunctionals. These are troubled people, regretful about their homosexuality, have difficulty in finding sexual partners and are unhappy about their sex lives.

5. Asexuals. These tend to be lonely and rate their sex appeal low; their lack of involvement with others is a major characteristic.

The main characteristics of each type are given in Table 1.5.

From this study it was noted that less than 20% of all the homosexual females had ever 'cruised' (the term 'cruising' means the purposeful search for a sexual partner) during the preceding year whereas nearly all the homosexual males had 'cruised' other males in that time (Bell & Weinberg 1978). Only one homosexual female had ever contracted a 'venereal disease' from a homosexual contact in contrast to the two-thirds of the males.

SEXUAL TECHNIQUES FAVOURED BY HOMOSEXUAL MEN AND WOMEN

In addition to classifying the diverse types Bell & Weinberg (1978) listed a range of sexual techniques favoured

Table 1.4 Heterosexual-homosexual rating scale (Kinsey et al 1948).

0. Exclusively heterosexual
1. Predominantly heterosexual, only incidentally homosexual
2. Predominantly heterosexual but more than incidentally homosexual
3. Equally homosexual and heterosexual (no strong preferences)
4. Predominantly homosexual but more than incidentally heterosexual
5. Predominantly homosexual but incidentally heterosexual
6. Exclusively homosexual

Table 1.5 Typology in homosexual males and females (data from Bell & Weinberg 1978). The main characteristics of each type are given in capital letters. The term 'cruising' means the purposeful search for a sexual partner. The letter x represents average findings respectively in the typical male or female respondent in the sample population studied; 201 of the 686 males (29%) and 82 of the 293 females (28%) could not be classified.

Type (Bell & Weinberg 1978)	Sex	Number	Percentage classifiable	Coupled	Regret over homosexuality	Sex problems	Number of sexual partners	Amount of 'cruising'	Sexual activity
Close-coupleds	M	67	14	yes	<X	low	low	low	>X
	F	81	38						
Open-coupleds	M	120	25	yes	>X	high	high	high	>X
	F	51	24						
Functionals	M	102	21	no	low	low	high	>X	high
	F	30	14						
Dysfunctionals	M	86	18	no	high	high	high	>X	high
	F	16	8						
Asexuals	M	110	23	no	>X	>X	low	low	low
	F	33	16						
Total classifiable:	M	485							
	F	211							

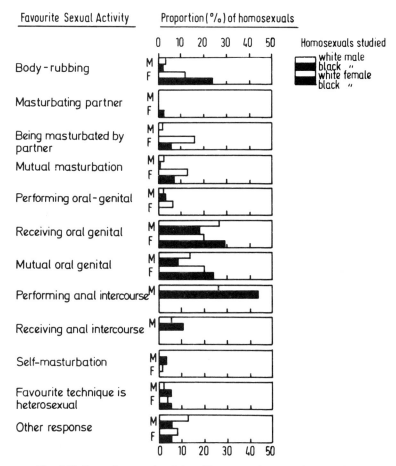

Fig. 1.12 Favourite sexual activity of homosexual men and women in the San Francisco Bay Area, USA (adapted from Bell and Weinberg, 1978, p 330).

by homosexual men and women (Fig. 1.12). Lowry & Williams (1983) add kissing and ano–lingual sex as being sexual habits usually practised. The sexual repertoire of minorities of homosexual males may now include the dangerous practice known as 'fisting' — the closed or clenched fist is introduced into the rectal ampulla, the upper rectum or sigmoid colon to achieve sexual gratification. Severe lacerations of the rectum and even perforation of the recto-sigmoid colon have resulted from this technique (Sohn et al 1977, Owen 1980). Other unusual habits include spitting, spanking, the use of enemas, urinating on partners (watersports). shaving body hair, bondage (use of ropes, etc., as restraints and whipping) (Lowry & Williams 1983). Such practices vary geographically and individuals will express a definite preference for one or another type of sexual activity.

Oral sex as a component of sexual behaviour in homosexuals and heterosexuals

Oral sex (Fig. 1.13) is important for gay men's satisfaction but it has also the potential to be disruptive for couples (Blumstein & Schwartz 1983); one or other partner may dislike performing or receiving oral-genital sex. In the case of lesbians the more often they have oral-genital sex the happier they are with their sex life and with their relationship with each other. In the case of heterosexuals, men who receive oral sex are

happier with their sex lives and with their relationships in general; men who perform oral sex are also happier. For heterosexual women oral sex, on average, neither contributes to nor detracts from the quality of their sex lives. More insight into the reactions of individuals to this and other sex acts is provided by Blumstein & Schwartz (1983) from extensive data collected in their study of American couples.

NUMBERS OF PARTNERS IN HOMOSEXUAL MEN AND WOMEN

Homosexual males tend to have large numbers of sexual partners, significantly more than heterosexual men; in Bell & Weinberg's study (1978) almost one-half of the white homosexual males and one-third of the black homosexual males said that they had had at least 500 different partners during the course of their homosexual careers. Although the numbers given might reflect exaggeration on the part of some, over 90% of their white male respondents reported having 25 or more partners. Most of the white homosexual males, as opposed to about one-third of the black homosexual males, said that more than half of their partners were persons with whom they had sex only once. In contrast lesbians have fewer partners (Fig.1.14); the majority had less than 10 sexual partners throughout the course of their homosexual career.

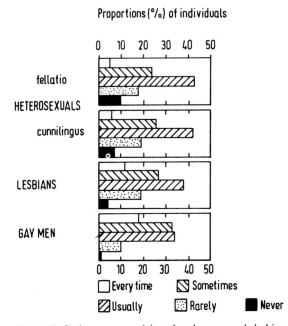

Fig. 1.13 Oral sex as an activity when heterosexual, lesbian and gay couples have sex. (Adapted from Blumstein & Schwartz 1983, p. 236.)

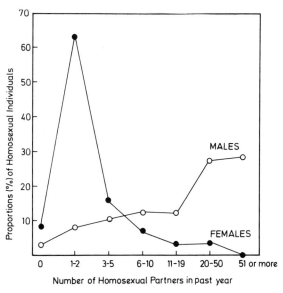

Fig. 1.14 Number of homosexual partners had by white homosexual men (N = 572) and women (N = 228) in the preceding year (San Francisco Bay Area, USA). (Derived from data in Bell & Weinberg 1978, p. 312.)

FURTIVE SEXUAL ENCOUNTERS IN HOMOSEXUAL MEN

Furtive, impersonal sexual encounters where participants may obtain sexual satisfaction anonymously without obligation or commitment are aspects of male homosexual behaviour which occur in public toilets or restrooms or, in the language of the homosexual subculture of the time, in 'tea rooms'. Most sexual encounters in these circumstances are of an oral–genital nature and in only 1% is anal intercourse the objective (Humphreys 1975).

NOTE TO CHAPTER 1

Note 1.1

If testicular weight is plotted against body weight for a whole range of primates, the ones with the largest testes are those with the highest copulatory frequencies and promiscuous mating systems, like the baboons, macaques and chimpanzees. In monogamous species, like the marmoset, or in polygynous species like the gorilla where copulation may occur as infrequently as once or twice a year, and even in man himself, the testes are extremely small relative to body weight (Short 1985).

Within the human species itself no relation has yet been found between testis size and copulatory frequency. Striking racial differences in testis size are to be found, with the mean testicular weight in Caucasians being about 20 g compared with less than 10 g in Chinese, for example. The trait appears to have correlates in the female, with the dizygotic twinning rate of Asians (3.9 per 1000 births) being about half that of Caucasians (7.9 per 1000 births). It has been suggested that there is strong selection against dizygotic twins in populations of small stature and slender build because of increased maternal and infant mortality (Diamond 1986).

REFERENCES

Alzate H 1978 Sexual behavior of Colombian female university students. Archives of Sexual Behavior 7: 1: 43–54

Alzate H 1984 Sexual behavior of unmarried Colombian university students: a five-year follow-up. Archives of Sexual Behavior 13: 2: 121–132

Anderson P, McPherson K, Beeching N, Weinberg J, Vessey M 1978 Sexual behaviour and contraceptive practice of undergraduates at Oxford University. Journal of Biosocial Science 10: 277–286

Bancroft J 1983 Human sexuality and its problems. Churchill Livingstone, Edinburgh, ch 6, p 165, 171

Barrett F M 1980 Sexual experience, birth control usage, and sex education of unmarried Canadian university students: changes between 1968 and 1978. Archives of Sexual Behavior 9: 5: 367–390

Beach F A 1979 Animal models for human sexuality. In: Sex, hormones and behaviour. Ciba Foundation Symposium 62 (New Series), p 113–143

Bell A P, Weinberg M S 1978 Homosexualities. A study of diversity among men and women. Mitchell Beazley, London, p 75, 79, 81–102, 118–119, 129–138, 312, 330, 346–347

Blumstein P, Schwartz P 1983 American couples. William Morrow, New York

Brown A, Kiernan K 1981 Cohabitation in Great Britain: evidence from the General Household Survey, Population Trends. Office of Population Censuses and Surveys, London, HMSO, p 4–10

Carstairs G M 1963 This island now. The BBC Reith Lectures, 1962. The Hogarth Press, London

Christensen H T, Gregg C F 1970 Changing sex norms in America and Scandinavia. Journal of Marriage and the Family 32: 616–627

Dann T C, Roberts D F 1973 End of the trend? A 12-year study of age at menarche. British Medical Journal 3: 265–267

Diamond J 1984 Evolution: DNA Map of the human lineage. Nature 310: 544

Diamond J M 1986 Ethnic differences. Variation in human testis size. Nature 320: 488–489

Doring G K 1969 The incidence of anovular cycles in women. Journal of Reproductive Fertility Suppl. 6: 77–81

Dunnell K 1976 Family formation 1976. Office of Population Censuses and Surveys. Social Survey Division, London, HMSO, p 57

Farkas G M, Sine L F, Evans I M 1978 Personality, sexuality and demographic differences between volunteers and non volunteers for a laboratory study of male sexual behavior. Archives of Sexual Behavior 7: 283–289

Ford C S, Beach F A 1952 Patterns of sexual behaviour. Eyre and Spottiswoode, London. Reprint of Edition published 1980 by Harper and Row, New York, available Greenwood Press, Westport, Connecticut

Freeland W J 1976 Pathogens and the evolution of primate sociality. Biotropica 8 (1): 12–24

Gagnon J, Simon W 1973 Sexual conduct: the social sources of human sexuality. Aldine, Chicago

Gebhard P H (ed) 1982 Prostitution. Encyclopaedia Britannica 15th edn. Encyclopaedia Britannica, Chicago, p 75–81

Gribbin J, Cherfas J 1982 The monkey puzzle. The Bodley Head, London

Harré R 1979 Social being. A theory of social psychology. Basil Blackwell, Oxford, p 1–36

Hobart C W 1979 Changes in courtship and cohabitation in Canada, 1968–1977. In: Cook M, Wilson G (eds) Love and attraction, An International Conference. Pergamon Press, 359–371

Humphreys R A Laud 1975 Tearoom trade (impersonal sex in public places). Aldine, Chicago

Kiernan K 1980 Patterns of family formation and dissolution in England and Wale in recent years. Occasional Paper 19/2. Office of Population Censuses and Surveys

Kinsey A C, Pomeroy W E, Martin C E 1948 Sexual behaviour in the human male. Saunders and Coy, Philadelphia, p 638, 639, 655, 671

Le Gros Clark W E 1971 The antecedents of man, 3rd edn. Edinburgh University Press

Lowry T P, Williams G 1983 What homosexuals do: a study of two homosexual subcultures in California. The British Journal of Sexual Medicine 10(102): 41–43

Marshall W A, Tanner J M 1974 Puberty. In: Davis J A, Dobbing J (eds) Scientific foundation of paediatrics. Heinemann, London, p 146

Notes and News 1982 The molecular clock and human evolution. Lancet i: 1137

Owen W E 1980 Sexually transmitted diseases and traumatic

problems in homosexual men. Annals of Internal Medicine 92: 805–808

Sarich V, Wilson A 1967 An immunological time scale for hominid evolution. Science 158: 1200–1203

Scarman, Sir Leslie 1974 English law — the new dimension. Stevens and Son, London

Short R V 1976a Definition of the problem: The evolution of human reproduction. Proceedings of the Royal Society of London, Series B: 3–24

Short R V 1976b Sexual selection and the descent of man. Reproduction and Evolution 4th International Symposium on Comparative Biology of Reproduction, Australian Academy of Science, Canberra. In: Calaby C and Tyndale-Bisco C H (eds) Reproduction and Evolution (1978). Australian Academy of Science

Short R V 1979 Sexual selection and its component parts, somatic and genital selection as illustrated in Man and the Great Apes. In: Advances in the Study of Behavior, ch 9, p 131–157

Short R V 1981 Sexual selection in Man and the Great Apes. In: Graham G E (ed) Reproductive biology of the Great Apes. Academic Press, London, p 319–373

Short R V 1985 Species differences in reproductive mechanisms. In: Austin C R Short R V (eds) Reproduction in mammals, Book 4. Reproductive fitness. Cambridge University Press ch 2, p 24–61

Sibley C G, Alquist J E 1984 The phylogeny of the hominoid primates, as indicated by DNA-DNA hybridization. Journal of Molecular Evolution 20: 2–15

Skegg D C G, Corwin P A, Paul C, Doll R 1982 Hypotheses. Importance of the male factor in cancer of the cervix. Lancet ii: 581–583

Sohn N, Weinstein M A, Gonchar J 1977 Social injuries of the rectum. American Journal of Surgery 134: 611–612

Tanner J M 1962 Growth at adolescence, 2nd edn. Blackwell Scientific Publications, Oxford

Tanner J M 1978 Foetus into Man. Open Books, London, p 152

Pathogens, actual or potential, in sexually transmissible diseases

Specific organisms causing specific disease, usually with an initial or primary lesion on the external genitalia developing after a short latent (hidden) or prepatent period of fixed limits, can be readily labelled sexually transmitted pathogens. If such organisms, known to be conventional pathogens, can be readily identified by easily available bacteriological means, e.g. *Neisseria gonorrhoeae* or *Treponema pallidum*, and also rendered inocuous by specific antibiotic or chemotherapy then the medical requirements for treatment and control can be identified and spelled out. In the case of organisms which produce less well-defined effects, and. which sometimes seem to be non-pathogenic, or nearly so, in certain individuals, there is often doubt in a given individual about the role of the organism being causal or merely casual, e.g. *Gardnerella vaginalis, Mycoplasma genitalium, Ureaplasma urealyticum*. In infections thought to be due to such organisms, management becomes more difficult and answers to questions of control more uncertain. Many infective agents, such as herpes simplex virus or cytomegalovirus, exist in their host without causing obvious ill-effects and are continuously transmitted by intimate, including sexual contact, with only certain individuals developing obvious lesions or disease in the clinical sense. With immunosuppression, as in the Acquired Immune Deficiency Syndrome (AIDS) viruses, prokaryotes and eukaryotes may become opportunistic pathogens producing serious disease.

Sexual habits (Ch. 1) are important in determining the class of organisms liable to be transmitted. Homosexual males with multiple contacts enable the transmission of enteric pathogens or potential pathogens as a result of faecal ingestion resulting from anal sexual contact e.g. *Entamoeba histolytica, Giardia intestinalis, Chilomastix mesnili* or bacteria such as *Shigella* or *Salmonella*.

The new high technology has brought about more understanding of the nature of human papillomavirus (HPV) and the subtlety of its persistence and transmission. The association of certain DNA-types with cancer of the cervix uteri and other malignancies, spells out a medical responsibility which extends far beyond clinics for genitourinary medicine or sexually transmitted disease. In the case of the Acquired Immune Deficiency Syndrome, the complexity and mode of transmission of the causative retrovirus is being unravelled also by the new high technology. The virus is apparently widespread in the population of Central Africa but it is probably one to which the populations of advanced societies are still as yet naive. Although it is understandable that in the West it should infect those to whom transmission is easiest, viz. promiscuous male homosexuals in particularly, spread to heterosexuals has occurred and infection eventually may become more general. The disease 'AIDS', is not only a problem for a minority group but, as Maddox writes (1984), 'casts a longer shadow' and is everybody's concern.

In this chapter the identity of pathogens, actual or potential in sexually transmissible diseases, are classified and considered briefly as a basis for the appreciation of their role and as a foundation for the study of the subject of this book.

PATHOGENICITY

Pathogenicity is referred to in terms defined by Parker (1984a).

Conventional pathogens cause similar diseases in healthy members of the general population and in hospital patients.

Conditional pathogens seldom give rise to clinical disease in healthy persons, but many invade the tissues in the presence of local predisposing factors that permit the organism to bypass the natural defences of the body surface.

Opportunistic pathogens very rarely cause systemic disease in the apparently healthy, but often do so in patients with severe depression of one or more of the body's general defence mechanisms, e.g. in immunodeficiency. This group may be sub-divided into two subgroups:

1. opportunistic pathogens which cause significant disease only in predisposed persons
2. opportunistic pathogens which occasionally cause systemic infections in apparently normal persons; some are common causes of mild or localized diseases in the general population.

CLASSIFICATION AND TAXONOMY

Viruses are listed in various groups, V1–V7; prokaryotes (Note 2.1) P1–P14; and eukaryotes (Note 2.2) E1–E4. The main species are grouped as in the text and listed for ease of reference in Table 2.1 for viruses, in Table 2.2 for prokaryotes and in Table 2.3 for eukaryotes.

Table 2.1 Main viruses listed in the groups considered in the text. The asterisk denotes that the virus is included in the list only because it may be an important opportunistic pathogen in the Acquired Immune Deficiency Syndrome (AIDS).

V1	Papillomavirus
	Miopapovavirus JC*
V2	Herpes simplex virus Types 1 & 2
	Varicella-zoster virus
	Cytomegalovirus
	Epstein-Barr virus
	Human herpesvirus 6*
	Molluscum contagiosum virus
V3	Hepatitis B virus
V4	Hepatitis A virus
V5	Non-A Non-B
	Delta agent
V6	Human immunodeficiency viruses
V7	Marburg virus
	Ebola virus

VIRUSES

A virus consists of genetic material enclosed in a protective coating and is one of the simplest entities able to reproduce. The ability to maintain genetic continuity, with the possibility for mutation, is the only basis for considering viruses to be alive (Hughes 1977). The fully formed, mature virus (or virion) consists of nucleic acid within a protein or protein and lipid coat. Nucleic acid is either DNA or RNA in animal viruses. The infectivity resides in the nucleic acid component which is released from the virion into the infected cell, where it initiates synthesis of more virions. Some viruses, however, contain a transcriptase enzyme that is essential for their infectivity. A few kinds of virion contain enzyme(s) involved in attachment and release of virus from the host cell (Abercrombie *et al* 1980).

Those viruses that may be sometimes or often sexually transmitted, together with those important in immunodeficiency, including the Acquired Immune Deficiency Syndrome (AIDS), are listed below and classified on the basis of Melnick's 1982 paper on taxonomy; reference has also been made to his 1971 study. For names of viruses in the text normal type has been used rather than the italics used for genus and species in the nomenclature of prokaryotes and eukaryotes.

V1: DNA-containing viruses with cubic symmetry and naked nucleocapsid
Family I: Papovaviridae
    Genus I: Papillomavirus (virion 55 nm; DNA mol.wt. 5×10^6)
        Papillomavirus (HPV), especially Types 6, 11, 16 & 18
    Genus II: Miopapovavirus (*mio*, Greek for smaller) (virion 45 nm; DNA mol. wt. 3×10^6
        Miopapovavirus JC
        Miopapovavirus BK
Family II: Adenoviridae

Papillomavirus
Human papillomavirus (HPV) consists of a heterogeneous group of DNA viruses which have been placed in the family of papova viruses (pa = papilloma; po = polyoma; va = vacuolating agent) although they do not appear to be related to the two other genera included in that family. Since papillomaviruses cannot be propagated in vitro progress, until recent years, has been difficult and unrewarding. Now that DNA from warts can be cloned in plasmids or in bacteriophage lambda sufficient quantities of DNA can be obtained for classifying HPV into separate types based on DNA hybridization studies (Pfister 1984; Note 2.3). On the basis of these nucleic acid studies more than 40 types have been reported of which at least four are specific to the urogenital tract viz. HPV-6, 11, 16 and 18 (Singer et al 1984). Malignant transformation of genital warts is rare (zur Hausen 1977) but in cancer of the cervix uteri and cervical intra-epithelial neoplasia HPV may have a role in the aetiology, although co-factors may also be important (Ch. 27).

Miopapovavirus
Progressive multifocal leucoencephalopathy (PML) is an uncommon central nervous system disease of humans due to an opportunistic infection in those with an immunodeficiency (as in AIDS [Ch. 31]). Two miopapovaviruses, JC virus and SV-40-PML virus, have been recovered from PML brain (Stroop & Baringer 1982).

V2: DNA-containing viruses with envelopes or complex coats

Family I: Herpesviridae
    Sub-family I: Alphaherpesvirinae (rapidly growing, cytolytic)
        Genus I: Simplexvirus
            Herpes simplex virus Type 1 (HSV-1) (Human alphaherpesvirus 1)
            Herpes simplex virus Type 2 (HSV-2) (Human alphaherpesvirus 2)
        Genus II: Varicellavirus
            Varicella-zoster virus (VZ) (Human alphaherpesvirus 3)
    Sub-family II: Betaherpesvirinae (slowly growing, cytomegalic)
        Genus: Cytomegalovirus
            Cytomegalovirus hominis (CMV) (Human betaherpesvirus 5)
    Sub-family III: Gammaherpesvirinae (replicate in lymphoblastoid cells)
        Genus: Lymphocryptovirus
            Epstein-Barr virus (EBV) (Human lymphocryptovirus 4)
    Sub-family: Not yet assigned
            Human herpesvirus 6 (closely related to CMV)
Family II: Poxviridae
    Sub-family: Chordopoxvirinae
        Genus: Unclassified
            Molluscum contagiosum virus (MCV)

For herpesviruses (Family: Herpesviridae) transmission is mainly by contact of moist mucosal surfaces. The viral envelope adsorbs to receptors on the plasma membrane of the host cell, ultimately fuses with the membrane and releases the capsid into the cytoplasm. A DNA-protein complex is then translocated to the nucleus. mRNAs generated from the transcripts are translated in the cytoplasm. Viral DNA is replicated in the nucleus and is spooled into immature nucleocapsids. Infectivity is acquired as capsids become enveloped by budding through the inner lamella of the nuclear membrane and sometimes through other membranes. Herpesviruses remain latent in their host for the lifetime of the host (Roizman et al 1981).

In the classification of the Herpesvirus Study Group of the International Committee on Taxonomy of Viruses (ICTV) herpesviruses are designated (bracketed name given in list) firstly by the name of the host's family, viz. human — the term human is used rather than hominid since humans are the sole living members of the family Hominidae; secondly by the sub-family name, which reflects their biological properties; and thirdly by an arabic number, which relates to the order in which they were discovered and carries no implied meaning about the properties of the virus (Roizman et al 1981, Melnick 1982).

As examples, the common name, herpes simplex virus Type 1 (HSV-l) as used in this book is replaced by the designation human alphaherpesvirus 1, and cytomegalovirus by the designation human betaherpesvirus 5.

Herpes simplex virus

Herpes simplex virus (HSV) consists of two types, HSV-1 causing predominantly herpes labialis and HSV-2 causing herpes genitalis, although the two types may be found in any site. The viruses are noted for their ability to evade the immunological system by developing persistent, often latent (hidden) infections. The natural history of the infection is discussed in Chapter 26 and its various stages defined viz. primary infection, initial infection, latency, re-activation, recurrence, axonal transport and asymptomatic virus shedding.

Varicella-zoster virus

Varicella-zoster infections are seen sporadically in clinics. In AIDS patients these infections appear to be more frequent than in the general population and some cases of herpes zoster are severe and prolonged; there is sometimes dissemination, although infections are not thought to be life-threatening in AIDS (Armstrong 1984).

Cytomegalovirus (CMV) of man

Since the first isolation of this virus in 1956 the spectrum of diseases associated with this virus has been continually expanding (Ch. 28). It is a large species-specific double-stranded DNA virus in the sub-family Betaherpesvirinae. The most significant and serious disease associated with it occurs with congenital infection of the newborn and is currently the most common viral cause of birth defects. In infants, older children and adults with normal immunity, infection with CMV is usually asymptomatic and becomes latent. Beyond the period of infancy, when the infection is spread from the breast milk of seropositive mothers, the acquisition of CMV diminishes in frequency until, with increased sexual activity in adolescents and young adults, there is again a higher rate of CMV transmission. During the acute infection CMV is excreted in the saliva, urine, milk and semen and may continue to be found in these fluids for many months (Spector & Spector 1984).

CMV can rarely cause pneumonia, hepatitis, heterophile antibody-negative mononucleosis, chorioretinitis or encephalitis in the apparently immunocompetent, but in the immunocompromised it is a dangerous pathogen (Spector & Spector 1984). Large volume (100 ml sterile isotonic saline) broncho-alveolar lavage has been introduced as a technique for the rapid diagnosis of CMV pneumonitis in the immunocompromised such as in AIDS cases, where *Pneumocystis carinii* may also be found in the respiratory tract (Griffiths et al 1984, Du Bois et al 1985).

In the Acquired Immune Deficiency Syndrome, although human immunodeficiency Viruses (HIV) (see V5) are the primary aetiological agent, infection with CMV probably enhances the immunosuppression and it may act alone as a cocarcinogen in transforming cells which then grow unchecked as a consequence of the severe immunological defect (Spector & Spector 1984). Retinitis due to CMV with widespread haemorrhage and exudate is common in AIDS (Armstrong 1984).

Epstein-Barr virus (EBV)

In Epstein-Barr virus infections only B-lymphocytes have been shown to have receptors for the virus and although immunity is established against reinfection the virus is harboured for life by the infected individual. A small number of circulating B-lymphocytes carry the virus genome and there is a productive infection in the oropharynx or nearby with shedding of virus into buccal fluid. The response to primary infection is age-related and if delayed until adolescence or young adult life there is a 50% chance it will be accompanied by the clinical manifestations of infectious mononucleosis (Mims & White, 1984) The pathogenesis of EBV-associated malignant disease such as Burkitt's lymphoma and nasopharyngeal carcinoma is not yet solved (Ch. 29).

Epstein et al (1964), discovered the EBV in electron-micrographs of Burkitt's lymphoma but the herpesvirus story in mankind is not ended since Zaki Salahuddin has now recorded a new B-lymphotropic herpesvirus obtained from an AIDS-related B cell tumour, a cutaneous T-cell lymphoma and an immunoblastic lymphoma (Weiss & Mulder 1986). This virus may be called 'Human herpesvirus 6' and although more closely' related to CMV, its sub-family has not yet been assigned (Roizman, personal communication).

Molluscum contagiosum virus (MCV)

MCV is a poxvirus which has not yet been cultivated in vitro and cannot yet be classified adequately. It is unique to man and spread by close skin or mucosal contact under moist conditions. The virus produces pearl-like umbilicated papules in the skin (Ch. 32).

V3: DNA-containing viruses with properties difficult to determine, not yet cultivable

Family Hepadnaviridae (hepatitis B-like viruses) (proposed)

    Genus: None established (Murphy, 1985a)

Hepatitis B virus (HBV)

In this virus a very short circular double-stranded DNA molecule, containing a single-stranded region of variable length, is associated with a DNA polymerase inside an icosahedral protein 'core' (HBcAg). This is in turn enclosed within a closely adherent 'envelope' containing cellular lipids, glycoproteins and 'surface' antigen (HBsAg). The 42 nm virion (Dane particle) is usually accompanied by excess 22 nm HBsAg particles. In addition to the polypeptides of HBsAg and HBcAg there is another, the 'e' antigen (HBeAg). Human hepatitis B virus, of which there are a number of subtypes, is transmitted principally by blood, saliva, semen and perinatally especially from chronic carriers. The infection may progress to chronic hepatic cirrhosis or hepatocellular carcinoma (Mims & White 1984).

'Such prodigious' numbers of HBsAg particles circulate in the serum that they can be extracted from volunteers and, after purification and precautionary inactivation to destroy any possible contamination with live virus, used as a vaccine. Since the cost of vaccine is high and will always be in short supply until the next generation of genetically engineered vaccines becomes more widely available, careful consideration is required in deciding priorities (Ch. 30) (White 1984).

V4: RNA-containing viruses with cubic capsid symmetry

Family: Picornaviridae
    Genus: Enterovirus
        Hepatitis A virus

Hepatitis A virus

Hepatitis A is one of the enteric infections that may be acquired more frequently by male homosexuals, particularly as a result of oral/anal sex (Corey & Holmes 1980). Now that the virus has unequivocally been cultured in vitro the way is open to develop a vaccine against this widespread disease (Mims & White 1984). Recombinant DNA technology offers an alternative approach to the production of viral antigens in the preparation of a vaccine.

V5: Non-A, Non-B hepatitis viruses and the delta agent

Non A, Non B hepatitis agent (NANB)

Classical reverse transcriptase, associated with particles, has been consistently obtained in sera at diagnosis of NANB hepatitis. The particles and their infectivity banded in sucrose at a density identical to that of HTLV-III, were additional findings consistent with the belief that NANB is probably caused by a retrovirus or retrovirus-like agent (Seto et al 1985). This virus, provisionally designated on epidemiological grounds 'blood (transfusion) transmitted' is not the only one to cause the hepatitis, diagnosed by exclusion of other viral causes (viz. hepatitis A virus, hepatitis B virus, hepatitis delta virus, cytomegalovirus and Epstein-Barr virus particularly) to be non-A, non-B hepatitis. Two others, 'coagulation-factor transmitted' and 'epidemic water-borne' viruses, have been given these descriptive provisional names (Tabor 1985).

Delta hepatitis virus
The delta virus, often referred to as hepatitis D virus or HDV, is unique in that infection is dependent on HBV replication, including synthesis of HBsAg. In blood the delta virus is surrounded by an HBsAg envelope. Disruption of the particle with detergent releases delta antigen and the RNA genome. In the liver the delta antigen is localized to hepatocyte nuclei that do not contain HBcAg (Hollinger 1985).

V6: RNA-containing viruses with architecture, asymmetric or unknown

Family: Retroviridae
    Sub-family: (Lentivirinae, possibly)
        Genospecies: Human immunodeficiency viruses (HIV)
            'Subspecies' HIV (geographically informative letter code — sequential number of isolate)

Retrovirus
A retrovirus (Fig. 2.1) consists of *genomic* RNA associated with a central core of *structural protein* and small amounts of *reverse transcriptase*. The core is surrounded by a *lipoprotein* membrane envelope which contains a glycoprotein which is needed for binding the virus to the host cell on infection. When a susceptible cell is infected, the reverse transcriptase present in the viral core synthesizes double-stranded DNA copies of the viral RNA. The viral DNA moves to the cell nucleus, where it can be found both in a linear and several circular forms. Within the nucleus viral DNA molecules become inserted into host chromosomes to form a *provirus* by a recombination event between viral and cellular DNA. The integrated DNA provirus serves as a template for the synthesis of RNA chains identical to those formed in the original virus particle (see Watson et al 1983).

Human immunodeficiency viruses (HIV)
Retrovirus isolates, present in blood, saliva, semen, breast milk and tears, recovered by separate research teams from the tissues of patients with the Acquired Immune Deficiency Syndrome (AIDS) and from patients with related conditions (Ch. 31) have been given various names:

a. lymphadenopathy-associated virus (LAV) by the Paris team (Barré-Sinoussi et al 1983);
b. human lymphotropic virus-III (HTLV-III) by the Bethesda team (Gallo et al 1984, Popovic et al 1984);
c. AIDS-associated retrovirus (ARV) by the San Francisco team (Levy et al 1984).

All three (LAV, HTLV-III and ARV) are variants of the same virus (Ratner et al 1985, Wain-Hobson et al 1985) whose nucleotide sequences differ generally by only 1% overall and whose genetic organization is identical. A subcommittee empowered by the International Committee on the Taxonomy of Viruses has now proposed that the retroviruses implicated in 'AIDS' should be officially designated as human immuno-deficiency viruses to be known in the abbreviated form as HIV (Coffin et al 1986).

All human retroviruses that have been extensively studied to date are lymphotropic, especially OKT-4 lymphotropic. The first two studied, HTLV-I and HTLV-II, were associated with T-cell malignancies and can transform T-cells in vitro and for this reason were first called human T-cell leukaemia viruses. The third group of viruses, isolated from patients with AIDS, has cytopathic effects rather than transforming activity so the term human T-lymphotropic retrovirus has been.used by the Bethesda team to refer to the whole 'family' of viruses and HTLV-III to refer to this third group (Hahn et al 1984). There is no nucleotide homology, however, between HTLV-III and HTLV-I or HTLV-II, and the genetic structure of HTLV-III does not resemble that of HTLV-I or HTLV-II.

Electronmicroscopy also shows that the protein cores of virus from patients with AIDS are condensed and cylindrical in shape whereas those of HTLV-I and HTLV-II are circular and symmetrically placed with respect to the shell protein. HIV is now considered to be a prototype of a new virus, possibly a lentivirus (Anonymous (New Scientist) 1985, Wain-Hobson et al 1985). The processes of organization and replication of the AIDS virus are summarized diagrammatically in Figure 2.1

In addition to the *gag*, *pol* and *env* genes, illustrated in Figure 2.1, others have been identified including *sor* (short open reading frame) and *tat* lying between the *pol* and *env* genes. The gene *tat* is able to mediate activation and its product is an absolute requirement for virus expression; specific inhibition of the activity of *tat* could be a 'novel and effective therapeutic approach to the treatment of AIDS' (Fisher et al 1986).

Individuals with AIDS show a unique loss of a single

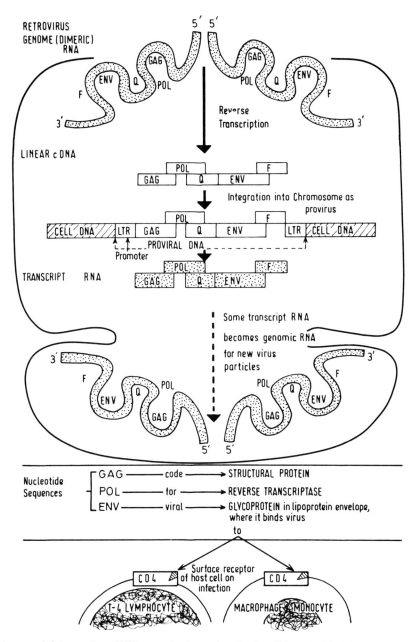

Fig. 2.1 Human immunodeficiency virus (HIV), organization and replication. When the RNA HIV (synonym LAV, HTLV-III, ARV) infects a susceptible cell, the *reverse transcriptase*, present in the viral core, synthesizes double-stranded DNA copies of the viral RNA. The viral DNA moves to the cell nucleus, where some viral DNA molecules become inserted into host chromosomes to form a *provirus* by a recombination event between viral and cellular DNA. As a result the integrated *provirus* has at both ends identical *long terminal repeats* (LTR) of several hundred base pairs. The proviral DNA serves as a template for the synthesis of RNA chains complementary to those found in the virus particle. The *promoter* for this transcription is to be found in the left-handed LTR sequence.

The main nucleotide sequences GAG, POL and ENV code for the specific viral proteins listed in the figure. The genes Q (*sor*) and F (3¹ *orf*) are located as shown; two other nucleotide sequences recognized, *tat* and *trs* are not included in the diagram. The protein cores of HIV are condensed and cylindrical (for further information see Watson et al 1983, Anonymous (New Scientist). 1985, Wong-Staal & Gallo 1985, Gallo 1987; see text also).

The *tat* gene (*tat*-III) is able to mediate activation and its product is an absolute requirement for virus expression (Fisher *et al* 1986).

cell type, the helper-inducer T4 lymphocyte. The CD4 (T4, OKT4) molecule that gives T4 cells their name is the HIV receptor and the interaction is mediated by the 100 kd glycoprotein of the viral envelope (gp110). When HIV infects T4 cells in vitro or in vivo, multi-nucleated giant cells (syncytia) appear in the population; the latter produce large quantities of virus then rupture and die. Infected cells fuse with each other and also with uninfected T4 cells; gp110 expressed on the surface of infected cells interacts strongly with CD4 molecules on uninfected cells 'gluing' normal and infected cells together to form syncytia. HIV infections are persistent, and not all cells infected are immediately killed and seem not to express the CD4 antigen unless they are induced to do so, say possibly, by some other antigen. In the case of brain infections HIV is to be found in multinucleated cells possibly derived from microglia (see review by Curtin 1986).

Isolates of the retrovirus associated with AIDS, in the United States and in western Europe, are currently designated as HIV-1 since analysis of the nucleotide sequences of the human retrovirus (HIV-2), associated with AIDS in West Africa, has shown that the latter is evolutionarily distinct. Both HIV-1 and HIV-2 cause AIDS, are cytopathic in vitro, have tropism for CD4-bearing cells and have elements transactivating expression of viral genes at the LTR (long terminal repeats) level (Guyader et al 1987).

In western urban society the Acquired Immune Deficiency Syndrome has appeared predominantly in male homosexuals, although others have been involved such as intravenous drug abusers and haemophilia patients infected by factor VIII contaminated by the retrovirus. Heterosexual spread also occurs, particularly in regular partners of those in at-risk groups, although spread between heterosexuals appears to occur less readily and from female to male less readily than from male to female. In tropical Africa south of the Sahara, however, heterosexual spread appears to be the rule. The syndrome is characterized by malignancies, particularly Kaposi's sarcoma and opportunistic infections due to, for example, *Pneumocystis carinii* and *Cryptosporidium* (see Ch. 31).

V7: RNA-containing, enveloped viruses, filamentous and of extraordinary length
Family: Filoviridae (Tentative family — Mims & White 1984)

     Marburg virus
     Ebola virus

Marburg and Ebola viruses
Marburg disease is a rare but dangerous infectious disease in which, whatever the original source, person-to-person transmission is the means by which outbreaks and epidemics progress. Patient care and contact with infected blood, secretions, excretions and tissues puts hospital personnel at risk. Isolation of patients and the use of barrier nursing procedures, including protective clothing and respirators have been sufficient to interrupt transmission (Brotherston 1977, Simpson, 1977).

Marburg virus infection was unknown until 1967 when it appeared in circumscribed outbreaks in the Federal Republic of Germany and in Yugoslavia among laboratory workers engaged in processing kidneys from vervet monkeys (*Cercopithecus aethiops*) from Uganda for cell culture production. Altogether 31 people were involved, and 7 of them died. The illness was characterized by fever, rash and haemorrhagic manifestations. The liver was particularly affected and there was involvement of the central nervous system.

The virus has a filamentous structure (665 nm in length) and each contains a molecule of RNA. The last case in the outbreak concerned a woman probably infected by the semen of her husband, which contained the virus, during his convalescence. Transmission is believed to have occurred in this way 83 days after the onset of his illness and involvement of his wife may have been favoured by her previous total hysterectomy for carcinoma of the uterus (Siegert 1970). Spread by sexual intercourse is not, however, the usual method of spread in this epidemic disease in which the search for reservoir hosts still continues.

A structurally similar but antigenically distinct virus has been isolated during epidemics in Sudan and Zaire, for which the name of Ebola virus has been given. In these dangerous diseases specimens for virus isolation and serology can be sent, *by prior arrangement*, to high security laboratories with optimum biocontainment facilities (Murphy 1985b).

PROCARYOTAE

In the classification of bacteria or more specifically of prokaryotic organisms (Kingdom Procaryotae) (Note 2.1) Bergey's Manual of Systematic Bacteriology volume 1 (Krieg & Holt 1984) has been used as the source of reference. Each section (P1 to P15) has been given a simple heading generally based on a few readily determined criteria; sometimes the section is given as the 'family'. The 'genus' and 'species' are usually given also and the terms 'biovar' and 'serovar' refer respectively to strains having special biochemical or physiological properties or, in the case of the latter, distinctive antigenic properties.

Eubacteria
The chromosomal material of eubacteria is in the form of haploid DNA (i.e. unpaired chromosomes) without

Table 2.2 Main prokaryotes listed in the groups considered in the text. The asterisk denotes that the organism is included in the list only because it may be important as an opportunistic pathogen in the Acquired Immune Deficiency Syndrome (AIDS).

P1	*Chlamydia trachomatis biovar trachoma*
	Chlamydia trachomatis biovar lymphogranuloma
P2	*Mycoplasma genitalium*
	Mycoplasma hominis
	Ureaplasma urealyticum
P3	*Clostridium difficile*
P4	*Bacteroides fragilis*
	Fusobacterium nucleatum
P5	*Shigella* spp
	Salmonella serovars
	Yersinia enterocolitica
	Haemophilus ducreyi
P6	*Calymmatobacterium granulomatis*
	Gardnerella vaginalis
	Eikenella corrodens
P7	*Streptococcus agalactiae*
P8	*Staphylococcus aureus*
P9	*Neisseria gonorrhoeae*
	Neisseria meningitidis
	Kingella kingae
	Moraxella osloensis
	M.branhamella catarrhalis
P10	*Legionella pneumophila**★*
P11	*Mycobacterium tuberculosis*
	*Mycobacterium avium**★*
P12	*Actinomyces israelii*
	Nocardia spp★
P13	*Lactobacillus* genotypes
	*Listeria monocytogenes**★*
	Corynebacterium minutissimum
P14	*Campylobacter fetus*
P15	*Treponema pallidum pallidum*
	Treponema pallidum pertenue
	Treponema pallidum 'endemicum'
	Brachyspira aalborgi

the important protein component found in eukaryotic chromosomes; it is not separated from the cytoplasm by a nuclear membrane (Note 2.2). The cell wall of prokaryotic organisms is unique in containing mureins (Abercrombie et al 1980).

P1: Family Chlamydiaceae

Genus I: *Chlamydia*
 Species:
  Chlamydia trachomatis
 (i) Biovar: *Chlamydia trachomatis biovar trachoma*
  a. Trachoma serovars A, B, Ba & C
  b. Genital serovars D, E, F, G, H, I, K
 (ii) Biovar: *Chlamydia trachomatis biovar lymphogranuloma*. LGV serovars L-l, L-2 & L-3

Within this family Chlamydiaceae (Moulder et al 1984), in the genus *Chlamydia* (*chlamydia*, Latin feminine diminutive for a cloak), there are two species, *Chlamydia psittaci* and *C.trachomatis*. The organism multiplies within membrane-bounded vacuoles in the

cytoplasm of host cells. The many striking and detailed phenotype resemblances in structure and behaviour of all chlamydial strains suggest a common evolutionary origin, but surprisingly the demonstrated DNA relatedness between the two species is very low (<10%). Insofar as sexually transmitted diseases are concerned *C.trachomatis* is the more important. Of three biovars known, one is found as a latent infection in mice and two, which concern man, have no animal reservoir, viz. *Biovar trachoma* (see Ch. 17) and *Biovar lymphogranuloma venereum* (LGV) (see Ch. 23). These two biovars show 100% DNA/DNA homology.

Biovar trachoma

In areas where blinding trachoma occurs *C.trachomatis biovar trachoma* is spread from child to child among family members having close contact. Serovars A, B, Ba and C are associated with this form of blinding endemic trachoma. In other communities the biovar is spread by sexual contact and causes diseases in the genital tract or in newborns exposed through an infected birth canal (serovars D, E, F, G, H, I and K are most commonly associated with this transmission pattern (see Ch. 17).

Biovar LGV

The *Biovar LGV* is sexually transmitted (serovars L-l, L-2 and L-3) and in contrast to the *Biovar trachoma*, which is pathogenic to the squamocolumnar cells of mucous membranes, it causes primarily a disease of lymphatic tissue although protean clinical manifestations occur: lymphogranuloma venereum is a disease characterized by marked invasion of the lymph nodes of the genito-anal region (see Ch. 33). All chlamydial infections tend to persist in chronic or clinically inapparent forms.

P2. Family Mycoplasmataceae

Genus I: *Mycoplasma*
 Species: (urogenital tract mucosae: pathogenicity not known)
  Mycoplasma genitalium
  Mycoplasma primatum
  Mycoplasma fermentans
 Species: (urogenital tract mucosae: pathogenicity, potential)
  Mycoplasma hominis
Genus II: *Ureaplasma*
 Species: *Ureaplasma urealyticum*
  Serovar group A: 2, 4, 5, 7, 8, 9, K2, U24
  Serovar group B: 1, 3, 6

Organisms within the family Mycoplasmataceae (Razin & Freundt 1984) are characterized by being totally devoid of cell walls and are bounded by a plasma membrane only. Two genera are accepted: *Mycoplasma* and *Ureaplasma*.

Mycoplasma

M. genitalium has been isolated from the human urogenital tract and its pathogenicity is under discussion (see below). *M. salivarium* is common in the oropharynx and pathogenicity is not known. There is a significantly higher incidence in the gingival sulci of those with periodontal disease. *M. primatum* is a common inhabitant of the oral cavity and urogenital tract of at least four primate groups and has been found once in the genital tract of man; its pathogenicity is unknown. *M. pneumoniae* is the aetiological agent of cold haemagglutinin associated primary atypical pneumonia of man; sometimes the organism involves the CNS and sometimes it causes pancreatitis, pericarditis, myocarditis, haemolytic anaemia and exanthemata. *M. orale* is a common inhabitant of the oropharynx; its pathogenicity is not known.

Chlamydia trachomatis accounts for a quarter to one half of all acute cases of pelvic inflammatory disease (PID). *Mycoplasma hominis* appears to be involved in about a quarter. In Great Britain and Scandinavia *N. gonorrhoeae* is also a cause (Mardh 1980). In the remainder the cause of acute PID is unknown.

In the case of *Mycoplasma genitalium* a significant change in antibody was found in 12 of 31 patients (31%) with acute salpingitis who were negative for antibodies to *C. trachomatis* and *M. hominis* — these data suggest an aetiological role for *M. genitalium* in infection of the upper genital tract. A clue about the possible cause of the pathogenicity of *M. genitalium* has been suggested by its adherence properties and structural features, which have been associated with pathogenicity in another human mycoplasma *M. pneumoniae* but which are absent in *M. hominis*. In grivet monkeys *M. genitalium* reaches the oviducts and induces endosalpingitis whereas *M. hominis* causes a parametritis and exosalpingitis (Möller et al 1984).

M. fermentans is a rare inhabitant of the urogenital tract of man and of uncertain pathogenicity. *M. faucium*, similarly, is a rare inhabitant of the human oropharynx with no known pathogenicity.

M. hominis is a very common inhabitant of the mucosae of the lower urogenital tract of humans; more rarely it is encountered in the oropharynx. It has been found also in these anatomical sites in non-human primates. *M. hominis* is potentially pathogenic and has been recovered from inflamed uterine tubes, tubo-ovarian abscesses and the blood of patients with postpartum fever and septic arthritis. Particularly strong evidence for the aetiological role of this species in inflammatory pelvic disease was provided by its isolation in pure culture, in 8% of cases of acute salpingitis, from samples collected from the uterine tubes by laparoscopy (Mardh & Westrom 1970a) and by serological studies (Mardh & Westrom 1970b).

Ureaplasma

Members of the genus *Ureaplasma* (Taylor Robinson & Gourly 1984) are distinguished by their ability to hydrolyse urea. This is the minimum requirement for assigning a new isolate to the genus. Arginine and the usual carbohydrates are not utilized. Ureaplasmas were termed 'T-strains' or 'T-mycoplasmas' originally so-named because of the production of small (tiny) colonies (15–60 μm) particularly on the agar medium used at that time. The optimum pH for growth (6 $\pm$ 0.5) and the relatively small number of organisms attained on growth in broth media are other features distinguishing ureaplasmas from mycoplasmas. Simple reliance on the detection of alkalinization of the culture medium, supplemented by 1% urea instead of glucose or L-arginine (which are not attacked by ureaplasmas), as a result of hydrolysis of urea to CO_2 and ammonia, has one deficiency in that arginine positive mycoplasmas, which do not possess urease activity, may cause alkalinization of the growth medium by hydrolysis of significant quantities of L-arginine present in the conventional mycoplasma medium. More specific tests for urease activity are therefore recommended. These include the flooding of the colonies with a manganous chloride solution. Urease positive colonies stain dark brown. A sensitive specific and quantitative test is based on breakdown and disappearance of radioactive urea added to the culture medium (Razin & Freundt 1984).

Some 14 serologically distinct serovars exist at present, of which Group A contains serovars 2, 4, 5, 7, 8, 9, K2, U24 and Group B contains serovars 1, 3, 6. The subdivision is consistent with the results of recent DNA hybridization.

Ureaplasmas occur predominantly in the mouth, respiratory tract and urogenital tract. *Ureaplasma urealyticum* may cause urethritis in man.

P3. Spore bearing anaerobes: Clostridium

Genus: *Clostridium*

    Species

        Clostridium difficile

The genus *Clostridium* consists of species which are anaerobic or aerotolerant rods producing endospores. *Clostridium difficile* is found in the faeces of 40% of normal infants but rarely in normal adults. This finding probably reflects a sparse presence rather than a restricted distribution (Larson et al 1978, Willis 1983).

The role of *C. difficile* in antibiotic-associated diarrhoea with or without pseudomembrane formation is well established. The organism has also been held responsible for relapse in some cases of ulcerative colitis. Positive *C. difficile* stool cultures may be obtained in some patients with the irritable bowel syndrome in which the organism may be also grown from a vaginal specimen (Tvede & Willumsen 1982).

P4. Anaerobic Gram-negative straight, curved and helical rods

Family I: Bacteroidaceae
    Genus I: *Bacteroides*
        Species
            Bacteroides fragilis
    Genus II: *Fusobacterium*
        Species
    Fusobacterium nucleatum
    Genus III: *Leptotrichia*
        Species
            Leptotrichia buccalis
    Genus IV: *Mobiluncus*
        Species
            Mobiluncus curtisii
            Mobiluncus mulieris

Bacteroides

Bacteroides fragilis and variants with overall morphological and phenotype similarities were all designated as subspecies, but DNA homology studies showed that these 'saccaroclastic bacteroides that grow well in bile' are to be regarded as separate subspecies. This species, sometimes with other organisms, has been isolated from various clinical specimens including appendicitis, peritonitis, heart valve infections, rectal abscesses and lesions of the urogenital tract; occasionally it is isolated from the urogenital tract. It is (99%) relatively resistant to penicillin, and many strains produce beta-lactamases, but the majority are susceptible to metronidazole (8 μ/ml in vitro).

Although *B. fragilis* is the most common species of anaerobic bacteria isolated from soft tissue infections and anaerobic bacteraemia it accounts for less than 1% of the normal human intestinal flora. *Bacteroides vulgatus*, *B. disasonis*, *B. multiacidus* and a number of other species are very common in human faeces (Holdeman et al 1984).

Fusobacterium

In the genus *Fusobacterium* (Latin, *fusus*, a spindle; Greek, *bakterion*, a small rod), '*Fusobacterium nucleatum* (nucleatum means having a kernal viz. nucleated) deserves mention as it is occasionally isolated from the gingival margin and sulcus and from infections of the upper respiratory tract and occasionally from other infections (the epithet synonymously used for this organism '*Fusobacterium fusiforme*' has no legitimate taxonomic standing (Moore et al 1984)).

Leptotrichia

Leptotrichia are straight or slightly curved rods, 0.8–1 μm wide, 5–15 μm long, with one or both ends pointed or rounded. In Gram-stained smears generally they appear as Gram-negative single cells or in pairs, end to end, with adjacent ends flattened and in a straw-like arrangement. *Leptotrichia buccalis*, generally considered apathogenic, has its habitat in the oral cavity and in dental plaque. This species is also to be found in the microflora of the periurethral region of healthy girls and has been reported from the cervix of a pregnant woman with premature rupture of the membranes (Hofstad 1984).

Mobiluncus

Interest in the aetiology of bacterial 'vaginosis' (Mardh & Taylor Robinson 1984) has focused attention on a recently described genus, *Mobiluncus*, a curved motile rod-shaped bacterium (Spiegel & Roberts 1984). *Mobiluncus* is more resistant to alkaline solutions than most bacteria in vaginal discharge. Isolations can be best achieved from vaginal discharge some 5–10 minutes after it has been diluted in a buffer of pH 12.0–12.6 (Pahlson & Forsum 1985).

P5: Facultatively anaerobic Gram-negative rods

Family I: Enterobacteriaceae
    Genus I: *Escherichia*
       II: *Shigella*
          Species
            Shigella dysenteriae — subgroup A
            Shigella flexneri — subgroup B
            Shigella boydii — subgroup C
            Shigella sonnei — subgroup D
    Genus III: *Salmonella* — many serovars and subserovars
    Genus IV: *Proteus*
        Species
            Proteus vulgaris
    Genus V: *Yersinia*
        Species
            Yersinia enterocolitica
Family III: Pasteurellaceae
    Genus: *Haemophilus*
        Species
            Haemophilus ducreyi

Shigella

The genus consists of the four species listed which are often referred to as the subgroups also listed above (Rowe & Gross 1984).

Shigella sonnei and *Shigella flexneri* have been found in outbreaks of shigellosis in men, of whom homosexuals formed a high proportion of those infected. Infection was probably acquired as a result of ingestion of faecal material (Bader et al, 1977).

Salmonella

Bacteria related by 70% or more on the basis of

DNA/DNA hybridization belong to the same 'geno-species' and the so-called 'genus' *Salmonella* is in fact one species. Because of the importance in pathology in this discussion the names such as *Salmonella typhi* have been retained as they continue to be used in clinical bacteriology (Le Minor 1984).

One homosexual male acquired acute typhoid fever caused by *Salmonella typhi*; his partner, with whom he shared neither housing nor food, was found to carry the same Vi type. In another similar pair, one developed typhoid due to phage type El and the partner was a carrier of the same phage type. After 6 weeks oral ampicillin, after cholecystectomy and after six consecutive negative tests (faeces and urine) for *S. typhi* they were 'freed' from the interdiction against working as food handlers (Dritz & Braft 1977, Dritz et al 1977).

Yersinia

Yersinia is a very homogeneous genus of Gram-negative straight rods or coccobacilli which are characteristically non-motile at 37 °C but motile with peritrichous flagella when grown below 30 °C, except for *Y. pestis* which is always non-motile. *Yersinia enterocolitica* is responsible for diarrhoea, terminal ileitis, mesenteric lymphadenitis, arthritis in man and animals. A number of biovars are known and are useful epidemiological tools (Bercovier & Mollaret 1984).

Haemophilus

Haemophilus ducreyi is named after Ducrey, the bacteriologist who first isolated the organism which causes chancroid or 'soft chancre' (see Ch. 34). A carrier state in healthy individuals has not been detected. In the tropics it is common. In Nairobi *H. ducreyi* accounts for over half of all cases of 'genital ulcer disease' (Nsanze et al 1981). It is uncommon in classically low endemic areas such as the United Kingdom (Forster et al 1983) and Belgium (Piot et al, 1983).

The organism may appear as a short rod with parallel sides and rounded ends staining evenly; or ovoid or navicular in shape with bi-polar staining or in pairs end-to-end having a dumb-bell appearance. It may be intra- or extra-cellular in position (Smith 1983).

Haemophilus equigenitalis is the name sometimes used for the causative organism of contagious equine metritis. Taylor et al (1979) found agglutinins to this organisms in 37.6% of 223 human patients with non-gonococcal urethritis, but advised caution in interpreting the finding.

P6: Facultatively anaerobic Gram-negative rods; not assigned to any family

Genus: *Calymmatobacterium*
    Species
        Calymmatobacterium granulomatis

Genus: *Gardnerella*
    Species
        Gardnerella vaginalis
Genus: *Eikenella*
    Species
        Eikenella corrodens

Calymmatobacterium

A number of genera not assigned to any family can be considered. The genus *Calymmatobacterium* contains the type species *Calymmatobacterium granulomatis* which is pathogenic for humans and causes donovanosis (granuloma inguinale; see Ch. 35). The infection is seen throughout the world, in some developing countries particularly; it appears to be found mainly in the dark-skinned races and occurs mostly in regions where the climate is warm and humid for several months of the year. Initial lesions may occur in skin areas other than the genital region and most researchers support the contention that donovanosis is not primarily sexually transmitted but is an infection resulting from intimate contact and poor hygiene (Dienst & Brownell 1984).

Gardnerella

The genus *Gardnerella* (Greenwood & Pickett 1984) appears to have a worldwide distribution and is found in the human genital/urinary tract; it is commonly present in 'bacterial vaginosis' or 'non-specific vaginitis' (see Ch. 20). The type species is *Gardnerella vaginalis* and all strains are fastidious in their nutritional requirements. The cell wall is unusual and DNA/DNA hybridization (Note 2.3) has shown that it is not closely related to many organisms in genera with which it has superficial resemblance e.g., *Actinobacillus*, *Haemophilus*.

Eikenella

The type species *Eikenella corrodens* occurs in the human mouth, intestine and urogenital tract and is so named because colonies of most strains appear to corrode the surface of the agar. It is non-haemolytic but causes slight greening of blood media around colonies. Although non-motile by conventional tests, observation of corroding strains, growing on agar surfaces, has shown that a 'twitching motility' occurs; this 'twitching' appears to be due to asymmetrically arranged pilus-like structures (Jackson & Goodman, 1984).

E. corrodens acts either as a conditional or opportunistic pathogen and has been recognized not only after human bites, crush and fist-fight injuries but also in cervical secretions in association with copper-tailed intrauterine contraceptive devices in patients with lower abdominal pain (Drouet et al 1987) and in a case of abscess of the greater vestibular gland (Bartholin's Abscess) (Riche et al 1987).

P7: Facultative anaerobic Gram-positive predominantly spherical or ovoid bacteria

Family Streptococcaceae
    Genus: *Streptococcus*
        Species
            Streptococcus pyogenes (beta-haemolytic*, Lancefield Group A)
            Streptococcus agalactiae (beta-haemolytic, Lancefield Group B)
            Streptococcus faecalis (beta- or non-haemolytic, Lancefield Group D)
            Streptococcus intermedius (*Peptostreptococcus*; anaerobic non-haemolytic)

*Beta-haemolytic — complete haemolysis resulting in a clear zone around the colony grown on blood agar. Alpha-haemolytic — a greenish discoloration around colony grown on blood agar.

Disease due to Group A streptococci has declined in importance in developed countries during the last 70 years. The progressive disappearance of rheumatic fever in Europe and North America has been related to improved living standards which have also led to a reduction in the total number of streptococcal attacks in children and adolescents (Parker 1978)

The epidemiological situation differs in three common diseases due to Group A streptococci: tonsillitis, impetigo and infection of wounds and the genital tract. In the first, spread is favoured by close proximity and large salivary particles from the mouth are more important than smaller dry particles; in impetigo minor, trauma may determine the site of infection; and although infections of wounds, burns and the female genital tract may occur sporadically in the general population, epidemics may occur in hospitals. The long-term throat carrier may be a source, but a person with an acute throat is the greatest danger. The perianal carrier, who may not harbour the streptococcus in the throat is rare but a carrier with the organism has been responsible for several outbreaks affecting the ano-genital area (Parker 1978).

Group B streptococci (*Streptococcus agalactiae*) are a serious cause of bacteraemia and other invasive infection in the newborn within the first few days of life. Dense vaginal colonization seems to make transmission more likely, and prematurity and a prolonged labour after rupture of the membranes are important risk factors. Promiscuity in the female or that of her male partner is one determinant of the organismal flora of the genital tract and in the case of Group B streptococci carriage rates of about 12–36% have been noted in the case of women attending STD clinics (Christensen et al 1974, Finch et al 1976). The organism is found on the penis and a presumptive case for its transmission sexually can be made out. In relation to the problem of the newborn, however, positive cultures during pregnancy (6–28% recorded) may be less at term and a few patients may acquire the organism at delivery. Invasive infections develop only in about 1% of colonized babies (Editorial (Lancet), 1984; see Ch. 20).

Peptostreptococcus is now regarded as a separate genus, anaerobic and able to metabolize peptone (Moore et al 1986).

P8: Facultatively anaerobic Gram-positive cocci: the genus staphylococci

Genus: *Staphylococcus*
    Species
        Staphylococcus aureus

Staphylococcus
Parker (1983) recognizes among the aerobic, catalase-positive, Gram-positive cocci a genus *Staphylococcus* that form irregular clusters, are facultative anaerobes and ferment glucose, and distinguishes it from the genus *Micrococcus*, consisting of organisms that are strictly aerobic and do not ferment glucose. Among the staphylococci *Staphylococcus aureus* is a 'reasonably defined species' and reference may be made to its capacity to develop resistance to antibiotics and the existence of multiple antibiotic-resistant strains. As a cause of boils and abscesses it is well known and reference is made in Chapter 20 to the toxic shock syndrome in menstruating young women using a certain type of intravaginal tampon continuously and changed infrequently in which toxin producing staphylococci are important in the aetiology (Parker 1984b).

P9: Gram-negative aerobic rods and cocci

Family Neisseriaceae
    Genus I: *Neisseria*
        Species (conventional pathogens)
            Neisseria gonorrhoeae
            Neisseria meningitidis
                Serovar
            Groupable A, B, C, W-135, X, Y, Z^1, Z.
                Non-groupable
        Species (mostly never pathogens)
            N.lactamica, N.sicca, N.subflava, N.mucosa, N.cinerea, N.elongata
    Genus II: *Acinetobacter* (contaminants probably; some strains formerly labelled '*Herellea vaginicola*' or '*Mima polymorpha*')
        Species
            Acinetobacter colcoaceticus
    Genus III: *Kingella*
        Species
            Kingella kingae
            Kingella denitrificans

Genus IV: *Moraxella*
   Species
     Moraxella osloensis
     M.branhamella catarrhalis

Neisseria

The genus Neisseria (named after Dr Albert Neisser who discovered the aetiological agent of gonorrhoea in pus cells of patients in 1889) contains only two species that are considered to be conventional pathogens for man: *N. gonorrhoeae* and *N. meningitidis*. The principal habitats of those Neisseria species isolated from humans are the mucous membrane surfaces (Vedros 1984).

In *Neisseria gonorrhoeae*, rearrangement of the genes within the genome leads to expression of altered surface proteins (Meyer et al 1982) and so enables the organism to evade the immune reaction of its host. Structures called 'pili' on the outer membrane of the organisms, in different clinical isolates, are antigenically distinct, that is, antibodies against one type of pilus from one isolate will not react with the pilus of another. This antigenic variability may be important in immune evasion by the gonococcus; this versatility of *N. gonorrhoeae* is analogous to the variable surface glycoproteins on African mammalian trypanosomes by which this protozoon escapes immune surveillance (Watson et al 1983). The antigenic diversity and variability of pili protein are the main obstacles to developing any effective pilus-based vaccine. Certain outer membrane proteins, particularly Protein II, have this variability and present the same difficulty (Gotschlich 1984).

Different 'African' and 'Asian' types of plasmid (Note 2.4) which code for penicillinase-production enable the gonococcus to escape the effect of penicillin therapy to a degree which varies widely geographically. A transfer factor also assists in the dissemination of some of these plasmids (Eisenstein et al 1977). In addition, certain serovars have a high degree of resistance to penicillin but do not contain plasmids nor produce penicillinase (Ch. 14).

In women with a gonococcal infection (in any anatomical site) the pharynx is more likely to be colonized with *N. meningitidis* than those without. They are more likely to be colonized by a groupable serovar than women without gonorrhoea. The suggestion is that mouth-to-mouth contact is more frequent in high-risk patients and that this leads to a higher risk of acquiring the *N. meningitidis* and groupable serovars in particular. The non-groupable serovars show no differences in rates and this finding suggests that non-groupable serovars of *N. meningitidis* may be spread by a means other than kissing viz. possibly by droplet spray. In the study it seemed that men would be placed in the high risk group (Young et al 1983) (Ch. 14).

N. lactamica is commonly found in the nasopharynx of infants and is rarely pathogenic. Genetic transformation and DNA/DNA hybridization have indicated a close relationship between *N. lactamica*, *N .meningitidis* and *N. gonorrhoeae* (Vedros 1984). *N. sicca*, *N. subflava*, *N. mucosa*, *N. cinerea* and *N. elongata* are all non pathogenic organisms found in the human nasopharynx.

Acinetobacter

In the family Neisseriaceae, the genus *Acinetobacter* (*akinetos*, Greek adjective — unable to move) (Juni 1984) contains strains which were formerly labelled '*Herellea vaginicola*' if capable of aerobic acidification of glucose medium whereas those unable to acidify the medium were referred to as '*Mima polymorpha*'. At present *Acinetobacter calcoaceticus* is the only species retained although there are two major phenetic groups (phenetic refers to classification based on maximum observable similarity) which differ in their ability to use a given set of carbon sources.

As a result of their evolution acinetobacters carry a large variety of surface antigens which may interact with antisera against Group B and Group C streptococci. An extract of antigen from the genus fixed complement when reacted with sera containing chlamydial antibodies. Although normally non-pathogenic, acinetobacters are causative agents of nosocomial infections, particularly in debilitated individuals (Glew et al 1977) and infections may occur as a result of hospital instrumentation. The genus occurs naturally in soil and water and may be present on the human host as contaminants rather than commensals.

Kingella and Moraxella

Both *Kingella kingae* and *Moraxella osloensis* can cause disseminated infection with similar clinical manifestations to those seen in disseminated gonococcal or meningococcal infections. Infections due to these species are, however, rare (Shanson & Gazzard 1984). *Branhamella* is a subgenus of *Moraxella* which requires to be differentiated from species of the genus *Neisseria*.

P10: Other Gram-negative rods
   Family: Legionellaceae
     Genus: *Legionella*
       Species
         Legionella pneumophila

Legionella

Legionella pneumophila was first recognized as a cause of serious pneumonia in 1976 when some 200 people attending an American Legion convention were affected. The organism is a short rod with tapering ends, 1–2 μm long $\times$ 0.5 μm in its greatest width and without a capsule. On electron microscopy fimbriae are seen to be arranged around the organism which also has a single polar or subpolar flagellum. It is sensitive in vitro to erythromycin at therapeutically attainable concentrations. Six serotypes exist (Wilson 1983b). The organism is of importance occasionally in AIDS (Ch. 31).

P11: Family Mycobacteriaceae
Genus: (sole genus) *Mycobacterium*
    Species (slowly growing)
        Mycobacterium tuberculosis
        Mycobacterium avium
        (*Mycobacterium avium intracellulare*, probably a variant of *M.avium*).
        Mycobacterium xenopi
    Species (rapidly growing)
        Mycobacterium fortuitum
        Mycobacterium smegmatis

Mycobacteria (Grange 1984) are characterized by their ability to resist decolorization by acid after being stained by an arymethane dye (*acid-fastness*), the chemical structure of their mycolic acids and their antigenic structure. The cultivable members of the genus are divisible into two major groups, the slow growers and the rapid growers which have other physical differences (e.g.. DNA relatedness).

Mycobacterium 'avium-intracellulare' is a common environmental contaminant that rarely caused disseminated disease until the advent of AIDS. Isolations have been made from lymph nodes, bone marrow, liver, spleen, urinary and intestinal tract of patients with the syndrome and also from blood culture (Macher et al 1983). The taxonomy is in doubt and it is believed to be a variant of *M. avium*, the causative organism of tuberculosis in birds (Grange 1984).

Mycobacterium xenopi, a slow-growing species originally isolated from the skin of a toad, has been frequently isolated from tap water. It may cause a granulomatous disease of the liver, lung, epididymis and elsewhere and a disseminated infection has been encountered in homosexual men with the Acquired Immune Deficiency Syndrome (AIDS) (Weinberg et al 1985) (see also Ch. 31).

M. fortuitum is one of the principal pathogenic species among the rapidly growing mycobacteria (Grange 1984). It used to be termed the 'tubercle bacillus of the frog'. Recorded as an opportunistic pathogen in AIDS there are other species also which can cause pulmonary disease in similar circumstances. *M. kansasii* is the most important opportunist mycobacterial pathogen in Britain and most sensitive to rifampicin. *M. avium* is usually partially resistant to most *anti-tuberculosis* drugs and at least four should be used (rifampicin, isoniazid, ethambutol, streptomycin) (Tyrrell et al 1979).

M. smegmatis is seldom seen in clinical specimens or in the natural environment (Grange 1984).

P12: Actinomyces and Nocardia
Genus I: *Actinomyces*
    Species
        Actinomyces odontolyticus
        Actinomyces viscosus
        Actinomyces israelii
Genis II: *Nocardia*
    Species
        Nocardia asteroides
        Nocardia brasiliensis

Actinomyces
Actinomyces are mould-like organisms which appear morphologically as Gram-positive jointed or unjointed filaments which frequently show branching. *Nocardia* is another genus with branched filaments whose primary residence is in the soil, whereas *Actinomyces* are strict parasites (e.g. *A. odontolyticus* occurs in human saliva and carious teeth; *A. viscosus* has been isolated from the mouth and produces plaque and periodontal disease).

Actinomyces israelii has been found in association with the long-term (more than 2 years) use of inert intrauterine contraceptive devices; conversely when copper-containing devices have been used there is a very low prevalence of actinomycetes, a finding which may be related to the bacteriostatic action of copper (Duguid et al 1984). Copper-containing IUCDs may however be associated with other infections e.g. *Eikenella corrodens* (see paragraph in Section P6 in this chapter).

Nocardia
Nocardia asteroides gives rise to abscesses and pulmonary disease in man and *N.brasiliensis* to mycetoma in man. The distinction between *Actinomyces* and *Nocardia* is based mainly on biochemical characters and cell-wall composition; the identity of many of these organisms may be hard to distinguish (Wilson 1983a). *Nocardia* may be a cause of focal or lobar pneumonia in AIDS (Ch. 31).

P13: Irregular non-sporing Gram-positive rods
Genus I: *Lactobacillus*
Genus II: *Listeria*
    Species
        Listeria monocytogenes
Genus III: *Corynebacterium*
    Species
        Corynebacterium minutissimum

Lactobacillus
Lactobacilli grow under anaerobic conditions, or at least under reduced oxygen tension. They decrease the pH

of their substrate by lactic acid formation to below 4.0 thus preventing, or at least delaying, growth of virtually all other competition except other lactic acid bacteria or yeasts. Lactobacilli occupy certain ecological niches such as the vagina and intestine which can be regarded as a natural habitat and where the organism are beneficial; there are many genotypes with low DNA-DNA homology even though they may have similar phenetic characteristics (Kandler & Weiss 1986)

Listeria

Listeria are Gram-positive coccoid to rod-shaped organisms with a tendency to form long filaments. Until recently the genus was usually said to contain only one species *Listeria monocytogenes* but different species, types, subtypes and serotypes have now been listed. Worldwide in distribution, regardless of climate, *L. monocytogenes* has been isolated from 50 species of wild and domestic animals as well as from fields and plants. Ordinarily saprophytic living in a plant-soil environment it is naturally pathogenic to a wide range of animals (Smith 1983). It is an uncommon cause of meningitis. In AIDS it is a rare cause of meningo-encephalitis which is curious since the T-lymphocyte has a crucial role in host defence and *L. monocytogenes* is excreted in the faeces of one person in 100 (Kernbaum and Francillon 1985).

Corynebacterium

The genus Corynebacterium (Greek *coryne*, a club; Greek *bacterion*, a small rod) comprise facultatively anaerobic heterogeneous organisms of which *C. diphtheriae* (Greek *diphthera*, leather — the disease in which a leathery membrane forms in the throat) is the best known for its production of a highly lethal endotoxin, the cause of death in diphtheria.

C. minutissimum colonies, when grown on certain rich media (e.g. 20% bovine fetal serum), show a coral red fluorescence; the organism may cause erythrasma (Collins & Cummins 1986).

P14: Microaerophilic spirally curved Gram-negative rods
Genus: *Campylobacter*
    Species
        Campylobacter fetus
            Subspecies
                intestinalis
                jejuni

Campylobacter

These slim Gram-negative rods — with some comma or S-shaped forms — are made motile by a polar flagellum. Growth is achieved in vitro in an atmosphere containing a partial pressure of oxygen at 2.5–6.0% and of CO_2 at 10%. Little or no growth occurs anaerobically. *C. fetus*

was the first member of the group to be isolated from the uterine exudate of aborting sheep (Parker & Smith 1983). *C. fetus* subsp. *intestinalis* and subsp. *jejuni* produce systemic infections and enteritis in man (Wilson & Smith 1984). This organism is sometimes of importance in homosexual males (Ch. 38).

P15. Family Spirochaetaceae
Genus I: *Treponema*
    Species (non-cultivable)
        Treponema pallidum subspecies *pallidum*
        Treponema pallidum subspecies *pertenue*
        Treponema pallidum 'subspecies' *endemicum*
        Treponema carateum
    Species (cultivable) from oral cavity, non-pathogenic
        Treponema denticola
        Treponema vincentii
        Treponema scolodontum
    Species (cultivable) from genitalia, non-pathogenic
        Treponema refringens
        Treponema minutum
        Treponema phagedenis
Genus II: (newly proposed) *Brachyspira*
    Species (newly proposed, cultivable)
        Brachyspira aalborgi

Treponema (non-cultivable 'species')

In the genus Treponema (Smibert 1984), the species or subspecies listed above have not been cultivated in artificial medium, a fact which has hampered studies including those of taxonomic classification. With DNA/DNA hybridization techniques (see Note 2.2) it has been shown however, that there is 100% homology between *Treponema pallidum* and *Treponema pertenue* (Miao & Fieldsteel 1980) so these two have been combined as two subspecies of *T. pallidum* albeit with different degrees of virulence and different ability to infect laboratory animals. *T. pallidum* subspecies *pallidum* causes venereal (sexually transmitted) and congenital syphilis and *T. pallidum* subspecies *pertenue* causes yaws in man. The causative organism of non-venereal syphilis of Africa, the Middle East, some areas of South-east Asia and certain parts of Yugoslavia, is spread by contact, considered also a variant of *T. pallidum*, and is designated 'subspecies' *endemicum*. All three are classed as the same species but each has different ability to infect various laboratory animals. In the case of *Treponema carateum*, the cause of a South American contagious disease of man, carate or pinta, it seems to be again a variant spread by contact but it does not produce skin lesions in rabbits, hamsters, mice or guinea pigs.

Treponema (cultivable species)

Anaerobic and cultivable treponemes from the oral cavity *T. denticola*, *T. vincentii*, *T. scolodontum* are found in the oral cavity of man. *T. refringens* is non-pathogenic and part of the normal flora of male and female genitalia of man or animals. *T. minutum* and *T. phagedenis* occupy a similar niche. *T. macrodentium* and *T. orale*, reported in the literature as being found in the gingival crevice of man are names that at present have no standing in nomenclature. *T. pallidum*, *T. phagedenis* and *T. refringens* are genetically distinct and show less than 5% DNA sequence homology (Miao & Fieldsteel 1978). Since oral treponemes can cause confusion in the diagnosis of oral lesions in early syphilis, diagnosis by dark ground examination (see Ch. 8) is not to be relied upon in lesions in this anatomical site.

Brachyspira (cultivable species)

Intestinal spirochaetosis, found particularly in male homosexuals (Ch. 38), is a condition where spirochaetes are to be found as a massive infestation of the luminal borders of the epithelium of the colon and rectum. The spirochaete is sigmoidal in shape with tapered ends, 2–6 μm long with a wavelength of 2 μm, flexible, with a maximum width of 0.2 μm. It is anaerobic, growing slowly at 37–38 °C in an atmosphere of 5% CO_2. The name proposed for the new species is *Brachyspira aalborgi* — the original biopsies studied were taken in the Danish town Aalborg (Hovind-Hougen et al 1982).

EUCARYOTAE

Eukaryotic organisms have one or more cells each with at least one well-defined nucleus of eukaryotic type,

where the nucleus is separated from the cytoplasm by a nuclear membrane and the genetic material borne on a number of chromosomes consisting of DNA and protein. Nuclear division is by mitosis.

Fungi (E1), protozoa, amoebae and flagellates (E2), nematodes (E3) and arthropods (E4) are considered in this group.

E1: Fungi

Classification

Fungi are eukaryotic organisms, classed with the protozoa and algae, but they differ fundamentally from the latter in that they have no chlorophyll and so are unable to photosynthesize their own carbohydrates from carbon dioxide. They are therefore of necessity obligate parasites or saprobes, dependent respectively on living or dead organic material for carbohydrates. Being larger and morphologically more complex than bacteria their classification and identification are based primarily on their appearance and only secondarily on their nutritional and biochemical differences.

Fungal spores may be produced sexually or asexually, the two types being quite distinct from one another. Should both the perfect (sexual) and imperfect (asexual) state of a given fungus be known they will almost certainly have been discovered at different times and will have been given different names (Note 2.5). Both the names are valid under the International Code of Botanical Nomenclature, but that of the perfect state takes precedence over that of the imperfect (English 1980).

The classification of Fungi is based on their mode of sexual reproduction, i.e. their perfect state (Note 2.8), but to clinicians many fungi, even those whose perfect state is described, will tend to be known by the more familiar names of their imperfect (or asexual) states (English 1980).

E1a: Fungi, ordinarily independent as saprobes, but sometimes occasional and/or opportunistic pathogens

Species (International Code of Botanical Nomenclature)
  Aspergillus fumigatus (Sartorya fumigata⋆)
  Cryptococcus neoformans (Filobasidiella neoformans⋆)
  Histoplasma capsulatum (Emmonsiella capsulatus⋆)
  Coccidioides immitis
  Thermoascus crustaceus⋆ (Dactylomyces crustaceus⋆)
  ⋆Name for perfect (sexual) state.

These saprobic fungi are primarily free-living, but they can and do multiply in mammalian tissue although this is for them an unnatural habitat. Transmission from a patient to a contact is almost unknown (Emmons et al 1977).

Table 2.3 Main eukaryotes listed in the groups considered in the text. The asterisk denotes that the eukaryote is included in the list only because it may be important as an opportunistic pathogen in the Acquired Immune Deficiency Syndrome (AIDS).

E1a	*Aspergillus fumigatus⋆*
	Cryptococcus neoformans⋆
	Histoplasma capsulatum⋆
	Coccidioides immitis⋆
	Thermoascus crustaceus⋆
E1b	*Candida albicans*
	Candida stellatoidea
	Candida tropicalis
	Torulopsis glabrata
E1c	Dermatophytes
E2a	*Entamoeba histolytica*
E2b	*Toxoplasma gondii⋆*
	Pneumocystis carinii⋆
	Isospora belli
	Cryptosporidium
E3	*Strongyloides stercoralis⋆*
	Enterobius vermicularis
E4	*Pthirus pubis*
	Sarcoptes scabiei

Aspergillus fumigatus is a fast-growing mould that thrives in the high temperatures of rotting vegetable matter. It produces enormous numbers of air-dispersed conidia on its mop-like sporing heads — *aspergillum* is a small brush used for distributing holy water. The conidia are ubiquitous but *A. fumigatus* cannot invade or colonize healthy lungs. The form of pulmonary aspergillosis seen in the patient, e.g. allergic aspergillosis or the aspergilloma, depends on the nature of the patient's primary lung condition. The fungus is not ordinarily invasive, behaving more as a saprobe than as a pathogen except in those gravely ill or immunosuppressed (English 1980), as in the Acquired Immune Deficiency Syndrome (AIDS), see Chapter 31.

Cryptococcus neoformans is widespread in nature and occurs in many parts of the world: it does not cause disease in pigeons but it shows a preference for pigeon droppings as a substrate in its saprobic phase (English 1980). The disease occurs only sporadically or in the immunosuppressed (e.g. AIDS), involving the lung, central nervous system and occasionally other organs. Histologically, *C. neoformans* is seen as spherical or oval thin-walled cells 2.5–20 μm in diameter surrounded by a mucoid polysaccharide capsule of varying thickness and best demonstrated by India ink preparations. With a mucicarmine stain the cell wall and capsule appear red (Frey et al 1979). In AIDS the capsule of *C. neoformans* seems to be defective and smaller than that in organisms seen in the cryptococcal meningitis of patients who do not have AIDS (Bottone et al 1985).

The perfect state or sexual state is now described and carries the name *Filobasidiella neoformans*, which takes precedence over the name given to the imperfect or asexual state viz. *Cryptococcus neoformans* (Kwon-Chung 1975). Clinicians may tend to use the more familiar name of the imperfect state.

Coccidioides immitis, again reported as an opportunistic infection in AIDS (Ch. 31), is seen as an infection, coccidioidomycosis, only in certain semi-arid desert areas where spores are adapted to survive the summer in the hot, dry, saline and very sandy soils, viz. south west USA, Central America and northern South America. The fungus does not exist in adjacent areas, where richer moist soils support its competitors (English 1980). In tissue, histological examination reveals diagnostic spherules containing endospores produced by the process, endosporulation (Frey et al 1979).

Atypical strains of *Thermoascus crustaceus* (*Dactylomyces crustaceus* is another name proposed for the perfect state) have been obtained from 6-week monocyte cultures from 3 patients with AIDS. Preliminary studies showed that mycelial extracts contained a cyclosporin-like material in high concentration which was observed to be immunosuppressive in vitro in mixed leucocyte culture (Sell et al 1983).

E1b: *Candida*, an artificial genus of medically important yeasts, normally a commensal of the digestive tract in man

'Genus' (able to produce pseudohyphae) *Candida*
    Species
        Class 1
        Candida albicans
        Candida stellatoidea
        Candida clausenii
        Candida tropicalis
        Class 2
        Candida parapsilosis
        Candida guilliermondii
        Class 3
        Candida pseudotropicalis (*Kluyveromyces fragilis*[*])
        Candida krusei (*Issatchenkia orientalis*[*])
'Genus' (unable to produce pseudohyphae) *Torulopsis* (now regarded as a synonym of *Candida*)
    Species
        Torulopsis glabrata
[*]Name for perfect (sexual) state.

Molecular studies have shown that the 'genus' *Candida* should be regarded as an artificial one in that its name does not imply descent from a common ancestor. The 'genus' is characterized by extreme diversity of its genetic material with base compositions (guanine + cytosine) ranging from 30–64 mol% and it is to be considered to be comprised of non-sexually reproducing forms of members of a variety of other genera, some of which have now been identified. Perfect forms of *C.pseudotropicalis* (*Kluyveromyces fragilis*) and *C.kreusei* (*Issatchenkia orientalis*) have been established or confirmed by DNA hybridization techniques. Similarly it has been shown by these techniques that *C.albicans* and *C.stellatoidea* are apparently synonymous. In recent years medically important *Candida* species have been studied further at the molecular level, and immunological data, in general agreement with DNA hybridization studies, has enabled the three main classes, as listed above, to be recognized. It remains something of a mystery, however, why the species *C.albicans* and *C.tropicalis*, which have low DNA homology, should be so similar in terms of their physiological and immunological properties (Riggsby 1985).

One classical group characteristic of the 'genus' *Candida* is its ability on certain laboratory media to produce pseudohyphae — germ tubes or elongated filaments which remain attached to the parent cells. It was believed that the 'genus' could, on the basis of this characteristic, be differentiated from *Torulopsis* spp which do not produce pseudohyphae (Odds 1979). The presence or absence of pseudohyphae, however, is now considered an inadequate basis for separating genera, and taxonomically *Torulopsis* spp are included within the genus *Candida* (Meyer et al 1984).

Many people harbour within them an ecosystem of commensal yeasts which have a potential to become pathogenic. The infective process seems to be linked with the ability to undergo conversion from yeast to the mycelial phase (Riggsby 1985). The distribution of species among yeasts in the vagina in subjects without vaginitis from Europe and North America resembles the distribution of yeasts in the faeces (percentages: *C.albicans*, 61.0; *Torulopsis glabrata*, 17.0; other or unidentified species, 7.8; *C.krusei*, 2.8; *C.tropicalis*, 2.4; *C.stellatoidea*, 2.3; *C.parapsilosis*, 2.0; *Rhodotorula* spp, 2.0; other *Candida* spp, 1.2; unspecified *Torulopsis* spp, 0.7; *C.guilliermondii*, 0.6; *C.pseudotropicalis*, 0.1). In Asia and South America the most prominent difference in distribution is the absence of *Torulopsis* spp. In general terms *C.albicans* must be regarded as the principal vaginal yeast pathogen (90% of cases of vaginitis) with *T.glabrata* the second most common cause of vaginitis (Odds 1979) (see Ch. 21).

Candida is a very versatile organism and may manifest itself as oral thrush in babies and adults, as vaginal thrush (Ch. 21), as infection of body folds in diabetes and in those on steroids, as nail-fold infections and corneal infection after trauma and steroids. Chronic mucocutaneous candidiasis is seen in immunodeficiency, circumstances when other organs may also be involved (English 1980). *Candida* infection of the oesophagus may be a warning sign of immunosuppression in AIDS (Ch. 31).

E1c: Dermatophytes

Species (anthropophilic)
Trichophyton interdigitale
Trichophyton rubrum
Epidermophyton floccosum
Species (zoophilic)
Microsporum canis (hosts: cats, dogs)
Trichophyton verrucosum (host: cattle)
Trichophyton mentagrophytes (host: rodents [feral, tame and laboratory])
Species (other)
Malassezia furfur

Dermatophytes are fungi which grow only in keratinized areas of the skin, hair and nails. *Trichophyton interdigitale* involves the feet and toe nails. *Trichophyton rubrum* spreads from these sites to involve the groin. *Epidermophyton floccosum* is found in both groin and feet. Six species are common in Britain and each have their distinctive behaviour pattern. In Third World countries anthropophilic species causing tinea pedis are far less common than in Britain and other more affluent areas (English 1980, p 30–33).

The skin lesions of *Malassezia furfur*, tinea versicolor, are often revealed by a suntan in those returning from holiday resorts of warmer climates. On direct examination skin scales of *M.furfur* show round budding yeast cells measuring up to 8 μm in diameter together with occasionally branched hyphal fragments of variable length. Direct findings are quite characteristic and although culture is possible it is not necessary for diagnosis (Emmons et al 1977, Frey et al 1979).

E2: Protozoa (a. Amoebae of digestive tract)

Order Amoebidae
Suborder I: Tubulinae
Genus: *Entamoeba*
Species
Entamoeba histolytica
Entamoeba hartmanni
Entamoeba coli
Genera (separate genera):
Species
Endolimax nana
Iodamoeba butschlii
Dientamoeba fragilis (resembles
Histomonas meleagridis lacking flagella
(McDougald & Reid 1978).

Amoebae of the digestive tract

The amoebae, commonly found in the human digestive tract, primarily the colon, are as follows:

1. three species in the genus *Entamoeba*, viz. *E.histolytica*, *E.hartmanni* and *E.coli*; and

2. three species of three different genera, viz. *Endolimax nana*, *Iodamoeba butschlii* and *Dientamoeba fragilis*. The latter protozoon, *D.fragilis* bears a strong resemblance to *Histomonas meleagridis* except for the absence of flagella (McDougald & Reid 1978). *Entamoeba histolytica*, although often a commensal, may be pathogenic and invasive both locally in the colon or extra-intestinally, particularly in the liver; all other intestinal amoeba are non-pathogenic (Albach & Booden 1978). Pathogenicity of *E. histolytica* is a complex subject to investigate. Progress has been made in characterizing these organisms by isoenzyme groups (zymodemes) and seeking to link symptomatic amoebiasis to specific isoenzyme markers (Sargeaunt & Williams 1980) but studies with controls, serology and biopsy will be required to make further advances. Insofar as sexually transmitted diseases are concerned, in areas of traditionally low endemicity intestinal amoebae are more commonly found in male homosexuals than in heterosexuals (Ch. 38). Although attention has been fixed on intestinal aspects destructive genital lesions due to *Entamoeba histolytica* are encountered (Peters & Gilles 1977a).

E2 Protozoa (b. Other protozoa)

Order: Eucoccidiida
Suborder: Eimeriina

Genus: *Toxoplasma*
    Species
       Toxoplasma gondii
Taxonomic position uncertain
    Species
       Pneumocystis carinii
       Isospora belli
       Cryptosporidium

Toxoplasma

Toxoplasma gondii (*toxon* means arc and *plasma*, form) is a common infection in humankind. It can be transmitted by the ingestion of raw meat; in Paris, where it is customary to eat raw meat, 80% of the adult population has antibody to *Toxoplasma*. It is spread by cats, which are the definitive hosts; the sexual phase of the parasite takes place in the small intestine of the cat. Oocysts are shed in the faeces and are infective after 1–5 days if ingested by any warm blooded animal, including humans. The fetus may also be infected when the woman becomes infected during pregnancy. In the congenital eye infection eye disease is a common sequela. *Toxoplasma* may proliferate in the retina. In the postnatally acquired infection lymphadenopathy is common (90%). Encephalitis occurs in the immunosuppressed (Dubey 1977) and the parasite is an important opportunistic pathogen in AIDS (Ch. 31).

Pneumocystis

Pneumocystis carinii is an unicellular eukaryote (Note 2.2) which develops extracellularly and undergoes encystment during one phase of its life cycle. It is the aetiological agent of pulmonary disease seen in the immunosuppressed as in the current epidemic disease, Acquired Immune Deficiency Syndrome (AIDS) in homosexual males and others (see Ch. 31). *P. carinii* is thus an opportunistic infection which exists ordinarily as a latent infection.

A useful laboratory animal model exists. If Sprague-Dawley rats, a commercially available strain of laboratory rats, are immunologically suppressed with corticosteroid and treated with antibiotic to suppress bacterial infection, gross pulmonary foci due to *Pneumocystis* appear in one month, to be followed later by pneumonic death (Seed & Aikawa 1977).

Isospora

Isospora belli infection has been reported in individuals suffering from AIDS. It is acquired by ingestion of oocysts (elongate, ellipsoidal and measuring 20–33 × 10–19 μm) in faeces. Sporulated oocysts contain two sporocysts which in turn contain four crescent-shaped sporozoites. The sexual cycle occurs in the upper intestinal epithelial cells. Infection causes fever, malaise, persistent diarrhoea, weight loss, steatorrhoea. Diagnosis is established by finding oocysts in the faeces or coccidian stages in duodenal biopsy (Dubey 1977).

Cryptosporidium

Cryptosporidia are coccidian parasites, probably of one species which can infect many species of mammal, bird and reptile. Spread by the faecal–oral route, the infection has been reported in cases of AIDS (Ch. 31). The endogenous stages of *Cryptosporidium* are small (2–6 μm) and characteristically they attach to the microvillous border of enterocytes in the large and small intestine. Diagnosis can be made by demonstrating the parasites in biopsy material or in the faeces stained by Giemsa or with dilute carbol fuchsin (Angus 1983, Snodgrass 1983). Cryptosporidiosis can cause severe and prolonged diarrhoea with wasting in patients with AIDS (Ch. 31). The disease has been recognized also in the United Kingdom in young adults working with calves imported from the USA and in such cases there may be no general or selective immune deficiency (Fletcher et al 1982). In addition it may be a cause of mild gastroenteritis, self-limiting in immunocompetent patients, with 4–6 watery mucoid and offensive motions a day lasting 1–2 weeks. Contact with farm animals may not be a feature and it is suggested that *Cryptosporidium* should be included routinely with those enteric pathogens sought in patients with diarrhoea (Hunt et al 1984).

E2c: Flagellates of the alimentary and urogenital tracts

Order 4: Retortamonadida
    Genus I: *Retortamonas*
       Species
          Retortamonas intestinalis
    Genus II: *Chilomastix*
       Species
          Chilomastix mesnili
Order 5: Diplomonadida
    Sub order 1: Enteromonadina
       Genus: *Enteromonas*
          Species
             Enteromonas hominis
    Suborder 2: Diplomonadina
       Genus: *Giardia*
          Species
             Giardia intestinalis
Order 7: Trichomonadida
    Genus: *Trichomonas*
       Species
          Trichomonas vaginalis
          Trichomonas tenax
          Pentatrichomonas hominis
    Genus: *Histomonas*

Species
'*Dientamoeba fragilis*' resembles *Histomonas meleagridis* lacking flagella (McDougald & Reid 1978).

Retortamonadae and Diplomonadae
Retortamonas intestinalis is generally a harmless intestinal commensal. *Chilomastix mesnili* may occasionally be a mild pathogen and be associated with diarrhoea. *Enteromonas hominis* is a harmless commensal. *Giardia intestinalis* may cause an asymptomatic infection but frequently causes diarrhoea, and malabsorption characterized by steatorrhoea may be seen. All are associated with ingestion of faecal material linked to water contamination by sewage. Interhuman transmission is probably the main process but host specificity in *G. intestinalis* requires re-appraisal (Kulda & Nohynkova 1978). Trophozoites are found in the jejunum and cysts in the faeces. In homosexual males infection is a frequent finding in the promiscuous as transmission by ingestion of cysts is made possible by ingestion of faecal material (Schmerin et al 1978). *Giardia* appears to be more common as an infection in homosexuals than *Chilomastix* (Ch. 38).

Trichomonadidae
Of the Trichomonadida, *Trichomonas tenax* occurs in the mouth, *Pentatrichomonas hominis* in the intestine and *Trichomonas vaginalis* in the urogenital tract. Diagnosis of the latter is most frequent in the female; it is a recognized cause of vaginitis (see Ch. 22). The first two species *T. tenax* and *P. hominis* are generally regarded as commensals (Honigberg 1978).

E3: Intestinal nematodes and other 'worms'
Species showing auto-infection by infective larvae.
    Strongyloides stercoralis
Species showing auto-infection by infective ova
    Enterobius vermicularis

Strongyloides
Although millions of people worldwide are infected with *Strongyloides stercoralis* (Note 2.6) the majority of infestations are asymptomatic or evoke minimal reaction. In the United States surveys from the southern and border states indicate a prevalence of 0.4–4% whereas in tropical countries prevalence may reach 85%. Symptoms may be cutaneous, pulmonary or intestinal and be related anatomically to the site reached by the migrating larvae; reinvasion of the host through the ileum or colon or perineal skin can occur and sometimes cause serious effects (e.g. haemorrhage) (Dellacona et al 1984). It is the only intestinal nematode where filariform *infective* larvae, rather than eggs are found in the faeces, which should be examined fresh to avoid confusion with other nematodes which may hatch into the larval form in the

stool (Ch. 38). In immunosuppression or after corticosteroid therapy systemic strongyloidiasis may be fatal as, for example, in a case reported in a man who had left an endemic area 30 years previously and who had been given dexamethasone following a head injury (Kimmelstiel & Lange 1984).

In Okinawa, Japan, it has been noted that there is a higher frequency of antibody positivity to human T-cell leukaemia virus (HTLV) in carriers of *S. stercoralis* (60%) compared with controls (20%). This may be due either to impairment of immunity in the host with such antibody which permits the proliferation and detection of the nematode. Alternatively long-standing nematode infection may promote infection or growth of HTLV in vivo resulting in the development of HTLV antibody (Nakada et al 1984). A similar situation may also exist in AIDS (Ch. 31).

Enterobius
Enterobius vermicularis is small, white and threadlike (length: males 2–5 mm, females 8–13 mm). The females emerge on to the perianal region where they lay 10 000–15 000 eggs then die. The embryonated eggs are directly infectious on ingestion and hatch in the duodenum. The larvae mature in the caecum.

Enterobius is a cause of pruritus ani, especially in children; reinfection occurs frequently from eggs under the fingernails. Bedding is a source of infection which tends to present in households and institutions. Homosexual males may acquire the infection more readily than others (Ch. 38) (see Note 2.6).

Taenia solium (the pig tapeworm), a cestode and not a nematode, may be conveniently mentioned here. It produces its serious effects when man becomes host to the 'bladder worms' (cysticerci). This may come about when he swallows the eggs (from food contaminated by human faeces or possibly by sexual oral/anal contact) (Bell 1984) as well as by internal auto-infection in which reverse peristalsis or upward migration of an adult worm leads to gravid proglottids releasing eggs in the upper gut.

E4: Arthropoda
Insecta
    Genus: *Pediculus*
        Species
            Pediculus humanus (var capitis; var corporis)
    Genus: *Pthirus*
        Species
            Pthirus pubis
Arachnida
    Genus: *Sarcoptes*
        Species
            Sarcoptes scabiei var *hominis*

Pediculus humanus is found in two forms, the head louse and the body louse, which can be considered as unstable environmental subspecies of one species (Clay 1973). As Busvine (1978) writes, however, the behavioural character which impels head lice to seek the scalp and body lice the garments is clearly a critical one but little is known about it. The smaller size of head lice, too, is advantageous in allowing them to slip easily through the dense hair of the scalp and escape capture. Head lice are more able to persist as a hygienic nuisance in communities of the developed world.

The human louse, which is cosmopolitan in its distribution, is of great importance as the vector of typhus fever (caused by *Rickettsia prowazeki*) and louse-borne relapsing fever (caused by *Borellia* (= Spirochaeta) *recurrentis*). *Pthirus pubis* is the correct name for the crab louse (Busvine 1978). The spelling 'Phthirus' is incorrect even although it has been hallowed in use in the important monograph on 'The Louse' by Professor P H Buxton (1947) and early work by G H F Nuttall FRS (1918). *Pthirus pubis* (Ch. 36) has not been incriminated as a vector of disease although it is suspected as a possible means of transmission in the case of hepatitis B.

The condition known as scabies or 'the itch' is caused by the invasion of the stratum corneum of man by the mite *Sarcoptes scabiei* var *hominis*. Although promiscuous behaviour may contribute to its spread, domestic or family outbreaks are more important within the community and some individuals may harbour very large numbers of *Sarcoptes* (Ch. 36).

NOTES TO CHAPTER 2

Note 2.1

Procaryotae (Greek *pro* before, implying primordial; *karyon* kernel, implying nucleus). In prokaryotic organisms the chromosomal material is in the form of haploid DNA (i.e. unpaired chromosomes) without the important protein component as in eukaryotic organisms, and is not separated from the cytoplasm by a nuclear membrane. The cell wall of prokaryotic organisms is unique in containing mureins (Abercrombie et al 1980).

Note 2.2

Eucaryotae. In contrast to prokaryotes, eukaryotic cells are the units of structure of all organisms except bacteria and blue-green algae. The nucleus of eukaryotes is separated from the cytoplasm by a nuclear membrane (Abercrombie et al 1980).

Note 2.3

Hybridization techniques are used to determine whether two specimens of DNA have blocks or segments of complementary base sequences and to what extent they may pair and rewind at their complementary regions.

Two specimens of DNA are mixed and heated to cause unwinding and separation of the strands at the melting point. On cooling, if they possess complementary base sequences, they will associate together to form *hybrid duplexes*. The extent to which hybrids form is easily determined if one specimen is labelled with ^{32}P; this gives their taxonomic relationship (Lehninger 1975).

The per cent homology is expressed as the amount of heterologous binding divided by the amount of homologous binding $\times 100$ (Johnson 1984).

Note 2.4

A plasmid is a small extrachromosomal piece of genetic material that can replicate autonomously and maintain itself in the cytoplasm of a bacterium for many generations; it is a circular piece of double-stranded DNA.

Note 2.5

Classification of fungi is based primarily on their mode of sexual reproduction, i.e. their perfect state. Fungi of medical importance belong to the following subgroups (English 1980):
1. Zygomycotina: fusion of the tips of two fertile hyphae with the formation of a zygospore.
2. Ascomycotina: formation of a sac or ascus containing eight sexually produced ascospores, e.g. *Emmonsiella capsulatum* (imperfect state: *Histoplasma capsulatum*).
3. Basidiomycotina: formation of four basidiospores borne on projections at tip of a club-shaped basidium, e.g., *Filobasidiella neoformans* (imperfect state: *Cryptococcus neoformans*).
4. Deûteromycotina or Fungi Imperfecti: Perfect (sexual) state not known, e.g. *Coccidioides immitis*).

Note 2.6

The life cycle of *Strongyloides stercoralis* has three main patterns (Peters & Gilles 1977b):
1. Free-living adult males and females have a sexual cycle in moist soil where rhabditiform larvae develop into infective filariform larvae.
2. Filariform infective larvae penetrate the skin of the new host (e.g. man) and the developing nematodes migrate via the lung to the jejunum. Parthenogenetic females only are ordinarily to be found in man and rhabditiform larvae developing from these also grow into infective filariform larvae before leaving the intestine.
3. Auto-infection can lead to severe creeping eruption, usually of the back, an eosinophilic lung infection or, if the patient is given immunosuppressive agents, the severe effects with haemorrhage into the colon referred to in the text.

REFERENCES

Abercrombie M, Hickman C J, Johnson M L 1980 The Penguin Dictionary of Biology, 7th edn. Penguin Books, Middlesex

Albach R A, Booden T 1978 Amoebae. In: Kreier J P (ed) Parasite protozoa vol.II. Intestinal flagellates, histomonads, trichomonads, amoebae, opalinids and ciliates. Academic Press, New York, p 455–506

Angus K W 1983 Cryptosporidiosis in man, domestic animals and birds: a review. Journal of the Royal Society of Medicine 76: 62–70

Anonymous 1985 Why the AIDS virus is not like HTLV-I or II. New Scientist 1442: 4

Armstrong D 1984 The Acquired Immune Deficiency Syndrome: Viral infections and etiology. Progress in Medical Virology 30: 1–13

Bader M, Pedersen A H B, Williams D C, Spearman J, Anderson H 1977 Venereal transmission of shigellosis in Seattle-King County. Sexually Transmitted Diseases 4: 89–91

Barré-Sinoussi F, Chermann J C, Rey F et al 1983 Isolation of a T-lymphotropic retrovirus from a patient at risk for Acquired Immune Deficiency Syndrome (AIDS). Science 220: 868–871

Bell D R 1984 Cysticercosis, a new hope. British Medical Journal 289: 857–858

Bercovier H, Mollaret H H 1984 Genus XIV Yersinia etc; *Yersinia enterocolitica* In: Krieg N R, Holt J G (eds) Bergey's manual of systematic bacteriology vol 1, p 498–503, 505

Bottone E J, Toma M, Johansson B E, Wormser G P 1985 Capsule-deficient *Cryptococcus neoformans* in AIDS patients. Correspondence, Lancet i: 400

Brotherston, Sir John 1977 Memorandum on Lassa fever. Scottish Home and Health Department, HMSO, Edinburgh

Busvine J R 1978 Evidence from double infestations for the specific status of human head lice and body lice (Anoplura). Systematic Entomology 3: 1–8

Buxton P A 1947 The Louse. Arnold, London

Christensen K K, Christensen P, Flamhole L, Ripa T 1974 Frequencies of streptococci of groups A, B, C, D and G in urethra and cervix swab specimens from patients with suspected gonococcal infection. Acta Pathologica et Microbiologica Scandinavica B 82: 470–474

Clay T 1973 Lice. In: Smith K G V (ed) Insects and other arthropods of medical importance. British Museum, Natural History, London, ch 9, p 395–397

Coffin J, Haase A, Levy J A, et al 1986 What to call the AIDS virus. Correspondence, Nature 321: 10

Collins M D, Cummins C S 1986 Genus Corynebacterium. In: Sneath P H A, Mair N S, Sharpe M E, Holt J G (eds) Bergey's manual of systematic bacteriology vol 2, p 1272

Corey L, Holmes K K 1980 Sexual transmission of hepatitis A in homosexual men. New England Journal of Medicine 302: 435–438

Curtin M E 1986 AIDS and the single cell. Microbiological Sciences 3: 274–275

Dellacona S, Spier N, Wessely Z, Margolis I B 1984 Massive colonic haemorrhage secondary to infection with Strongyloides stercoralis. New York State Journal of Medicine 84: 397–399

Dienst R B, Brownell G H 1984 Genus Calymmatobacterium etc. In: Krieg N R, Holt J G (eds) Bergey's Manual of systematic bacteriology, vol 1, Williams and Wilkins, Baltimore, p 585–587

Dritz S K, Braft E H 1977 Sexually transmitted typhoid fever. New England Journal of Medicine 296: 1359–1360

Dritz S K, Ainsworth T E, Garrard W F, Back A, Palmer R D, Boucher L A, River E 1977 Patterns of sexually transmitted enteric diseases in a city. Lancet ii: 3–4

Drouet E, De Montclos H, Boude M, Denoyel G A 1987 Eikenella corrodens and intrauterine contraceptive device. Correspondence, Lancet ii: 1089

Dubey J P 1977 Toxoplasma, Hammondia, Besnoitia, Sarcocystis and other cyst-forming coccidia of man and animals. In: Kreier J P (ed) Parasitic protozoa, vol III, Gregarines, Haemogregarines, Coccidia, Plasmodia, and Haemoproteids. Academic Press, London, p 101–237

Du Bois R M, Griffiths P D, Prentice H G 1985 Rapid diagnosis of cytomegalovirus infection. Correspondence, Lancet i: 171

Duguid H L D, Duncan I D, Parrat H D, Taylor D 1984 Risks of intrauterine contraception devices. Correspondence, British Medical Journal 289: 767

Editorial 1984 Prevention of early onset Group B streptococcal infection in the newborn. Lancet i: 1056–1057

Eisenstein B I, Sox T, Biswas G, Blackman E, Sparling P F 1977 Conjugal transfer of the gonococcal penicillinase plasmid. Science 195: 998–1000

Emmons C W, Binford C H, Utz J P, Kwon-Chung K J 1977 Medical mycology, 3rd edn. Lea and Febiger, Philadelphia, p 35–37, 174–180

English M P 1980 Medical mycology. The Institute of Biology's Studies in Biology No 119, Edward Arnold, London, p 1–4, 10, 24, 30–33, 34

Epstein M A, Achong B G, Barr Y M 1964 Virus particles in cultured lymphoblasts from Burkitt's lymphoma. Lancet i: 702–703

Finch R G, French G L, Phillips I 1976 Group B streptococci in the female genital tract. British Medical Journal 1: 1245–1247

Fisher A G, Feinberg M B, Josephs S F et al 1986 The trans-activator gene of HTLV-III is essential for replication. Nature 320: 367–371

Fletcher A, Sims T A, Talbot I C 1982 Cryptosporidial enteritis without general or selective immune deficiency. British Medical Journal 285: 22–23

Forster G E, Karim Q N, White K B, Harris J R W 1983 Isolating Haemophilus ducreyi. Lancet ii: 909–910

Frey D, Oldfield R J, Bridges R C 1979 A colour atlas of pathogenic fungi. Wolfe Medical Publications p 21, 78, 79, 80–81

Gallo R C 1987 The AIDS virus. Scientific American 256: 38–48

Gallo R C, Salahuddin S Z, Popovic M et al 1984 Frequent detection and isolation of cytopathic retroviruses (HTLV-III) from patients with AIDS and at risk for AIDS. Science 224: 500–503

Glew R H, Moellering R C, Kunz L J 1977 Infections with Acinetobacter calcoaceticus (Herrellea vaginicola): Clinical and laboratory studies. Medicine 56: 79–97

Gotschlich E C 1984 Development of a gonorrhoea vaccine; prospects, strategies and tactics. Bulletin of the World Health Organization 62 (5): 671–680

Grange J M 1984 The mycobacteria. In: Wilson Sir Graham, Miles Sir Ashley, Parker M T, Smith G R (eds) Topley and Wilson's Principles of bacteriology, virology and immunity, vol 2, Systematic bacteriology. Edward Arnold, London, p 60–93

Greenwood J R, Pickett M J 1984 Genus Gardnerella etc. In: Krieg N R, Holt J G (eds) Bergey's manual of systematic bacteriology, vol 1, Williams and Wilkins, Baltimore, p 587–590

Griffiths P D, Panjwani D D, Stirk P R, Ball M G, Ganezakowski M, Blacklock H A, Prentice H G 1984 Rapid diagnosis of cytomegalovirus infection in immunocompromised patients by detection of early antigen fluorescent foci. Lancet ii: 1243–1245

Guyader M, Emerman M, Sonigo P, Clavel F, Montagnier L, Alizon M 1987 Genome organization and transactivation of the human immunodeficiency virus type 2. Nature 326: 662–669

Hahn B H, Shaw G M, Suresh K A, Popovic M, Gallo R C, Wong-Staal F 1984 Molecular cloning and characterization of the HTLV-III virus associated with AIDS. Nature 312: 166–169

Hofstad T 1984 Genus IV Leptotrichia etc. In: Kreig N R, Holt J G (eds) Bergey's manual of systematic bacteriology, vol 1. Williams and Wilkins, Baltimore, p 637–641

Holdeman L V, Kelley R W, Moore W E C 1984 Genus I Bacteroides etc. In: Krieg N R, Holt J G (eds) Bergey's manual of systematic bacteriology, vol 1. Williams and Wilkins, Baltimore, p 604–631

Hollinger F B 1985 Part III Non-A, non-B hepatitis viruses and the delta agent. In: Fields B N, Knipe D M, Chanock R M, Melnick J, Roizman B, Shope R (eds) Virology. Raven Press, New York, p 1407–1415

Honigberg B M 1978 Trichomonads of importance in human medicine. In: Kreier J P (ed) Parasitic protozoa, vol II. intestinal flagellates, histomonads, trichomonads, amoebae, opalinids and ciliates. Academic Press, New York, p 275–454

Hovind-Hougen K, Birch-Andersen A, Henrik-Nielsen R, Orholm M, Pedersen J O, Teglbjaerg P S, Thaysen E H 1982 Intestinal spirochaetosis: Morphological characterization and cultivation of the spirochete Brachyspira aalborgi gen. nov., sp. nov. Journal of Clinical Microbiology 16: 1127–1136

Hughes S S 1977 The virus: A history of the concept. Heinemann Educational Books, London

Hunt D A, Shannon R, Palmer S R, Jephcott A E 1984 Cryptosporidiosis in an urban community. British Medical Journal 289: 814–816

Jackson F L, Goodman Y 1984 Genus Eikenella Jackson and Goodman, 1972. In: Krieg N R, Holt J G (eds) Bergey's manual of systematic bacteriology, vol 1. Williams and Wilkins, Baltimore, p 591–597

Johnson J L 1984 Bacterial classification III, nucleic acids in bacterial classification. In: Krieg N R, Holt J G (eds) Bergey's Manual of systematic bacteriology, vol 1, Williams and Wilkins, Baltimore p 8–11

Juni E 1984 Genus III Acinetobacter etc. In: Krieg N R, Holt J G (eds) Bergey's Manual of systematic bacteriology, vol 1. Williams and Wilkins, Baltimore, p 303–30

Kandler O, Weiss N 1986 Section 14, Regular, nonsporing Gram-positive rods. In: Sneath P H A, Mair N S, Sharpe M E, Holt J G (eds) Bergey's Manual of systematic bacteriology, vol 2. p 1208–1219

Kernbaum S, Francillon A 1985 Meningoencephalitis due to Listeria monocytogenes in a patient with AIDS. Unreviewed reports. British Medical Journal 290: 606

Kimmelsteil F, Lange M 1984 Fatal systemic strongyloidiasis following corticosteroid therapy. New York State Journal of Medicine 84: 399–401

Krieg N R, Holt J G 1984 Bergey's Manual of systematic bacteriology, vol 1. Williams and Wilkins, Baltimore

Kulda J, Nohynkova E 1978 Flagellates of the human intestine and of intestines of other species. In: Kreier J P (ed) Parasitic protozoa, vol II, Intestinal flagellates, histomonads, trichomonads, amoebae, opalinids and ciliates. Academic Press, New York, p 1–138

Kwon-Chung K J 1975 A new genus, Filobasidiella, the perfect state of Cryptococcus neoformans. Mycologia 67: 1197–1200

Larson H E, Price A B, Honour P, Borriello S P 1978 Clostridium difficile. Lancet i: 1063

Lehninger A L 1975 The hybridization techniques: Sequence homologies in DNA of different species. In: Lehninger A L (ed) Biochemistry, 2nd edn. Worth Publishing, New York, ch 31, p 882–890

Le Minor L 1984 Genus III Salmonella etc. In: Krieg N R, Holt J G (eds) Bergey's manual of systematic bacteriology, vol 1. Williams and Wilkins, Baltimore, p 427–458

Levy J A, Hoffman A D, Kramer S M, Landis J A, Shimabukuro J M, Oshiro L S 1984 Isolation of lymphocytopathic retroviruses from San Francisco patients with AIDS. Science 225: 840–842

Macher A M, Kovacs J A, Gill V et al 1983 Bacteriuria due to Mycobacterium intracellulare in the Acquired Immuno-deficiency Syndrome. Annals of Internal Medicine 99: 782–785

Maddox J 1984 AIDS casts a longer shadow. News and Views. Nature 312: 97

Mardh P-A 1980 An overview of infectious agents of salpingitis, their biology and recent advances in methods of detection. American Journal of Obstetrics and Gynecology 138: 933–951

Mardh P-A, Taylor-Robinson D (eds) 1984 Bacterial vaginosis. Almqvist and Wiksell International, Stockholm

Mardh P-A, Westrom L 1970a Tubal and cervical cultures in acute salpingitis with special reference to Mycoplasma hominis and T-strain mycoplasmas. British Journal of Venereal Diseases 46: 179–186

Mardh P-A, Westrom L 1970b Antibodies to Mycoplasma hominis in patients with genital infections and in healthy controls. British Journal of Venereal Diseases 46: 390–397

McDougald L R, Reid W M 1978 Histomonas meleagridis and relatives. In: Kreier J P (ed) Parasitic protozoa, vol II, Intestinal flagellates, histomonads, amoebae, opalinids and ciliates, Academic Press, New York, p 142

Melnick J L 1971 Classification and nomenclature of animal viruses. Progress in Medical Virology 13: 462–484

Melnick J L 1982 Taxonomy and nomenclature of viruses. Progress in Medical Virology 28: 208–221

Meyer S A, Ahearn D G, Yarrow D 1984 Genus 4 Candida Berkhout. In: Kreger-van Rij N J W (ed) The yeasts, a taxonomic study, 3rd revised and enlarged edition. Elsevier, Amsterdam, p 841–843

Meyer T F, Mlawer N, So M 1982 Pilus expression in Neisseria gonorrhoeae involves chromosomal rearrangement. Cell 30: 45–52

Miao M, Fieldsteel A H 1978 Genetics of Treponema: Relationship between Treponema pallidum and five cultivable treponemes. Journal of Bacteriology 133: 101–107

Miao M, Fieldsteel A H 1980 Genetic relationship between Treponema pallidum and Treponema pertenue, two non-cultivable human pathogens. Journal of Bacteriology 141: 427–429

Mims C A, White D O 1984 Viral pathogenesis and immunology. Blackwell Scientific Publications, p 16, 214–216, 298

Møller B R, Taylor-Robinson D, Furr, P M 1984 Serological evidence implicating Mycoplasma genitalium in pelvic inflammatory disease. Lancet i: 1102–1103

Moore W E C, Holdeman L V, Kelley R W 1984 Genus II Fusobacterium etc. In: Krieg N R, Holt J G (eds) Bergey's manual of systematic bacteriology, vol 1. Williams and Wilkins, Baltimore, p 631–637

Moore L V, Johnson J L, Moore W E C 1986 Peptostreptococcus. In: Sneath P H A, Mair N S, Sharpe M E, Holt J G (eds) Bergey's manual of systematic bacteriology, vol 2. Williams and Wilkins, Baltimore p 1083–1086

Moulder J W, Hatch T P, Kuo C-C, Schachter J, Storz J 1984 Genus I Chlamydia etc. In: Krieg N R, Holt J G (eds) Bergey's manual of systematic bacteriology, vol 1. Williams and Wilkins, Baltimore, p 729–739

Murphy F A 1985a Virus taxonomy. In: Fields B N, Knipe D M, Chanock R M, Melnick J L, Roizman B, Shope R E (eds) Virology, Raven Press, New York, ch 2, p 15

Murphy F A 1985b Marburg and Ebola viruses. In: Fields B N, Knipe D M, Chanock R M, Melnick J L, Roizman B, Shope R E (eds) Virology. Raven Press, New York, ch 47, p 1111–1118

Nakada K, Kohakura M, Komoda H, Hinuma Y 1984 High incidence of HTLV antibodies in carriers of Strongyloides stercoralis. Correspondence, Lancet i: 633

Nsanze H, Fast M V, D'Costa L J, Tukei P, Curran J, Ronald A 1981 Genital ulcers in Kenya: Clinical and laboratory study. British Journal of Venereal Diseases 57: 378–381

Nuttall G H F 1918 The biology of Phthirus pubis. Parasitology 10: 383–405

Odds F C 1979 Candida and candidosis. Leicester University Press, p 68–69, 101–112

Pahlson C, Forsum U 1985 Rapid detection of Mobiluncus species. Lancet i: 927

Parker M T 1978 The pattern of streptococcal disease in men. In: Skinner F A, Quesnel L B (eds) Streptococci. The Society of Applied Bacteriology Symposium No 7.

Academic Press, London, p 71–106

Parker M T 1983 Staphylococcus and Micrococcus; the anaerobic gram-positive cocci. In: Wilson Sir Graham, Miles Sir Ashley, Parker M T, Smith G R (eds) Topley and Wilson's Principles of bacteriology, virology and immunity, vol 2, Systematic bacteriology. Edward Arnold, London, p 218–245

Parker M T 1984a Hospital-acquired infections. In: Wilson Sir Graham, Miles Sir Ashley, Parker M T, Smith G R (eds) Topley and Wilson's Principles of bacteriology, virology and immunity, vol 3. Bacterial diseases, Edward Arnold, London, p 192–224

Parker M T 1984b Staphylococcal diseases. In: Wilson Sir Graham, Miles Sir Ashley, Parker M T, Smith G R (eds) Topley and Wilson's Principles of bacteriology, virology and immunity, vol 3. Bacterial diseases. Edward Arnold, London, p 254–278

Parker M T, Smith G 1983 Campylobacter. In: Wilson Sir Graham, Miles Sir Ashley, Parker M T, Smith G R (eds) Topley and Wilson's Principles of bacteriology, virology and immunity, vol 2. Systematic bacteriology. Edward Arnold, London, p 148–155

Peters W, Gilles H M 1977a Amoebic balanitis. Colour atlas of tropical medicine and parasitology. Year Book Medical Publishers, Chicago, p 258

Peters W, Gilles H M 1977b Strongyloidiasis. Colour atlas of tropical medicine and parasitology. Year Book Medical Publishers, Chicago, p 168–169

Pfister H 1984 Biology and biochemistry of papillomaviruses. Review of Physiology, Biochemistry and Pharmacology 9: 111–181

Piot P, Slootmans L, Nsanze H, Ronald A R 1983 Isolating Haemophilus ducreyi. Correspondence. Lancet ii: 909–910

Popovic M, Sarngadharan M G, Read E, Gallo R C 1984 Detection, isolation and continuous production of cytopathic retroviruses (HTLV-III) from patients with AIDS and pre-AIDS. Science 224: 497–500

Ratner L, Gallo R C, Wong-Staal F 1985 HTLV-III, LAV, ARV are variants of the same AIDS virus. Scientific correspondence. Nature 313: 636–637

Razin S, Freundt E A 1984 Family Mycoplasmataceae etc. In: Krieg N R, Holt J G (eds) Bergey's Manual of systematic bacteriology, vol 1. Williams and Wilkins, Baltimore, p 742–770

Riche O, Vernet V, Megier P 1987 Bartholin's abscess associated with Eikenella corrodens. Correspondence, Lancet ii: 1089

Riggsby W S 1985 Some recent developments in the molecular biology of medically important Candida. Microbiological Sciences 2(9): 257–263

Roizman B, Carmichael L E, Deinhardt G de-The et al 1981 Herpesviridae, definition, provisional nomenclature and taxonomy. Intervirology 16: 201–217

Rowe B, Gross R J 1984 Genus II. Shigella etc. In: Krieg N R, Holt J G (eds) Bergey's Manual of systematic bacteriology, vol 1. William and Wilkins, Baltimore, p 423–427

Sargeaunt P G, Williams J E 1980 The epidemiology of Entamoeba histolytica in Mexico City, a pilot survey 1. Transactions of the Royal Society of Tropical Medicine and Hygiene 74: 653–656

Schmerin M J, Jones T C, Klein H 1978 Giardiasis: association with homosexuality. Annals of Internal Medicine 88: 801–803

Seed T M, Aikawa M 1977 Pneumocystis. In: Kreier J P (ed) Parasitic protozoa, vol IV. Babesia, Theileria, Bartonellaceae, Anaplasmataceae, Ehrlichia and Pneumocystis. Academic Press, New York, p 329–357

Sell K W, Folks J, Kwon-Chung K J, Coligan J, Malloy W L 1983 Cyclosporin immunosuppression as the possible cause of AIDS. Correspondence, The New England Journal of Medicine 309: 1065

Seto B, Gerety R J, Coleman W G, Iwarson S 1985 Non-A, non-B hepatitis agent. Correspondence, Lancet i: 169–170

Shanson D C, Gazzard B G 1984 Kingella kingae septicaemia with a clinical presentation resembling disseminated gonococcal infection. British Medical Journal 289: 730–731

Siegert R 1970 The Marburg virus. In: Health R B, Waterson A P (eds) Modern trends in medical virology-2. Butterworths, London, p 204–240

Simpson D I H 1977 Marburg and Ebola virus infections: A guide for their diagnosis, management and control. World Health Organization Offset Publication No 36, Geneva

Singer A, Walker P G, McCance D J 1984 Genital wart virus infections; nuisance or potentially lethal. British Medical Journal 288: 735–737

Smibert R M 1984 Genus III Treponema. In: Krieg N R, Holt J G (eds) Bergey's manual of systematic bacteriology, vol 1. Williams and Wilkins, Baltimore, p 49–57

Smith G 1983 Erysipelothrix and Listeria. In: Wilson Sir Graham, Miles Sir Ashley, Parker M J (eds) Topley and Wilson's Principles of bacteriology, virology and immunity, vol 2. Systematic bacteriology. Edward Arnold, London, p 50–57

Snodgrass D R 1983 Cryptosporidiosis. Communicable Diseases in Scotland, Weekly CDS Report 83/32a, CDS Unit, Ruchill Hospital, Glasgow G20 9NB, p vii

Spector D H, Spector S A 1984 The oncogenic potential of human cytomegalovirus infection. Progress in Medical Virology 29: 45–89

Spiegel C A, Roberts M 1984 Mobiluncus gen nov, Mobiluncus curtisii sp nov, Mobiluncus curtisii subsp holmesii subsp nov, and Mobiluncus mulieris sp nov, curved rods from the human vagina. International Journal of Systematic Bacteriology 34: 177–184

Stroop W G, Baringer J R 1982 Persistent slow and latent viral infections. Progress in Medical Virology 28: 1–43

Tabor E 1985 The three viruses of non-A, non-B hepatitis. Occasional Survey. Lancet i: 742–745

Taylor C E D, Rosenthal R O, Taylor-Robinson D 1979 Preliminary communication. Patients with non-gonococcal urethritis to causative organism of contagious equine metritis. Lancet i: 700–701

Taylor-Robinson D, Gourly R N 1984 Genus II Ureaplasma etc. In: Krieg N R, Holt J G (eds) Bergey's manual of systematic bacteriology, vol 1. Williams and Wilkins, Baltimore, p 770–775

Tvede M, Willumsen L 1982 Clostridium difficile in patients with irritable bowel syndrome and ulcerative colitis. Correspondence, Lancet i: 1124

Tyrrell D A J, Phillips I, Goodwin C S, Blowers R 1979 Microbial disease: the use of the laboratory in diagnosis, therapy and control. Edward Arnold, London, p 92

Vedros N A 1984 Genus I Neisseria etc. In: Krieg N R, Holt J G (eds) Bergey's manual of systematic bacteriology, vol 1. Williams and Wilkins, Baltimore, p 290–296

Wain-Hobson S, Alizon M, Montagnier L 1985 Relationship of AIDS to other retroviruses. Scientific correspondence. Nature 313: 743

Watson J D, Tooze J, Kurtz D T 1983 Recombinant DNA; A short course. Scientific American Books, Freeman, New York, p 127–139, 147–149

Weinberg J R, Dootson G, Gertner D, Chambers S T, Smith H 1985 Disseminated *Mycobacterium xenopi* infection. Lancet i: 1033–1034

Weiss R, Mulder C 1986 Virology, news and views. A new human herpesvirus. Nature 323: 762

White D O 1984 Antiviral chemotherapy, interferons and vaccines. In: Melnick J L (ed) Monographs in virology 16. Karger, Basel, p 68–85

Willis A T 1983 *Clostridium*: The spore bearing anaerobes In: Wilson Sir Graham, Miles Sir Ashley, Parker M T (ed) Topley and Wilson's Principles of bacteriology, virology and immunity, vol 2, Systematic bacteriology. Edward Arnold, London, p 442–475

Wilson G 1983a *Actinomyces, Nocardia* and *Actinobacillus*. In: Wilson Sir Graham, Myles Sir Ashley, Parker M T (eds) Topley and Wilson's Principles of bacteriology, virology and immunity vol 2. Systematic bacteriology. Edward Arnold, London, p 31–49

Wilson G 1983b Legionella. In: Wilson Sir Graham, Myles Sir Ashley, Parker M T (eds) Topley and Wilson's Principles of bacteriology, virology and immunity vol 2. Systematic bacteriology. Edward Arnold, London, p 481–483

Wilson G, Smith G 1984 Campylobacter infections. In: Smith G R (ed) Topley and Wilson's Principles of bacteriology, virology and immunity, vol 3. Bacterial diseases. Edward Arnold, London, p 161–169

Wong-Staal F, Gallo R C 1985 Human T-lymphotropic retroviruses. Nature 317(6036): 395–403

Young H, Harris A B, Robertson D H H, Fallon R J 1983 Ano-genital gonorrhoea and pharyngeal colonisation with meningococci: a serogroup analysis. Journal of Infection 6: 49–54

zur Hausen H 1977 Human papillomaviruses and their possible role in squamous cell carcinomas. Current Topics of Microbiology and Immunology 78: 1–30

3

Nature and incidence of sexually transmissible infections

Within the compass of a few pages it is feasible to present only an incomplete and perhaps impressionistic picture on the nature and incidence of sexually transmissible disease throughout the world. Some points, however, can be made usefully in this context with regard to infections due to *Treponema pallidum*, *Neisseria gonorrhoeae* and *Chlamydia trachomatis*, but it is in other parts of this book that detailed reference will be made to infections due to those prokaryotes less surely and regularly transmitted by sexual intercourse. Sexual spread of *Pthirus pubis* and *Trichomonas vaginalis* is familiar but the spread of enteric organisms as a result of homosexual intercourse in males may not receive necessary consideration by clinicians. Insofar as virus infections are concerned vaccination is only available at present against hepatitis B, and chemotherapy is as yet only practicable and useful for herpes simplex. The advent of disease due to human immunodeficiency viruses (HIV) brings new dimensions to the subject that are profoundly difficult to contain. Human papillomavirus infections (HPV) and their uncertain relationship to cervical cancer turn straightforward management and follow-up, seen as practice in the case of, say, gonorrhoea and syphilis, into problems of securing advanced virological services, probably lifetime follow-up, with costly colposcopy and other gynaecological facilities.

The nature and incidence of sexually transmissible infections are considered in this chapter under the various headings, viz. infection due to 1. prokaryotes, 2. eukaryotes and 3. viruses.

1. INFECTIONS DUE TO PROKARYOTES

SYPHILIS

Syphilis is worldwide in its distribution but, as in the case of gonorrhoea, it is difficult to compare the incidence of the disease from one country to another. The extent to which available statistics reflect the incidence of the disease depends upon the efforts made in case finding, the variations in notification practices and social factors which may limit, increase or reduce the interaction between infected individuals and health services. If errors in reporting in each country are assumed to be consistent the data provided by the World Health Organization (Fig. 3.1) suggest that few countries have been able to reduce the incidence of syphilis over the past two or so decades (World Health Organization 1982).

Before the advent of antibiotic and chemotherapy the impact of the prokaryotic venereal diseases, particularly syphilis and gonorrhoea, was profound and continues to remain so in populations with no access to medical treatment. The miraculous change attributable to modern antibiotic treatment is shown by the situation in the United Kingdom, for example, where congenital syphilis virtually disappeared as a cause of death in infants under the age of one year (Fig. 3.2); the death rate started to decline when arsenical treatment became widely available and accelerated with the advent of penicillin. Some 70 years ago about 1200 infants died each year from congenital syphilis whereas today the discovery of the disease in the newborn is a rare event. Congenital syphilis accounted for 12% of the blindness in the UK in the 1930s but by the mid-1950s for less than 1% and the numbers continued to fall.

Again, in the United Kingdom, syphilis affected about 10% of the total population in 1913. If untreated, about 40% of those with acquired disease developed late-stage disease viz. gummatous, cardiovascular or central nervous system syphilis. Acquired syphilis accounted for 6% of the blindness in adults aged 30–49, but 30 years later less than 0.1%. A striking decline occurred in late-stage syphilis, particularly in neurosyphilis where the decline accelerated after World War II (Fig. 3.3); in cardiovascular syphilis, less easy to detect or reverse by treatment, death rates declined more slowly (Fig. 3.4).

The number of new cases of cardiovascular and central nervous system syphilis has continued to fall, but the other category of late syphilis (i.e. other late and

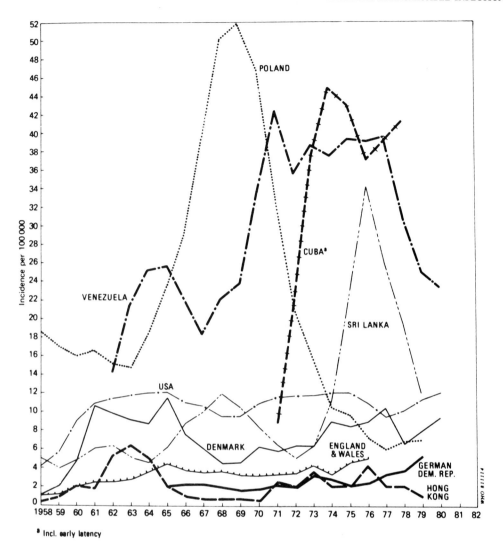

Fig. 3.1 Reported incidence of primary and secondary syphilis per 100 000 population, 1958–1980. (World Health Organization 1982.)

latent) has not followed this pattern (Fig. 3.5). The very sensitive and specific serological test for syphilis, the *Treponema pallidum* Haemagglutination Assay (TPHA), used widely both inside and outside clinics has without doubt contributed to the increase by enabling the detection of 'latent' infections, often among the elderly who may or may not have had previous antibiotic treatment for this or an unrelated infection.

The universal serological testing of pregnant women in antenatal clinics has been important in eliminating congenital syphilis and remains an important facet of preventive medicine. An infection detected and treated early in pregnancy — in the first six months — with penicillin is most effective in preventing infection of the fetus.

The impact of syphilis in a country with good access to antibiotic treatment, used both widely in general practice as well as a specific therapy for syphilis, is clearly different from effects seen in the pre-antibiotic era (Figs. 3.2, 3.3, 3.4). Without antibiotics uncertain cure, transmission of possibly incurable venereal disease to a partner, and involvement of the fetus or newborn were serious causes of social and medical morbidity. Response to treatment in syphilis is so good that its social impact is now much less profound. The potential menace remains, however, and health education and ease of access to facilities for diagnosis and treatment are essentials that are important to maintain.

Trends for syphilis in the United Kingdom for the period 1965–1980 (Figs. 3.5, 3.6, 3.7) reached a peak

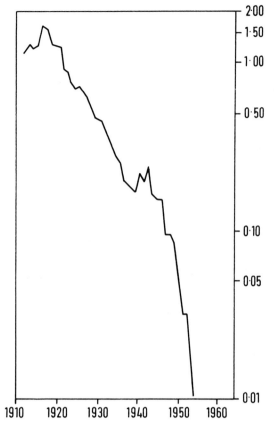

Fig. 3.2 Infant mortality per 1000 live births. Congenital syphilis, England and Wales 1911–1962. (Office of Health Economics 1963). Death rates per 1000 infants for years after 1954*–1954 0.003; 1955 Nil; 1956 Nil; 1957 Nil; 1958 0.004; 1959 0.003; 1960 Nil; 1961 Nil; 1962 0.001.

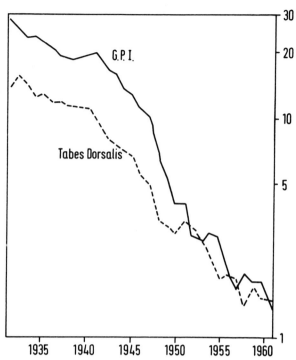

Fig. 3.3 Death rates per million population for neurosyphilis, England and Wales 1931–1961. (Office of Health Economics 1963.)

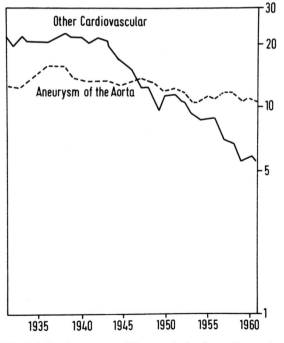

Fig. 3.4 Death rates per million population for cardiovascular syphilis, England and Wales 1931–1961. (Office of Health Economics 1963.)

of 4886 in 1978 but this was less than one-fifth of the post-war peak of 27 761 in 1946. The increase in the detection of early syphilis (Fig. 3.5) may have been partly due to the increased use of serological tests, more sensitive and specific than the older methods, such as the Wasserman Reaction and partly to the number of tests carried out, particularly in male homosexuals (PHLS Communicable Disease Surveillance Centre et al 1982).

The rise in numbers of infections in homosexual males was probably another factor because of the tendencies of 'open coupled' or 'functional' members in this group to casual and often numerous sexual contacts. In a large-scale survey in 1977, 54% of syphilis infections were reported as homosexually acquired compared with 42% in 1971 (British Co-operative Clinical Group 1980). Marked differences existed, however, between clinics within London: for example 372 (70.9%) of 525 cases of primary and secondary syphilis were treated at five clinics within the West End, where the proportion

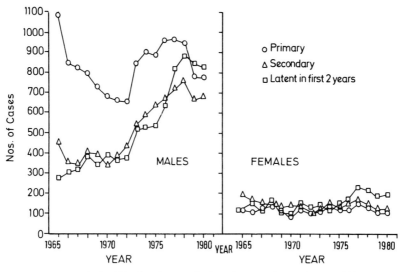

Fig 3.5 Syphilis, United Kingdom 1965–1980, showing trends for primary and secondary syphilis and latent syphilis in first two years of infection.

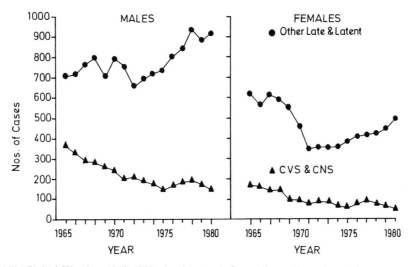

Fig. 3.6 Syphilis, United Kingdom 1965–1980, showing trends for cardiovascular and central nervous system syphilis (late-stage) and other late or latent forms of disease.

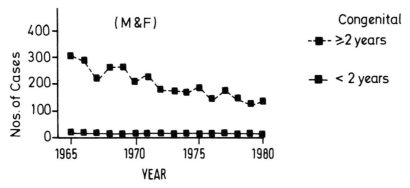

Fig. 3.7 Syphilis, United Kingdom 1965–1980, showing trends for congenital syphilis in the less than 2 years age group and in the age group 2 years and over.

of homosexually acquired infections was 76.9% compared with 37.9% in London clinics elsewhere.

In the USA the increase in infectious syphilis observed between 1969 and 1976 was almost exclusively among men; at the same time the proportion of men with early-stage syphilis who named other men as sexual partners increased by about 200% (Henderson 1977). In Australia similarly as many as 73% of primary and secondary infections occurred in homosexual men (Garner 1976). In Edinburgh in 1984 20 of 25 cases of early syphilis were acquired by homosexual activity in males. Since a number of males may be bisexual, females may also become involved.

The sudden fall in incidence since 1978 is not yet explained. Fear of the Acquired Immune Deficiency Syndrome (AIDS) which began in the United States in 1979 and soon reached epidemic proportions, may have had an impact, modifying behaviour and reducing promiscuity.

GONORRHOEA

Gonorrhoea, again a disease worldwide in distribution, shows trends in incidence, (Fig. 3.8), that are difficult to interpret as methods of reporting vary. It is mainly a disease of young adults, most cases being found within the 15–24 year age group. For example, in the USA in the age group 20–24 the incidence per 100 000 for 1956, 1960 and 1978–1980 is shown in Table 3.1. The reported incidence in males previously was much greater than in females but the overall male:female ratio shows a greater trend towards unity. In contrast, the rate for girls under 16 years is about four times that for boys of the same age group and reflects their earlier sexual maturation.

In many countries single-dose single antibiotic treatment is sufficient to ensure cure rates of over 95%. In Bangkok, however, the high proportion (42%) of gonococci producing beta-lactamase and the high

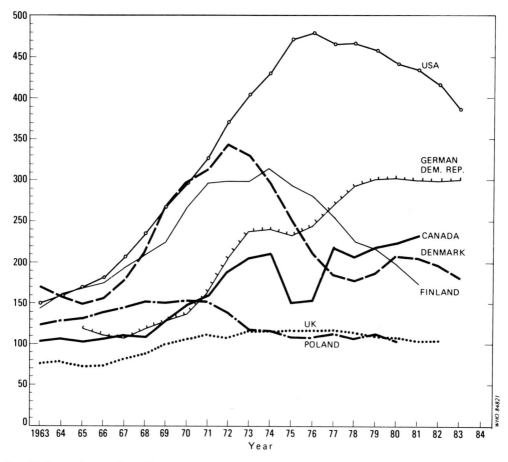

Fig. 3.8 Reported gonorrhoea (1963–1983) incidence per 100 000 population (World Health Organization data).

Table 3.1 Gonorrhoea in the United States. Rates of reported gonorrhoea cases per 100 000 in 20–24 year age group (US Department of Health and Human Services 1982).

Year	Males	Females	M:F ratio
1956	1255.8	406.8	3.09
1960	1354.4	443.7	3.05
1978	2409.9	1568.7	1.54
1979	2308.9	1532.2	1.51
1980	2102.2	1458.6	1.44

proportion showing high-level resistance to a wide range of antibiotics indicated that the gonococcus had adapted to the antimicrobial selective pressures in that city and suggested that single drug treatments were no longer appropriate and that much more costly 'combination therapies' were needed to delay emergence of further antimicrobial resistance (Brown et al 1982). The proportion of isolates of *N. gonorrhoeae* in various localities and in recent years showing beta-lactamase production are listed in Table 3.2.

Oro-genital sexual contact has apparently become more common as a practice in recent years and this has been reflected in our locality in the number of gonococcal infections of this site (Fig. 3.9).

With promiscuous homosexual activity in men, spread of the traditionally named venereal diseases — syphilis and gonorrhoea — increased, often markedly. The spread of enteric organisms, such as *Shigella* spp

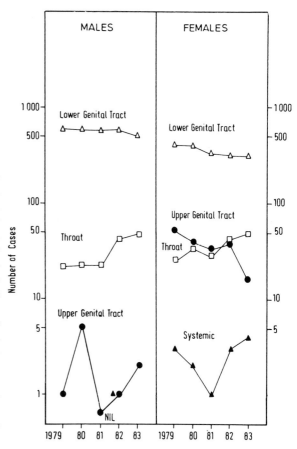

Fig. 3.9 Gonorrhoea in adults, Department of Genito-Urinary Medicine, Edinburgh Royal Infirmary 1979–1983. Cases according to anatomical site of infection. (The figure given for cases of lower genital tract infection in males includes those with homosexually acquired anorectal infections.) Numbers are shown on logarithmic scale.

Table 3.2 Proportion of isolates of *Neisseria gonorrhoeae* producing beta-lactamase (penicillinase) in various countries.

Country	Beta-lactamase producing *N.gonorrhoeae* (percentage)	City	Year
Australia	3, 8	(Melbourne, Perth)	1984
Thailand	49	(Bangkok)	1982
Korea	25	(Seoul)	1982
Netherlands	4, 23	(South Holland, Den Haag)	1982
Switzerland	3	(Zurich)	1982
Malaysia	35	(Singapore)	1982
Zimbabwe	12	(Harare)	1983
Italy	<1	(Rome)	1981
India	<1	(Varanasi)	1979–1982
Philippines	40		1981
Indonesia	17	(Surabaya)	1981–1982
Indonesia	25	(Jukarm)	
Hong Kong	32		1981
Japan	15	(Fukuoka)	1981
Zambia	3		1980–1981
S. Arabia	12	(Riyadh)	1979–1980
United Kingdom	<1		1981

and *Salmonella* serovars, created new clinical problems. Behaviour enables spread of these and other prokaryotes by the faecal–oral route.

Immunosuppression, as in the Acquired Immune Deficiency Syndrome (AIDS, see Ch. 30) enables opportunistic prokaryotes to cause systemic disease, e.g. *Nocardia* spp, *Mycobacterium avium*, *Listeria monocytogenes*.

INFECTIONS DUE TO *CHLAMYDIA TRACHOMATIS*

Surveys based on the detection of anti-*Chlamydia* antibodies show evidence of considerable exposure to chlamydial infection among sexually active groups. The greater prevalence in women in comparison to men may be due to the longer duration of infection or the involvement of a larger anatomical surface area producing a greater immunological stimulus. In such an infection its epidemiology is complex and difficult to assess. Urethritis, pelvic inflammatory disease and perihepatitis may be overt manifestations but latency and difficulty in isolating chlamydia from genital sites are also characteristic. There is no reasonable doubt, however, that at the clinical level in the case of the female patient and her partner laboratory diagnosis is highly desirable so that principles of control may be applied (Oriel & Ridgway 1982). In *C.trachomatis* infections the 'carrier' state will ensure its persistence in a population.

2. INFECTION DUE TO EUKARYOTES

The prevalence of enteric protozoa, whether pathogenic or not, is an interesting marker for promiscuous male homosexuals (Table 3.3) in urban settings in developed countries where transmission by the faecal–oral route is prevented in the general population by a clean drinking water supply and proper sewage disposal. The situation may be sometimes described as 'hyperendemic' as this term has been defined as 'the persistence of a fourfold or greater prevalence of infection in a sub-population, as compared with the background level in the community' (Phillips et al 1981).

In the immunocompetent individual *Trichomonas vaginalis, Entamoeba histolytica, Enterobius vermicularis, Pthirus pubis* and *Sarcoptes scabiei*, among the eukaryotes will cause usually remediable problems. In the Acquired Immune Deficiency Syndrome (Ch. 31) *Strongyloides stercoralis* is a serious danger and a wide range

Table 3.3 Intestinal protozoa in men and women attending a sexually transmitted diseases clinic in Edinburgh 1984.

Species	Number (%) of infected individuals		
	Men		Women
	Homosexual	Heterosexual	
	(n = 345)	(n = 105)	(n = 68)
Retortamonas intestinalis	0	1 (1.0)	0
Chilomastix mesnili	1 (0.3)	0	0
Giardia intestinalis	23 (6.7)	0	0
Entamoeba histolytica	48 (13.9)	0	0
Entamoeba hartmanni	2 (0.6)	0	0
Entamoeba coli	36 (10.4)	1 (1.0)	1 (1.5)
Iodamoeba butschlii	13 (3.8)	0	0
Endolimax nana	39 (11.3)	2 (1.9)	1 (1.5)

of opportunistic protozoa may become pathogens, e.g. *Toxoplasma gondii, Pneumocystis carinii, Isospora belli, Cryptosporidium*. Ordinarily not pathogenic, the fungi like *Aspergillus fumigatus, Cryptococcus neoformans, Histoplasma capsulatum, Coccidioides immitis* and *Thermoascus crustaceus* become so.

3. INFECTION DUE TO VIRUSES

The interaction of viruses with permissive cells leads ordinarily to productive infection and cell death and this is reflected in an individual as an acute infection against which an immune response is mounted. In virus infections which persist, however, an equilibrium is established between virus and host, but this equilibrium may break down with resultant cellular injury and disease. To persist and to ensure its replication and spread the virus has developed a number of strategies (Mims 1982). Those viruses which ensure shedding to the outside world or, more specifically, on skin or mucosal surfaces of the mouth or genital tract are those that concern us here. In contrast to infections with prokaryotes or eukaryotes, medical intervention with the administration of antibiotic or chemotherapy is much more limited in value in virus infections. In herpes simplex virus infection a latent infection of the cells of the sensory ganglion develops with sporadic symptomatic or asymptomatic virus shedding at the periphery. In hepatitis B there is a prolonged carrier state with persistent viraemia. Papillomavirus exhibits the tendency to produce persistent infection of epithelial sites and warts which remain infective for long periods of time. In infection with human immunodeficiency viruses (HIV) viral reverse transcriptase enables the formation of a DNA copy with its integration into the chromosomes, mainly of the T4 lymphocyte. Once infected, latency may be prolonged but the facility for further transmission in body fluids containing lymphocytes, particularly by semen or blood, persists for life. Medical advice is directed to the problematical task of promoting a behavioural change in both those at risk and those already infected with HIV. Behavioural change is required both with respect to the nature of individual sexual acts practised and with respect to life style. The medical idiom, organismal diagnosis followed by specific treatment of patient and contact-tracing, valid in relation to prokaryotes and eukaryotes, is no longer effective and dialogue with the patient has to become more intrusive and more deeply personal. In the long term, in the individual patient such 'counselling' is unpredictable in its result whether the HIV antibody status of the patient is positive, negative or not known.

In the case of the Herpesviridae (Ch. 2) all are spread

by mucosal contact and all produce a latent infection for life with the new host either constantly or sporadically producing virus at the periphery. In herpes simplex and Epstein Barr virus infections host response in adolescence or early adulthood to a primary infection is pronounced, whereas in childhood infection may be acquired sub-clinically. In this way severe primary infections occur mainly in 'developed' countries and among those whose socio-economic status has enabled them to escape primary infection in childhood. Non-immune adolescents or young adults thus acquire primary EB virus infection by kissing or primary HSV infection by intercourse or orogenital contact.

In a study of flying civil airline personnel (Swissair) hepatitis A immunity (anti-HA) was found to be similar to that of the blood-donor population but the most outstanding feature was that *male* flight attendants (employees and candidates) significantly more often had anti-HBs and/or anti-HBc antibodies (20–33%) than either flying personnel (1.4–5.6%) or Swiss blood donors (4–8%). Furthermore, the high incidence of acute manifest hepatitis B, viz. 5 cases per 1000, was mainly among male flight attendants. In contrast, in Switzerland only 0.5–0.8 cases per 1000 are recorded for the general population per year. It was thought that homosexuality was the most realistic explanation. The authors concluded that for male cabin attendants on recruitment, as for other individuals with a high risk life style, immunization would be warranted (Holdener & Grob 1981).

PAPILLOMAVIRUS INFECTION, GENITAL CONDYLOMATA ACUMINATA AND CANCER OF THE CERVIX UTERI

The high prevalence, high infectivity, long prepatent periods and poor response to treatment in genital warts make control of papillomavirus infection by therapy and contact-tracing possible only to a limited extent. Warts have been considered until recent years to be wholly benign growths which regress spontaneously but evidence accumulates to show that human papilloma-viruses are not solely causes of benign tumours of the skin and mucosa but may in the longer term, possibly in association with herpes simplex virus and/or other co-factors such as smoking, play a part in the aetiology of the cervix uteri. The increasing incidence of HPV infection (Fig. 3.10) leads to problems in the care of patients who may require multiple attendances for treatment of limited effectiveness and who, in the case of women, are faced with lifetime follow-up on at least an annual basis on account of co-existing dysplasia which may be either evanescent or progressive leading to cancer of the cervix uteri (Ch. 25).

THE ACQUIRED IMMUNE DEFICIENCY SYNDROME (AIDS)

Its impact in the USA
In 1981, in the United States, previously healthy young

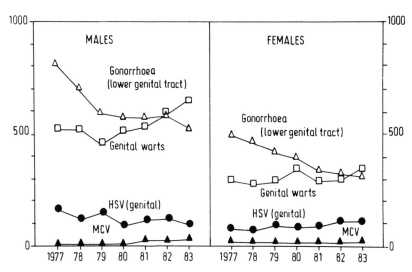

Fig. 3.10 Gonococcal infections (lower genital tract infections including rectal infections in the case of males) compared with papillomavirus (HPV), herpesvirus (HSV) and molluscum contagiosum virus (MCV) infections in adults, Department of Genito-Urinary Medicine, Edinburgh Royal Infirmary 1977–1983. Diagnoses were based upon culture results in the case of gonococcal and HSV infections and in molluscum contagiosum on confirmation by electron microscopy.

men began to die in large numbers from an unknown disease. They developed rare tumours and unusual systemic infections, and studies indicated that those affected had suddenly and inexplicably lost their normal immunity to disease. The first cases of the new syndrome reported in the Morbidity and Mortality Weekly Report of 5th June 1981, involved 5 young men, all active homosexuals, who had been treated in Los Angeles Hospitals for a rare infection, *Pneumocystis carinii* pneumonia (PCP). 2 of the 5 had died and all had evidence of other infections and a defective immune system. To this disease was given the name, Acquired Immune Deficiency Syndrome — or AIDS (Cahill 1984). At about the same time an uncommon malignant disease in the United States, Kaposi's sarcoma, was diagnosed in 26 homosexual men. A task force was established by the Centers for Disease Control (CDC) of the US Public Health Service to characterize the syndrome, and epidemiologists identified a subset of homosexual men who were more likely to have many anonymous sexual partners, to have a history of a variety of sexually transmitted diseases and to engage in sexual practices that increased the risk of exposure to small amounts of blood or faeces (Foege 1984). By the autumn of 1981, PCP and other opportunistic infections were being seen also in heterosexual men and women who abused intravenous drugs. Tuberculosis often appeared as the harbinger for even more serious disease in Haitian patients, recent immigrants to the United States, notably of Miami and New York City (Landerman 1984). Early in 1982 there followed the first reported death, due to PCP, in a patient with haemophilia. By December deaths due to AIDS had occurred in other haemophilia patients, known to be heterosexual in orientation, all of whom had received Factor VIII concentrate, a product with individual batches prepared from the plasma of as many as 20 000 donors (Foege 1984).

The CDC definition of AIDS at this time required the presence of a disease at least moderately indicative of defective cell-mediated immunity in an individual who has no known underlying cause for diminished resistance to that disease. Such diseases included Kaposi's sarcoma (KS), PCP and other opportunistic infections, but excluded less well-defined manifestations (fever, weight loss, generalized or persistent lymphadenopathy). By 5th April 1983, 1306 cases had been reported, but 80% of these cases were concentrated in six metropolitan areas of the East and West Coasts including New York City, San Francisco, Miami, Newark and Los Angeles. By 13th January 1986 16 458 cases had been recorded — 16 227 adults and 231 children — and of those 8361 (51%) of adults and 59% of children were reported to have died, including 71% of patients diagnosed before July 1984. In those with AIDS PCP was

Table 3.4. Clinical manifestations of the Acquired Immune Deficiency Syndrome (AIDS) in the USA, 1986.

Manifestation	Percentage
Pneumocystis carinii pneumonia	63
Kaposi's sarcoma	24
Candida oesophagitis	14
Cytomegalovirus infection	7
Cryptococcosis	7
Chronic herpes simplex	4
Cryptosporidiosis	4
Toxoplasmosis	3
Other opportunistic infections	3

Totals: 1982–747; 1983–2124; 1984–4569; 1985–8406

the most common (43%) and opportunistic infection and Kaposi's sarcoma comprised 13% of reported diagnoses (Morbidity and Mortality Weekly Report 1986a). In AIDS patients a wide range of syndromes developed after incubation periods up to 7 years (Table 3.4).

The impact of the epidemic (Fig. 3.11) had other serious social dimensions recorded with sensitivity by physicians involved in its control (Cahill 1984). The tragedy was sharpened by the youth of its victims, the

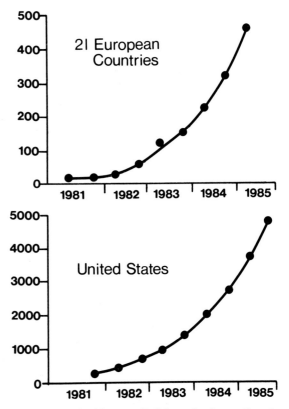

Fig. 3.11 Acquired Immune Deficiency Syndrome. Cases by 6-month period in 21 European countries and in the United States, 1981–1985. (Data from Morbidity and Mortality Weekly Report 1986a, b.)

prolonged debility and often fatal outcome of untreatable conditions. Each at-risk group, male homosexuals, some immigrant Haitians and intravenous drug abusers, outside the mainstream of society either racially or through social behaviour, suffered effects of discrimination in employment and other contexts. New problems, including those of communication, also faced health workers, unfamiliar as they were with life styles and practices of those groups at risk (Sencer 1984).

AIDS in Europe

Before 1981 a few AIDS cases were seen in Denmark, Switzerland, France, Federal Republic of Germany and the United Kingdom, but subsequently increasing numbers were seen in Europe and by 31st December 1984, 762 cases had been reported to the World Health Organization (WHO) with death in 376 (49%) cases. By 30th September 1985 the number reported had reached 1573, of whom 792 (50%) were reported to have died. The highest rates were noted in Switzerland, Denmark and France; these rates are low compared with the US rate in January 1986 of 69.5 per million (Fig. 3.12). Males accounted for 92% of cases. There were 36 cases in children under 15 years of age, of whom 24 had parents with AIDS or belonging to a group of high risk for AIDS. In addition there were 10 paediatric patients, of whom 5 had haemophilia and 5 had received a blood

transfusion. In 2 no risk factors were noted. Of 1330 European patients 78% were homosexual or bisexual; 7% were intravenous drug abusers and 2% both homosexual and intravenous drug abusers. There were 39 (2%) Carribeans, of whom 4 were homosexual, and 157 (10%) Africans, of whom 63% were from Zaire and 10% from the Congo (Morbidity and Mortality Weekly Report 1986b).

Patients not belonging to any of the at-risk groups (male homosexuals, IVDA, recipients of blood and blood products) contributed the second largest number of cases. In four countries a high proportion of patients originated from regions where most AIDS patients have not belonged to any of the at-risk groups and where heterosexual transmission is thought to be a major factor. In Belgium 72% of patients originated from equatorial Africa; in France 11% were from Africa and 8% from Haiti; and in Switzerland 12% were from equatorial Africa.

AIDS virus and other retrovirus infections in Africa

AIDS virus infection and the Acquired Immune Deficiency Syndrome are epidemic in Central Africa. The occurrence of AIDS is well documented for Zaire (Piot et al 1984); Rwanda (Van de Perre et al 1984); Uganda and Zambia (Bayley et al 1985). Neither bisexuality nor homosexuality in males nor intravenous drug abuse are

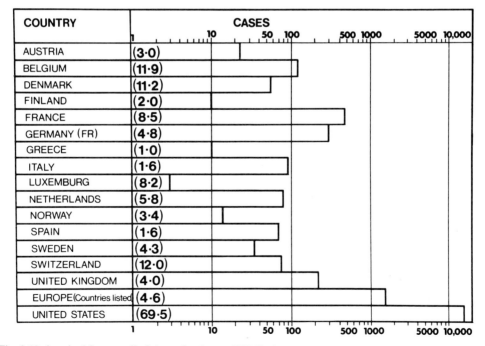

Fig. 3.12 Acquired Immune Deficiency Syndrome (AIDS). Cases in Europe reported to the World Health Organization European Collaborating Centre on AIDS 1985 compared with those recorded for the United States of America. Rates per million population are shown in the brackets and numbers of cases are represented in a logarithmic scale. Nil returns were made for Czechoslovakia, Hungary, Iceland and Poland. (Data mainly from Morbidity and Mortality Weekly Report 1986a, b.)

risk factors in this African region, whereas heterosexuality, promiscuity and contact with prostitutes in urban areas are associated with transmission of this retrovirus (Clumeck et al 1985). In contrast, in Johannesburg, South Africa, male homosexuality is a very important risk factor (Sher & Dos Santos 1985): in this city about 15% of the male homosexual population were thought to have been exposed to the virus. The situation in Central Africa is highlighted by the high female:male ratio for AIDS patients viz. 1:1 in Zaire, compared with 1:16 in the United States of America (Kreiss et al 1986). Now the infection has been found to involve East Africa, where in Nairobi, Kenya, a high prevalence of antibody to HTLV-III has been discovered in female prostitutes; in those of low socio-economic status 66% were positive and in those of higher, with activities involving tourists particularly, 31% were positive (Kreiss et al 1986).

The implications of an epidemic of HIV virus in Africa are sobering. Urban migration of men particularly, on a massive scale, has brought about disruption of family units; involvement of women and the likelihood of perinatal transmission with high rates of infection among infants and children make the outlook bleak in a serious disease where control is dependent on counselling and education programmes directed at modifying sexual behaviour and limiting sexual contact with persons at high risk.

Parenteral transmission through contaminated needles used for intramuscular injections of medication is another possible route for spread, but heterosexual intercourse is likely to be the main route in tropical Africa. Antibody to human T-cell leukaemia virus (HTLV-I) is also found in the sera of African populations — 1–2% of people from Kenya (Hunsmann et al 1983) and in nearly 4% of blood donors in Nigeria (Fleming et al 1983). A high prevalence of antibody to HTLV-III in relatively low titres in sera collected from people of the West Nile district of Uganda in 1972–1973 suggested that either a predecessor, HTLV-II or HTLV-III itself existed at that time (Saxinger et al 1985). The direct ELISA used in this study, however, is suspected of giving false-positive results with sera from areas where parasitic infection is common and more recent results with the competitive ELISA (Wellcome) did not support the suggestion, and on the contrary indicated that the AIDS arrived in Uganda in recent years (Carswell et al 1986). Of 716 healthy adults in Kampala in this study 110 (15.4%) were seropositive whereas none of 96 old people were found to be so.

REFERENCES

Bayley A C, Dowing R G, Cheingsong-Popov R, Tedder R S, Dalgleish A G, Weiss R A 1985 HTLV-III serology distinguishes atypical and endemic Kaposi's sarcoma in Africa. Lancet i: 359–361

British Co-operative Clinical Group 1980 Homosexuality and venereal disease in the United Kingdom, a second study. British Journal of Venereal Diseases 56: 6–11

Brown P, Warnissorn T, Biddle J, Panikabutra K, Traisupa A 1982 Antimicrobial resistance of Neisseria gonorrhoeae in Bangkok: Is single-drug treatment passé? Lancet ii: 1366–1368

Cahill K M 1984 The evolution of an epidemic. In: Cahill K M (ed) The AIDS epidemic, Hutchinson, London, p 1–6

Carswell J W, Sewankambo N, LLoyd G, Downing R G 1986 How long has the AIDS virus been in Uganda? Correspondence, Lancet ii: 1217

Clumeck N, Van de Perre P, Carael D, Rouvroy D, Nzaramba D 1985 Heterosexual promiscuity among African patients with AIDS. Correspondence, New England Journal of Medicine 313(3): 182

Fleming A F, Yamamoto N, Bhusnurmath S R, Maharajan R, Schneider J, Hunsmann G 1983 Antibodies to ATLV (HTLV) in Nigerian blood donors and patients with chronic lymphatic leukaemia or lymphoma. Lancet ii: 334–335

Foege W 1984 The national pattern of AIDS. In: Cahill K M (ed) The AIDS epidemic, Hutchinson, London, p 7–17

Garner M F 1976 An analysis of 340 cases of syphilis diagnosed in six months in 1973. Medical Journal of Australia 1: 735–737

Henderson R H 1977 Improving sexually transmitted diseases health service to gays: A national perspective. Sexually Transmitted Diseases 4: 58–62

Holdener F, Grob P J 1981 Hepatitis virus infections in flying air line personnel. Lancet ii: 867–868

Hunsmann G, Schneider J, Schmitt J, Yamamoto N 1983 Detection of serum antibodies to adult T-cell leukemia virus in non-human primates and in people from Africa. International Journal of Cancer 32(3): 329–332

Kreiss J K, Koech D, Plummer F A et al 1986 AIDS virus infection in Nairobi prostitutes: spread of the epidemic to East Africa. The New England Journal of Medicine 314: 414–418

Landerman S H 1984 The Haitian connection. In: Cahill K M (ed) The AIDS epidemic, Hutchinson, London, p 28–37

Mims C A 1982 Role of persistence in viral pathogenesis. In: Mahy B W J, Minson A C, Darby G K (eds) Symposium 33 Virus persistence. Published for the Society of General Microbiology, Cambridge University Press, Cambridge, p 1–13

Morbidity and Mortality Weekly Report, Centers for Disease Control 1986a Update: Acquired Immunodeficiency Syndrome, USA, 35(2): 17–21

Morbidity and Mortality Weekly Report, Centers for Disease Control 1986b Update: Acquired Immunodeficiency

Syndrome, Europe, 35(3): 35–38, 43–46

Office of Health Economics 1963 The venereal diseases. OHE 195, Knightsbridge, London SW7

Oriel J D, Ridgway G L 1982 Genital infection by *Chlamydia trachomatis*. Current Topics in Infection Series. Edward Arnold, London, p 99–112

Phillips S C, Mildvan D, William D C, Gelb A M, White M C 1981 Sexual transmission of enteric protozoa and helminths in a venereal-disease clinic population. New England Journal of Medicine 305: 11: 603–606

PHLS Communicable Disease Surveillance Centre and the Communicable Diseases (Scotland) Unit, with the assistance of the Academic Department of Genito-Urinary Medicine, Middlesex Hospital Medical School 1982 Epidemiology, sexually transmitted disease surveillance: 1980. British Medical Journal 284: 124

Piot P, Quinn T C, Taelman H et al 1984 Acquired Immunodeficiency Syndrome in a heterosexual population in Zaire. Lancet ii: 65–69

Saxinger W C, Levine P H, Dean A G et al 1985 Evidence for exposure to HTLV-III in Uganda before 1973. Science USA 227: 1036–1038

Sencer D J 1984 Tracking a local outbreak. In: Cahill K M (ed) The AIDS epidemic, Hutchinson, London, p 18–27

Sher R, Dos Santos L 1985 Prevalence of HTLV-III antibodies in homosexual men in Johannesburg (Correspondence). South African Medical Journal 67(13): 484

US Department of Health and Human Services 1982 Sexually transmitted diseases statistical newsletter, calendar year 1980 (Issue No 130). Centers for Disease Control, VD control Division, Atlanta, Georgia 30333, p 5

Van de Perre P, Rouvroy D, Lepage P et al 1984 Acquired Immunodeficiency Syndrome in Rwanda. Lancet ii: 62–65

World Health Organization 1982 Treponemal infections. Technical Report Series 674. World Health Organization, Geneva

4

Health education and sexually transmitted diseases

CONSIDERATIONS FOR SCHOOLS

Profound changes both in attitudes to sex and in sexual behaviour itself (see Ch. 1) have produced a situation where education on sex and sexually transmitted diseases should not continue to be omitted from health education. An outline of the problems involved and a reasoned theme for consideration are discussed in detail in this chapter.

EDUCATION: COUNCIL OF EUROPE AND ITS INFLUENCE

Introducing sex education into schools may often bring controversy and unease to parents and teachers alike. Accepting that it is an essential component of education is but a first step. In Denmark, for example, 'integrated' and hence compulsory sex education was introduced by an Act of Parliament on 27th May 1970. Later Kjeldsen, Busk Madsen and Pedersen (1976) raised an objection in the European Court of Human Rights because they considered that sex education raised ethical questions and so preferred to carry out themselves their children's instruction in this sphere. Their requests, however, to have their children exempted from such education had been refused by the competent authorities in Denmark.

In making the decision on this case the European Court of Human Rights (1976) examined the legislation complained of mainly in the light of Article 2 of Protocol 1 of the European Convention on Human Rights (The European Convention on Human Rights 1983) which reads as follows:

> No person shall be denied the right to education. In the exercise of any functions which it assumes in relation to education and to teaching, the State shall respect the right of parents to ensure such education and teaching in conformity with their own religious and philosophical convictions.

In fulfilling these educational functions the State —

referring to those Governments being Members of the Council of Europe — must take care that 'information is conveyed in an objective, critical and pluralistic manner'. The State is forbidden to pursue an aim of indoctrination that might be considered as not respecting parents 'religious and philosophical convictions'.

The Court (ECHR) found the Danish legislation in question to be principally intended to give pupils better information to enable them when the time comes 'to take care of themselves and show consideration for others in that respect', and 'not . . . . . [to] land themselves or others in difficulties solely on account of lack of knowledge'. Whilst the Court believed that these considerations were indeed of a moral order, they were very general in character and did not entail overstepping the bounds of what in a democratic state may be regarded as the public interest. The Danish legislation complained of, according to the Court, in no way amounted to an attempt at indoctrination aimed at advocating a specific kind of sexual behaviour and did not affect the rights of parents to enlighten and advise their children.

At an earlier date, in 1974, the Committee of Ministers, Council of Europe, adopted a resolution on the control of sexually transmitted diseases in which, among other principles and practices, newer approaches to health education and psycho-social care were to be promoted to the fullest extent. These newer approaches were specified in Appendix A, paragraph 7, as follows:

a. Introduction in schools of programmes allowing children to acquire progressive knowledge of human sexuality in its biological, behavioural and other aspects, and information on STD in association with discussions of behavioural relationships which depend on varying cultural and social patterns in different countries: integration of parent instruction in such educational programmes so as to avoid disapproval and obtain co-operation:

b. Financing by governments or state-assisted

agencies of health education programmes using modern mass media techniques, lectures, debates, group discussions, and various audio-visual aids, aiming particularly at young people and at other special STD risk groups, such as tourists, migrants, seafarers and members of the armed forces: promotion by these agencies of teaching activities for information disseminators, like teaching staff, medical and nursing personnel, social and welfare workers.

More recently, in a declaration on cultural objectives, the European Ministers for Cultural Affairs accepted among other objectives an obligation (1984):

4. To ensure that each individual has open access to education and training necessary for full personal development and proper integration into society.

With reference also to human sexual variability, the subject of homosexuality, particularly in males, may arouse strong prejudices but education about such minority problems should not be omitted on this account. Sir Vincent Evans, a judge in the European Court of Human Rights (ECHR) at Strasbourg, has drawn attention (1983) to principles, outlined in judgements of this court, characterizing a 'democratic society' which are relevant to our discussion on education: 'freedom of expression' constitutes one of the essential foundations of such a society and is a principle (Article 10 European Convention of Human Rights; see Note 4.1), applicable not only to 'information' or 'ideas' that are favourably received or regarded as inoffensive or as a matter of indifference, but also to those that offend, shock or disturb the State or any sector of the population. The importance of 'pluralism, tolerance and broadmindedness' is again and again emphasized. Any restrictions to these principles must be proportionate to the legitimate aim pursued or conducive to the 'protection of morals' (Handyside v. United Kingdom 1976). Again, in 1981, the Court (Young, James and Webster v. United Kingdom 1981) continued 'although individual interests must on occasion be subordinated to those of a group, democracy does not simply mean that the views of a majority must always prevail; a balance must be achieved which ensures the fair and proper treatment of minorities and avoids any abuse of a dominant position'.

Human rights are a common topic today and, as Paul Sieghart explains (1985), for the first time in history, how a state treats its own citizens is no longer a matter for its own exclusive determination but a matter of legitimate concern for all other states and for their inhabitants. The formal product of this revolution is a detailed code of international law defining the legal rights of individuals. In Europe, particularly, many states have had to modify their laws and administrative practices following authoritative and reasoned findings, particularly of the European Commission or Court of Human Rights. Paul Sieghart clarifies the meaning of the term 'human rights' and explains how these become lawful and guaranteed under the European Convention. Human rights are by their nature vested in the individual and have three characteristics viz. inherence, inalienability and equality. To these is added a further distinction, that of duty. In the subject of this discussion, clearly, if an individual has a 'right' to sex education, someone else, namely the State, must have the 'correlative duty' to provide it.

Although rights to health education, and indeed sex education, can be claimed from the European Convention of Human Rights (1983) and judgements of the European Court of Human Rights, reference has already been made to bounds that may be set. Teaching material should not contain 'sentences or paragraphs that young people, at a critical stage of their development could have interpreted as an encouragement to indulge in precocious activities harmful for them or even to commit criminal offences'. It was in these terms that a 'schoolbook' published on the subject was considered likely to have 'pernicious effects on the morals of many children and adolescents who would read it' (Handyside v. United Kingdom 1975).

VARIABILITY IN SEQUENCE OF EVENTS OF PUBERTY: A FACTOR IN SEX EDUCATION

'Puberty', in older literature, was used as a term to denote the appearance of the pubic hair, but now it can be used interchangeably with 'adolescence' to denote the period at which testes, prostate gland and seminal vesicles or the uterus and vagina suddenly enlarge. The sequence of these and other events in puberty show enormous variability; in boys and girls at the ages of 13, 14 and 15 years this variability in development is, in Tanner's words, 'an ineluctable fact of biology' (Tanner 1962, 1978) which raises difficult social and educational problems. With an early menarche among the well-nourished of developed countries both sexuality and fertility will frequently be developed at an age well in advance of a girl's intellectual maturity and ability to cope — psychological features which are more dependent than sexual maturity on chronological age (see Ch. 1).

SURVEYS TO OBTAIN DATA

Farrell (1978, p. 54) identifies two main areas of difficulty in obtaining good data in surveys relating to infancy, childhood and adulthood. The first relates to the problem of faulty recall or inaccurate memories. The second relates to 'existentialist insight' so that 'instead of the past determining the character of the present, the present significantly reshapes the past as we reconstruct our biographies in an effort to bring them into greater congruence with our current identities, roles, situations and available vocabularies'.

THE WAY PEOPLE LEARN

The way young people in the United Kingdom learn about sex and reproduction, including the topic of sexually transmitted diseases, is illuminated by the study by Christine Farrell with her collaborator, Leonie Kellaher (1978). The source of information encountered during the period 1974–1975 by young people (16–19 year age group) in their early years which helped or hindered them in the acquisition of knowledge about sex are spelled out in the results of their detailed survey. As a preliminary to an examination of that part of a health education project dealing with sexuality and reproduction or any proposal for change, the study provides valuable insights. Gagnon & Simon (1973) have pointed out that, in their American studies, the primary source of sex education is generally the peer group, but Farrell (1978) showed, however, that although the peer group does have an important part to play it is not considered to be a satisfactory source of information nor do young people consider it to be the 'best' way to learn about sex (Farrell 1978, p. 163). Most felt that an authoritative source such as school or parent was the best way to learn the 'facts' which could then form the basis for later discussion with their friends or other adults.

Parents may often see themselves as sex educators but fail usually to carry out the task (Farrell 1978, Ch. 6); often they are positively embarrassed about discussing with their children any aspect of sex. Freudian psychologists relate these difficulties to the incest taboo which means not only that erotic attachments within the nuclear family are repressed but also that its revival is permitted only outside the family (Farrell 1978, p. 82). Parents too may not agree about their respective roles as teachers and the matter is either shelved or the responsibility shifted on to the teachers.

BARRIERS TO SEX EDUCATION

Barriers to sex education in schools vary geographically, within the United Kingdom, for example, according to prevailing attitudes. In a number of schools in Scotland visited, the HM Inspectors of Schools commented 'head teachers did not conceal their reluctance to develop a policy on sex education and some teachers were disinclined to touch on the physical aspects of human relationships in groups of children of very different sensitivity and maturity'. At early stages of primary education it was usual for the birth of babies to be explained in simple terms but at the later stages in many schools there was a lack of contexts for studying reproduction and birth. There was no sure study of the human body which would have enabled pupils to consider reproduction as one of the body systems, and relate physical development to changes taking place, or about to take place, in the pupils themselves. Only a few schools related menstruation to physical and emotional development of girls as was suggested in an earlier (1965) memorandum. Their evidence suggested that menstruation might be less effectively and sympathetically discussed than it once was. In the rather sombre report (Scottish Education Department 1979) several instances were brought to light where outside contributors were ineffective. This was usually the result of poor communication between school and visitors, or lack of association of class teachers with the visitor, or inability on the part of the visitor to present material at the right level. Regional variation has been commented on by Reid (1982) in a review on school sex education. In the National Child Development Study in 1974 it was evident that 22% Scottish, 12% Welsh and 5% English teenagers were attending schools where no such lessons were given. Reid (1982) thought, however, that provision of basic sex education had greatly increased in recent years.

In a background paper prepared for the World Health Study Group on Young People and Health for All by the Year 2000 in Geneva, Paxman (1984) touches on laws, which in a number of countries expressly authorize them to gain access to treatment. These laws take three general forms:

1. the enabling of minors irrespective of age to consent to treatment for sexually transmitted diseases;

2. allowing minors of a certain age to seek out and consent to treatment; and

3. requiring parental approval before receiving treatment.

The aim of these laws is the same — the detection, early treatment and prevention of sexually transmitted diseases, although the underlying philosophies may be different. In some localities access to facilities may be made difficult when parental consent is insisted upon for the young. The problems of access to these and other facilities relating to reproductive health care and education are important, are often ignored and extend into the implications of contraception, pregnancy and abortion in the adolescent (Bury 1984). Paxman (1984) draws attention to the estimate, on a world scale, that-three-quarters of adolescents under 15 years of age and half of those over this age have no access to reproductive health information and education programmes.

FARRELL'S SURVEY (1978)

In Farrell's survey (p. 57) the mean age for boys learning about reproduction was 10.3 years and for girls 10.0 years (ages mentioned ranged from 5–15, with a peak at 11), some 2 years earlier than the boys and girls in Schofield's study 10 years previously (Schofield 1965). In spite of this trend, over a quarter (28%) of the 16–19-year-old boys and girls did not learn about reproduction till they were 12 or older. The mean age for learning about sexual intercourse (11.6 years) was later than the age of learning 'where babies come from' and furthermore, it was common for parents and teachers to talk about reproduction without mentioning the act of intercourse. Evidence suggested that the peer group was still the most frequent source of information particularly for boys.

In connection with sexually transmitted diseases, Farrell (1978) found this to be a subject most parents approached with enthusiasm; 97% believed it should be taught. A teacher was suggested as the appropriate source by 44%. More mothers (41%) than fathers (25%) thought children should learn from parents, but daughters should not be taught by fathers alone (p. 95). STD were seen as a sanction against permissiveness and promiscuity. Fulfilment of sexual relationships and pleasure involved were rarely mentioned anywhere, but the vigour with which parents commented on VD suggested a persisting Victorian morality.

80% of young people knew more or less how venereal diseases were transmitted. When asked about symptoms there was much uncertainty, due possibly to embarrassment and not wanting to name genitalia but mostly due to lack of precise knowledge. In this survey 66 boys and 29 girls said that they might have had VD (STD) at some point, that is 8% of the boys and 4% of girls. Of these only 8 (3 boys and 5 girls) said that VD had actually been diagnosed. The disturbing point was made that half of the boys (52%) and a quarter of the girls (24%) who thought that they might have had VD did nothing about it and reported that their symptoms disappeared. The figures on action taken contrast with what all the young people in the sample said they would do if they thought that they had VD. In answer to that question (Farrell 1978, p. 52) 53% said that they would go to their own doctor, 44% said they would go to a VD clinic and 1% would have asked a friend or panicked. Nobody said they would 'do nothing and wait and see if the symptoms disappeared' which was what nearly half (43%) of those who had thought they had VD had

done. Intentions, as the author emphasizes, are often coloured by what people think they should do, and are not always translated into action. Knowledge about VD is widespread but generalized; in sex education accurate information and practical advice are needed rather than unspecified and dramatic warnings.

The project on health education (Schools Council/Health Education Council 1982) to be described provides a valuable information base for young people and deserves consideration for inclusion in the curriculum. Sex education is an important part of child, adolescent and adult education; it offers first information and then opportunity, as adolescence develops, to use this information in understanding personal feelings and actions in relation to others. With the bewildering choice of behaviour norms offered and publicized in the media, such education can help to reduce confusion of young people, their families and the rest of society (Spicer 1981). Within its context contraception, abortion, sexually transmitted diseases are discussed, and anxieties concerning, for example, homosexuality or masturbation should be accommodated. Such programmes need, however, to be subjected to external critical scrutiny as too quickly they can become 'empty rituals that serve to lessen the anxieties of parents and educators and, at the same time, only reinforce the children's and adolescent's already well developed belief in the unhealthy and hypocritical posture of adults towards sex' (Farrell 1978).

Clearly the barriers to health education including sex education have not been overcome. The most constructive outcomes appeared to occur when schools had worked out their policies, approached parents with specific proposals, discussed with them the content of the programme, respected the rights of parents to withdraw their children, and encouraged them to watch any television programmes they proposed to use. It did seem that schools were not wholly facing their responsibilities in health education of their pupils (Scottish Education Department 1974, 1979).

Farrell's national survey of teenagers in England and Wales (Farrell 1978) in 1974, revealed that only a small proportion (9%) of boys and girls remembered having any kind of sex education in primary school and in secondary school only one in four had birth control lessons which included discussions of specific contraceptive methods. Farrell considers (1980) that medical intervention or health education per se are unlikely to bring change to established adult behaviour which results from a complex set of experiences and beliefs developed during childhood and adolescence, which are then proscribed by environmental and personal circumstances. There are serious difficulties, even ethical problems in devising ways to bring about long-term behavioural change. The individual right to choose is sacrosanct in a democracy and the role of health education is to provide and reinforce information to enable individuals to assess risks to health and to use the health and social services when appropriate. Clearly this process includes and extends beyond schooldays (Farrell 1980).

OBJECTIVES IN SEX EDUCATION

The objectives in sex education in Sweden (Linner 1967, Bergstroom-Walan 1977), are still to be commended.

1. Acquire knowledge about anatomy, physiology, psychology, ethics and sociology.

2. Acquire an objective and comprehensive orientation about various norms and attitudes of importance for sexual life, both the accepted and controversial.

3. Develop the ability to perceive sexuality as an integrated part of human life.

4. Acquire increased consciousness and thereby a better chance for personal judgement on different levels of maturity and sexual experience.

Principles of democracy, equality and respect for the individual are stressed; traditional double standards of morality by which certain sexual modes of behaviour are acceptable for males but condemned for females are to be avoided. Tolerance and an understanding view of the various forms of sexuality are encouraged, as well as an acceptance of the right to a sexual life for the handicapped, the elderly and the mentally ill. Different life forms are discussed objectively but the risks in a too early sexual debut emphasized, namely unwanted pregnancy, sexually transmitted diseases, superficial and disharmonious relationships.

In respect to sexually transmitted diseases (STD) the following should be stressed:

1. Duty to protect yourself and others against STD.
2. Hasty sexual contact can lead to infection.
3. Avoid casual sexual relationships.
4. Consult a doctor or clinic — make sure that the facilities in each locality are well known — if infected or a risk has been taken.
5. The sooner the condition is treated the sooner cured.
6. A condom, properly used, offers a substantial defence.
7. Do not let a sense of shame deter you from such help.

The propositions outlined in the Swedish theme aim to help the individuals to reach their own decisions and to make their own judgements. The objectives given are simple but important. Campbell (1975) considers that one basic goal in health education is to enhance the capacity of individuals to form relationships, a more complex aim than those outlined. Much has been written on the subject and many teaching aids have been developed (The Schools Council 1979). A recently published project (Health Education 13–18, 1982) is recommended and described in some detail.

HEALTH EDUCATION IN SCHOOLS: THE SCHOOLS COUNCIL'S PROJECT

The Schools Council's publication 'Health Education 13–18' (1982), to which the reader is advised to refer, opens with the proposition that health problems in present-day society are more associated with life style than with environmental health and infectious diseases. Acknowledging inspiration from such definitions of health as World Health Organization's 'a state of complete physical mental and social well being, not merely the absence of disease and infirmity' and ideals of individual growth and fulfilment, the concerns of Health Education in Schools and Colleges are:

1. Giving young people a basic health knowledge and an understanding of human development.

2. Helping young people to adapt to change in themselves and their environment.

3. Helping young people to explore and understand the feelings, attitudes and values of themselves and others.

4. Helping young people to determine where they have control over their health and where they can by conscious choice determine their future health and life styles.

Emphasis is placed on helping young people to make informed choices in matters relating to their health, as in smoking, and development of self-esteem is clearly emphasized. Health education is seen as an integrated part of different courses and different departments. Reference is made to the importance of the influence of other adults as well as peers. The course under discussion is made up of attractively titled units, a number of which are illustrated in Figure 4.1.

Level 1 (13–14 years) — Health is what you make it
                        — Calculating the odds
                        — Coming of age
                        — Life styles
                        — Road sense
                        — Smile please
Level 2 (14–15 years) — What would you do about STD (sexually transmitted diseases)?
                        — Finding out about fluoride
                        — Pressure points
                        — Happy eating I

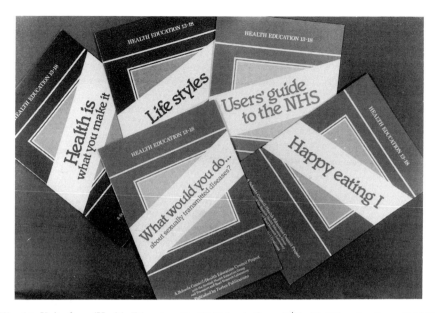

Fig. 4.1 Units from 'Health Education 13–18' (Schools Council/Health Education Council 1982).

— Happy eating II
— Happy eating III
— Under the influence
— Coping with accidents
— You in a group
Level 3 (16+ years) — Health and self
— Dilemma
— Users' guide to the NHS
— Accident

In the unit 'What would you do . . . about sexually transmitted diseases?,', teachers in England and Wales are reminded that their local education authority has a duty to inform parents of the nature and contents of sex education under The Education (School Information) Regulations 1981 (Note 4.2). In addition reference is made to the publication of the Department of Education and Science (1981) 'The School Curriculum' where advice is also given on the sensitive nature of sex education (Note 4.3). Since the publication of the titled units discussed the Department of Education and Science (1987) issued to all Local Education Authorities a circular on 'Sex Education at School'. This dealt with a number of important matters; the control over the content and organization of sex education; the place of sex education within the 5–16 curriculum; a moral framework for sex education; teaching about AIDS; advice to pupils under 16; and gave details on the action to be taken by those involved in developing the policy on the subject.

Advice that this particular unit (Schools Council 1982), should be conducted by a teacher who knows the students well is coupled with a reminder that the whole subject of STD is value laden and raises questions of morality and responsibility. The unit aims are summarized:

1. To enable students to grasp a simple outline of symptoms, treatment and courses of action by combining their own knowledge with any further information.
2. To enable students to explore their own attitudes towards STD and those of the people around them.
3. To enable the students to make decisions about STD, when and if necessary, which will further their own health and that of the community.

In regard to STD it is noted:

a. The harm that can be caused by non-specific genital infection (NSGI) is perhaps underrated and pushed into the shade by the emotional reaction of syphilis and gonorrhoea. The symptoms of NSGI in the male can be similar to those of gonorrhoea but are much more likely to be missed.
b. The major point is that there is an increase in the incidence of symptomless STD and that both boys and girls — but particularly girls — are very likely not to notice any symptoms.

This emphasizes the need for a check at the clinic when there is a risk of infection, rather than waiting for symptoms to appear (for detailed comments on p. 3, see unit on STD). In the Unit (p. 3) the major treatment of almost all STD is described as being a large dose of antibiotic, usually injected, with repeated checks to ensure that the infection has cleared. (The emphasis on 'large' and 'injection' appears to the authors to be unduly threatening and it would be better to say that antibiotic treatment by mouth or injection may be required.) The problem of antibiotic resistance in gonococci is discussed and conclusions are listed:

1. There are a number of factors which stand in the way of efforts to control STD but two major ones are:
   a. Commonly held attitudes towards the infections — shame, disgust an a refusal to talk or think about them.
   b. The large reservoir of girls or women or some men who have no symptoms and therefore do not present themselves for treatment but who are infected and can infect others.
2. The main points which need emphasis and re-emphasis are:
   a. The understanding that many girls and some boys may be infected but appear to have no symptoms.
   b. The importance of a check if there is any possibility of infection — i.e. after any casual sex or contact.
   c. The need for and importance of repeat visits to a clinic after treatment to check that the infection has been cleared.

Reference is made to the role of the contact tracer (Worksheet 2). Further background information on STD is recorded as being available in the form of regularly updated Fact Sheets from the Family Planning Information Service, 27/35 Mortimer Street, London WlN 7RJ (Tel. 01–636–7866).

A sequence of units suggested for the 4th–5th year (S3–S4) in the 14–16 year age group is as follows: 1. Pressure Points; 2. You in a Group; 3. Under the Influence; 4) What would you do . . . . about sexually transmitted diseases? In the unit 'Users Guide to the NHS' for the 16-year age group, reference is also made to STD (Worksheet 1). With current pressures on departments of genito-urinary medicine young people should learn not to be discouraged by difficulties in securing immediate appointments. In the event of dissatisfaction individuals should feel confident to seek advice from their own general practitioners, who can help the individual as well as exert influence on the health service of the locality.

CONCLUSIONS

Although sex education appears to be increasingly perceived as a component of social education whose aims include: improving decision making skills; raising self esteem and clarifying values; becoming aware of the consequences of one's own actions and increasing one's sensitivity to the needs of others (Reid 1982), it is important not to allow the subject to become too narrowed. Many present-day sexual issues may bring no comfort and the increased prevalence of STD, for example, is a fact of life. Although teaching may be more comfortable and untroubled when discussing ideals and values, the factual situation needs to be appraised. New difficulties, particularly those with persistent virus infections (e.g. herpes simplex virus, human papillomavirus and hepatitis B virus) involving increasing numbers, bring not only morbidity in the short term but problems of coping with possible or certain effects in the longer term. The newly discovered retrovirus associated with the Acquired Immune Deficiency Syndrome (Ch. 31) has brought great danger, particularly to homosexual males, and there is now proof of its heterosexual transmission and wider dissemination in the community. Knowledge of these new hazards is important in the modern world; geographical isolation has ceased to be one firm protection against infection.

Human sexual behaviour is infinitely variable within the range of cultural restraints imposed upon it — either polyandry, polygamy, monogamy, serial monogamy, promiscuity or celibacy may be regarded as a norm for a particular community (Short 1981). Mankind's sexual behaviour requires study for its comprehension (Ford & Beach 1952) and cannot be learned by mere introspection (Ch. 2). Within existing norms infection is an inevitable and important factor which cannot with safety be disregarded as a subject in education.

There is a continual problem of maintaining impetus and securing standards in sex education. Reluctance to deal with these subjects tends to persist; to overcome this tendency once does not mean that the teaching programme will be accepted and promoted for all time. There are often objections based upon sexual ethical norms; attitudes of what may or may not be considered to be desirable may assume more importance than knowledge of the norms in human sexual behaviour as revealed by research (Kosnik et al 1977) (see also Ch. 1). The health educator will wish to prepare the individual to cope with the present-day problems of humanity as well as to encourage self-regarding virtues and consideration for others. It is an essential aim that those taught will not develop feelings of guilt that will make them fear to surface for medical help when needed.

MASS PUBLICITY AND AIDS

The pandemic of HIV infection and AIDS continues to produce widespread alarm, and massive 'public education' programmes have been mounted with the primary purpose of preventing its spread. In Britain, for example, in November 1986 £20 million was made available for the first year's programme in which emphasis is to be placed on the need for individuals to modify their sexual behaviour and which is to be couched in universally understood language. The campaign of newspaper advertisements; posters appearing in 1500 sites around Britain; approaches to young people by magazines, radio and cinema; advertising by radio and television has been backed up by a national leaflet sent to all 23 million households and by a distribution of another informative leaflet 'AIDS, what everybody needs to know' to all pharmacies for collection by the public (Notes and News (Lancet) 1986).

The epidemic curves for the Acquired Immune Deficiency Syndrome in the United States, (Figs. 4.2, 4.3, 4.4) for Britain, or elsewhere are seen to show an annual increase which follows roughly an exponential rise and therefore, if expressed on a logarithmic scale, the plotted points form almost a straight line. Temptation to extrapolate this line to estimate numbers of cases in future years should be resisted since for such predictions to be statistically valid it must be assumed that the factors influencing the course of the epidemic will remain constant. The spread of epidemic infection is related to the number of susceptible people and the aim of mass education of the public is that these numbers should diminish and the epidemic wane. In HIV infection symptomless cases are very much more numerous than AIDS itself and other factors may also influence the disease (McEvoy & Tillett 1985).

To determine prevalence of seropositivity it would be necessary to make assays of HIV antibodies in random samples of the population. Such sampling, if repeated at intervals, would provide data on the pace at which seropositivity was increasing, the rate of involvement of the general heterosexual population and its geographical pattern (Leading Article (Lancet) 1987). Notifications of AIDS alone are not reliable enough nor timely

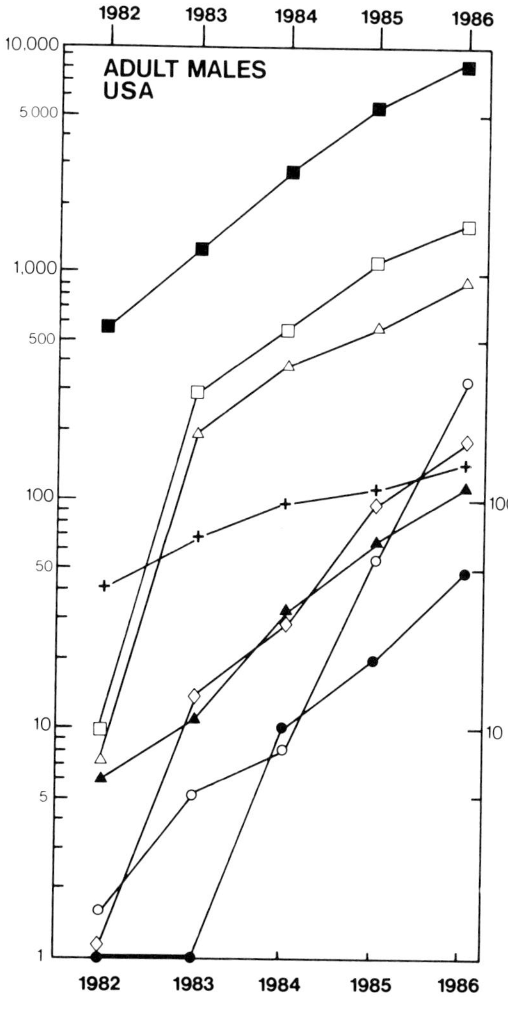

Fig. 4.2 Numbers of AIDS cases in adult males, plotted on a logarithmic scale and categorized by means of transmission for the period from before 12th August 1982 and in the years ending 12th August for 1983, 1984, 1985 and 1986. The numbers of AIDS cases continue to increase; the proportions amongst most 'transmission' categories have remained relatively constant. Homosexual or bisexual men who are not known to have misused intravenous drugs (IVDA) represent 70% of all reported male cases. Homosexual or bisexual IVDA comprise 8% of cases in males. Heterosexual IVDA comprise 15% of cases in males. Persons with haemophilia/coagulation disorders represent 1% of cases in males. Heterosexual sex partners of persons with AIDS or at-risk of AIDS represent 2% of males. Recipients of transfused blood or blood components account for 1% of males. For 3% of AIDS cases in males the means of acquisition of the disease was not determined. The total cases of AIDS in the USA up till 12th August 1986 was 28,098, comprising 1870 cases in women (6.66%); 27 704 cases in men (98.6%); and 394 cases in children under the age of 13 years (1.4%). (Figure constructed from data in Centers for Disease Control 1986.)
Key
■ Homosexual/bisexual only
□ IVDA
△ Homosexual + IVDA
○ Undetermined
◊ transfusion
+ Heterosexual (non US-born)
△ Haemophilia/coagulation disorders
● Heterosexual (US-born)

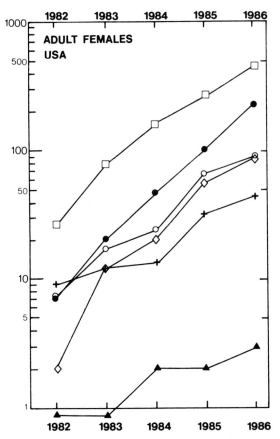

Fig. 4.3 Numbers of AIDS cases in adult females, plotted on a logarithmic scale and categorized by means of transmission for the period from before 12th August 1982 for 1983, 1984, 1985 and 1986. The number of AIDS cases continues to increase; the proportions amongst 'transmission' categories have remained relatively constant except with regard to numbers of cases of AIDS in those with a coagulation disorder. Heterosexual women who have misused intravenous drugs (IVDA) comprise 51% of cases in females. Persons with coagulation disorders represent 0.4% of cases in females. Heterosexual sex partners of persons with AIDS or at-risk of AIDS represent 27% of cases in females. For 11% of AIDS cases in females the means of acquisition of the disease was not determined. (Figure constructed from data in Centers for Disease Control 1986.)

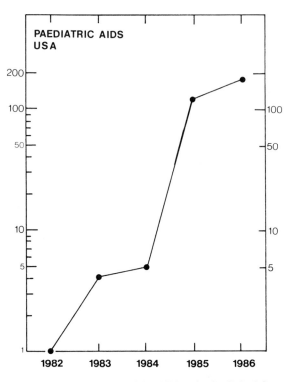

Fig. 4.4 Most cases of AIDS in children in the United States (79%) came from families in which one or both parents had AIDS or were at increased risk of developing AIDS. 6% had haemophilia and 13% had received blood or blood components before the onset of the illness. Risk factors could not be determined in 3%. Perinatal transmission is the most important factor in young children. Only 62 cases occurred within the very large population of children of the ages 5–15 years comprising 16% of the total US population. The total cases of AIDS in the USA up till 12th August 1986 was 28 098, comprising 1870 cases in women (6.66%); 27 704 cases in men (98.6%); and 394 cases in children under the age of 13 years (1.40%). (Figure constructed from data in Centers for Disease Control 1986.)

enough to give the information required, since the onset of disease follows infection acquired three or more years earlier. Sir Richard Doll (1987) as chairman of the epidemiological subcommittee of the Medical Research Council's working party on AIDS, recognizing the difficulties inherent in random sampling, has sought support for a plan for random samples of blood taken for other purposes, say at antenatal clinics or casualty departments, to be tested in such a way that the individual is unidentified except for sex, age and residential district.

The testing of such unidentified blood samples is the only way to determine the progress of the epidemic in Britain at a stage when there is a hope to stem the epidemic. British Medical Association's working party (1987), however affirm in this connection, inter alia, that: the population as a whole should not be screened for HIV infection; that AIDS and HIV infection should not be made notifiable diseases; and that tests for HIV antibodies should only be carried out with the individual's consent. Support for these principles arises from concern for the individual; perhaps also for the difficulties in securing anonymity of the samples to be tested; and an awareness of a human tendency to break any code to improve the value of the epidemiological information.

Although in western urban communities the overt

disease AIDS at present has been to a very great extent confined to groups at risk, notably homosexual and bisexual men and intravenous drug misusers, there is a fear that it will engulf the general heterosexual population unless all people modify their sexual behaviour and, in the case of intravenous drug misusers, avoid using another's needle or syringe. Since there is evidence of widespread HIV infection in the heterosexual population of tropical Africa south of the Sahara, however, and also undoubted proof of incidents of spread by heterosexual intercourse, public health policy in Britain, for example, has at present been based on the fact that both heterosexual men and women may also be at risk (Acheson 1986). Outside Africa there is as yet, however, little evidence of a heterosexual epidemic of AIDS. In the United States by December 8th 1986 there were 28 000 cases, of whom 93% were men, and in adults 97% of cases belonged to recognized at-risk groups, a figure which has remained constant for several years. In Britain, where the disease is still relatively rare, no outbreak of HIV infection has yet been detected in those without at-risk factors.

In addition to specific advice about the nature of infection and the means of its avoidance emphasis in the mass publicity campaign has been placed on the safety of the supply of blood for transfusion and of products derived from blood. In this connection endeavour has been made by blood transfusion services to select a subpopulation of donors by excluding any who might have even a remote risk of being infected with HIV (McClelland 1986). In May 1987 the following rules were applied by the Scottish National Blood Transfusion Service:

SNBTS MESSAGE
AIDS — PEOPLE WHO MUST NOT GIVE BLOOD

1. Anyone who has AIDS or the AIDS antibody.
2. Any man who has had sex with another man since 1977.
3. Anyone who has EVER injected themselves with drugs.
4. Anyone who has lived in or visited Africa South of the Sahara at anytime since 1977 and has had sex with men *or women* living there.
5. Anyone who has had *regular* treatment with blood products since 1977.
6. Anyone who is, or has been, a prostitute.
7. Anyone who has ever had sex with a person in the above groups *even on a single occasion*.
MUST NOT GIVE BLOOD

In addition it is aimed to exclude any donor who admitted heterosexual intercourse with 'multiple part-

ners' and was uncertain if any of their partners fell into category 5. This policy is framed to diminish as far as possible the risk of accepting HIV infected blood. The strategy of collecting the patient's own blood before an elective operation and transfusing it to him during the operation, if necessary, offers an alternative suitable for some instances (Kay 1987). This practice, known as autologous blood transfusion, even with its logistical difficulties is likely to be more actively considered in the future.

In Britain by January 1987 the blood of 3 million donors had been tested for anti-HIV and 65 were found to be positive — giving a prevalence of 1 : 46 154; most were found to be male homosexuals and only 6 denied being in at-risk groups (Contreras 1987). At present (January 1987) the risk of a patient receiving blood contaminated with HIV through the National Blood Transfusion Service is less than 1 : 10^6 and guidelines to donors combined with testing safeguard the position (AIDS: Joint statement by DHSS and BMA 1987). In Edinburgh where HIV infection is very prevalent among intravenous drug abusers (Robertson et al 1986) it has been found that even with the use of exclusion criteria the prevalence of HIV-infected blood donations, as judged by the antibody test, is 1 : 10 000 compared with the UK prevalence of 1 : 46 154. Most of this excess was attributable to individuals who did not at the time of donation inject drugs but who became infected during past experimentation which included needle-sharing (Gillon, personal communication).

Clearly, the use of exclusion criteria in seeking blood donors who are free from infection is not without danger. The deepest human motive is to seek the respect of others (Harré 1979) and donation of blood is one activity in which this may be achieved. A donor may fear contempt by being rejected as a donor and this may well induce a person to withhold the information which is being sought.

The Standard Life Assurance, Scotland's largest life and pensions group, like others, is now to act against applicants who are considered at risk of AIDS (Short 1987). The questions asked in proposal forms vary but they leave no moral nor legal loophole for the applicant. The words 'Have you ever received or considered you ought to seek medical advice regarding AIDS? If the answer is 'YES' give details' are included, for example, in present proposal forms for full life insurance cover (Scottish Widow's Fund and Life Assurance Society). Some organizations within the homosexual community recommend that homosexual men should not come forward for testing until arrangements have been made which ensure that persons with positive tests are not subject to financial detriment. The Government in Britain has set up an interdepartmental Ministerial

Committee to examine these and other issues (Acheson 1986) but it is difficult to envisage how they could be overcome by government intervention.

The first part of this chapter outlines an approach based on that prepared by the Health Education Council before the threat of AIDS sufficiently sharpened the argument. It is clearer than ever to present authors that health education including sex education should be mandatory and integrated into the school curriculum. Individuals must receive sufficient biological and psychological insights to comprehend their own nature, including their sexuality, as well as the nature of infection. Education on sex cannot omit reference to sexual orientation nor to the dangers of HIV infection.

The second part of the chapter outlines the result of a very recent change in public health policy in which the communication media are used to a much greater extent than ever before. Information is plentiful but it now reaches many who are ill-prepared educationally and emotionally to receive it. Although the media, perhaps the radio to a greater extent than television, are able to assist, it is one-to-one counselling services which are highly desirable but not easy to provide sufficiently. Many people at very low risk are being made anxious; more effort should be directed to the clearly defined at-risk groups.

NOTES TO CHAPTER 4

Note 4.1: The European Convention on Human Rights, Strasbourg 1984

ARTICLE 10

1. Everyone has the right to freedom of expression. This right shall include freedom to hold opinions and to receive and impart information and ideas without interference by public authority and regardless of frontiers. This Article shall not prevent States from requiring the licensing of broadcasting, television or cinema enterprises.

2. The exercise of these freedoms, since it carries with it duties and responsibilities, may be subject to such formalities, conditions, restrictions or penalties as are prescribed by law and are necessary in a democratic society, in the interests of national security, territorial integrity or public safety, for the prevention of disorder or crime, for the protection of health or morals, for the protection of the reputation or rights of others, for preventing the disclosure of information received in confidence, or for maintaining the authority and impartiality of the judiciary.

Note 4.2: Statutory Instruments 1981 no. 630 Education, England and Wales

THE EDUCATION (SCHOOL INFORMATION) REGULATIONS 1981

Made	15 April 1981
Laid before Parliament	1 May 1981
Coming into Operation	25 May 1981

Information as respects individual schools to be published by education authorities or school governors.
4.-(1) The information to be published in pursuance of section 8(5)(1) of the Act of 1980:
    a. in the case of a school other than an aided or special agreement school, by the relevant education authority;
    b. in the case of an aided or special agreement school, by the governors thereof or, in pursuance of section 8(6) of that Act, on their behalf by the relevant education authority, shall be the information specified in Schedule 2.

SCHEDULE 2 (extract)

Information relating to individual schools to be published by an education authority or by or on behalf of the governors of an aided or special agreement school
4. Particulars of the school curriculum including, in particular inter alia:

c. of the manner and context in which education as respects sexual matters is given;

Note 4.3: Department of Education and Science Welsh Office

DEPARTMENT OF EDUCATION AND SCIENCE (1981) THE SCHOOL CURRICULUM

24. Moral education in schools seeks to promote integrity, considerate behaviour and the pupil's understanding of the relationship between action and beliefs. It has to recognise the critically important influence of the home and society upon children's moral development and the formation of moral attitudes. It is occasionally taught on its own: more often it is most effectively achieved as a significant aspect of other subjects, in particular — but not exclusively — of literature and of religious and health education. Awareness of moral values is also encouraged by appropriate and well planned assemblies, as well as by good pastoral care. The school needs to make explicit to parents, pupils and the local community its aims in moral education: and the head teacher and his staff need to keep curricular, pastoral and other provision under review so as to ensure that these aims are translated into effective practice.

25. Health education, like preparation for parenthood, is part of the preparation of the individual for personal, social and family responsibilities. Health education should give pupils a basic knowledge and understanding of health matters both as they affect themselves and as they affect others, so that they are helped to make informed choices in their daily lives. It should also help them to become aware of those moral issues and value judgements which are inseparable from such choices. Preparation for parenthood and family life should help pupils to recognise the importance of those human relationships which sustain, and are sustained by, family life and the demands and duties that fall on parents.

26. Schools are responding in a variety of ways to the need for sound sex education. Sex education is one of the most sensitive parts of broad programmes of health education and the fullest consultation and cooperation with parents are necessary before it is embarked upon. In this area offence can be given if a school is not aware of, and sensitive to, the cultural background of every child. Sex education is not a simple matter and is linked with attitudes and behaviour. The regulations to be made under Section 8 of the Education Act 1980 will require LESAs to inform parents of the ways and contexts in which sex education is provided.

REFERENCES

Handyside v. United Kingdom 1976 European Human Rights Reports 1976 vol 1, p. 737–766

Kjeldsen, Busk Madsen and Pedersen v. Denmark 1976 European Court of Human Rights. Judgement of 7 December 1976, Strasbourg

Young, James and Webster v. United Kingdom 1981 European Human Rights Reports 1982 vol 1, p. 38–63 (especially p 57)

Acheson E D 1986 AIDS: A challenge for the public health. Lancet i: 662–666

AIDS: Joint statement by DHSS and BMA 1987 British Medical Journal 294: 192

Bergstroom-Walan M 1977 Sex education — Sweden's experiences — success and failure. British Journal of Sexual Medicine 4: 18

British Medical Association's working party 1987 BMA's AIDS working party. British Medical Journal 294: 192–193

Bury J 1984 Teenage pregnancy in Britain. Birth Control Trust, 27–35 Mortimer Street, London W1N TRJ

Campbell A V 1975 moral dilemmas in medicine Churchill Livingstone, Edinburgh, p 190

Centers for Disease Control 1986 Acquired immunodeficiency syndrome. Morbidity and Mortality Weekly Report. Update, United States 35: 757–760; 765–766

Contreras M 1987 Who may give blood? Correspondence, British Medical Journal 294: 176

Council of Europe, Committee of Ministers 1974 Resolution (74)5 on the Control of Sexually Transmitted Diseases (STD). Adopted by the Committee of Ministers on 27 February, 1974 at the 229th Meeting of the Minister's Deputies.

Department of Education and Science 1981 The school curriculum. HMSO, paragraphs 24–26, p 7–8

Department of Education and Science 1987 Sex Education at School. Circular No. 11/87 of 25:9:87. Department of Education and Science, Elizabeth House, York Road, London SE1 7PH

Doll Sir Richard 1987 A proposal for drug prevalence studies of AIDS. Correspondence, British Medical Journal 294: 244

European Convention of Human Rights 1983 The European Convention on Human Rights: First Protocol to the Convention, Article 2, Council of Europe, Strasbourg, p 28

European Ministers for Cultural Affairs 1984 Resolution No. 11 on European Declaration on Cultural Objectives (23–25 March 1984). Information Sheet No.16, Human Rights (H/INF(84)3) p 203–206

Evans Sir Vincent 1983 Information Conference, The European Convention on Human Rights and the Law in Scotland 14 November 1983. University of Edinburgh

Farrell C in collaboration with Kellaher L 1978 My mother said . . . The way young people learned about sex and birth control. Routledge and Kegan Paul, London (page numbers given in text)

Farrell C 1980 Health Education. In: Farrell C, Robinson D (eds) Health education and self help. Kings Fund Centre, 126 Albert Street, London NW1 7NF

Ford C S, Beach F A 1952 Patterns of sexual behaviour. Eyre and Spottiswoode, London. Reprint of Edition published 1980 by Harper and Row, New York, available

Greenwood Press, Westport, Connecticut

Gagnon J H, Simon W 1973 Sexual conduct. Hutchinson, London, p 117

Gillon J 1986 quoted in Dinwoodie R. Drs fight to keep blood off the floor. Scotsman, 6/1/1987, p 9

Harré Rom 1979 Social being: A theory for social psychology. Basil Blackwell, Oxford

Kay L A 1987 The need for autologous blood transfusion. Leading article, British Medical Journal 294: 137–139

Kosnik A, Carroll W, Cunningham A, Modras R, Schulte J 1977 Human sexuality. New directions in American Catholic thought. Paulist Press, New York, ch 3, p 53–77

Leading Article 1987 HIV Seroepidemiology. Lancet i: 259–260

Linner B 1967 Sex and society in Sweden. Jonathan Cape, London

McEvoy M, Tillett H 1985 AIDS for all by the year 2000? British Medical Journal 290–463

McClelland D B L 1986 quoted in Dinwoodie R. Drs fight to keep blood off the floor. Scotsman, 6/1/1987, p 9

Notes and News 1986 Fighting AIDS. Lancet ii: 1291

Paxman J M 1984 Laws and policies, affecting health services for young people: problems, practicalities and possibilities. Background paper prepared for WHO Study Group on Young People and Health for All by the Year 2000, Geneva, June 4–8, 1984

Reid D 1982 School sex education and the causes of unintended teenage pregnancies — a review. Health Education Journal 41: 4–11

Robertson J R, Roberts J J K, Buchnall A B V, Welsby P D, Brettle R P, Inglis J M, Peutherer J F 1986 Epidemic of AIDS-related virus (HTLV-III/LAV) infection among intravenous drug abusers. British Medical Journal 292: 527–529

Schofield M 1965 The sexual behaviour of young people. Longman, London

Schools Council 1979 Relationships and sexuality, resource list 1979. Schools Council/Health Education Council, 78 New Oxford Street, London WC7A 7AH

Schools Council/Health Education Council 1982 'What would you do . . . . about STD?' from 'Health education 13–18'. Forbes Publications, London

Scottish Education Department 1974 Health education in schools, curriculum paper 14. HMSO, Edinburgh

Scottish Education Department 1979 A report by H.M. Inspectors of Schools. Health education in primary secondary and special schools in Scotland. HMSO, Edinburgh

Short R V 1981 Sexual selection in Man and the Great Apes. In: Graham G E (ed) Reproductive biology of the Great Apes. Academic Press, London, p 319–373

Short E 1987 Assurance group to act on AIDS-risk applicants. Financial Times 30/1/1987

Sieghart P 1985 The lawful rights of mankind: an introduction to the international legal code of human rights. Oxford University Press, Oxford

Spicer Faith 1981 Sex education. In: Duncan A R, Dunstan G R, Welbourn R B (eds) Dictionary of medical ethics. Darton, Longman and Todd, London, p 387–389

Tanner J M 1962 Growth at adolescence, 2nd edn. Blackwell Scientific Publications, Oxford, p 28–39

Tanner J M 1978 Foetus into man. Open Books, London, p 60–77

5

Some social, ethical and medico-legal aspects of sexually transmitted diseases

A number of social, ethical and medico-legal aspects of sexually transmitted diseases are given consideration in this chapter:

a. Confidentiality and sexually transmitted diseases
b. Medical advice and treatment in young persons
c. Tracing of contacts and the case against compulsion; lessons from history.
d. Child abuse and sexually transmitted disease
e. Persistent virus infections (including that due to human immunodeficiency viruses) and control of their spread
f. Testing for antibody to human immunodeficiency viruses (HIV) (limitations, indications and restraints)
g. Homosexuality in males
h. Prostitution in females
i. Self-help groups
j. Companionship, marriage and divorce
k. Dilemma of a name.

A. CONFIDENTIALITY AND SEXUALLY TRANSMITTED DISEASES

Consent and confidentiality

In medical practice in sexually transmitted diseases two ethical principles, namely voluntary consent to medical investigation and treatment and medical confidentiality, deserve special attention. The argument against legal compulsion, if applied to investigation and treatment, is discussed in a historical context in Section (c) of this chapter and it again receives attention in relation to testing the blood of individuals against human immuno-deficiency viruses (HIV) where explanation to the patient beforehand and obtaining truly informed consent to the test are regarded as essential preliminaries (Section (f)). These ethical principles can only be maintained under circumstances where respect for the individual is given its due importance.

In both law and ethics medical confidences are regarded as sacred, with certain exceptions. It is a complicated subject with an extensive bibliography including the following: Lord Mansfield's ruling in The Duchess of Kingston Case of 1776 in Melville (1927); AB v. CD (1851); Garner v. Garner (1920); Birkenhead (1922); Riddell (1929); Henley v. Henley (1955); Bernfeld (1967; 1972); Mason & McCall Smith (1983).

The question is what the exceptions are (Riddell 1929) and 'when may the doctor tell, when should he tell and when must he tell?'. In the case of sexually transmitted infections, eminently treatable conditions, such as syphilis and gonorrhoea, often present a dilemma to doctors. Although 'to tell' without the consent of a patient in this case may well secure virtually certain cure to a given partner, medical secrecy from the points of view of both the index patient and prospective patients, however, should not be broken without consent and confidentiality should be secure. Otherwise doubt and fear of its breach might dissuade those needing medical attention from attending as patients in the first place. Mere statement of this viewpoint, however, and a negative attitude with lack of concern about the sexual partner of the index patient may lead to omission and development of preventive action by tracing of contacts. Such action should be based on persuasion and encouragement to patients. Legal coercion has no place as it leads to unwanted changes in attitudes to patients (see Section (c)). Confidentiality, in England and Wales, is expressly demanded in two Ministerial Regulations (Notes 5.1 and 5.2); to encourage the tracing of contacts information may be passed in confidence to those responsible for the process.

In the case of infection with immunodeficiency viruses (HIV) continued unprotected sexual intercourse with a sexual partner as yet uninfected may bring to the latter catastrophic illness, even more serious in pregnancy, when there is also involvement of the fetus. The view that has gained acceptance is based on the value and effectiveness of persuasion tempered with respect for individual privacy. Failure to persuade should be a rare event which is not made rarer by the availability of a legal threat. The doctor cannot escape the nature of a moral dilemma. Professor Emmett (1979) in her book 'The Moral Prism' clarifies the nature of the dilemma and in her opening chapter writes, 'Ideally moral judgement might be a white light showing clearly what action would be best in any situation but just as light coming through a prism is refracted into a spectrum of different colours, so our moral thinking shows a range of different features, and attention can fasten now on one and now on another'. Morality is clearly a contestable concept. Respect for the patient, the value of persuasion and concern are likely to continue to yield more than the use of legal coercion which so profoundly alters the clinical atmosphere. Legal compulsion or threats, we maintain, should have no place in the tracing of contacts. These measures are discredited and were first rejected in England by the repeal of the Contagious Diseases Acts in 1886; later such measures in the United Kingdom were proved useless again by the failure more than 45 years ago of Regulation 33B (Defence Regulations 1939) described in Section (c) of this Chapter.

Relaxation of the rule of medical secrecy is permissible with the patient's consent, but how much information and to which members of the clinical team it may be released is a complex question. Release of information may be permissible within a department but not to other hospital staff outside. To act on occasions in the patient's interests when consent to communicate information has not been specifically obtained may be justified. Consent from the patient certainly should be sought whenever possible. If 'dysplasia' is reported in a cervical cytology smear and a patient fails to return, it is proper, if the patient cannot be found and asked for permission directly, to communicate the results to her general practitioner. In this epidemic of genital papillomavirus infection, with the as yet uncertain outcome for an individual, it is our policy now to enter the patient's name and address on the request form unless the patient expresses a particular wish to the contrary. The concept of informed consent, however, is a good one, and together with the giving of explanations is an ever increasing and necessary part of present-day medical practice.

Young people must be encouraged to attend if they have run risks of acquiring STD. In those under the age of 16 it is important to ask if they have told one or other parent and to suggest to them that they should do so. If they decline to confide in parents then confidences should be kept although they may agree to have a letter sent to their general practitioner. At no age should legal rules prevent the doctor from examining the patient, with his or her consent, in the manner indicated as necessary by the medical history or from treating an infection, provided the patient is capable of understanding the situation. If a girl is under 12 years of age the doctor has a responsibility to report what may have been a serious crime. In all cases the doctor's acts should be governed by what is considered to be best for the patient and medical attitudes should be protective avoiding disclosures which may be damaging.

Disclosure of confidential medical information may be required by statute as in the requirements for reporting by the doctor of infectious diseases. In the context of genito-urinary medicine and since 1968 it has been a statutory obligation in the United Kingdom for all doctors to notify the Home Office of any person whom they consider to be addicted to a drug appearing on a list of mainly opiates (cocaine, dextromoramide, diamorphine (heroin). dipipanone, hydrocodone, hydromorphone, levorphanol, methadone, morphine, opium, oxycodone, pethidine, phenazocine, piritramide) (Stimson & Oppenheimer 1982). Again no immunity is granted to the doctor when a statutory duty is imposed on 'any person' to provide information in relation to the Prevention of Terrorism (Temporary Provisions) Act 1976, Section II and the doctor must provide on request any evidence which he has which may lead to the identification of a driver involved in an accident. Courts of law are empowered to order disclosure as they see fit either to the applicant, the applicant's legal advisers, or to his medical advisers. Medical confidences will always be broken in British courts of law in the interest of securing justice although in Belgium and France such confidences are absolute and are protected by their respective penal codes (Mason & McCall Smith 1983).

Confidences, however, are protected in a British court of law where they are part of a discourse between a person and his advocate or solicitor in connection with legal proceedings (Birkenhead 1922, Riddell 1929). Privilege is also given to those acting as conciliators in a matrimonial dispute (Henley v. Henley 1955) on the basis that the State is more interested in reconciliation than divorce. The case of Garner v. Garner (1920) is important with regard to 'venereal diseases'. In this case the petitioner was 'praying for the dissolution of her marriage' and relied on the fact that 'syphilis had been communicated to her by her husband'. The doctor, called to give evidence, claimed that his knowledge of the case had been obtained in the course of treatment of a venereal disease under the Public Health (Venereal Diseases) Regulations and was therefore confidential and not to be disclosed in a court of law. These Regulations expressly provided that 'all information obtained in regard to a person treated under the scheme approved by the Board in pursuance of the Regulations shall be regarded as confidential'. The doctor concerned was, however, being called as a witness by the woman upon whom he had attended; no question of 'privilege' therefore arose and Mr Justice McCardie decided that evidence must be given.

The provision of the Regulations of 1916 did not affect the question of medical privilege. Any attempt to treat and control venereal diseases, or using the term sexually transmitted diseases to include infections due to agents from viruses to eukaryotes, is often bedevilled by fear of disclosure of information on the part of those who might need such treatment. For this reason confidentiality has always been accorded great importance and at the present time when irrational fears of infection with the human immunodeficiency viruses (HIV) are prominent in the minds of the public confidentiality is very important to maintain. In British courts of law such confidentiality may be broken but, in contrast, in French law no witness is obliged in a civil case to give evidence against his will and by Article 378 of the Penal Code a doctor who does so in a case of any sort is guilty of an offence and is liable to punishment. What action would be best in many situations is contestable and the matter of medical confidentiality is no exception. Professor Ian Kennedy, Director of the Centre for Medical Law and Ethics, King's College, London, it is reported (*The Independent*, 26th March, 1987), gave to members of the Social Services Select Committee as his belief that if doctors have an HIV-infected patient and fail to inform a wife or husband then they may be open to challenge in the courts. Clearly the doctor must make every endeavour to persuade an HIV-infected patient to bring his or her sexual partner, but the need for special coercive legislation in this regard is questionable. There is a view, however, that the criminal law might play a small part in protecting those at risk from a carrier. In the case where an individual, fully aware of the danger and nature of his infection, wilfully continues to put his sexual partner at risk then it is possible, in present English law, that a prosecution might be brought under the Offences Against the Persons Act 1861 — if transmission of HIV-infection were covered by section 23 'maliciously administering any poison or destruction or noxious thing'. If any such prosecution were to be brought and were to succeed the victim would then have the possible additional benefit of access to the Criminal Injuries Compensation Board (Forlin & Wauchope 1987).

B. MEDICAL ADVICE AND TREATMENT IN YOUNG PERSONS

At puberty, and particularly when sexual intercourse takes place at an early age, the questions of providing necessary advice on contraception and on sexually transmitted diseases inevitably arise and bring with them problems such as the validity of consent to medical examination and treatment. In England and Wales for girls over the age of 16 no legal problem arises as the Family Reform Act 1969 provides by Section 8(1) that a person of 16 years can give his or her own consent to medical treatment. For those under 16 it was considered that if the girl understood the nature of the treatment then she could validly consent to contraceptive advice. This view was specifically confirmed by a court of law for the first time (Norrie 1983) when Mr Justice Woolf decided the case of Gillick v. West Norfolk and Wisbeck Area Health Authority 1983. Mrs Victoria Gillick had sought a declaration from the court that advice, given by the Department of Health and Social Security to area health authorities, that contraceptive and abortion advice and treatment might exceptionally be provided for children under the age of 16, at a doctor's clinical discretion and without parental consent, was illegal. Mr Justice Woolf rejected her claim on the ground that there was nothing in law to show that a person under the age of 16 could not give personal consent to medical treatment and that the validity of such consent depended upon the person's intelligence and understanding of the proposed treatment. The Court of Appeal overruled the decision and granted Mrs Gillick the declaration asked for (Norrie 1985a, b, c. Brahams 1985). In October 1985, however, the decision of the Court of Appeal was reversed by the House of Lords. Lord Fraser considered (Times Law Report 18/10/1985 House of Lords):

The only practical course was '. . . . .to entrust the doctor with a discretion to act in accordance with his view of what was in the best interests of the girl who was his patient.

He should, of course, always seek to persuade her to tell her parents that she was seeking contraceptive advice, and the nature of the advice that she received. At least he should seek to persuade her to agree to the doctor's informing the parents.

But there may well be cases where the girl refused either to tell the parents herself or to permit the doctor to do so and in such cases, the doctor would . . . be justified in proceeding without the parents' consent or even knowledge, provided he was satisfied that:
1. the girl would although under 16 years understand his advice;
2. he could not persuade her to inform her parents or to allow him to inform the parents that she was seeking contraceptive advice;
3. she was very likely to have sexual intercourse with or without contraceptive treatment;
4. unless she received contraceptive advice or treatment her physical or mental health or both were likely to suffer; and
5. her best interests required him to give her contraceptive advice, treatment or both without parental consent.'

In Scottish law the concept of parental rights over children is fundamentally different and follows Roman law in distinguishing between the pupil child and the minor child. The pupil child is the girl below 12 and the boy below 14, the minor child is one above those ages and below 18. Although the parent of a pupil has power both over the person and property of the pupil the traditional long accepted view in Scots law is to the effect that the parent of a minor has no power over the actual person of a minor and only certain powers of consent over the minor's dealing with his or her own property. Medical treatment concerns one's own body and the minor child — the girl over 12 and the boy over 14 — therefore needs no consent from her or his parent before accepting medical treatment, contraceptive or otherwise. A doctor must of course be very wary about treating a very young patient without parental consent, for he may only do so if convinced that the patient understands the nature of the treatment, otherwise the patient's own consent will not be valid. The determination of the girl's understanding is a matter for the doctor's judgement. It is the Secretary of State for Scotland's opinion that the provision of contraceptive abortion advice and treatment to patients under the age of 16 is a matter which 'rests with the doctor concerned, in light of the individual patient's needs and circumstances' (Norrie 1985a, b).

C. TRACING OF CONTACTS AND THE CASE AGAINST COMPULSION; LESSONS FROM HISTORY

Although males may have an asymptomatic gonococcal infection, the majority (85–90%) tend to develop an obvious urethral discharge which makes them seek medical help. In contrast, in females the infection is frequently inapparent or asymptomatic (75–85%) so it is essential to ensure that the female consort is investigated and treated. The process of securing the attendance of a sexual contact is known as contact-tracing and to be successful depends upon the trust of the patient and contact(s) in the confidentiality of the process.

The necessary interviewing of the index patient is a matter of great delicacy; it is time-consuming and it must be carried out in privacy. It depends essentially upon the regard and respect of the interviewer for the patient. There is no place for hostility and everything must be done to encourage rapport. Gently, the patient must be persuaded that he or she is the only person who can ensure that the one or more consorts are treated. It is explained how effective treatment is and how helpful it would be for all concerned if the sexual partner could attend. Irrespective of the length of the list of recent consorts, irrespective of the varied character of those involved and irrespective of the form of sexual behaviour, the patient must not be allowed to feel stigmatized or allowed to feel unworthy. If the patient's memory is faulty and the relationship has been casual, details are often hazy. At the best a note giving the index case number, date, diagnosis in code (Note 5.3) and clinic address, can be delivered by the patient to a consort to bring as an introduction to the clinic. If the patient fears to make the approach, the person responsible for contact-tracing, say a health visitor, involved also in the clinic with counselling and all aspects of health education, will take the necessary steps. Sometimes, but not often, the description of a tattoo, a scar or a dress may help in the tracing. Information about haunts, about friends, or about work may also be of value. The patient must be assured of the tact and experience of the staff involved and of their skills in avoiding embarrassing situations. A good guide to the essentials of contact tracing containing useful reference material was published jointly by the Health Education Council and The Department of Health and Social Security (Hunter et al 1980). Reference has been made in Section (a) of this chapter to the two Ministerial Regulations (Notes 5.1 and 5.2) which demand confidentiality in the contact tracing process.

In Edinburgh it has been found generally that about half of the female contacts acknowledged by male patients with gonorrhoea as possible sources of infection (source contacts), are unknown and therefore untraceable. The other half of source contacts are mostly traced and treated without great difficulty unless belonging to a floating population or changing their address frequently. The secondary contacts with whom the index patient may have a long-term relationship and who may have been infected are traced and treated in nearly every case. In spite of the nature of the careful approach needed in contact-tracing and the few, known insufficiently to be described, who are missed, some still feel that legal compulsion is necessary. In the authors' opinion such compulsory measures are inappropriate and the power to use them inevitably changes attitudes of those working in clinics and discourages attendance in those whose need is greatest; persuasion and voluntary compliance are keywords to the procedures.

History is revealing. In the British Army of the middle of the nineteenth century, more than 90% of the soldiers were unmarried as they were not permitted to marry until they had seven years service and had one good conduct badge. Many in the lower socio-economic groups married early, but breakdown due to poverty was common. Women were particularly vulnerable as it was generally impossible for them to find employment and, if a servant, for example were sacked without a 'character' because she became pregnant, prostitution was often the only alternative to destitution or the harsh environment of the workhouse. There was, too, an excess of women over men because of the higher death rate of male children.

In 1860 about 25% of soldiers in London suffered from syphilis, and the Contagious Diseases Acts (1864, 1866 and 1869) were introduced with the object of checking the spread of venereal disease in the Armed Forces. These Acts applied to garrison towns and provided for the examination of prostitutes and their detention in hospital if diseased. The regulations were oppressive and extraordinarily bureaucratic in form; every move in the appalling process required a certificate, duly listed in the Acts which were administered by officers drawn from the Metropolitan Police.

Josephine Butler opposed and vigorously campaigned against these Acts, forming a Ladies National Association for the repeal of the Contagious Diseases Acts. Her case was based on the fact that certain women, usually poor, were robbed of their civil rights and this violated the constitution. Among other objections she showed how these Acts were designed for the benefit of soldiers or sailors but applied only to civilian women who could be unjustifiably persecuted by officials administering the Acts. The opening shots in the campaign against the Contagious Diseases Acts include a protest in the Daily News, 31st December 1869, signed by Harriet Martineau, Florence Nightingale, Josephine Butler, and more than one hundred other women. Although the statement provoked much abuse it effectively launched the vigorous debate which led, 17 years later, to the repeal of the Acts (Blom-Cooper & Drewry 1976). Although medical opinion of the day supported the legislation it provided no evidence that the diseases were checked in any way. The main attack was directed also against the double standard of morality in a male dominated society which condoned the sexual activities of the male and persecuted the female, applied legislation against the prostitute but ignored her client. The evils of prostitution, including recruitment of girls to the trade, were under attack at a time when a virgin could be bought for a few shillings and the age of consent to sexual intercourse (up till 1885) was only 12 years (Bell 1962, Rover 1967, Petrie 1971). The Acts were finally repealed in 1886.

Further attempts to introduce coercive Acts have been made in the United Kingdom. In 1917 a Criminal Law Amendment Bill was introduced in the House of Commons by which it was proposed to make it penal for a person suffering from venereal disease in a communicable form to have sexual intercourse with any other person. The maximum penalty provided was two years imprisonment with hard labour. Power was to be given to the court to order a medical examination of the person charged. As the existence of the infection could only be provable by medical evidence it was a matter

of close concern to doctors. By November the opposition to the Bill in the House of Commons, which preferred a policy of persuasion to a policy of penalty, led to its being abandoned.

As the Criminal Law Amendment Bill failed to reach the statute book because of opposition inside and outside Parliament and as there was a demand from Dominion Armed Forces' representatives, the Army Council in May 1918 passed Regulation 40D (Defence of the Realm Act 1917) imposing punishment for the offence of communicating venereal disease to soldiers, although the Regulation did not proceed as far as to make it compulsory for women arrested for this offence to subject themselves to a medical examination. The basis of the Regulation was similar to that of the Contagious Diseases Acts of 1864, 1866 and 1869, in that it was directed against civilian women with the intention of protecting soldiers (Venereal Disease and the Defence of the Realm Act 1917).

The Regulation was not effective as a public health measure and women against whom no charge had been established were arrested, imprisoned and remanded for examination (201 prosecutions, 101 convictions). By the end of 1918 Regulation 40D was suspended as valueless and other more helpful measures were being suggested by the Royal Commission on Venereal Diseases, 1913–1916 (Cd 8189 & 8190 1916), at a time when an estimated 300 000 men, still infectious, of the Navy and Army were actually under treatment and might be due to return to their homes. As a result of these enlightened recommendations the Local Government Board developed an organization with clinics providing for the free diagnosis and treatment of persons suffering from venereal disease (Leading Article (Lancet) 1917).

Compulsory powers were sought unsuccessfully by the Edinburgh Corporation Bill 1928 (Statement for the Corporation 1928). The proposers believed that it was those who discontinued treatment while still infective who were the chief cause for the failure of medical control of these diseases.

Regulation 33B (Defence Regulations 1939) was brought in during the fourth year of World War II. It extended its compulsion, as a war-time measure only, to a group of persons, small in number, who refused to attend voluntarily. In this Regulation specialists were required to pass on to the Medical Officer of Health the name of the contact thought by a patient to be responsible for passing on the venereal infection. The Medical Officer of Health would serve a notice on the contact if he received two or more notifications relating to him (or her) requiring him (or her) to attend a specialist and submit to an examination. If infected he (or she) would be required to have treatment.

Inevitably the Regulation restarted the controversy which raged at the time of the Contagious Diseases Acts and its inefficiency was shown by a reply given by the Minister of Health in Parliament (see Note 5.4) (Results of Regulation 33B 1943, Shannon 1943).

In 1962 and again in 1967 attempts were made to restore the provisions of Regulation 33B in Bills introduced by Mr Richard Marsh and Sir Myer Galpern respectively.

Proposals of this kind are no doubt well meaning but legislation of this kind is an ineffective, discredited public health measure. It is the policy of persuasion backed up by a humane approach, careful techniques in clinics and good antibiotic and chemotherapy with contact-tracing that is the mainstay of control. In the case of persistent virus infections, such as that of the human immunodeficiency viruses, when neither curative treatment nor vaccination are available, the problem of control is more complex but the present authors believe that legal compulsion is not likely to be successful as a means of applying any control measures. In Japan AIDS is to become a notifiable disease but it is claimed that the new law will protect the privacy of AIDS sufferers as long as they follow the doctor's advice (Swinbanks 1987).

In practice, a very small proportion of contacts, less than 1% who are found, refuse or fail to attend and about half of female contacts of men attending with gonorrhoea cannot be traced due to a genuine lack of information. In the case of homosexually acquired infection the propotion of contacts seen is often very low (about 14% in a recent study), probably because, in some individuals at least, the hostility of society makes the individual fearful to surface for help.

Although international action is envisaged by Resolution (74)5, adopted by the Committee of Ministers at Strasbourg in 1974, the greater the distance involved and the larger the number of administrative, political or geographical barriers the less effective is contact-tracing. The concept of international contact-tracing would, to be effective, depend upon confidence that a humane system free from threats would be used to secure the necessary high standard of medical investigation and treatment. In the case of early syphilis and gonorrhoea, efforts to achieve these aims on an international basis are laudable (Willcox 1973), but when a patient knows a contact sufficiently to give an adequate description more can often be achieved at a personal level by letter.

D. CHILD ABUSE AND SEXUALLY TRANSMITTED DISEASE

In industrialized countries in the last two decades there has been a huge increase in the number of documented cases of child abuse, much of it occurring within the home, and an increasing proportion of this abuse is sexual. In developing countries too there are specific patterns of sexual abuse to children and worldwide there is much concern about the many facets of the problem (Lancet (Leading Article) 1987). Recognizing that boys are more likely to be physically injured or fail to thrive and that girls are more likely to be sexually abused (Lancet (Notes and News) 1986, Creighton 1987) it is necessary for doctors to take steps, beyond those required for making a diagnosis of sexually transmitted disease, administering specific antibiotic or chemotherapy and ensuring follow-up with tests of cure: sexual abuse may include anal penetration with or without resultant injury (Hobbs & Wynne 1986) and in prepubertal girls *Neisseria gonorrhoeae*, for example, may be shown to be the cause of vulvovaginitis. When sexual abuse is considered to be possible the following approach, based on Clayden (1987) is recommended.

1. A history should be obtained and if this includes that of emotional disturbance or if the child hints or states that sexual abuse has happened this should be regarded as a warning symptom.

2. The detection or exclusion of sexually transmissible disease is important. An organismal diagnosis must be substantiated in the laboratory (see Ch. 15) and if an isolation of *N. gonorrhoeae* is made this should whenever possible include serogroup and serovar analysis, since these findings may have important medico-legal significance (see p. 195). Insofar as other sexually transmitted infections are concerned, restriction endonuclease patterns of the DNA of herpes simplex virus make fingerprinting of the HSV isolate possible (see p. 331–332): in papillomavirus infections similarly, typing by DNA/DNA hybridization may also be useful from the medico-legal point of view (see Ch. 27).

3. It is a warning sign if the child lies passively on the examining couch and does not resist anal inspection by tightening the levator ani or external sphincter muscles.

4. Signs of anal relaxation in the absence of abdominal distension are suspicious, especially if anal relaxation diminishes when a child is away from the abusing suspect.

5. Excoriation or bruising around the anus or inner aspects of the buttocks or thigh suggests assault.

The absence of anal signs cannot exclude sexual abuse (Clayden 1987) and gaping of the anal canal is seen in children with significant constipation. Referral of the child for early expert paediatric assessment is mandatory in those where sexual abuse is either suspected or proved (Hey et al 1987) and in response to the whole problem of non-accidental injury to children guidelines for action have been put together for use of practitioners in the various disciplines concerned. These guidelines have been developed in various geographical localities

(Lothian Regional Review Committee 1983) in response to the problem and include a number of important points. In the case of hospitals medical staff should take immediate action *to safeguard the child*. Firstly the family doctor should be informed and the hospital social worker notified who will in turn in this locality inform the social work area officer. The latter will call a case conference when the circumstances indicate that this is necessary. Consideration should also be given to reporting the circumstances to the police who will report all cases of non-accidental injury (NAI) giving rise to concern to the Procurator Fiscal.

When the clinical investigations are completed they should be signed by the examining doctor giving the date and time of examination and witnessed by a qualified nurse or doctor.

In the case of children who have been abused or are at risk of being abused 'NAI at risk' registers have been set up. These are maintained centrally by the social work departments and access for the purposes of consultation and registration is limited to those professions which require information as a necessary part of their responsibility to prevent or treat child abuse (Lothian Regional Review Committee 1983).

Allegations of sexual abuse in children are easy to make but difficult to prove. There is difficulty too in obtaining disclosure from a child who may have been long silenced by guilt or fear. The child abuse clinic at Great Ormond Street Hospital for Sick Children, led by the psychiatrist Bentovim, has pioneered an interview technique to overcome this problem using anatomically correct dolls to help to tease out details from a child who may lack the words to describe her experiences. The growing use of the technique, not just for treating victims but for diagnosing whether abuse has happened, has sparked off controversy. There is conflict, clearly, between the needs of clinical and therapeutic methods and the 'evidential' requirements of the courts in legal proceedings. The use of video-recording and full transcripts in the case of the diagnostic interviews and expert evidence, together with limitation in the use of leading questions at the interviews are modifications which are being added to what is seen as a constructive attempt to enable the courts to grapple with the problem of handling an allegation of sexual abuse (Douglas & Willmore 1987, Dyer 1987). It has been considered, too, that protection of the child from further abuse and his or her future care are more in the interests of justice than the prosecution of the abuser.

In the case of children considered to be 'in need of compulsory measures of care' there has been in Scotland a break with the traditional law court setting since 1971 when a system based on 'Children's Hearings' was set up by the Social Work (Scotland) Act 1968. Under this Act the post of Reporter to the Children's Panel was

established with the basic task to decide whether or not cases notified should be brought before a Children's Hearing. If the reporter initiates proceedings he has to satisfy a lower standard of proof which is 'the balance of probabilities' rather than the high standard of proof, viz. 'that of beyond reasonable doubt', required by the Procurator Fiscal when a person is accused in criminal proceedings (Lothian Regional Review Committee 1983). Child–adult sexual contact is a complex subject deserving attention. Additional informed and fully referenced discussion is available in the report of a working party of the Howard League for Penal Reform (1985).

E. PERSISTENT VIRUS INFECTIONS (INCLUDING THAT DUE TO HUMAN IMMUNODEFICIENCY VIRUSES) AND CONTROL OF THEIR SPREAD

When there are no effective vaccines or anti-viral agents the means of controlling the spread of sexually transmissible persistent virus infections are limited, problematical and uncertain. In both the infected and in those at risk prevention consists of health education and counselling and is aimed at producing behavioural change. In relation to hepatitis B, for example, in those at high risk, but as yet uninfected, as in the case of promiscuous homosexual men, vaccination is an effective preventive. In the chronic carrier state, however, lifelong restrictions on the individual in regard to his sexual life and number or nature of contacts are difficult to secure. In herpes simplex virus infection the sporadic shedding of virus at the periphery, both in those with recurrences and in those who remain asymptomatic, enables further spread of the virus but the consequences do not have the gravity seen in the case of the human immunodeficiency viruses (HIV), where both in those infected and in those at risk there are very serious problems to be faced.

The AIDS related retrovirus (HIV) has been recovered from semen, blood and saliva (Curran et al 1985); tears (Fujikawa et al 1985); breast milk (Thiry et al 1985); cervical and vaginal secretions (Vogt et al 1986, Wofsy et al 1986) but only with semen, blood and blood products has transmission been clearly associated apart from, in one case report, a presumptive infection of an infant as a result of breast feeding (Ziegler et al 1985). In the latter a mother had been transfused after delivery with blood from a male donor infected with HIV and subsequently the baby was found to have been infected. In the case of virus from saliva and tears successful attempts at isolation are infrequent and the virus is probably at a very much lower titre than in the blood. In 83 saliva samples obtained from 71 homosexual men seropositive for HIV, isolation of the retrovirus was successful in only one (1%) compared with 28 of the 50 blood cultures (56%) which yielded the virus (Ho et al 1985). The isolation of HIV from the tears of one of seven patients with AIDS (Fujikawa et al 1985) has raised the issue of the possible transmission of the virus during contact lens fitting sessions. It is recommended (Centers for Disease Control 1985a) that operators should wash their hands immediately after performing eye examinations and disinfect the lenses with hydrogen peroxide. Epidemiological data suggest that those who are household contacts but not sexual partners of, or born to, patients infected with HIV are not at risk of the infection (Friedland 1986).

A public health policy can be derived logically from this knowledge and of known mechanisms of spread (Acheson 1986) but attempts at its promotion, however, can be confounded by human tendencies and by difficulties such as those 'in conveying sexually explicit information without offence' as well as in evaluating the response, both in the individual and in the public at large. Outside tropical Africa relative risks are much higher in homosexual males, particularly those who practise receptive anal intercourse and who have many partners, than in the heterosexual male practising vaginal intercourse. In sub-Saharan Africa, however, transmission appears to be linked to heterosexual promiscuity and prostitution in females (Clumeck et al 1985). The general message is nevertheless clear: it is to avoid 'risky' sexual behaviour viz. casual sex, multiple partnerships and anal intercourse. In the positive sense forms of 'safe sex' will require to be explained and the proper use of condoms promoted (Note 5.5) in those unable to limit their practice of penetrative sexual intercourse. Condoms may have a substantial failure rate as a contraceptive, presumably because of tears, slippage or because they have not been used properly. In penetrative anal intercourse the failure rate is likely to be as high or higher and in sexually active groups at special risk of HIV infection penetrative anal intercourse should be discouraged (Kelly & St Lawrence 1987). It is important for individuals to have insight into the risks of their own behaviour and to be encouraged to seek medical advice early. Among homosexuals concurrent or recent sexually transmitted diseases (viz. early syphilis, gonorrhoea, non-gonococcal urethritis and primary HSV infection) are apparently an important factor in developing antibody to HIV and in progression of infection to persistent generalized lymphadenopathy (see Ch. 31) (Weber et al 1986). It is self-evident that such consultations with regard to HIV infection must include the investigations and follow-up necessary for the exclusion or detection of other sexually transmissible diseases and when appropriate the tracing of sexual contacts. If adopted, the guidelines for

homosexual males, promoting a behavioural change, produced by the American Physicians for Human Rights (Note 5.6) should limit the spread of HIV.

An addict, say on a heroin maintenance regimen, with a regular supply of pure drug who uses sterile injection technique and who takes good care of food and health may live out a normal lifespan (Stimson & Oppenheimer 1982) but contamination by sharing syringes with or without the added effects of impure and illicitly manufactured heroin produces a scenario of disaster. In relation to the transmission of the HIV the prevalence of antibody among intravenous drug abusers attending a general practice in a deprived area of Edinburgh has been given as 51%, well above that reported elsewhere in Britain and Europe and approaching that observed in New York City; in the Edinburgh group of intravenous heroin abusers needle and syringe sharing practices and numbers of injections with contaminated needles are extreme aspects of behaviour and responsible for the epidemic of HIV seropositivity (Robertson et al 1986). In Amsterdam three measures have been taken to prevent the spread of HIV among drug addicts — 1. a publicity campaign; 2. an exchange system for syringes and needles; and 3. the distribution of condoms among addicted prostitutes. In the exchange system addicts receive a sterile syringe and needle free of charge when they return a used syringe and needle; in 1985 some 100 000 syringes and needles were provided (Buning et al 1986).

Experiments in injection of drugs by adolescents, as well as its continued practice, are clearly highly dangerous.

Body fluid (blood, milk, semen) donation and testing for antibody to HIV

Voluntary donation of blood without monetary reward is highly regarded worldwide from a social point of view. The proposition has often been made that individuals will offer themselves as donors in order to secure a 'blood test' without having to admit openly to their sexual orientation or to anxiety about a sexual risk. The exclusion of syphilis and hepatitis B has long been routine and now, in the belief that the antibody test will exclude most with infection by AIDS related virus, this test too has been introduced by many blood transfusion services. In the attempt to ensure that donations do not contain anything harmful to the patient receiving them, e.g. medicines or viruses, an extensive health check for new donors has been developed. In the Scottish National Blood Transfusion Service prospective donors are shown rules which will, it is hoped, eliminate as donors those even at remote risk of acquiring HIV infection. It is explained that although HIV testing (meaning antibody testing) has been introduced the individual must not volunteer to give a blood donation if he or she belongs to any of the listed categories, recently revised and shown in Chapter 4 (see p. 65).

When an individual comes to the donor session the prospective donor is asked to sign a health check form which includes a statement that the important new message has been read and understood ('Mass Publicity and AIDS', see also Ch. 4). Those who do not wish to have their blood tested for HIV antibody are asked not to donate blood at any session.

The technique of 'self-exclusion' may not be, however, wholly effective and screening tests on serum are essential additional safeguards. Much human social activity may be explained on the hypothesis that individuals will undertake activities to secure the respect of others. This 'search for honour' as well as the tendency of most individuals to prefer short-term expressive advantage to long-term practical gains (Harré 1979) may be a psychological explanation in those known to have presented themselves as blood donors but who, nevertheless, may have briefly experimented with drugs taken intravenously in the past or have had homosexual experiences. In spite of this they nevertheless see themselves, and wish to be seen, as honourable people acting honourably.

The prevalence of antibody to HIV from apparently healthy male and female donors in England and Wales who have been asked not to donate if they belonged to high risk groups is very low (16 confirmed positive tests among 845 497 donations; 0.02 per 100 000); of the 16 positives all were found to have been at risk either as homosexual males or as drug abusers (Acheson 1986). The Blood Transfusion Service secures the agreement of prospective donors to testing of their blood for antibody to HIV with a prime purpose of rendering blood transfusion as safe as possible; the response of the individual who is told of a positive result is a secondary consideration, although donors have a right to expect help and protection so that their generous gift does not lead to a personal disaster (Osterholm et al 1985). The ethical issues surrounding the introduction of the test are profound and the question whether the donor should or should not be informed of the result has been debated at length. The continued guidance and counselling of increasing number of antibody-positives in the long term has to be provided for (Jeffries 1986) as well as for the family.

Testing for HIV antibody in patients or others at high risk

'To test or not to test?' that is the question. In those with or without symptoms but revealed as HIV antibody positive the knowledge has far-reaching and deeply felt psychological aspects as well being possibly financially detrimental (e.g. life assurance). It involves

breaking the news, and the resultant shock to the individual. Access to medical help will require to be constantly available. Specific information has to be given. A consistent and humane approach in counselling can achieve much (Miller & Green 1985) but the consequences of infection are grave.

A view has been expressed that serotesting should be encouraged in genitourinary medicine clinics for men who may be bisexual, for women who are partners of men at risk, and for drug abusers (Acheson 1986). In the case of the bisexual he may infect his female partner who then can transfer the HIV infection to a subsequently conceived child. Knowledge of seropositivity can give the individual an opportunity to make an 'informed choice' and measures can be taken to limit spread of infection. The question whether knowledge of HIV antibody positivity induces a change of sexual behaviour of the individual in the long term is not likely to be easily answered. At-risk patients may drift away from clinics where testing is known to have become virtually mandatory or if the patient is not given every opportunity to consider in the light of his own situation the advisability or otherwise of the test. Essentially in at-risk groups the advice to both infected and uninfected is the same.

In 1983 the Centers for Disease Control, US Department of Health and Human Services, recommended that members of high risk groups reduce the numbers of their sexual partners to avoid acquiring or transmitting HIV (Centers for Disease Control 1983). Surveys subsequently showed substantial reduction both in the average number of reported sexual partners and in the number of sexually transmitted infections in homosexual men. For example, rates for rectal and pharyngeal gonorrhoea for New York City males in the 15–44 year age group declined from 129 per 10^5 males in 1980 to 74 per 10^5 males in 1983 (Centers for Disease Control 1984). Again in Denver, Colorado, marked reduction in numbers of cases of gonorrhoea was recorded for homosexual men but not for heterosexual men and women (Judson 1983). In regard to the number of sexual partners within the past 30 days reported by homosexual men, means diminished from 6.8 in 1982 to 3.2 in 1983. In addition there was a doubling of the proportion of men reporting only a single partner (Golubjatnikov et al 1983). In Vancouver, Canada, in a cohort study between 1982 and 1984, the proportion of men reporting no more than five partners per year rose from 21 to 37%. Specific sexual practices (anal intercourse, oro-anal contact and fisting) also were more likely to have decreased than increased except for orogenital contact during the study period (Schechter et al 1984).

The risk of transmission of HIV infection and of AIDS to infants born to infected mothers is substantial but not yet quantified. Women who have clinical, epidemiological or serological evidence of this infection should postpone or avoid pregnancy. Infants when infected require humane and considered policies during their development.

Other aspects of prevention

Precautions directed towards the prevention of spread of blood-borne infections to individuals exposed to the risk have been detailed, particularly with respect to the hepatitis B model of transmission. The infectivity of the human immunodeficiency viruses, however, is less than that of hepatitis B, the titre of circulating virus substantially lower and perhaps only one in 10^4 infected T4 lymphocytes produces complete virus (Zuckerman 1986) but nevertheless the application of the recommendations in prevention of spread of hepatitis B will also prevent the transmission of the HIV. For detailed guidelines in specific situations consultation of published recommendations is necessary. There is much public concern about the problem and anxieties require to be relieved. Deep and problematical issues nevertheless remain and are not soluble in absolute terms.

In those responsible for providing personal services viz. hairdressers, barbers, manicurists, massage therapists, and where non-sterile instruments might be used. viz. tattooing, ritual scarification, ear piercing, circumcision, risks will vary from trivial to high and instrument sterilization, care of puncture wounds, and avoidance of contamination by exudates or other body fluids will require consideration. For health care workers precautions necessary in relation to blood-borne infectious disease should be standard practice and regularly enforced whether or not the patient or the health care worker is or is not known to be infected. In the care, education and fostering of children there are issues of confidentiality, ethics and civil rights to consider although transmission by casual person to person contact, as would occur among school children, appears to pose no risk although epidemiological information of the kind desirable is very limited. Children infected with HIV should be educated and cared for in settings which minimize exposure of other children to blood or body fluids (Centers for Disease Control 1985 a, b, c, d).

With respect to dentistry both patient and health care workers have the potential of transmitting infections to each other. Protective attire and barrier techniques are necessary and everything should be done to minimize the formation of droplets and aerosols when dealing with potentially infective materials. Routine sterilization of instruments is highly desirable (Centers for Disease Control 1986). The British Dental Association is conducting a campaign to promote hepatitis B vacci-

nation among dental clinic staff. Among recommendations to prevent cross infection are included personal protection by the use of gloves and by vaccination. Autoclaving of instruments is recommended, and the taking of careful medical histories to identify high risk patients is another precaution given in a recent report (British Dental Association Dental Health and Science Committee Workshop 1986, Notes and News (Lancet) 1986).

F. TESTING FOR ANTIBODY TO HUMAN IMMUNODEFICIENCY VIRUSES (HIV) (LIMITATIONS, INDICATIONS AND RESTRAINTS)

A confirmed positive result in the HIV antibody test is a marker of a previous infection of the retrovirus. The antibody response and seroconversion usually develops 2–3 months after exposure to the virus. The test does not measure infectiousness although the potential for this must be assumed. False-negative and false-positive results occur and necessitate further tests for confirmation. In B-cell lymphomas the test may establish the diagnosis of AIDS.

Counselling beforehand and informed consent are essential before testing. There are number of contexts in which the use of the test is considered medically valuable (Miller & Green 1985, Miller et al 1986):

1. In the case of donations of tissue or body fluid for the *benefit of the recipient* testing the donor's blood is important to ensure that HIV negative materials are used, e.g. in proposed donations of blood for transfusion or the manufacture of blood products such as factor VIII; organs for transplant (kidneys, livers, hearts, lungs, cornea, bone marrow); semen (see Stewart et al 1985); milk; or post-menopausal urine for the manufacture of follicle stimulating hormone. In the case of Factor VIII concentrates heating may inactivate HIV but further experience of this and other methods are required before conclusions can be drawn (Leading Article (Lancet) 1984).

2. In the case of *patients* the result of the test has a *medical benefit* in determining treatment in specific instances such as in recipients of haemodialysis where the therapeutic use of immunosuppressive drugs may bring risk of clinical deterioration in HIV positive patients.

3. In the case of 'high-risk' women (intravenous drug abusers, partners of IVDA, partners of bisexual men or men known to be positive for HIV antibody) in reproductive age groups, contemplating pregnancy or in early pregnancy, antibody testing is indicated because preg-

nancy is a definite co-factor in expression of maternal disease and there is a high risk of HIV infection in infants of seropositive women. Those born in sub-Saharan Africa should be considered at risk since heterosexual transmission plays a major role in many localities.

As antibodies to HIV may not be detectable in the serum for months after exposure, repeat testing may be indicated in pregnant women in high risk groups in whom the initial antibody test is negative. In seropositive women, pregnancy should be delayed until the risks of perinatal transmission of the virus are more clearly defined. Advice on contraception must be given to the woman and her partner. The questions of termination of pregnancy and sterilization require consideration. Infected women should avoid breast feeding (Centers for Disease Control 1985).

4. In the case of patients with or suspected as having AIDS the test is indicated. To confirm infection with HIV or to reassure in connection with non-infection the HIV antibody tests are available; antigen tests are to be more widely accessible soon.

5. In the case of individuals at high risk some advocate the use of this test as a stimulus to changing sexual behaviour. Advice about 'safe sex techniques' should, however, be given irrespective of whether individuals are seropositive or seronegative (Note 5.6). Considerable psychological and emotional morbidity may occur in a patient on learning that he or she is seropositive to HIV, particularly when the test has been conducted without consent or pre-counselling. Psychological shock, uncertainty over prognosis and the reaction of others may lead to severe anxiety, depression, obsessive disorder and sometimes suicidal acts. Broken relationships, unemployment and social dysfunction add to these burdens. Specific difficulties have been encountered — difficulties in obtaining dental or medical treatment, dismissal or premature retirement, financial and accommodation problems — in Saudi Arabia, for example, compulsory screening for immigration and employment has been introduced.

6. Anxious patients frequently refer to their wish for testing and counselling and a negative result may relieve the anxiety. Time must be allowed for a patient to make a decision whether or not to have a test.

In syphilis routine screening is justifiable as effective antibiotic remedy is to hand. In HIV infection no vaccine is available and positive results of the test have profound consequences on the individual in a situation when supporting services are limited and individual response to information of this kind may have serious consequences. Essentially counselling and education on 'safe sex' and positive behavioural change are necessary to limit spread of the retrovirus infection.

G. HOMOSEXUALITY IN MALES

Homosexuality is often a 'stigma label' (Plummer 1975). To be called homosexual is to be degraded, denounced, devalued or treated as different. It may well mean shame, ostracism, discrimination, exclusion or physical attack. It is the knowledge of the cost of being publicly recognized as homosexual that leads many to conceal their sexual identity.

In western society hostility towards the homosexual male by the heterosexual majority has ancient origins; in the first century AD the sin of Sodom (Genesis; XIX, 5) became closely identified with homosexual behaviour (Bailley 1955). Later in the sixth century Justinian admonished homosexuals and a thousand years later, in the England of Henry VIII, buggery was deemed a felony punishable by death. After repeals and re-enactments Queen Elizabeth fixed death as the penalty which remained on the statute book until 1861, when it was replaced by a term of imprisonment of seven years liable to be extended to penal servitude for life. Later in more modern times, the well-known Labouchere amendment (named after a Member of Parliament), to the Criminal Law Amendment Act 1885, brought homosexual acts in private expressly within the scope of the criminal law. A less repressive approach developed with time and in 1944 in Sweden, for example, homosexual acts between consenting adults in private ceased to be criminal offences. A reasoned view that this should be so also in England and Wales was set out in the Report of the Committee on Homosexual Offences and Prostitution, chaired by Sir John Wolfenden and known by his name (1957). An important issue in jurisprudence was raised in this Report, namely that 'unless society made a deliberate attempt to equate the sphere of crime with that of sin, there must remain a realm of private morality which is, in brief and crude terms, not the law's business'. In the high level debate that followed, Lord Devlin (1959), a Judge of the Queen's Bench, believed, on the one hand, that the law should indeed enforce morality, whereas Professor Hart (1963) maintained that deviations from sexual morality such as homosexuality did not harm others and were therefore not a matter for the law. The liberal argument was based on the theme set out by John Stuart Mill in his famous essay 'On Liberty', published in 1859, in which he gave reasoned defence of individualism as an element of permanent importance to society and opposed coercion to enforce moral values. The Wolfenden Committee recommended 'that homosexual behaviour between consenting adults in private be no longer a criminal offence'. Ten years later the Sexual Offences Act 1967 came into force and laid down that a homosexual act in private shall not be an offence 'provided

behaviour and concluded that it was simply a natural variation of sexual expression (Bell & Weinberg 1978).

That a homosexual — man or woman — is neither a sinner nor a sick person is the thesis of Bancroft's paper (1975). 'Homosexuality is not an illness but an alternative life style which may be and often is compatible with normal health and with those interpersonal and social values that we hold most high'. There is, as Bancroft writes, a duty for the right-minded, and for the medical practitioner in particular, to encourage a climate of opinion, more positive and less repressive than that which has unjustly given rise to the social stigma associated with homosexuality, the repression that stems from it and the suffering that often results.

From the individual patient's point of view his sexual identity is crucially important to his adjustment and that whether he sees himself as homosexual or heterosexual is more important than, say, his place in the Kinsey scale. Bancroft (1981) goes on to identify three ways in which an individual with homosexual problems may need help from doctors: 1. facilitating the individual's adaptation to a homosexual role; 2. assisting those who have either a homosexual or uncertain sexual preferences to explore and establish heterosexual relationships; and 3. helping the individual to gain control over certain aspects of behaviour which may bring him into conflict with the law. Although the help given is not necessarily medical, the medical profession is one of the important sources of such help. To these undoubtedly important issues there is also added the important matter of prevention and treatment of sexually transmitted disease.

Bell & Weinberg (1978) admit that although they have taken a step forward in delineation of types of homosexuals their study failed to capture the full diversity that must be understood if society is ever fully to respect and appreciate the way in which individual homosexual men and women live their lives. In the lives of all, as in the most distinguished, there is much to reflect upon (Hodges 1983).

H. PROSTITUTION IN FEMALES

Sexually transmitted disease is an indisputable occupational hazard in prostitution. Figures for infection rates have been collected, as for example, about 20% in Atlanta, Georgia, USA (Conrad et al 1981) and 9% in Singapore (Khoo et al 1977) but clearly these will vary geographically according to prevailing circumstances. Infection rates in particular will tend to be greater in prostitutes in areas, particularly of the third world, where access to medical care and specific therapy is poor. The number with sexually transmitted disease will be a function of the frequency with which they are tested, the sensitivity and specificity of the diagnostic tests used and the effectiveness of the therapy given, as well as the number of unprotected exposures they have, the prevalence of disease in their partners and the rates of transmission from hosts to susceptibles (Willcox 1976).

Prostitution in women is defined most precisely by Paul Gebhard (1982) who emphasizes its two essential elements: 1. the exchange of money or valuable materials in return for sexual activity with physical contact; and 2. the relatively indiscriminate availability of such a transaction to individuals other than spouses or friends. Sexual activity with strangers or with persons for whom there is no affectionate feeling does not itself constitute prostitution if the economic element is absent. The definition represents one end of a continuum ranging from the socially-accepted arrangement of marriage, where one male is morally and legally entitled to sexual gratification in exchange for support, to the other extreme where the arrangement is of a very brief duration and involves numerous males.

The complexity of modern life, with accelerated cross-cultural diffusion made possible by rapid transportation, makes a brief description of prostitution in any given nation quite impossible. With reference to the nature of the sexual interaction itself, Gebhard (1982) comments that in female prostitution the prostitute rarely or never reaches orgasm whereas the client almost invariably does; in contrast, in male homosexual prostitution the prostitute almost invariably reaches orgasm but the client frequently does not.

Cunnington (1980) was able in 1979 to study in London the circumstances of 30 women convicted of soliciting at Bow Street Magistrates' Court close to the West End and the street walkers' beats off Soho and Mayfair. In contrast to those in escort agencies and the like, street walkers could make contact with and choose clients quickly and, as accommodation was normally provided by the client, overheads were low. Half of the women had procurers, euphemistically called boyfriends, mostly from an ethnic sub-culture other than their own, who had a role partly personal and partly as business managers and would generally 'manage' several women. For the prostitute, her work is described as hard, negotiating with a dozen or so men daily, getting them into a hotel room, avoiding sadists, having sex and avoiding the police. A secondary category of the women interviewed (Cunnington 1980) did not think of themselves as prostitutes and had other jobs as barmaids, waitresses or shop assistants. This second category were part-time and included those who engaged in isolated acts of prostitution.

On conviction leading to imprisonment the prostitute would often be abandoned by the procurer and precipitated into seeking female companionship with the more experienced and later into habitual prostitution. Cunnington's views (1980) were that penalties were ineffective, probation effective only when the order was in force and a prison sentence inappropriate, tending itself to produce serious effects on the family and an embittered victim.

Elsewhere in the series of reports, Trott (1980) refers to the fact that prostitution is grossly under-researched. Studies involving the rich and transient population of large hotels, gaming clubs with satellite illegal or semi-legal entertainments bring risks also to a researcher. Reference is also made to the fact that the Street Offences Act 1959 (Note 5.10) clears prostitutes off the streets but drives prostitution underground into the clutches of criminal elements. In another context, the cohabitation ruling in the UK, denying state support in the case of a single woman, may drive her into prostitution (Vickers 1980). Little is known of the lives of former prostitutes because those who have adequately coped with the transition back into society are anxious to conceal their past; one tends to see the failures rather than the successes (Gebhard 1982).

There exists a socio-economic demand for prostitution among travellers and military personnel, for example, who may have temporary difficulty in obtaining relationships. There are those, too, who do not wish to become emotionally involved or who may wish to enjoy techniques that their customary partners refuse them — oral–genital contact being a prime example. It appears impossible to suppress prostitution in a complex society particularly one in which sexual gratification is made difficult by mores and law. In large urban centres anonymity is easily achieved and many are temporary visitors. In a small community, however, where secrecy is difficult and where life depends upon mutual co-operation, social sanctions, say in the form of ridicule and ostracism, are extremely effective in controlling prostitution (Gebhard 1982).

Toleration with some degree of stigma is a common posture in many societies. In such, prostitution is often the resort of disadvantaged females for whom it may be a solution to the economic problem of survival without husbands.

In the context of modern times sex tourism has become targeted on a number of eastern countries such as Thailand, the Philippines and South Korea. In Bangkok for example, some 100 000 are engaged in prostitution, and sexually transmitted diseases are a massive problem. Women arriving from impoverished rural areas are often forced into the prostitution business and Japanese and European men appear to be among the large number of tourists who exploit the situation (Change International Reports 1980).

I. SELF-HELP GROUPS

Among the options in health care available for example, in Britain, to individuals, Kelnan (1984) identified three main sectors, viz. popular, folk and professional. Choices are, however, restricted by law (Venereal Diseases Act 1917 — see Note 5.11), insofar as the legally defined *venereal diseases* are concerned, to the professional sector. In the case of the wider range of diseases, covered by the term sexually transmissible disease, there may be no legal prohibitions but open discouragement against self-diagnosis and self-medication is one facet of health education generally agreed as correct. Among components of the popular sector is a wide range of self-help groups — 335 groups have been listed for the year 1982 — which can be classified on the basis of why people join them. The long list includes associations such as Alcoholics Anonymous, Lesbian Line, Gay Switchboard, National Council for the Single Woman and her Dependants, Womens Health Concern, Rape Crisis, Back Pain Association, Psoriasis Society, Herpes Club. These self-help groups undertake a number of activities: 1. information and referral; 2. counselling and advice; 3. public and professional; 4. political and social activity; 5. fund-raising for research or services; 6. providing therapeutic services under professional guidance; 7. mutual supportive activities. Many groups are 'communities of suffering' where experience of a type of misfortune is a credential for membership. The reasons for the growth in number of these groups include: the perceived failure of existing medical and social services to meet people's needs; the recognition by members of the value of mutual help; and the role of the media in publicising the extent of specific difficulties. These groups also have a role as a coping mechanism for individuals with conditions which carry a 'stigma' and provide a means of combating the latter difficulty (Kelnan 1984).

The Terence Higgins Trust, another self-help group, was first formed and so named following the death of Terence Higgins from the Acquired Immune Deficiency Syndrome (AIDS). Saddened and alarmed at that time by the failure of official services and by the ignorance in the community of the threat of this disease, a group of his friends banded together to form this Trust. The activities of the Trust, now a registered charity, range from working with people with AIDS, through health education, to advising government, trade unions and professional groups. There are over three hundred people working as volunteers for the Trust as well doctors, nurses and health advisers that are part of the medical group of the Trust. With the objectives to inform, advise and help on AIDS the Trust prepared a number of booklets (An introduction to the Trust; AIDS and HTLVIII, Medical Briefing; AIDS — HTLVIII Antibody; To Test or not to Test? AIDS — The facts; Your chance of getting AIDS; More facts for gay men); Address: The Terence Higgins Trust, Ltd., BM A.I.D.S., London WClN 3XX — telephone helpline 01833 2971 or 01 278 8745.

A comparable organization (The Scottish AIDS Monitor, 23 Dublin Street, Edinburgh. — tel. 031 558 1167) has provided booklets 'Safe Sex Guide'; 'AIDS, The latest facts'. In addition the Scottish Aids Monitor provides AIDS information. A phone line was started in an attempt to answer questions from the general public about AIDS and HIV. This was provided to counteract the fear they considered was being instilled due to misinformation and rumour, often presented by communications media. Confidential advice and/or information is also available.

J. COMPANIONSHIP, MARRIAGE AND DIVORCE

It is clearly important for the doctor to avoid adding to a patient's difficulties by an approach which might upset the relationship between one partner and the other. The doctor must not divulge the confidences of one partner by giving information to the other although there are clearly difficulties, not insurmountable, when he is responsible for the medical care of both. An attempt must be made to elicit what one partner has told the other and to determine the attitudes of the patient to his or her situation. An individual patient has a right to know the nature of any infection discovered and if asked directly the doctor should not prevaricate further but tell the truth, although he can do this in a re-assuring and conciliatory way emphasizing the good parts of a relationship. Often a patient will convey without words an attitude to the situation and the doctor should try to interpret his patient's feelings and match his approach to them.

In divorce proceedings the acquisition of gonorrhoea or syphilis has implications regarding adultery and as such the doctor should know something about the law of marriage and divorce and, as in both England and Scotland, its recent changes (Grant & Levin 1973, Keith & Clark 1977). In companionate relationships, as well as in marriage, sexually transmitted diseases including gonorrhoea and syphilis may contribute to a breakdown and the doctor should not feel he is entitled to be more considerate to married partners and less to those who are not.

Essentially marriage is maintained by the continued consent of each partner. The law itself does not necessarily help in maintaining such person-to-person relationships and in childless marriages the interest of the secular state is clearly more limited than in those with children. Tensions and difficulties are common, and counselling and family services are more important than legalities provided there is a willingness to use such services. In Scotland, at least, where safeguards to individual rights are necessary, in companionate childless relationships, so common among young people today, recognition might become possible by the Scottish method where 'by habit and repute' the legal validity of such marriages can be established (Willock 1974).

The grounds for divorce in Scotland until lst January 1977, were adultery, cruelty, desertion, incurable insanity, sodomy and bestiality. In the case of the first four grounds the courts were in effect looking to see whether 'matrimonial offences' had been 'committed'. In recent times attempts have been made to get away from ideas of fault and guilt, and the new Act allows divorce by consent after two years separation (Keith & Clark 1977). There is still a clear difference between Scotland and England at the present time in regard to divorce. In England and Wales (Divorce Reform Act 1969) 'irretrievable breakdown' of marriage is the only reason for dissolving it. Although such a description has a complex meaning the lawyer tends to look for evidence or a clear definition. For example, if the respondent has committed adultery and the petitioner finds life with the respondent intolerable as a result then this is a ground for divorce. A petitioner cannot now have an impulsive divorce on sole proof of adultery.

In the case of Scotland, Divorce (Scotland) Act 1976, although 'irretrievable breakdown' of marriage is the sole ground for divorce, proof of adultery establishes this 'irretrievable breakdown' and it is therefore still possible to have an 'impulsive divorce' in Scotland.

From the point of view of the events leading up to divorce proceedings solicitors may seek information from STD clinics to be used as evidence of adultery. Generally such an imputation from the legal point of view may be made only in the case of gonorrhoea or syphilis, acquired after marriage. The doctor is required to give whatever information a solicitor may ask for on behalf of the client regarding the client's medical findings. He is not entitled to be given information about the client's partner without the consent of the party concerned unless the doctor receives an order by the Court, that is, in Scotland, the Court of Session at Edinburgh. It is important to maintain these safeguards and to avoid passing on information which the doctor is not entitled to give. Records on contact-tracing information are probably a separate issue to be excluded from case records.

Medical evidence in the United Kingdom is not privileged and the doctor must divulge his information if ordered to do so in court. Where litigation is imminent, however, between a husband and wife, as soon as a doctor or other counsellor is asked by either the wife or husband to act as an intermediary between them with a view to reconciliation, any statement written or oral made by either party is privileged. The law favours reconciliation and a person acting as a conciliator will not be compelled to give evidence as to what was said in the course of negotiation (Henley v. Henley 1955).

K. DILEMMA OF A NAME

The very nature of a moral dilemma is typified in the controversy over the name for the specialty that includes as a main interest the sexually transmitted diseases. In making a choice there are a range of different points to consider and attention can fasten now on one and now on another (Emmet 1979, see also Section (a)). The question is not new, and study of the Appendix to the Final Report of the Royal Commission on Venereal Diseases (1916) is revealing. The distinguished physician, Sir William Osler is asked the question: 'Do you think that every general hospital should establish an out-patient clinic, for dealing with these diseases?' — 'Yes', he replied, 'but I would not have it specially for venereal diseases, I would have it a genito-urinary clinic. There are certain advantages in that, because then you do not taboo it. A great many people who would not go to a special venereal clinic would willingly to a genito-urinary clinic'. He went on to say that the clinic at John Hopkins medical school was called 'a genito-urinary clinic' (Cd 8190 1916).

Sir William Osler's way of looking at the question is crucial, as he viewed it from the patient's point of view; he believed then, as many believe now, that patients would not like to attend a clinic labelled 'Venereal Diseases'. They are likely to feel a stigma and would suffer unnecessarily as a consequence.

In 1971 the Department of Health and Social Security in its statistical returns abandoned the term 'venereal diseases' (although it continues to have legal significance; see Note 5.11) and substituted 'sexually transmitted diseases' but continued to report the same wide range of genital infections. Oriel (1978) advanced the cause of the name 'genito-urinary medicine' and showed the wide range of genital disorders which could not be regarded as sexually transmitted. He felt that the new name symbolized a more mature and realistic view of the subject and strongly supported the abandonment in 1975 of the term venereology by the Department of Health and the Royal College of Physicians in London (Editorial (British Medical Journal) 1975). Controversy followed with a large following not wishing to accept the change (Cohen et al 1976). In the Faculty of Medicine, University of Edinburgh, the department hitherto named as the 'Department of Venereal Diseases' following the setting up in 1920 of the appointment of Dr David Lees as lecturer, was changed to that of the 'Department of Genito-Urinary Medicine'. This was agreed by the Senate of the University at their meeting of 7 May 1980.

The point is made that the name used for a department should reflect the work done and should not allow the patient to feel stigmatized. The term 'genito-urinary medicine' enables a general practitioner to explain to his patient that facilities exist for the diagnosis of a wide variety of infections and conditions and that the patient need feel no shame in being referred. Confirmation in the United Kingdom of the acceptance of the name is to be found in the changed title of the journal 'British Journal of Venereal Diseases to 'Genitourinary Medicine' (McMillan 1984).

NOTES TO CHAPTER 5

Note 5.1: National Health Service (VD) Regulations

(Applicable only to England and Wales.) 1968: (1968 No. 1624) National Health Service (Venereal Diseases) Regulations 1968 (coming into operation December 1, 1968).

The Minister of Health, in exercise of his powers under Section 12 of the National Health Service Act 1946 and of all other powers enabling him in that behalf, hereby makes the following regulations:

3. Every Regional Hospital Board and every Board of Governors of a teaching hospital shall take all necessary steps to secure that any information obtained by officers of the Board with respect to persons examined or treated for venereal disease in a hospital for the administration of which the Board is responsible shall be treated as confidential except for the purpose of communicating to a medical practitioner, or to a person employed under the direction of a medical practitioner in connection with the treatment of persons suffering from such disease or the prevention of the spread thereof, and for the purpose of such treatment or prevention.

Note 5.2: National Health Service (VD) Regulations

1974: (1974, No. 29) National Health Service (Venereal Diseases) Regulations 1974 (coming into operation April 1, 1974)).

Confidentiality of information

2. Every Regional Health Authority and every Area Health Authority shall take all necessary steps to secure that any information capable of identifying an individual obtained by officers of the Authority with respect to persons examined or treated for any sexually transmitted disease shall not be disclosed except:
a. for the purpose of communicating that information to a medical practitioner, or to a person employed under the direction of a medical practitioner in connection with the treatment of persons suffering from such a disease or the prevention of the spread thereof, and,
b. for the purpose of such treatment or prevention.

Note 5.3

Reference numbers used for diagnoses in this locality in contact-tracing in sexually transmitted diseases; the equivalent reference numbers from the International Classification of Diseases (ICD) may be useful for travellers (World Health Organization 1977).

	Local ref. no.	ICD number	
Syphilis	A1	091.0	Acquired, primary (genital)
	A1	091.1	Acquired primary (anal)
	A2	091.3	Acquired, secondary

	Local ref. no.	ICD number	
Syphilis (cont'd)	A3	092	Acquired, latent in first two years of infection
	A4	093	Acquired, cardiovascular
	A5	094	Acquired, neurological
	A6	096	Acquired, all other late or latent stages
	A7/A8	090	Congenital
Gonorrhoea	B1.1	098.0	With lower genito-urinary tract infection
	B1.2	098.6	With throat infection
	B1.3	098.4	With eye infection
	B1.4	098.1	With upper genital tract complications
	B1.5	098.8	With systemic complications
	B3	098.4	Gonococcal ophthalmia neonatorum
	C1	099.0	Chancroid
	C2	099.1	Lymphogranuloma venereum
	C3	099.2	Granuloma inguinale
	C4	099.4	Non-specific genital infections
	C5	099.3	Non-specific genital infections with arthritis
	C6	131.0	Trichomoniasis
	C7	112.1	Genital candidosis (female)
	C7	112.2	Genital candidosis (male)
	C8	133.0	Scabies
	C9	132.2	Pubic lice (*Pthirus pubis*)
	C10	054.1	Genital herpes simplex
	C11	078.1	Warts (condylomata acuminata)
	C12	078.0	Molluscum contagiosum
	D1	102	Other Treponemal diseases (yaws)
	D1	103	Other Treponemal diseases (pinta)
	D1	104	Other Treponemal diseases (other)

A3: This applies to cases presenting no clinical sign of syphilis but considered (e.g. by rapid reversal of serum VDRL or treatment or epidemiological evidence) to have contracted this disease within the preceding 24 months.
A4: Includes patients with cardiovascular syphilis who are also suffering from syphilis of any other system.
A7/A8: A7 refers to those aged under 2 years and A8 to those aged 2 years and over.
B1.1–B1.5: B1.1–B1.5 refer to post-pubertal gonorrhoea.
C4: Includes also all chlamydial infections, genital or ophthalmic.

Note 5.4: Results of Regulation 33B (1943)

'In England and Wales 36 men and 475 women had been reported to a Medical Officer of Health as alleged sources of venereal infection of which 1 man and 27 women have been the subject of more than one report. Of these 28 persons two women have refused treatment, one expressly, and one by default, and have been prosecuted and imprisoned. No civilian voluntarily undergoing treatment for venereal disease is subject to compulsion to complete it.'

Note 5.5

INSTRUCTIONS FOR CONDOM USERS (POPULATION REPORTS 1986)

For maximum protection, condoms must be used correctly. Health workers should not assume that people know how to use condoms. All condom users should receive very clear and explicit instructions.

1. Use a condom every time you have intercourse.
2. Always put the condom on the penis before intercourse begins.
3. Do not pull the condom tightly against the tip of the penis. Leave a small empty space — about one or two cm — at the end of the condom to hold semen. Some condoms have a nipple tip that will hold semen.
4. Unroll the condom all the way to the bottom of the penis.
5. If the condom breaks during intercourse, withdraw the penis immediately and put on a new condom.
6. After ejaculation, withdraw the penis while it is still erect. Hold onto the rim of the condom as you withdraw so that the condom does not slip off.
7. Use a new condom each time you have intercourse.
8. If a lubricant is desired, use water-based lubricants such as contraceptive jelly. Lubricants made with petroleum jelly may damage condoms. Do not use saliva because it may contain virus.
9. Store condoms in a cool, dry place if possible.
10. Condoms that are sticky or brittle or otherwise damaged should not be used.

CONDOMS AND HIV INFECTION

Although it is argued that only a radical change in sexual mores will substantially reduce the spread of HIV infection, it must be recognized that a substantial proportion of homosexual men practise anal intercourse (Ch. 1) and are unlikely to give it up. Without a sheath the risk of infection has been estimated as about 1% for each act of anal intercourse with an HIV-antibody positive partner (Peto 1986). Estimates of use-effectiveness of the condom as a contraceptive range from 0.8 to 4.8 per 100 women per year, and to enhance this effectiveness condoms should be used with a spermicide. The compound nonoxynol-9, present in concentrations of 5–12% in several spermicides in Europe (Thiery 1987), has been shown to inactivate HIV in vitro in a concentration of 0.05% (Hicks et al 1985) and together with the condom may be expected to reduce the spread of HIV. Sheaths, tested to British Standard 3704, and thick enough to withstand anal intercourse should be put on with care, and when used in this way with a water-based lubricant containing nonoxynol the risk of infection with HIV is likely to be reduced (Tovey 1987). Penetrative sex, particularly receptive, cannot be regarded as safe, however, and efforts should be made to encourage non-penetrative sex (Kelly & Lawrence 1987).

Note 5.6

The American Association of Physicians for Human Rights has a number of specific suggestions to reduce the risk of acquiring AIDS.

1. Decrease the number of different partners with whom one has sex, and avoid men who have many different sex partners.
2. Do not inject *any* drugs not prescribed and avoid sexual contact with intravenous drug users.
3. Avoid one-time encounters with anonymous partners and/or group sex.
4. Avoid oral-anal contact ('rimming').
5. Avoid 'fisting' (both giving and receiving).
6. Avoid active or passive rectal intercourse (use of condoms may be helpful).
7. Avoid faecal contamination through scat.
8. An additional probable risk factor may be mucous membrane (mouth or rectum) contact with semen or urine.
9. Take care of your general health (get adequate rest, good food, physical exercise, reduce stress, and reduce toxic substances such as alcohol, cigarettes).
10. If you know or suspect that you may have any transmissible disease do not risk the health of others.
11. Sexually active homosexual men should *not* donate blood for blood transfusion.
12. If you need help attend or telephone a clinic.

Note 5.7: Definition of 'privacy' and other restrictions in the Sexual Offences Act 1967, applicable to England and Wales

An act which would otherwise be treated for the purposes of this Act as being done in private shall not be so treated if done —
a. when more than two persons take part or are present; or,
b. in a lavatory to which the public have or are permitted to have access, whether on payment or otherwise.

There are important exceptions to these provisions:
(i) If one of the individuals is suffering from severe mental subnormality (Mental Health Act 1959) then his consent in law cannot be valid.
(ii) If one of the individuals is on the staff of the hospital having responsibility of the other then he would be excluded.
(iii) Members of the Armed Forces are excluded.
(iv) The homosexual acts among individuals on merchant ships are excluded also.

Note 5.8

54% of the males studied by Humphreys (1975, p. 105) were married and living with their families.

Note 5.9: Effect of conviction (Sexual Offences Act 1967)

a. N County Council v. B (1978) Industrial Relations Law Reports, 7, 252–255

A school teacher for almost 30 years was convicted after a plea of guilty of an offence of gross indecency with a man in a public lavatory and was as a result dismissed in accordance with the decision of a disciplinary committee. Although an Industrial Tribunal found in his favour that he had been unfairly dismissed, the local education authority appealed to the Employment Appeal Tribunal who set aside the decision of the Industrial Tribunal. The conviction provided evidence of homosexual inclinations which the teacher was not always able to resist or control and was the basis of the decision by the Disciplinary Sub-Committee. This body, acting on behalf of the Education Committee was entrusted with power of decision to dismiss or not to dismiss.

b. B v. X Police Authority (1978) Industrial Relations Law Reports, 7, 283–285

A chef in a canteen used by police and civilians admitting to being bi-sexual, was arrested and charged with two acts of gross indecency. Prosecution failed on technical grounds and he was acquitted. He had been arrested and charged in 1976 following police investigation into homosexual activities in the locality when a large number of people were interviewed and ultimately 15 or 16 of them faced prosecution at a Crown Court. Following discovery of his homosexual activities he was dismissed from his employment but he appealed to the Industrial Appeal Tribunal (B v. X Police Authority 1978), who decided that his dismissal was unfair on a number of counts including the tribunal's expressed surprise that it had been apparently accepted that 'seven police officers should all feel so strongly on the subject of homosexuality that they were not prepared to eat food cooked by a homosexual'.

Note 5.10

Street Offences Act (applicable to England and Wales) (1959) S1(1) makes it an offence for a common prostitute to loiter or solicit in a street or public place for the purpose of prostitution.

Note 5.11: Venereal Diseases Act 1917 (7 & 8 Geo. 5 Ch. 21).

Excerpts from the Act: 7 & 8 Geo. 5 Venereal Diseases Act 1917, Section 4. In this Act the expression 'venereal disease' means syphilis, gonorrhoea and soft chancre.

Prevention of the treatment of venereal disease otherwise than by duly qualified persons
   1.(1) In any area in which this section is in operation, a person shall not, unless he is a duly qualified medical practitioner, for reward either direct or indirect, treat any person for venereal disease or prescribe any remedy therefor, or give any advice in connection with the treatment thereof, whether the advice is given to the person to be treated or to any other person.

Restriction on advertisements & c.
   2.(1) A person shall not by any advertisement or any public notice or announcement treat or offer to treat any person for venereal disease, or prescribe or offer to prescribe any remedy therefor, or offer to give or give any advice in connection with the treatment thereof.
   2.(4) In this Act the expression 'venereal disease' means syphilis, gonorrhoea, soft chancre.

REFERENCES

A. CONFIDENTIALITY AND SEXUALLY TRANSMITTED DISEASES
AB v. CD 1851 Cases decided in the Court of Session. Scotland 177–180
Bernfeld W K 1967 Medical professional secrecy with special reference to venereal diseases. British Journal of Venereal Diseases 43: 53–59
Bernfeld W K 1972 Medical secrecy. The Cambrian Law Review 3: 11–26
Birkenhead Viscount, Lord Chancellor of England 1922 Should a doctor tell? Hodder and Stoughton, London, vol 1: 33–76
Emmet D 1979 The moral prism. MacMillan Press, London
Forlin G, Wauchope P 1987 AIDS and the criminal law. The Law Society Gazette 25/3/87, p 884–885
Garner v. Garner 1920 In: Medico-legal, medical professional privilege. British Medical Journal 1: 135–136
Henley v. Henley 1955 Law reports, Probate Division 202–204
Mason J K, McCall Smith R A 1983 Medical confidentiality. In: Law and medical ethics. Butterworth, London, p 95–110
Melville L (ed) 1927 Trial of the Duchess of Kingston. Hodge, Edinburgh, p 243
Results of Regulation 33B 1943 British Journal of Venereal Diseases 19 : 92
Riddell Lord 1929 The law and ethics of medical confidences. In: Medico-legal problems. H K Lewis, London, p 45–69
Stimson G V, Oppenheimer E 1982 Heroin addiction.

Treatment and control in Britain. Tavistock Publications, London, p 207

B. MEDICAL ADVICE AND TREATMENT OF YOUNG PERSONS
Brahams D 1985 Parental consent — does doctor know best after all? The Gillick case. New Law Journal 135: 8–10
Norrie K McK 1983 Contraceptives, consent and the child. The Scots Law Times, 16/12/1983, p 285–288
Norrie K McK 1985a A comment on the Gillick case. The British Journal of Family Planning 11: 1–4
Norrie K McK 1985b The Gillick crusade ill-conceived under Scots law. Scotsman, 23/3/1985, p 7
Norrie K McK 1985c The Gillick case and parental rights in Scots Law. The Scots Law Times: 157–162
Times Law Report, House of Lords 1985 DHSS contraceptive guidance to doctors is lawful. Times, 18/10/1985

C. TRACING OF CONTACTS AND THE CASE AGAINST COMPULSION, LESSONS FROM HISTORY
Bell E M 1962 Josephine Butler, Flame of fire, Constable, London
Blom-Cooper L, Drewry G (eds) 1976 Law and morality. In: Human sexuality 4.7, 4.8, 4.9. Duckworth, London, p 114–121
Cd 8189 & 8190 1916 Final Report and Appendix to Final Report of the Commissioners, Royal Commission on Venereal Diseases. London, HMSO
Contagious Diseases Acts (1864, 1866 and 1869) respectively:

27 & 28 Victoriae, Cap 85. An Act for the Prevention of Contagious Diseases at certain Naval and Military Stations (1864) 29 Victoriae, Cap 35. An Act for the better Prevention of Contagious Diseases at certain Naval and Military Stations (1866) 32 & 33 Victoriae, Cap 80. An Act to amend the Contagious Diseases Act (1866, 1869)

Hunter I, Jacobs J, Kinnell H, Satin A 1980 Handbook on contact tracing in sexually transmitted diseases. Health Education Council, 178 New Oxford Street, London WC1A 1AH

Leading Article 1917 The control of venereal disease. Lancet i: 309

Petrie G 1971 A singular iniquity: the campaigns of Josephine Butler. Macmillan, London

Results of Regulation 33B 1943 British Journal of Venereal Diseases 19: 92

Rover C 1967 Love, morals and the feminists, Routledge and Kegan Paul, London

Shannon N P 1943 The compulsory treatment of venereal diseases under Regulation 33B. British Journal of Venereal Diseases 19: 22–23

Statement for the Corporation 1928 Edinburgh Corporation Bill 1928 (Venereal Diseases). City and Royal Burgh of Edinburgh

Swinbanks D 1987 AIDS becomes a notifiable disease in Japan despite protests. News, Nature 326 : 232

Venereal Disease and the Defence of the Realm Act 1917. Lancet ii : 23

Willcox R R 1973 International contact tracing in venereal disease. WHO Chronicle 27 : 418

World Health Organization 1977 International Classification of Diseases, injuries and causes of death, based on the recommendations of the Ninth Revision Conference, 1975, vol 1, World Health Organization and HMSO, London

D. CHILD ABUSE AND SEXUALLY TRANSMITTED DISEASE

Clayden G 1987 Anal appearances and child sex abuse. Correspondence, Lancet i: 620–621

Creighton S 1987 Child abuse in 1985 — initial findings from NSPCC register research. Family Law 17: 117–118

Douglas G, Willmore C 1987 Diagnostic interviews as evidence in cases of child sexual abuse. Family Law 17: 151–154

Dyer C 1987 The dolls of Great Ormond Street. The Law Magazine, 1/5/1987, p 22–24

Hey F, Buchan P C, Littlewood J M, Hall R I 1987 Differential diagnosis in child sexual abuse. Correspondence, Lancet i: 283

Hobbs C J, Wynne J M 1986 Buggery in childhood — a common syndrome of child abuse. Lancet ii: 792–796

Howard League for Penal Reform 1985 Unlawful sex. The Report of a Howard League Working Party. Waterlow Legal and Social Policy Library

Lancet, Notes and News 1986 Increase of abuse in children. Lancet ii: 1473

Lancet, Leading Article 1987 I11-treatment of children. Lancet i: 367–368

Lothian Regional Review Committee 1983 Non-accidental injury to children (abused or at risk to abuse). Guidelines, 3rd edn (with addenda of 1984 and 1987)

E. PERSISTENT VIRUS INFECTIONS (INCLUDING THAT DUE TO HUMAN IMMUNODEFICIENCY VIRUSES) AND CONTROL OF THEIR SPREAD

Acheson E D 1986 AIDS: A challenge for the public health. Lancet i: 662–666

British Dental Association Dental Health and Science Committee Workshop 1986 British Dental Journal 160: 131–134

Buning E C, Coutinho R A, van Brussel G H A, van Santen G W, van Zadelhoff A W 1986 Preventing AIDS in drug addicts in Amsterdam. Correspondence, Lancet i: 435

Centers for Disease Control 1983 Prevention of acquired immune deficiency syndrome (AIDS): report of inter-agency recommendations. Morbidity and Mortality Weekly Report 32: 101–103

Centers for Disease Control 1984 Declining rates of rectal and pharyngeal gonorrhea among males — New York City. Morbidity and Mortality Weekly Report 33: 295–297

Centers for Disease Control February 1985a Update: Prospective evaluation of health-care workers exposed via the parenteral or mucous-membrane route to blood or body fluids from patients with acquired immunodeficiency syndrome — United States. Morbidity and Mortality Weekly Report 34: 101–103

Centers for Disease Control 1985b Summary: Recommendations for preventing transmission of infection with human T-lymphotropic virus type III/lymphadenopathy-associated virus in the workplace. Morbidity and Mortality Weekly Report 34: 681–686; 691–695

Centers for Disease Control 1985c Education and foster care of children infected with human T-lymphotropic virus type III/lymphadenopathy-associated virus. Morbidity and Mortality Weekly Report 34: 517–521

Centers for Disease Control 1985d Current trends: Recommendations for assisting in the prevention of perinatal transmission of human T-lymphotropic virus type III/lymphadenopathy-associated virus and acquired immunodeficiency syndrome. Morbidity and Mortality Weekly Report 34(48): 721–732

Centers for Disease Control April 1986 Recommended infection control practices for dentistry. Morbidity and Mortality Weekly Report 35: 237–242

Clumeck N, Van de Perre P, Carael M, Rouvroy D, Nzaramba D 1985 Heterosexual promiscuity among African patients with AIDS. New England Journal of Medicine 313 : 182

Curran J W, Morgan W M, Hardy A M, Jaffe H W, Darrow W W, Dowdle W R 1985 The epidemiology of AIDS. Current status and future prospects. Science 229: 1352–1357

Friedland G H, Saltzman B R, Rogers M F, Kahl P A, Lesser M L, Mayers M M, Klein R S 1986 Lack of transmission of HTLV-III/LAV infection to household contacts of patients with AIDS or AIDS-related complex with oral candidiasis. New England Journal of Medicine 314: 344–349

Fujikawa L S,. Salahuddin S Z, Palestine A G, Masur H, Nussenblatt R B, Gallo R C 1985 Isolation of human T-lymphotropic virus type III from tears of a patient with acquired immunodeficiency syndrome. Lancet ii: 529–530

Golubjatnikov R, Pfister J, Tillotson T 1983 Homosexual promiscuity and the fear of AIDS. Correspondence, Lancet ii : 680

Harré R 1979 Social being, a theory for social psychology. Basil Blackwell, London, p 1–36

Hicks D R, Martin L B, Getchell J P et al 1985 Inactivation of HTLV-III/LAV-infected cultures of normal human lymphocytes by nonoxynol 9 in vitro. Lancet ii: 1422–1423

Ho D D, Byington R E, Schooley R T, Flynn T, Rota T R, Hirsch M S 1985 Infrequency of isolation of HTLV-III virus from saliva in AIDS. Correspondence, New England Journal of Medicine 313 : 1606

Jeffries D 1986 3. Virology. In: Miller D, Weber J, Green J (eds) The management of AIDS. Macmillan, London, p 53–63

Judson F N 1983 Fear of AIDS and gonorrhoea rates in homosexual men. Lancet ii: 159–160

Kelly J A, Lawrence J S St 1987 Cautions about condoms in prevention of AIDS. Lancet i : 323

Miller D, Green J 1985 Psychological support and counselling for patients with acquired immune deficiency syndrome (AIDS). Genitourinary Medicine 61: 273–278

Notes and News 1986 Preventing transmission of viral infection in dentistry. Lancet i : 1049

Osterholm M, Bowman R J, Chopek M W, McCullogh J J, Korlath J A, Polesky H F 1985 Screening donated blood and plasma for HTLV-III antibody. Facing more than one crisis? New England Journal of Medicine 312: 1185–1189

Peto J 1986 AIDS and promiscuity. Correspondence, Lancet ii : 979

Population Reports 1986 AIDS — a public health crisis. Population reports, Series L No.6 July–Aug 1986. Issues in world health. The John Hopkins University, Hampton House, 624 North Broadway, Baltimore, Maryland 21205 USA

Robertson J R, Bucknall A B V, Welsby P D, Roberts J S K, Inglis J M, Peutherer J F, Brettle R P 1986 Epidemic of AIDS related virus (HTLV-III/LAV) infection among intravenous drug abusers. British Medical Journal 292: 527–529

Schechter M T, Jeffries E, Constance P et al 1984 Changes in sexual behaviour and fear of AIDS. Lancet i : 1293

Stimson G V, Oppenheimer E 1982 Heroin addiction. Treatment and control in Britain. Tavistock Publications, London, p 4

Thiery M 1987 Condoms and prevention. Correspondence, Lancet i : 567

Thiry L, Sprecher-Goldberger S, Jonckheer T et al 1985 Isolation of AIDS virus from cell-free breast milk of three healthy virus carriers. Lancet ii: 891–892

Tovey S J 1987 Condoms and AIDS prevention. Correspondence, Lancet i : 567

Vogt M W, Witt D J, Craven D E, Byington R, Crawford D F, Schooley R T, Hirsch M S 1986 Isolation of HTLV-III/LAV from cervical secretions of women at risk of AIDS. Lancet i: 525–527

Weber J N, McCreaner A, Berrie E, Wadsworth J, Jeffries D J, Pinching A J, Harris J R W 1986 Factors affecting seropositivity to human T cell lymphotropic virus type III (HTLV-III) or lymphadenopathy associated virus (LAV) and progression of disease in sexual partners of patients with AIDS. Genitourinary Medicine 62: 177–180

Wofsy C, Cohen J, Hauer L B, Padian N, Michaelis B, Evans L, Levy J A 1986 Isolation of AIDS-associated retrovirus from genital secretions of women with antibodies to the virus. Lancet i: 527–529

Ziegler J B, Cooper D A., Johnson R O, Gold J 1985 Post-natal transmission of AIDS-associated retrovirus from mother to infant. Lancet i: 896–898

Zuckerman A J 1986 AIDS and insects. Leading article, British Medical Journal 292: 1094–1095

F. TESTING FOR ANTIBODY TO HUMAN IMMUNODEFICIENCY VIRUSES (HIV) LIMITATIONS, INDICATIONS AND RESTRAINTS

Centers for Disease Control 1985 Current trends: Recommendations for assisting in the prevention of perinatal transmission of human T-lymphotropic virus type III/lymphadenopathy-associated virus and acquired immunodeficiency syndrome. Morbidity and Mortality Weekly Report 34(48): 721–732

Leading Article 1984 Blood transfusion, haemophilia in AIDS. Lancet ii: 1433–1435

Miller D, Green J 1985 Psychological support and counselling for patients with acquired immune deficiency syndrome/AIDS. Genitourinary Medicine 61: 273–278

Miller D, Weber J, Green J (ed) 1986 The Management of AIDS patients, Macmillan Press, Basingstoke, p 131–173

Stewart G J, Tyler J P P, Cunningham A L et al 1985 Transmission of human T-cell lymphotropic virus type III (HTLV-III) by artificial insemination by donor. Lancet ii: 581–584

G. HOMOSEXUALITY IN MALES

Bailley D S 1955 Homosexuality and the Western Christian tradition. Longmans, London

Bancroft J 1975 Homosexuality and the medical profession: a behaviourist's view. Journal of Medical Ethics 1: 176–180

Bancroft J 1981 Human sexuality and its problems. Churchill Livingstone, Edinburgh, ch 6, p 165, 171

Bell A P, Weinberg M S 1978 Homosexualities. A study of diversity among men and women. Mitchell Beazley, London, p 229–231

Crane P 1983 Gays and the law. Pluto Press, London, p 8–39

Devlin P 1959 The enforcement of morals. Oxford University Press, London, ch 1, p 1–25

D. v. U.K. Judgement of 22/10/81. European Court of Human Rights (ECHR)

Finnie W 1983 Domestic effects of the European Convention on Human Rights. Background paper. Information conference. Edinburgh University.

Galloway B 1983 The Police and the courts. In: Galloway B (ed) Prejudice and pride. Routledge and Kegan Paul, London, p 102–106

Hart H L A 1961 The Concept of law. Oxford University Press, London, p 168–176

Hart H L A 1963 Law, liberty and morality. Oxford University Press, London.

Hodges 1983 Alan Turing: the enigma. Burnett Books

Honoré T 1978 Sex law. Duckworth, London, p 84–110

Humphreys R A Laud 1975 Tearoom trade (impersonal sex in public places). Aldine, Chicago

Humana C 1983 World human rights guide. Hutchinson, ISBN 0 09 153490 9

Jacqué Jean-Paul 1983 Forum. Council of Europe: 2/83 p VII–IX

Jowell R, Witherspoon S, Brook L 1986 British social attitudes, the 1986 report. Gower, Vermont, USA, p 151–156

Mill J S 1859 On liberty. In: On liberty, representative government and the subjection of women. 1912 edn. The World's Classics, Oxford University Press, p 15

Plummer K 1975 Sexual stigma: an interactionist account. Routledge and Keegan Paul, London

Walmsley R 1978 Indecency between males and the Sexual Offences Act 1967. The Criminal Law Review (July) p 385–452

Walmsley R, White K 1979 Sexual offences, consent and sentencing. Home Office Research Study No. 54 Her Majesty's Stationery Office, p 38–46

Wolfenden Report 1957 The Report of the Committee on Homosexual Offences and Prostitution, Cmnd.247 Her Majesty's Stationery Office, London, p 131–137

H. PROSTITUTION IN FEMALES

Change International Reports 1980 Providence and prostitution. Image and reality for women in Buddhist Thailand. Women and Society, 62 Chandos Place, London CC2

Conrad G L, Kleris G S, Rush B, Darrow W 1981 Sexually transmitted diseases among prostitutes and other sexual offenders. Sexually Transmitted Diseases 8: 241–244

Cunnington S 1980 Some aspects of prostitution in the West End of London in 1979. In: West D J (ed) Sex offenders in the criminal justice system. Cropwood Conference Series No. 12. Institute of Criminology, Cambridge, p 121–130

Gebhard P 1982 'Human sexuality' Encyclopaedia Britannica 15th edn. Encyclopaedia Britannica, Chicago, p 75–81

Khoo R, Sng E H, Goh A J 1977 A study of sexually transmitted diseases in 200 prostitutes in Singapore. Asian Journal of Infectious Diseases 1: 77–79

Trott L 1980 On understanding prostitution and its problematic sources of information, with particular reference to Mayfair, London. In: West D J (ed) Sex offenders in the criminal justice system. Cropwood Conference Series No. 12 Institute of Criminology, Cambridge

Vickers J 1980 Prostitution in the context of the Street Offences Act. In: West D J (ed) Sex offenders in the criminal justice system. Cropwood Conference Series No. 12. Institute of Criminology, Cambridge, p 114–120

Willcox R R 1976 What are the chances of catching VD? Medical Times 104: 53–58

I. SELF-HELP GROUPS

Kelnan C 1984 Culture, health and illness. Wright PSG, Bristol, p 54–57

J. COMPANIONSHIP, MARRIAGE AND DIVORCE

Grant B, Levin J 1973 Family law. Sweet and Maxwell, London

Henley v. Henley 1955 Law reports probate. Incorporated Council of Law Reporting in England and Wales, London, p 202

Keith R M, Clark G V 1977 The layman's guide to Scots law, vol 2, Divorce. Gordon Bennett, Edinburgh

Willock I D 1974 A new approach to divorce; irreconcilable break-up. Journal of the Law Society of Scotland 223–225

K. DILEMMA OF A NAME

Cd 8190 1916 Final Report and Appendix to Final Report of the Commissioners, Royal Commission on Venereal Diseases. London, HMSO

Cohen L, McCann J S, Couchman J M et al 1976 Venereology or genito-urinary medicine? Correspondence, British Journal of Venereal Diseases 52: 355–356

Editorial, British Medical Journal 1975 Genitourinary medicine. British Medical Journal 1: 51–52

Emmet D 1979 The moral prism. MacMillan Press, London

McMillan A 1984 Editorial, genitourinary medicine. British Journal of Venereal Diseases 60 : 213

Oriel J D 1978 Genitourinary medicine. British Journal of Venereal Diseases 54: 291–294

6

Clinical investigation of the patient

Under the circumstances of rising demand for clinical, laboratory and other services, coupled with restrictions on the availability of these resources, clear objectives have to be defined for out-patient departments particularly. To secure minimum standards appropriate to the economies of the society being served and to avoid omissions of important steps it is necessary to develop a structured approach to history-taking and clinical examination. Although inappropriate for some patients this will involve focus of attention on those anatomical sites where implantation of the infecting organism or agent is likely to occur, viz. the lower urogenital tract, the oropharynx and ano-rectum. Extension of history-taking and physical examination may be necessary for those with more serious disease, and underlying psychosexual difficulties should not be ignored.

It has been clear for a very long time that the straightforward immensely successful idiom in medicine, and particularly in genito-urinary medicine, viz. identify the cause and remove it, is no longer adequate (De Bono 1985). Although its extension to involve tracing and treatment of contacts is successful in immediately curable disease such as gonorrhoea it is clear that progress in STD medicine is slowed and made more complex by a number of interacting factors. First and foremost is the increasing incidence of persistent viral infection due, for example, to papillomavirus, herpes simplex virus and human immunodeficiency viruses (HIV). In all of these medical intervention is not curative and there is likely to be a long-term, often lifetime follow-up requirement. The first step outlined in this Chapter will be effective when it is possible to identify the cause, remove it, and trace and, if necessary, treat contacts. In dealing with the persistent infections, however, all cannot be offered within the context of a single specialty and indeed the problems can surface in almost any medical setting. Thus it will not be enough to focus solely on the patient's immediate problem but, in many cases it will be necessary to plan for follow-up and care in the long term. The potential need for help is staggering in its size but realizable goals can be defined and

will always need resources outside the confines of the clinic.

In designing the approach the clinical and laboratory investigations undertaken must be in proportion to 1. the degree of risk in the individual patient, and 2. the likelihood of investigations bringing benefit. In relation to the first the assessment will depend to a great extent upon the sexual behaviour of the individual, viz. sexual orientation, sexual practices and degree of sexual mixing (promiscuity). 'At-risk' grouping of patients will take into account also the geographical location of the sexual encounter(s) and the practice or otherwise of drug abuse whether intravenous or not. In relation to the second it is clear that the detection or exclusion of hepatitis B surface antigen (HBsAg), for example, will enable decisions to be made on vaccination whereas the detection or exclusion of antibody to the human immunodeficiency viruses in the serum will not. Specific diseases will vary geographically and in any given locality data keeping is necessary for the design of services (Fig.6.1).

RECEPTION

The quality of reception is important and peremptoriness is to be deplored at all stages. Privacy is highly desirable for patients when personal details are being recorded for registration; reassurance about the confidentiality of the consultation may be given at the same time. Reception of patients is always important but particularly so in departments of genito-urinary medicine, specializing in sexually transmissible infections. Those responsible for design of out-patient departments have often failed to give these matters sufficient consideration.

OBJECTIVES OF CLINICAL INVESTIGATION

In any clinic six main objectives should form the framework for investigation of the patient.

1. Detect or exclude early syphilis: if the patient is infected arrange *immediate* specific treatment and inter-

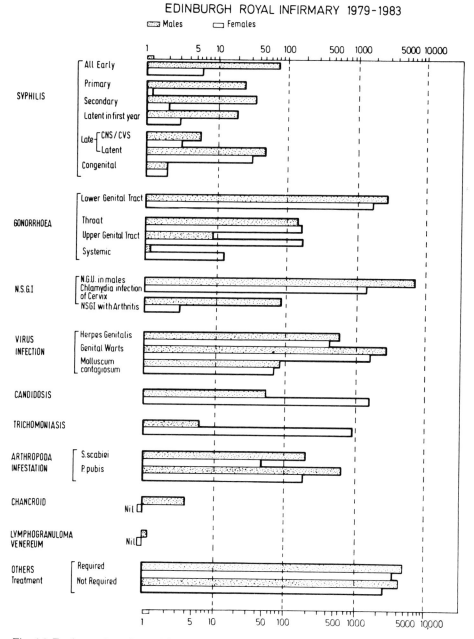

EDINBURGH ROYAL INFIRMARY 1979-1983

Fig. 6.1 Total cases in males and females for the Department of Genito-Urinary Medicine, Edinburgh Royal Infirmary 1979–1983. The totals are shown on a logarithmic scale.

view the patient to obtain sufficient information to trace sexual contact(s).

A high standard of serological testing for syphilis is an essential service for every clinic.

2. Detect or exclude gonococcal infection: if the patient is infected arrange *immediate* specific treatment and interview the patient to obtain sufficient information to trace the sexual contact(s).

The ability to detect gonococci by culture methods is a *sine qua non* for every clinic.

3. Make a clinical and microbial diagnosis of the wide variety of specific sexually transmissible infections, based on the isolation of the organism or agent considered to be causative. Limitations in resources may set limits to these investigations and some selection in the use of tests may often have to be imposed. In clinics

of the 'developed' countries laboratory tests for isolation of organisms or agents should be available for the following infections:

- *Chlamydia trachomatis*
- *Trichomonas vaginalis*
- *Candida albicans* and other yeasts
- *Gardnerella vaginalis*
- Hepatitis B virus (HBV)
- Herpes simplex virus (HSV)
- *Giardia intestinalis*
- *Entamoeba histolytica*

Within this objective will lie the detection or exclusion of lymph node enlargement and other clinical features seen in the infection due to HIV or in the Acquired Immune Deficiency Syndrme (Ch. 31).

Contact-tracing will be important in some infections, e.g. *Chlamydia trachomatis* but much less so in others, e.g. *Gardnerella vaginalis*.

4. The fourth objective will cover the detection of other medical problems and their resolution when possible. Some of the main aims may be summarized as follows:

a. The encouragement in the use of contraception in those at risk of unwanted pregnancy.
b. The detection of pregnancy.
c. Arrangement for antenatal care when necessary.
d. Assistance of those seeking help or advice in connection with continuation or termination of pregnancy.
e. Detection of psychosexual dysfunction.
f. Other medical issues which can conveniently be described as falling within the primary medical care of adolescents and young adults.

5. The fifth objective involves the clinic in medico-social work such as the detection and search for relief or remedy in homelessness, marital stress and poverty. Those with problems and difficulties in establishing and maintaining relationships are of special concern to the clinician. As well as knowing the patient's sexual orientation an understanding of typology is important (Ch. 1).

Offering to put individual patients in touch with self-help groups may be appropriate. The doctor-patient relationship is an important one. Patients may fear that the stigma of a venereal disease will lower them in the opinion of their fellows. Doctors particularly must look at persons from the point of view of their whole personality. They must not allow deviance, deformity or difference to overshadow the fact that patients are human beings with qualities and faults similar to those in whom no stigma is recognized. It is in hospitals, and in clinics in particular, that doctors are privy to the sexual behaviour of the individual. Doctors are, or should be, 'wise persons — before whom the individual

with a fault need feel no shame nor exert self control, knowing that in spite of his failing he will be seen as an ordinary other' (Goffman 1963).

6. A sixth objective has to be introduced now and relates to infection or risk of infection by human immunodeficiency viruses (HIV). Although this is discussed more fully in Chapter 5, sections (e) and (f) and in Chapter 31 it will be necessary in localities of low incidence of infection both in at-risk groups and in those anxious about their own situation to begin the process of giving explanations and counselling before raising the question of testing for antibody to HIV.

HISTORY TAKING

History-taking is an extension of clinical skills required in any branch of medicine. A patient attending a clinic on his own account, on advice from a sexual contact, or after an explanation and referral by his general practitioner, will generally expect a series of questions relating to his or her recent sexual contacts: in some cases, however, the doctor might best ask first about his or her main complaints and their duration or, in the case of females, begin to consider and record the menstrual history and contraceptive practice of the patient. Information on antibiotic or chemotherapy received during the last month or longer will be relevant, particularly as it may obscure diagnosis or, at least, diminish the effectiveness of techniques for the isolation of specific organisms.

Data about sexual intercourse are best obtained after the doctor has obtained rapport with the patient. Information on sexual orientation in the case of the male is essential to obtain. The date of last coitus is noted. Record this as 'LC' in the unmarried, as last marital coitus 'LMC' or as last extramarital coitus 'EMC' in the married. An assessment may be made simply by recording in a given individual:

a. sexual orientation whether heterosexual, homosexual, or bisexual;
b. the number of sexual partners of either sex in the last month, and
c. the number in the last year.

Fuller details of a more complex and detailed nature can be obtained later and recorded separately by health personnel responsible for tracing contacts.

For convenience, and to ensure that the main medical objectives are secured in every case, a proforma is important in busy clinics; this enables a framework for history-taking and examination to be constructed. Examples of these are shown in Figures 6.2 and 6.3 respectively for males and females and will be sufficient in the average case. Main details, therefore, will be

Referred by	Age	Diagnosis	First Attendance		Case No
			M S D Sep		

Date of recent contact and duration of relationship:
if married L.M.C.   1)   2)   3)

HISTORY

Contact(s)   M   F

Contraception   Antibiotic or Chemotherapy   Drugs

Previous History

Hepatitis   Eczema

Previous Penicillin   Penicillin Reaction   Asthma   Hay Fever   Other Sensitivity

Examination   Mouth   *P pubis*

Skin   *S scabiei*

Abd.

Ur. meatus

Testes   Scrotum

Penis   Anus

Inguinal nodes   Proctoscopy

Blood

Glucose

Urine   1)   2)   Hours held   Protein

Provisional diagnosis	STS		Treatment	Next attendance
	Ur. Sm.			
	Cultures	Ur.		
		T		
		R		
	HBsAg			

1.   Primary Contact   Known   Unknown

Contacts	Relationship	No.	Diagnosis	Date	Notes
	1				
	2				
	3				

Locality acquired	HV	
	Referred	
	Not referred	

Fig. 6.2 Framework for initial history and examination in the male.

Referred by	Age	Diagnosis	First Attendance		Case No
			M S D Sep.		

Date of recent contact and duration of relationship:
if married L.M.C.   1)   2)   3)

HISTORY

		Antibiotic or Chemotherapy	Drugs
Menarche			Contraception
L.M.P.			Adviser
Menstruation			Duration

Previous History

Hepatitis					Eczema
Previous Penicillin	Penicillin Reaction	Asthma	Hay Fever		Other Sensitivity

Pregnancies				E.D.C.

Examination	Mouth	P. pubis
Skin		P. capitis
		S. scabiei
Abdomen		

Inguinal nodes

Vulva		Vagina
		Cervix
Urethra		
		P.V.
Introitus		
Bart R.	L.	
Anus		
Urine:	Protein Glucose Blood	

HSV (isolation)		Cultures	T	STS			Cytology
HCFT			Ur				
Chlamydia			Cx				
			R				

Contacts		Relationship	No.	Diagnosis	Date	Locality acquired	HV
	1						Referred
	2						
	3						Not referred

Provisional diagnosis

Fig. 6.3 Framework for initial history and examination in the female.

rapidly apparent in the follow-up of the case by the doctor, who will not be necessarily the same one on every occasion.

In connection with the past history, information should be obtained about previous sexually transmitted diseases as well as previous illness of a medical or surgical nature. A history of hepatitis should be noted. Overseas visits whether recent or remote are relevant. The patient should be asked about past or present drug abuse and whether or not these drugs have been taken intravenously.

Family history is often restricted in the male to those questions of sexual relationships, unless more detail on social background is required. Narrowing of the scope of the investigation is often a result of limited time and a patient's apparent wish to be cured quickly with the least possible intrusion into personal affairs. In the case of patients with symptoms but no objective signs the possibility of psychosexual difficulties should be remembered and questions asked in explicit terms about matters such as premature ejaculation in the male and absence of orgasm in the female. In the case of the female, her children's needs may make her attendances difficult. Judicious questions will often elicit symptoms of family stress.

CLINICAL EXAMINATION: SPECIAL FEATURES

Initial examination in both male and female can conveniently include inspection of the skin surface above the waist. This can be carried out having due regard to the patient's sense of privacy and feelings. Examine the cervical, axillary and epitrochlear and inguinal lymph nodes. The axillary region and scalp should be inspected. Careful examination of the wrist creases, the webs between the fingers, and the back of the elbow is necessary for the detection of scabies. The presence of old self-inflicted scars, marks of intravenous injections, tattoo marks and uncleanliness should be noted.

Examination of the male
In the inspection of the skin surface below the waist and of the ano-genital region in particular, attention should be paid to the abdomen, inguinal lymph nodes, liver and spleen.

1. Penis. Retract the prepuce and note the extent it can move freely over the glans. Examine in particular the urethral meatus (note if there are meatal warts, ulcer or stricture), glans, frenum, coronal sulcus, prepuce, shaft and median raphe.

2. Scrotum and contents. Testes, epidydimes and spermatic cords and coverings.

3. Pubic region. Look for evidence of the crab louse (*Pthirus pubis*) and the lesions of molluscum contagiosum. Examine the inguinoscrotal fold for tinea cruris.

4. Anus and perianal skin. Look for warts, anal chancre or fissure.

Examination of the ano-genital region with gloved hands is the correct procedure and is mandatory where moist infective or potentially infective lesions are present. Disposable vinyl examination gloves are satisfactory (e.g., Triflex, Travenol Laboratories Ltd., Thetford, Norfolk, England). An attempt should be made to milk any discharge from the penile urethra. If a discharge is present, the urethral meatus should be cleansed with a saline-soaked gauze swab and the discharge obtained by means of a disposable plastic inoculating loop. The 10 μl loop, blue in colour (Nunc products, Kamstrup, DK–Roskilde, Denmark), is inserted past the everted lips of the meatus and gently passed for 2–3 cm within the urethra. Where even minor urethral symptoms are present in the male a scraping should be taken and plated directly on to a selective medium for the gonococcus even if there is no visible discharge. If direct placing is impossible transport medium should be used (Ch. 15). It is a useful procedure in such cases to ask patients to return the following morning after retaining urine overnight. The patient should empty his bladder late at night before retiring and come to the clinic in the early morning. Such early morning urethral smears, examined by microscopy and culture, are useful in the detection of minimal degrees of urethritis, whether non-gonococcal or gonococcal. To avoid missing asymptomatic cases, there is a strong case for the routine culture of urethral scrapings in all cases where there has been a risk of acquiring gonorrhoea. Facilities may, however, be restricted, in which case contacts should be examined to exclude the presence of the gonococcus.

In contacts of gonorrhoea or in those with gonorrhoea, a cotton-wool swab should be passed over the pharynx and both tonsils or tonsillar beds and plated directly on medium selective for the gonococcus.

In the male an endo-urethral swab (Medical Wire and Equipment Co., Ltd.,) is passed into the anterior urethra for 5 cm and withdrawn and agitated in a container of 2SP (see Note 6.1). Excess fluid is removed by rotating the swab while gently pressing against the inside of the container. After moistening, the swab can be passed gently along the anterior urethra for 5–10 cm. On final removal the swab may be cut off with disposable scissors. Since the non-gonococcal urethritis in the male will receive appropriate antibiotics, tests for *Chlamydia* may be omitted for economy.

Alternatively, and when the numbers examined are few, the use of fluorescein-labelled monoclonal antibodies in the form of a direct specimen test provides a rapid easy-to-perform diagnostic method for the detection of *Chlamydia trachomatis*. In such a test in the form of the 'Microtrak' *C.trachomatis* direct specimen test (Syva, California, USA) chlamydial antigens are detectable with a sensitivity of over 90% and a specificity of 98%. In this test a urethral swab is rolled on to a slide and fixed. Slides are then stained with a reagent containing fluorescein-labelled monoclonal antibody and counterstain. After rinsing *Chlamydia*-positive specimens show under a fluorescence microscope apple-green elementary or reticulate bodies contrasted by the red background of counterstained cells.

Urine
Direct visual examination of the urine is necessary in every case, but particularly so in the male as the urine will contain exudate from the urethra in the case of urethritis. In anterior urethritis, the initial 20 ml of urine passed will contain many pus cells, causing a turbidity, not cleared by the addition of 10% acetic acid, which will be less in the second portion of urine passed. This crude test has value in detecting obvious urethritis. In subacute or chronic urethritis, casts consisting of mucopus from urethra and urethral glands, may sink as threads and deposits in the specimen. In anterior urethritis exudate will tend to be passed mainly in the first urine voided; in posterior urethritis or prostatitis the first and second specimens may contain such deposit.

Examination of urine for protein, sugar and blood is essential. The most widely used tests for these are the stick tests (Fuller details are given in Whitby et al 1984).

Glucose. Qualitative test, based on glucose oxidase, that is practically specific for glucose.

Reducing substances. Semi-quantitative test which detects reducing sugars (e.g. glucose, galactose, lactose, fructose).

Protein. Semi-quantitative test, most sensitive for detection of albumin (Note 6.2). Very insensitive for Bence-Jones protein.

Blood. Semi-quantitative test for haem derivatives. The test does not differentiate between haematuria, haemoglobinuria and myoglobinuria. A false-positive result can be seen when the urine is contaminated (1/1000) with povidone-iodine (Betadine). For the investigation of microscopic haematuria see Note 6.3.

Blood
A specimen of venous blood is taken in every case for serological tests for syphilis and for herpes complement fixation and hepatitis B when appropriate. Venepuncture is conveniently carried out when the patient's examination is completed. In all tests it is *important* to keep to the guidelines laid down for safety at work (Note 6.4).

Examination of the homosexual male
As in cases of gonorrhoea among homosexuals the urethra may be involved in 60%, the ano-rectum in 40% and the pharynx in about 7%, sampling from *all* these sites should be a routine in every case. In gonococcal urethritis there are generally, but not always, symptoms; in ano-rectal gonorrhoea symptoms may be present only in one-third of cases and in the pharynx the infections tend to be asymptomatic. It is recommended that samples are taken from these sites as follows:

a. Urethral smear and culture.

b. Ano-rectal cultures. Because the lubricants used contain anti-bacterial agents, proctoscopy should be postponed until after the ano-rectal culture has been taken by passing a swab, moistened if necessary with sterile saline, through the anal canal towards the rectum. On proctoscopy, when there is evidence of inflammation with erythema, mucosal oedema, mucopus and blood, it may be possible to obtain a sample of pus in which the gonococcus can be seen on microscopy although diagnosis will require confirmation by culture.

c. Pharyngeal cultures. A swab is passed over the tonsillar area and the back of the pharynx and plated directly on to medium selective for the gonococcus. The microscopic examination of smears from the pharynx for the gonococcus is not useful as a diagnostic procedure.

Two sets of samples from ano-rectal and pharyngeal sites at consecutive follow-up attendances are required before a gonococcal infection is discounted.

Proctoscopy should always be undertaken at the initial clinic attendance of a man who has been the recipient partner during anal intercourse. Symptomless lesions of the anal canal such as warts will be readily identified and the appearance of the distal 5 cm of the rectum should be recorded. As the number of polymorphonuclear leucocytes in a Gram-stained smear of rectal material is highly variable (Ch. 38), we do not recommend enumeration of these cells in the diagnosis of proctitis. Inflammatory changes associated with gonococcal, chlamydial and herpetic infection are generally limited to the distal 10 cm of the rectum, whereas those caused by *Entamoeba histolytica*, *Shigella* spp, *Campylobacter* spp and *Salmonella* spp are seen at sigmoidoscopy to extend more proximally. As a routine diagnostic procedure, we do not advocate sigmoidoscopy unless there has been unexplained rectal bleeding or an organismal cause has not been found for altered bowel habit, ano-rectal discharge, a sensation of incomplete defaecation or pain. With the exception of infection with *C. trachomatis* LGV immunovars, the histology of the proctitis associated with the sexually transmissible enteric pathogens is non-specific, and rectal biopsy is unlikely to be helpful in diagnosis. This procedure which is only rarely complicated by haemorrhage or perforation, may, however, be indicated if the patient's symptoms do not resolve after successful anti-microbial therapy. In the investigation of patients with symptoms of proctitis, in addition to obtaining material for culture for *N. gonorrhoeae*, samples should be taken from the rectal mucosa, preferably by curette (the urethral curette described by Dunlop et al 1964 is suitable for this purpose) for culture for chlamydiae and herpes simplex virus. A stool sample should be examined for bacterial pathogens and protozoa (Ch. 38). Infection with *Giardia intestinalis* is usually symptomless but can produce diarrhoea without evidence of proctitis. In the case of patients with symptoms suggestive of protozoal infection, at least three stool samples should be examined before the diagnosis is excluded. It should be remembered that the use of anti-microbial agents, kaolin and other anti-diarrhoeal preparations may suppress the excretion of cysts.

Venepuncture for serological tests for syphilis (STS) should be carried out at the first visit after the culture tests have been taken. Serological tests for hepatitis B should be carried out in homosexual males, in cases of intravenous drug misuse, in those with tattoos and in those engaging in prostitution.

Examination of the female
As the initial examination above the waist may be carried out while the patient is seated, the taking of a throat culture and venepuncture for STS may be conveniently performed at this stage. Examination below the waist may be completed when the patient is in the semi-lithotomy position.

The abdomen should be examined first by inspection and palpation. The female ano-genital region can only be examined properly for inflammatory disease in the semi-lithotomy position. Disposable plastic gloves should be worn by the examiner.

Inspection and palpation, where necessary, of the anus and external genitalia should be systematic and include:

• Mons veneris and pubic hair
• Inguinal lymph nodes
• Perineum and anus
• Vulva — labia majora, labia minora, vestibule and fourchette
• External urethral meatus

A finger should be inserted into the vaginal orifice and the contents of the urethra and its para-urethral glands massaged towards the orifice. Smears and cultures are taken from this site in all cases.

Orifices of the distal pair of para-urethral glands open on either side of the urethral meatus (Skene's glands).

Smears and cultures can be taken from this site specifically or added to the urethral swab when pus is seen at the duct orifice.

The orifices of the greater vestibular glands (Bartholin's gland) open external to the hymen on the inner side of the labia minora. The gland (1–1.5 cm in diameter) may be examined by passing a finger into the vagina and hooking it behind a point in the substance of the labium majus at the junction of the anterior two-thirds and posterior one-third. It cannot be palpated unless enlarged or fibrotic. By gently massaging the gland and expressing the mucous secretion towards the duct orifice, material may be collected in a loop or cotton-wool applicator for the immediate preparation of a smear and culture.

The next step in the pelvic examination is to pass a self-retaining bivalve speculum of the Cusco type gently into the vagina so that the vaginal walls and cervix may be inspected. The presence and character of any vaginal discharge is noted and a record made concerning its odour, appearance and consistency. A swab is swept along the posterior fornix to collect the vaginal discharge. Specimens are taken routinely from this site as follows:

a. Vaginal film (dry) for Gram-staining is taken to describe the appearance of the bacterial flora and to detect *Candida*. Culture methods are available for *Candida*, *Gardnerella vaginalis*, *Trichomonas vaginalis* and anaerobes.

b. Vaginal film (wet). The discharge is suspended in a drop of saline and covered with a cover-slip for immediate microscopic examination (× 40 objective) for *Trichomonas vaginalis*. Again culture methods may be available to the clinician (Ch. 22).

When appropriate, a swab may be inserted into the cervical canal and swept across the upper part of the vagina, particularly the posterior fornix, to obtain secretions for examination for bacteria which can be isolated by special methods (e.g. *Gardnerella vaginalis*, *Candida* spp, *Trichomonas vaginalis* and anaerobes). The swab may be broken off into a bijou bottle containing Amies' transport medium.

Discharge is removed from the upper vagina and the external os is cleansed with a pledget of wool held in dressing forceps. A plastic bacteriological loop or suitable cotton-wool applicator is passed into the endocervix to obtain endocervical secretions from which a smear is made; this is stained with Gram stain and further secretions obtained with a second swab for plating on selective medium for the gonococcus.

Further samples of secretions and scrapings may be required from the endocervical canal, the os or the vaginal portion of the cervix for the isolation of *Chlamydia* (Ch. 17) or herpesvirus (Ch. 26).

A cervical smear for cytological examination should

be taken before touching the cervix. Using Ayre's method, a special wooden spatula is then used to scrape the superficial cells from the external os and lower end of cervix. The scrapings from the squamocolumnar junction are taken throughout an arc of 360° and a slide prepared and fixed immediately in 95% industrial methylated spirit. The detection of carcinoma of the cervix is discussed in Chapter 25.

After withdrawing the Cusco speculum, a swab is passed gently into the ano-rectum to obtain a sample for immediate plating on selective medium. If skin tags or haemorrhoids make this process difficult a child's proctoscope may be slightly lubricated with saline and passed into the rectum. The swab may now be passed beyond the tip of the proctoscope which is then itself withdrawn and the swab withdrawn gently afterwards.

A bimanual vaginal examination should be carried out gently. The lubricated (K-Y water-soluble lubricating jelly) index and second finger of the right hand are used to separate the labia and are then passed into the vagina. Gently pressing backwards the fingers are gradually passed towards the anterior fornix when the uterus can be palpated by the fingers of the left hand placed well above the symphysis pubis. The fundus of the retroverted uterus can be felt through the posterior fornix. The uterine appendages may be examined through the lateral fornix and a swelling outlined between the fingers of the two hands.

Tenderness in the fornices, with or without swelling of the Fallopian tubes or on movement of the cervix, are signs elicited in inflammatory disease such as in gonococcal infections of the upper genital tract. Inflammatory swellings may also be felt in the rectovaginal pouch (pouch of Douglas).

In the case of the female the urine may be examined after the pelvic examination. Pronounced dysuria or frequency tends to be more often associated with a urinary tract infection due to coliform organisms, than to the gonococcus. Pregnancy tests are often required and a clear understanding of these tests is important (Note 6.5).

Examination of ulcers (see Ch. 37)
Syphilis must be excluded as a cause of any sore in the anal or genital region. After cleansing the surface with a swab soaked in sterile saline, serum is squeezed by gentle pressure from the depth of the lesion. This serum may be collected directly on a cover-slip or, if this is difficult, in a capillary tube. If collected in a glass capillary, one end of the capillary can be sealed in a gas microburner: the column of air beyond the seal is then heated to expel fluid neatly on to the centre of a cover-slip which is then positioned on a slide. After firmly pressing the glass cover-slip and slide between pieces of filter paper, the preparation can be examined by dark

ground illumination. It is useful in a clinic to have the microscope arranged with an automatic focusing device so chances of damaging the oil-immersion lens may be minimized, and rapid examination made easy (the Zeiss research microscope with automatic focusing handle has given excellent service in this busy clinic for many years).

Dark ground examination of serum from all ulcers on genital mucosa or at mucocutaneous junctions is a policy which should be adopted routinely so that a diagnosis of early syphilis may not be missed. Three sets of tests should be taken if syphilis is suspected. The administration of co-trimoxazole tablets (sulphamethoxazole 5 parts, trimethoprim 1 part) 960 mg by mouth twice daily for 5 days will often reduce sepsis sufficiently, without affecting the treponeme, to achieve reduction of the phimosis and to obtain direct access to the ulcer. Lymph node puncture may occasionally yield *Treponema pallidum*. Monoclonal antibodies directed against a specific surface exposed antigen of *T. pallidum* should facilitate the development of diagnostic tests which may supplement or, in the interests of laboratory safety, replace dark-ground examination (see Ch. 8, p. 133; New technological approaches to diagnosis and control).

In homosexuals, typical anal chancres are uncommon, although dark ground examination of radial linear anal fissures, seen in early syphilis in such cases, will often reveal *T. pallidum*.

Culture of fluid from ulcers may yield herpes simplex virus although such a finding does not exclude the possibility of coexisting syphilis.

TRACING OF CONTACTS

It is essential that personnel involved in the tracing of contacts are adequately trained for their task. It is the authors' view that this aspect of the clinical task should fall on those who have had training in the care of patients as well as in community health. In the interviewing of patients a deep appreciation of the medical and social consequences of the various sexually transmissible diseases is essential. An ability to give reasoned explanations about health matters which the patient may have been unable to comprehend when seen by the doctor, is one of the essential educational priorities of this type of work. An open mind, knowledge of sexually transmitted disease and an awareness of the varied nature of human sexuality are essential. Experience in the local community and in the homes of patients are the leavening of experience which will help to prevent or mitigate the sometimes serious social catastrophes. Where appropriate, conciliation should be possible in difficult situations which arise between partners, whether married or not. The diagnosis of gonorrhoea and syphilis, and by implication the diagnosis of other STD may be regarded as defamatory, so there are legal and social obligations requiring the exercise of care and consideration. It is the patient's co-operation which must be sought, and everything should be done to mitigate not only the medical but the social consequences arising from the diagnosis.

In the tracing of contacts, as in the United Kingdom, it is useful to have some procedures common to all clinics in the country although methods of approach acceptable in one city may not be appropriate in another. At its simplest, a patient may be asked to give his or her consort a personal note, usually called a contact slip, to bring to the clinic. This note may be headed with the name of the clinic and contain a record of the patient's case number, his or her diagnosis in the code used in the locality or that to be found in the International Classification of Diseases (see Note 5.3) and the date of the diagnosis. Such a personal note can be readily interpreted in any clinic using the code, and the patient's anonymity is secure in the event of its loss.

If a contact is to be looked for in another part of the United Kingdom then a special contact tracing form (e.g. Special Clinic Contact Report; Department of Health & Social Security) may be sent to the physician in charge of the clinic serving the area concerned. When the name and address of the contact is known, limited additional details of description are needed. If only a forename is known and descriptions are inadequate, successful contact-tracing is rare. Recognizing that these forms together with the searching to be undertaken may be regarded as defamatory, personnel responsible for the process, including the medical staff, must exercise care and judgement in every case. In the process of tracing contacts the patient may be persuaded to help but it is not permissible to use any form of trick or coercion to obtain information. It is essential to treat individuals with respect and make sure that confidential information is not communicated to others. Threats are never justified; the exercise demands persuasion by explanation, kindness and tact. Initial failures may be rewarded by patience, and delays are preferable to the harmful effects of threats.

In the context of this Chapter an attempt has been made to put together a working guide as an indicator of priorities in the tracing of contacts (Table 6.1).

Table 6.1 Some priorities in tracing contacts. *See text; Chapter 5(a), (c), (e) & (f) especially.

Diagnosis	Degree of danger to a sexual partner (+ to +++)	Degree of priority for rapid contact-tracing (+ to +++)	Comment on priority
Acquired early-stage syphilis	+++	+++	Essential
Acquired late-stage syphilis	0	0	Except in a long-term partner.
Gonorrhoea	+++	+++	Essential
Non-gonococcal urethritis in the male. Chlamydial infection in male/female	++	++	Highly desirable
Lymphogranuloma venereum	++	++	Highly desirable
Trichomoniasis	+	+	Desirable in regular partner.
Candidosis	+	+	Desirable in regular partner if patient has recurrent infection.
Scabies	+	+	Treatment of household or family mostly advisable.
Pthirus pubis	+	+	Desirable in partner(s).
Herpes genitalis	Uncertain	Varies	Regular cervical cytology smears encouraged. If partner is pregnant examination justified; isolations important during six weeks before term.
Cytomegalovirus infection	+	+	Primary infection in pregnancy may be a danger to the fetus.
Genital warts	+	++	Highly desirable
Hepatitis B virus infection	+++	+++	Tracing of contacts justified, particularly in pregnancy. Vaccination available. Counselling in carrier and others.
Molluscum contagiosum	+	+	Desirable in regular partner.
Marburg disease, Lassa and Ebola fever	+++	+++	Essential to prevent spread of these rare epidemic diseases with a high mortality. Sexual intercourse is not the main method of spread.
HIV infection (AIDS)	+++	*	Counselling essential to prevent spread of this dangerous infection.

SOCIAL ASPECTS

Those involved in helping patients to resolve their social and personal problems which arise as a regular feature of STD clinical work, whether the clinician or health visitor, should be alert to possible needs of the patient, particularly financial or interpersonal which may fall within the ambit of medical social work. Specific matters are given fuller consideration in Chapter 5 but, in particular, all patients of 16 years of age or less require special attention in every case and an endeavour should be made to allow young patients to reconsider their life-style in relation to the risks that are taken. It gives opportunities to individuals to express their anxieties and problems as well as for the tendering of advice.

NOTES TO CHAPTER 6

Note 6.1: Transport medium for *Chlamydia*

'2SP' is 2.4 ml of a sucrose-phosphate solution i.e. 0.2 M sucrose in 0.02 M phosphate buffer pH 7.2 with 50 μg/ml of streptomycin, 100 μg vancomycin, and, except for 2SP to be used for conjunctival specimens, 25 units/ml of nystatin. Specimens may be stored at $-70°$ C before culture (Gordon et al 1969).

Note 6.2: Proteinuria

The urine 'stick' test (e.g. the multiple reagent strips, Multistix — Ames, Stoke Poges) is good for screening for proteinuria; the strip is impregnated with tetrabromphenol blue and buffered at pH 3.5. Based on the 'protein error of indicators' principle, the presence of protein results in the development of a green colour. The test yields negative results with normal urines, so any positive result greater than 'trace' indicates significant proteinuria. Clinical judgement is necessary in the interpretation of 'trace' results which may occur in urines of high specific gravity with non-significant proteinuria. The 'trace' result corresponds to 0.05–0.2 g per litre albumin but the test is less sensitive to globulin, Bence-Jones protein and microproteins, so that a negative result does not rule out the presence of these proteins. False-positive results may occur with alkaline, highly buffered urines or in the presence of contaminating quaternary ammonium compounds. Contamination of the urine sample with chlorhexide antiseptic will give false positive reading for protein (manufacturer's data). Although the rate of protein excretion rather than the urinary concentration is more relevant in determining pathological states, and the sensitivity of the 'stick' test depends upon the rate of urinary flow, the discovery of a positive result greater than the 'trace' necessitates referral for fuller renal investigation. Late effects of a nephropathy include hypertension and impaired renal function, but the discovery of symptomless mesangial IgA nephropathy may often depend upon the detection of abnormalities of the urine on routine testing (Kincaid-Smith 1985).

Note 6.3: Symptomless microscopic haematuria

Urine 'stick' tests for the presence of blood in the urine are very sensitive; they (e.g. the multiple reagent strips, Multistix — Ames, Stoke Poges) detect 150–620 μg/l free haemoglobin (or 5–20 $\times 10^6$ intact red blood cells per litre) in urines with a specific gravity of 1005 and ascorbic acid concentrations of less than 0.28 mmol per litre. They are less sensitive in urines with higher specific gravity or greater ascorbic acid content. The test is slightly more sensitive to free haemoglobin and myoglobin than to intact red cells. The appearance of green spots on the reacted reagent used indicates the presence of intact red cells in the urine. Certain oxidizing contaminants, such as betadine lotion, hypochlorite and microbial peroxidase associated with urinary tract infection, may cause false-positive results. Blood is often, but not always found in the urine of menstruating females.

The test is based on the peroxidase-like activity of haemoglobin which catalyses the reaction of cumene hydroperoxide

and 3, 3', 5, 5'-tetramethylbenzidine. The resulting colour ranges from orange through green to dark blue. When using the 'stick' test, all reagent areas on plastic strips should be immersed in a freshly voided, well-mixed, uncentrifuged urine specimen collected in a clean container. If testing is not possible within one hour after voiding, the urine should be refrigerated and returned to room temperature before testing. After immersion the edge of the strip should be tapped against the side of the container to remove excess urine and afterwards the strip should be held horizontally to prevent possible mixing of chemicals from adjacent reagent areas and soiling of the hands. The test areas should then be compared with corresponding colour charts on the bottle label at the reading times specified for each area. The strip should be held close to the colour blocks, the colours matched carefully. *Accurate timing is essential for reliable quantitative results.* All reagent areas may be read between 1 and 2 minutes for qualitative results. The reagent strips should be stored at temperatures under 30 °C only in the original bottles containing the desiccant which should not be removed (manufacturer's data, Ames Division, Miles Laboratories Ltd., Stoke Poges, Slough, SL2 4LY, England).

Microscopy of centrifuged urine sediment will reveal some red cells in all specimens of urine (Freni et al 1977) and this reflects the small but continuous loss of blood from the urinary tract (viz. less than 0.5×10^6 red blood cells per litre: Kesson et al 1978). In many laboratories it is usual to express haematuria as the number of cells seen per high power field (HPF) but the HPF covers a variable volume of urine, and Kesson et al (1978) showed that this method failed to reveal half of their cases of microscopic haematuria in patients with known renal disease. To obtain accurate results the urine should be centrifuged in tubes with pointed bottoms, the sediment resuspended in a known volume of fluid and the cells counted in a counting chamber.

With respect to the 'stick' test, any positive result is indicative of microscopic haematuria well above the suggested normal count. Occasionally the blood will be a contaminant from the vagina, hyperplastic intrameatal warts or in some cases in urethritis. Although in patients under the age of 40 years only 2% of those with symptomless microscopic haematuria will have a lesion that is life-threatening or requires major surgery, full investigation is essential.

Preliminaries will have included examination of the urethral meatus and of any urethral discharge. Tests will have been taken to exclude *Neisseria gonorrhoeae* and, when facilities are readily available, also *Chlamydia trachomatis*. Inspection of the urine microscopically for white cells and culture of a clean-catch specimen of urine are necessary at this stage. Subsequently examination for malignant cells and casts should follow. A full clinical examination should follow and include the taking of the blood pressure. For the patient under the age of 40 years the following will be considered.

Bacteriuria. The subject of bacteriuria has been discussed in Chapter 24 and its discovery in a young man is an indication for full investigation including urography and cystoscopy. In the young woman with haematuria, signs and symptoms of cystitis and a positive urine culture treatment should be given for the cystitis and, if on follow-up urinalysis is normal, no further investigation is needed (Benson & Brewer 1981). Evaluation will be needed should the haematuria persist after antibiotic or chemotherapy.

EXERCISE-RELATED HAEMATURIA

A specific syndrome '10 000 metre haematuria' has been described by Blacklock (1977) in the long-distance runner, involved in distances of 10^5 metres or longer. It occurs at the first voiding of urine after completion of the run and is typically profuse, sometimes with the passage of clots. Usually painless, there is sometimes suprapubic discomfort with some reference of pain to the tip of the penis. Cystoscopy within 48 hours reveals localized contusions with loss of epithelium and fibrinous exudate on the interureteric bar with extension laterally overlying the intramural ureter on each side. The posterior rim of the internal meatus has shown similar changes. The 'mirror image' lesions seen suggest that repetitive impact, minor in itself, produces the injury during a long run and it has been postulated that if there is sufficient urine within the bladder its cushioning effect prevents the apposition of the posterior bladder wall and the trigone. The lesion is superficial injury and theoretically could be preventable by the intake of fluid before running or the omission of bladder emptying before each run commences. Neither recommendation is easily acceptable by the dedicated athlete for fear of interfering with running performance (Blacklock 1977).

In sports, including those involving minimal trauma (e.g. swimming, lacrosse, track-running, football and rowing), haematuria is directly related to the duration of exercise and the energy consumed. During exercise blood is shunted from the splanchnic area and other organs including the kidney, and reduction in its blood flow may lead to hypoxia (Alyea & Parish 1958). It has been described as the renal response to exercise (Woodhouse 1982).

This exercise-related haematuria appears to be a frequent (9 of 50 marathon runners tested) self-limiting and benign condition and patients should be spared invasive testing unless its occurrence persists beyond 48–72 hours (Siegel et al 1979).

Haemoglobinuria occurs with prolonged trauma to the feet or hands in those susceptible. There is a raised serum haemoglobin, lowered serum haptoglobin and methaemalbuminaemia. If the haemolysis is sufficient to exceed the haemoglobin-binding capacity of the haptoglobins haemoglobinuria results. This 'march' haemoglobinuria may be prevented by wearing thick-soled shoes (Spicer 1970).

SCHISTOSOMIASIS

Haematuria, often at the end of micturition, is a characteristic early feature of infection with *Schistosoma haematobium*. The principal means of diagnosing all human schistosome infections remains the detection of ova in urine and faeces. In *Schistosoma mansoni* infection diagnosis is reached by demonstrating the ova in the stool, but intestinal biopsy through a proctoscope or sigmoidoscope is also an effective means of finding eggs; such biopsy may also be positive in *S. haemotobium* or *S. japonicum* infections. In *S. japonicum* infection eggs are more commonly deposited in ectopic sites than those of other schistosome species (Peters & Gilles 1977).

Immunological methods are available and the circumoval precipitation technique (COPT) remains popular. Competitive micro-enzyme linked immunosorbent assay (micro-ELISA) and radioimmunoassay (RIA) are additional techniques available. Attempts to develop and standardize antigen and improve stage, strain and species specificity proceed (Sturrock 1985).

HAEMOGLOBINOPATHIES

Unexplained haematuria in West Africans may be associated with haemoglobin SC disease, detected readily in the laboratory by starch gel electrophoresis of haemoglobin.

MORPHOLOGY OF ERYTHROCYTES IN HAEMATURIA

Glomerulonephritis

Although patients with proteinuria and accompanying haematuria — discovered by the stick test — are likely to be investigated for glomerular disease, those with haematuria and normal urinary protein may be subjected to extensive urological investigations when a more appropriate line of investigation would be renal function testing and renal biopsy.

In recent years it has been reported that the morphology of red cells found in the haematuria due to glomerular injury differs from that of non-glomerular bleeding (Chang 1982, Fairley & Birch 1982, Fassett et al 1982). Damage to the erythrocytes in glomerular disease may be due to a distortion during passage through the glomerular basement membrane or, more likely, due to osmotic changes in the distal nephron (Hauglustaine et al 1982). Red cells in urine in non-glomerular diseases (NG) have normal erythrocyte morphology, whereas those in glomerular disease (G) are markedly dysmorphic. The dysmorphism ranges widely; for example red cells may show extruded phase-dense blobs of cytoplasm; there may be granular deposits of phase-dense material around the inner aspect of the cell membrane; or red cells may have the appearance of 'doughnut cells' with cytoplasm extrusions (Fairley & Birch 1982). Morphological changes can be seen by phase-contrast microscopy, but staining techniques have been advised as useful simpler routine procedures (Iseghem et al 1983).

The site of urinary bleeding has been predicted in 85% of patients for whom a definite diagnosis was possible; in 11% haematuria was mixed, and an incorrect assessment of the site of bleeding was made in only 4%. The assessment of urinary red-cell morphology by means of phase-contrast microscopy can add importantly to clinical information and, together with the presence of red-cell casts and protein in the urine, can help the clinician decide on initial investigations in patients with haematuria (Fasset et al 1982). In patients presenting with gross haematuria, changes in red-cell morphology may not be clear cut and repeated examination of the urinary sediment may be necessary to avoid unnecessary urological investigations (Iseghem et al 1983). Examination of urinary casts for immunoglobulins, complement and fibrin provides a further non-invasive method for distinguishing patients with active glomerular disease (Fairley & Birch 1982).

The phase-contrast microscopy required for determining red-cell morphology in urine requires individual skill and experience, and as a result is not easy to set up as a service. It has been shown that a urinary-cell-size distribution curve can be obtained with speed and clarity with the use of an autoanalyser (Coulter counter S-plus II; Coulter Electronics Inc., Hialeah, Florida, USA). In this procedure about 10 ml of urine (from a midstream urine sample) is centrifuged at $600 g$ for 5 min. The supernatant is removed and the resuspended deposit analysed by means of the Coulter counter with the X-Y recorder attachment. Large differences in size distribution are seen in glomerular and non-glomerular cells. Patients with glomerular-cell-size distribution can be spared needless urological examinations and can be directly referred to a renal physician for consultation about renal biopsy. Those with a non-glomerular distribution can be referred for the essential urological investigations (Shichiri et al 1986).

Calculi, congenital anomalies, tumour, damage to renal papillae

In those with haematuria, apart from proven cystitis in the female; proven glomerulonephritis; and in young patients with haematuria that is clearly exercise-related, an excretion urogram is mandatory. If there is doubt concerning renal function a serum creatinine measurement should precede the excretion urogram.

The finding of congenital anomaly or stone necessitates referral since surgical judgement is required regarding further investigation and management. Retrograde ureteropyelogram will enable delineation of a filling defect in the renal pelvis or ureter, whether due to tumour, blood clot, sloughed renal papilla or non-opaque stone, and a cystoscopy will enable a co-existent bladder lesion to be excluded. Ultrasound, arteriograms and computed axial tomography (CAT) scanning are other techniques available to the urological surgeon (Benson & Brewer 1981).

Note 6.4: Hepatitis B virus (HBV) and human immunodeficiency viruses (HIV)

INFECTION CONTROL GUIDELINES

Virus infections, particularly hepatitis B, are an occupational hazard for health workers, who are at greater risk of contracting hepatitis B from their patients than vice versa. In clinics dealing with sexually transmissible infections, staff are repeatedly exposed to the risk of accidental infection so those who routinely carry out venepunctures or who handle other secretions should adhere scrupulously to sound hygienic measures. They should wear gloves and avoid, for example, touching their mouth or eyes with their hands; procedures for the safe handling of all clinical specimens should be meticulous. Vaccination with hepatitis B vaccine should be made available to all staff.

Although hepatitis B is infective, effective steps are available to protect anyone who has pricked herself or himself with a needle used to obtain blood from an infected person. In the case of HIV, the causative agent of the Acquired Immune Deficiency Syndrome (AIDS), transmission to health personnel by a needle prick is as yet known only in four cases when there was accidental injection of a small amount of blood; in contrast to hepatitis B there is no effective counter measure against the infection once acquired.

SPECIMENS FOR LABORATORY TESTS

Rules should be adopted for the taking and sending of all specimens for laboratory investigation (blood, specimens of mucus or discharge in 2SP or virus transport medium and, in fact, all bacteriological samples).

The nurse in the clinic *must* be told, before specimens are taken, that they specimens from a patient within the high risk group.

HIGH RISK SPECIMENS

These include those taken from the following patients.

1. Known or suspected carriers of hepatitis B.
2. a. Persons with opportunistic infections that are not associated with other underlying immunosuppressive disease or therapy.
   b. Patients under 60 years of age with Kaposi's sarcoma.
   c. Patients with chronic generalized lymphadenopathy.
   d. Patients with unexplained weight loss or prolonged unexplained fever.
   e. Patients with AIDS or increased risk of AIDS viz. homosexual/bisexual males; IV drug abusers; haemophilia patients; or heterosexual contacts of bisexual males or IV drug abusers.

It is the responsibility of the doctor to determine whether the patient's specimen is in the 'high risk' category.

TAKING VENOUS BLOOD SAMPLES

1. The arm should rest on a towel covered with a paper sheet.
2. The paper sheet should be discarded, preferably every time or at least at intervals, and particularly when contaminated with blood. If contamination with blood occurs, both towel and paper sheet should be discarded; the former should be placed with the soiled linen and the latter with soiled dressings into a plastic sack designated for that purpose (e.g. yellow in colour), or into the CINBIN (a rigid wall puncture-resistant container).
3. When a patient is considered to be in an *at risk group, then gloves must be worn* by the person carrying out the venepuncture, and the patient's arm laid on a plastic sheet. This plastic sheet should be discarded afterwards, whether contaminated or not.
4. The blood sample should be emptied *gently* into the screw-capped container, to avoid frothing which generates droplets and aerosols. Caps must be firmly in place. Screw-topped containers with overhang are much the safest. Label the specimen bottle 'Risk of Infection'.
5. The container and contents are then sealed in a plastic bag labelled 'High Risk Specimen' for transmission to the laboratory for serological testing.
6. A supply of Cidex is to be kept in the clinic and activated when require This activated Cidex is used for cleaning away any blood spillage from metal or other surfaces.
7. Any person who sustains a needle prick (or where contamination of the face, mouth, nose or eyes has occurred), should inform the doctor and sister, who will record the event. A blood sample should be taken from the patient for an urgent examination for hepatitis B surface antigen. Generally advice is available from the virologist.
8. After taking blood remove needle carefully. *Do not resheath needle after use.* To avoid risk of injury the needle and syringe should be placed carefully in a CINBIN for incineration.

TAKING OTHER SAMPLES

Good technique is important (Collins 1983). Plastic loops ($0.1 \mu l–1.0 \mu l$) are preferred to Nicrome wire, but if the latter used the internal diameter the loop should be 2–3 mm completely closed, with a shank not longer than 5–6 mm and secured in a proper aluminium or alloy loop holder. Replace the loop when bent or encrusted with carbonized material. Care and gentle handling are needed, as droplets and aerosols are made if the loop is wielded energetically when withdrawn. Bottles of sterile saline or buffered isotonic salts solution should be available in single packs as otherwise *Pseudomonas* and algae may grow, and contamination is frequent.

All specimens being stored at −70 °C or −20 °C should be placed in a *closed plastic bag*, the high risk specimens in a high risk bag.

PRECAUTIONS TO BE TAKEN BY STAFF DEALING WITH PATIENTS WHOSE SAMPLES ARE IN HIGH-RISK CATEGORY

1. Gloves should be worn by persons in contact with blood, blood specimens, any body fluids, excretions, articles or surfaces potentially contaminated by them. After any such contact hands should be washed immediately with soap and water.

2. Bench or other surfaces contaminated with blood or other body fluid should be cleaned immediately with activated Cidex.

3. Protective eye wear (goggles) should be worn only in situations where splatter with blood, blood-contaminated secretions or body fluid is expected.

4. Linen and fomites of contaminated disposable items considered as soiled should be identified as infectious waste and placed in a plastic sack designated for that purpose (e.g. orange in colour). The plastic sack and contents can then be sent for incineration.

5. Lensed instruments, e.g. the fibre optic fitting for the anoscope, should be cleaned and disinfected with ethylene oxide after each use.

6. Out-patients with AIDS or hepatitis B may use common waiting areas and bathroom facilities.

7. Gowns are recommended for those likely to have direct contact with patient's secretions, excretions or blood.

NOTES ON SUPPLIERS, ETC

A number of references are available on the subject of infection control: Finegold 1983, San Francisco Task Force 1983. Further details are discussed in Chapters 30 and 31.

'Cestra' clinical sheets (absorbent non-woven fabric) 45 × 27 cm, code no.101405; Robinsons, Chesterfield, England.

CINBIN, Metal Box Ltd., Labco, 54 Marlow Bottom Road, Marlow, Buckinghamshire, SL7 3NF, England. Bins can be incinerated.

Cidex (Ethicon) A 2% solution of glutaraldehyde, to which an activating powder is added before use to make a buffered solution, which is stable for 14 days. The activator acts as a corrosion inhibitor and gives optimum activity to aqueous solutions.

Note 6.5: Pregnancy tests

Tests for pregnancy (Hobson 1974) are required when there is a need for immediate information concerning the existence or otherwise of pregnancy. Early diagnosis depends upon the measurement of chorionic gonadotrophin (Heap & Flint 1984)

and makes it easier to secure the social and medical support required in antenatal care. If pregnancy exists, termination may be necessary for social or therapeutic reasons and the earlier in the pregnancy this is undertaken the less danger there is to the woman. Tests are carried out on urine and the immunological test (IPT) ordinarily used is the latex agglutination test.

Immunological tests for pregnancy react positively when chorionic gonadotrophin (hCG) is present in the urine. A positive result indicates the secretory activity of trophoblastic tissue usually associated with the presence of a viable fetus. There is close parallelism between trophoblastic mass and hCG levels in the maternal serum which double every 36–48 hours during early pregnancy. hCG is produced before the missed but expected menstrual period and in increasing amounts until a peak is reached about 8 weeks after conception. There is a dramatic fall after this peak but the hormone is excreted throughout normal pregnancy and into the post-partum period. Latex agglutination tests do not distinguish between pituitary luteinizing hormone (LH) and hCG, but results of these tests are correctly positive in the absence of a fetus when a hydatidiform mole, chorioadenoma or choriocarcinoma is present. Similarly, urine from men with testicular tumours containing trophoblastic tissue will evoke a positive reaction. To exclude pregnancy as a cause of secondary amenorrhoea, particularly in women approaching the menopause, quantitative determination of whole hCG and free beta-subunit in serum should be used since such women may excrete enough LH to produce a false-positive result with the latex agglutination test whereas such cross reaction does not occur with the former test. In disturbed or ectopic pregnancy the results of the tests may either be positive or negative, indicating the secretory activity of the trophoblast and not necessarily the viability of the fetus.

The majority of false negative results with the latex test are due to tests being done too soon after the missed but expected period or during the second or third trimester of pregnancy when urinary hCG levels are low. Whereas a latex agglutination test in urine gives a positive result in only 50% of ectopic pregnancies, the hCG beta-subunit radioimmune assay is positive in 95% (Leading Article (Lancet) 1980). With the recently developed magnetic immunoradiometric assay quantitative determination of hCG and its beta-subunit (hCG MAIA-CLONE kit, Serono Diagnostics, Woking, Surrey) can be carried out in 15 minutes on serum, plasma, or urine (Rattle et al 1984) and pregnancy can be detected 6 days after implantation — or 3–4 weeks after the last menstrual period — compared with the 5–6 weeks after the last menstrual period in the case of the latex agglutination urine tests (manufacturer's data). Although referral to a gynaecologist is indicated when ectopic pregnancy is being considered as a possibility, the hCG measurement is a useful initial step to rule out the non-pregnant patient viz. when hCG levels are lower than 6000 mIU/ml. Besides recognizing risk factors for ectopic pregnancy in the patient (e.g. the use of a intrauterine contraceptive device, infertility in those undergoing various treatments for sterility including tubal surgery, a previous ectopic pregnancy and salpingitis) ectopic pregnancy is to be suspected in those with the classic triad of abdominal pain, uterine bleeding and the presence of an adnexal mass. The desirable approach to diagnosis entails early recognition before rupture and in any case before 14 weeks from the last menstrual period: final diagnosis depends on the use of techniques including ultrasonography, serial hCG measurements and diagnostic laparoscopy.

REFERENCES

Alyea E P, Parish H H 1958 Renal response to exercise — urinary findings. Journal of the American Medical Association 167: 807–813

Benson G S, Brewer E D 1981 Haematuria, algorithms for diagnosis. II Haematuria in the adult and haematuria secondary to trauma. Journal of the American Medical Association 246: 993–995

Blacklock N J 1977 Bladder trauma in the long-distance runner: '10,000 metres haematuria'. British Journal of Urology 49: 129–132

Chang B S 1982 RBC morphology in glomerular (G) and non-glomerular (NG) haematuria. Abstracts. The American Society of Nephrology, Washington DC. Kidney International 21: 147

Collins C H 1983 Laboratory-acquired infections. Butterworth, London, p 62–63

De Bono E 1985 Conflicts, a better way to resolve them. Harrap, London (ISBN 0 245-54322-8) p 39–41 and throughout book

Dunlop E M, Jones B R, Al-Hussaini K 1964 Genital infection in association with TRIC virus infection of the eye. III Clinical and other findings, preliminary report. British Journal of Venereal Diseases 40: 33–42

Fairley K F, Birch D F 1982 Haematuria — a simple method for identifying glomerular bleeding. Kidney International 21: 105–108

Fassett R G, Horgan B A, Mathew T H 1982 Detection of glomerular bleeding by phase contrast microscopy. Lancet i: 1432–1434

Finegold S M 1983 Protecting health personnel. In: Cahill K M (ed) The AIDS epidemic. Hutchinson, London, p 133–134

Freni S C, Dalderup L M, Oudegeest J J, Wensveen N 1977 Erythrocyturia, smoking and occupation. Journal of Clinical Pathology 30: 341–344

Goffman E 1963 Stigma: Notes on the management of spoiled identity. Prentice-Hall, New Jersey, and Penguin Books, Harmondsworth, p 28, 160, 175, 189, 193

Gordon F B, Harper I A, Quan A L, Treharne J D, Dwyer R St C, Garland J A 1969 Detection of Chlamydia (Bedsonia) in certain infections of man. 1. Laboratory procedures: Comparison of yolk sac and cell culture for detection and isolation. Journal of Infectious Diseases 120: 451–462

Hauglustaine D, Bollens W, Michielsen P 1982 Detection of glomerular bleeding using a simple staining method for light microscopy. Correspondence, Lancet ii: 761

Heap R B, Flint A P F 1984 Pregnancy. In: Austin C R,

Short R V (eds) Reproduction in mammals. 3: Hormonal control of reproduction, 2nd edn. Cambridge University Press, Cambridge, p 153–194

Hobson B M 1974 Bibliography (with review) on advances in human pregnancy testing. Reproduction Research Information Service Ltd., 141 Newmarket Road, Cambridge CB5 8HA, England, p 1–2; 111–112

Iseghem Ph Van, Hauglustaine D, Bollens W, Michielsen P 1983 Urinary erythrocyte morphology in acute glomerulonephritis. British Medical Journal 287: 1183

Kesson A M, Talbott J M, Gyory A Z 1978 Microscopic examination of urine. Lancet ii: 809–812

Kincaid-Smith P S 1985 Mesangial IgA nephropathy. Leading article, British Medical Journal 290: 96–97.

Leading Article 1980 Removing the guesswork from diagnosis in ectopic pregnancy. Lancet i: 188

Peters W, Gilles H M 1977 Color atlas of hospital medicine and parasitology year book. Medical Publishers Inc., Chicago, p 180–207

Rattle S J, Purnell D R, Williams P I M, Siddle K, Forrest G C 1984 New separation method for monoclonal immunoradiometric assays and its application to assays for thyrotropin and human choriogonadotropin. Clinical Chemistry 30(9): 1457–1461

San Francisco Task Force on the Acquired Immunodeficiency Syndrome 1983 Infection-control guidelines for patients with the acquired immunodeficiency syndrome AIDS. The New England Journal of Medicine 309: 740–744

Shichiri M, Oowada A, Nishio Y, Tomita K, Shiigai T 1986 Use of autoanalyser to examine urinary-red-cell morphology in the diagnosis of glomerular haematuria. Lancet ii: 781–782

Siegel A J, Hennekens C H, Solomon H S, van Boeckel B 1979 Exercise related haematuria. Findings in a group of marathon runners. Journal of the American Medical Association 241: 391–392

Spicer A J 1970 Studies on march haemoglobinuria. British Medical Journal 1: 155–156

Sturrock R F 1985 Schistosomiasis: control programmes and related studies. Tropical Diseases Bulletin 82(9): R1–R13

Whitby L G, Percy-Robb I W, Smith A F 1984 Lecture notes on clinical chemistry, 3rd edn. Blackwell Scientific Publications, Oxford, p 31–33

Woodhouse C R J 1982 Symptomless abnormalities microscopic haematuria. British Journal of Hospital Medicine 27: 163–168

7

Syphilis: introduction

Syphilis is an infectious disease caused by the bacterium *Treponema pallidum*. It is spread principally by sexual intercourse but may also be acquired congenitally, that is to say, by the fetus infected in utero by the mother. The disease is systemic from the onset and fluctuates between short symptomatic and prolonged asymptomatic stages. The natural course of infection may span several decades.

Syphilis is conveniently divided into stages, early infectious and late non-infectious (Table 7.1). In the early infectious stage of the disease lesions occur on the moist mucocutaneous parts of the body, particularly the genitalia. These lesions contain many treponemes and enable transmission to occur by sexual intercourse. Even if untreated, these lesions tend to heal but may recur during the first 2–4 years, after which they heal and the disease becomes latent or hidden. The latent form or the non-infectious late stage of the disease may persist for decades without producing obvious clinical changes, but a proportion of patients will unpredictably develop active involvement of the cardiovascular system (about 10%), the central nervous system (about 10%), or localized gummatous destructive lesions which can affect the musculo-skeletal system (about 10%), the

Table 7.1 Classification of stages of syphilis. A patient whose serological tests for syphilis are positive, but in whom there are no clinical signs of the disease, no abnormality of the cerebrospinal fluid, and no past history of treatment of syphilis, is said to be suffering from latent syphilis. The distinction between early latent and late latent syphilis is an arbitrary one. Early latent syphilis refers to infection, diagnosed on serological grounds, and acquired within the preceding two years.

Acquired syphilis:
1. Early stage
   a. Primary
   b. Secondary
   c. Early latent
2. Late stage
   a. Gummatous ('benign')
   b. Cardiovascular
   c. Central nervous system
   d. Late-stage latent

viscera and mucous membranes (about 15%).

In both early and late stages of syphilis an infected mother can communicate the disease to her unborn fetus. Although the disease can be transmitted to the fetus transplacentally long after a mother has ceased to be sexually infectious, the longer she has had the disease the less likely is this to occur.

If treated in the early stage clinical cure can be achieved by penicillin treatment and with certain other antibiotics. In the late stages curative effects are often spectacular in some forms of neurosyphilis and in gummatous syphilis. In cardiovascular forms of the disease the effects of antibiotic therapy are not easy to define.

AETIOLOGY

The causative organism of syphilis, *Treponema pallidum*, is a delicate spiralled filament 6–20 μm in length. Members of the genus *Treponema* (treponemes) are found in the oral cavity, intestinal tract, and genital areas of man and animals. Whereas commensal species of treponeme can be cultured by employing appropriate cell-free culture media, the treponemes which are pathogenic to man cannot. Inability to cultivate these pathogenic treponemes has hindered our understanding of their biology but applications of modern methods, such as electron microscopy (Hovind-Hougan 1976) and DNA reassociation assays have enabled progress to be made. Miao & Fieldsteel (1980) demonstrated 100% homology between DNA of *T. pallidum* and *T. pertenue* and as a result of this finding and other similarities both are now considered to be the same species: because of the different degrees of virulence and clinical symptoms in man and their different ability to infect various laboratory animals, *T. pertenue* is considered as a subspecies of *T. pallidum* (see also Ch. 2).

The main differential characteristics of the non-cultivable treponemes are given in Table 7.2.

Diseases caused by the three subspecies of *T. pallidum* and *T. carateum* are referred to collectively as the treponematoses (see Ch. 13).

Table 7.2 Characteristic features of infection by non-cultivable 'subspecies' of the genus *Treponema* (modified from Smibert 1984).

Feature	*Treponema pallidum*			*T.carateum*	*T.paraluiscuniculi*
	subsp *pallidum*	subsp *pertenue*	subsp *endemicum*		
Natural host:					
Homo sapiens	+	+	+	+	−
Oryctolagus cuniculus (rabbit)	−	−	−	−	+
Nature of infection, potential to affect:					
skin, bone, viscera and CNS	+	−	−	−	−
skin and bone only	−	+	+	−	−
skin only	−	−	−	+	+
Transmission:					
sexual intercourse	+	−	−	−	+
close contact, mainly in childhood	−	+	+	+	
Geographical distribution:					
worldwide	+	−	−	−	
restricted (Middle East, SE Asia, previously in Yugoslavia)	−	−	+	−	
tropical, W and E hemispheres	−	+	−	−	
tropical, W hemisphere	−	−	−	+	
Cutaneous lesions produced experimentally in:					
O.cuniculus	+	+	+	−	
Mesocricetus auratus (hamster)	−	+	+	−	
Mus musculus (mouse)	−	−	−	−	
Cavia porcellus (guinea pig)	−	−	+	−	

T. pallidum subspecies *pallidum* is the only pathogenic treponeme indigenous to Britain. It is the cause of venereal and congenital syphilis in man. It is the most virulent with the capacity to cause pathological effects in the skin, bone, viscera and central nervous system.

T. pallidum subspecies *pertenue* is the cause of yaws, a non-venereal but communicable disease, found in tropical countries. It is regarded as intermediate in virulence of the three subspecies with the capacity to involve the skin and bone.

T. pallidum subspecies '*endemicum*' is the cause of non-venereal endemic syphilis known as 'bejel' in the Middle East.

T. carateum is the cause of pinta, a mild contagious disease similar to yaws but confined to the Central and South Americas. It is regarded as the least virulent of the three species with the capacity to involve only the skin.

T. paraluiscuniculi produces benign venereal spirochaetosis (rabbit spirochaetosis or rabbit syphilis) in rabbits.

Many commensal species of *Treponema* occur in the mouth (e.g. *T. denticola*, *T. vincentii*, *T. scolodontum*) and on the mucous surfaces of the genitalia (e.g. *T. refringens*, *T. minutum*, *T. phagedenis*) where their differ-entiation is important in the diagnosis of primary syphilis (see Ch. 2).

Treponema pallidum

Morphology and staining
T. pallidum is a delicate tightly coiled spiralled filament 6–10 μm (average 10–13 μm) by 0.1–0.18 μm in diameter (average 0.13–0.15 μm) with 6–12 regular coils: the wavelength of the coils is 1.1 μm and the amplitude 0.2–0.3 μm. The ends of the cells are pointed and covered with a sheath.

T. pallidum is feebly refractile and too narrow to be seen well by ordinary light microscopy. Dark ground illumination is normally used to examine the organism and this was the technique described by Fritz Schaudinn and Erich Hoffmann in 1905 to demonstrate that *T. pallidum* was the cause of syphilis: details relating to this discovery can be found in a brief biography of Schaudinn (Thorburn 1971). Special techniques such as silver impregnation may be used to demonstrate the organism, particularly in tissue, but this tends to alter the morphology. Immunofluorescent techniques can now be used to demonstrate the organism in tissues and body fluids. The presence of a capsular or slime layer has been observed occasionally on the surface of *T*.

pallidum and this may explain the lack of serological reactivity of organisms freshly isolated from animal tissues. *Treponema*-associated mucopolysaccharides may be part of the capsular layer or may be derived from tissue constituents of the host.

T. pallidum, like other spirochaetes comprises a central protoplasmic cylinder consisting of cytoplasmic and nuclear regions enclosed by a cytoplasmic membrane and a cell wall containing peptidoglycan. When isolated, the peptidoglycan retains a helical configuration indicating that it determines the shape of the cell.

Between the cell wall and the outer envelope lie the axial filaments or internal flagella which are presumed to be responsible for motility although there is no direct evidence for this. There are three movements that propel spirochaetes: slow undulation, corkscrew-like rotation and a sluggish backwards and forwards motion. *T. pallidum* often displays a characteristic tendency to bend at right angles near its midpoint. Spirochaetal motion persists at high viscosity which blocks the flagellar motion of ordinary bacteria, suggesting a possible basis for the evolution of the complex structure of spirochaetes.

A multilayered membrane, referred to as the outer envelope or outer membrane, encloses the cell. This outer envelope contains lipid, protein and carbohydrate and is similar to the outer membrane of Gram-negative bacteria. Cardiolipin, present in the lipid fraction of treponemes, brings about the production of an antibody which cross-reacts with host tissue antigens. This is important in the diagnosis of treponemal infection (Ch. 8).

Propagation and in vitro cultivation

Pathogenic treponemes can grow in the testicular tissue of rabbits, and this is the normal way of maintaining them in the laboratory. Apart from ethical considerations intratesticular inoculation and weekly passage is a difficult, expensive and time-consuming process. These factors, while limiting basic studies on the biology of *T. pallidum*, have produced strong incentives to elucidate the appropriate requirements for in vitro cultivation.

Most experiments with pathogenic treponemes employ Nichols strain of *T. pallidum* subspecies *pallidum*: this strain was isolated in 1913 from the cerebrospinal fluid of a patient with neurosyphilis and is still virulent for man.

The discovery that *T. pallidum* is microaerophilic, rather than a strict anaerobe like the cultivable treponemes, greatly aided culture studies. Successful replication of Nichols strain of *T. pallidum* was reported by Fieldsteel et al (1981). Treponemes were shown to attach and replicate on the surface of tissue culture cells of cottontail rabbit epithelium (Sf1Ep) growing as conventional monolayers. Extract of rabbit testis and selection of appropriate batches of fetal bovine serum were key factors in successful multiplication. The number of treponemes increased reaching a plateau between days 9 and 12 of incubation, with increases ranging up to 100-fold and averaging 49-fold. Organisms harvested after 7 days incubation remained virulent for rabbits with the inoculation of an average of 6–7 organisms producing erythematous, indurated treponeme-containing lesions.

Cultivation of *T. pallidum* under the conditions described above was independently corroborated by Norris (1982): although total increase in treponemes was lower (8.9 to 26.2-fold) treponemes retained motility and virulence over a 12 day incubation period. The doubling time (30 to 33 hours) approached that observed in vivo in rabbits. Further work by Fieldsteel et al (1982) suggests that *T. pallidum* is not as fastidious as was formerly believed, treponemal replication occurring over a fairly wide range of temperature and oxygen concentrations. The extent of treponemal multiplication was dependent on the initial inoculum: it was greatest when the inoculum was 10^6 and least at 10^8. For all inocula the maximum ceiling of multiplication was 2×10^8. It seems likely that the ceiling of multiplication is due to a combination of factors including exhaustion in the medium of some essential components, the accumulation of toxic products and exhaustion of oxygen, which both cells and treponemes need for survival and replication.

It may be necessary for *T. pallidum* to attach to a cell surface before the treponemes can divide. If this is the case, one of the newly divided treponemes will remain attached to one end, while the other end will be set free or will be attached to another site on the host cell after division. This process may be the method by which *T. pallidum* multiplies in vivo and in vitro, making tissue culture essential for successful in vitro propagation.

Although these observations of up to 100-fold increase of *T. pallidum* numbers with retention of virulence for at least seven days are most encouraging, serial in vitro cultivation has not yet been achieved.

ORIGIN OF SYPHILIS

The first recognizable epidemic of sexually transmitted syphilis in Europe occurred at the end of the 15th century. There are two main theories regarding the appearance of the disease.

Columbian theory

The outbreak is attributed to the importation of syphilis to Spain in 1493 by the crews of Christopher Columbus on their return from the West Indies where they acquired the infection. Some members of the crew later became mercenaries in 1494 at the siege of Naples where a great epidemic broke out. It was not called syphilis (see Note 7.1) at that time but referred to as the 'French disease' by the Italians and the 'Italian disease' by the French.

Social conditions, the abundance of wars and resulting mobility of armies and associated camp followers largely contributed to the spread of the infection throughout Europe. Protagonists of the Columbian theory base their arguments on the lack of description of any disease that can be clearly identified as syphilis, in Europe prior to this period. The Columbian theory, however, does not take account of the origin of syphilis on a worldwide scale.

Unitarian theory

This evolutionary theory put forward mainly by Hackett (1963) suggests that all the present-day treponemal diseases (treponematoses) have a common ancestor, a free-living saprophytic treponeme. The free-living organism came to be carried commensally by man as are the dental treponemes today. Disease syndromes then developed as natural selection favoured the survival of mutants most likely to produce the lesions best suited to transmission from host to host in the prevailing environment (Willcox 1974). The overwhelming similarity between the pathogenic treponemes (Table 7.2) makes this an attractive theory.

According to this theory, pinta was the first treponematosis to evolve within the Afro-Asian land mass, from where it gained worldwide distribution, finally persisting among the underprivileged people in the remoter areas of the Central Americas and the northern part of the South American continent.

Yaws evolved from pinta as a humid warm environment developed in Afro-Asia; the local moisture from sweating favoured the production of exuberant skin lesions containing vast numbers of treponemes characteristic of yaws. The absence of clothes and person-to-person contact of sweaty skins in a tropical environment facilitated its spread amongst primitive communities making it a disease predominantly of childhood.

Endemic syphilis (called bejel in the Middle East) probably evolved in a warm dry climate with colder nights: the wearing of clothes would prevent skin-to-skin transmission and only organisms producing lesions of the mucous membranes could survive, presumably due to transfer by kissing and sharing of eating and drinking utensils. Infection would tend to occur before puberty and sexual spread would be a rare occurrence.

Venereal syphilis developed from endemic syphilis as social advance limited transmission between children; as the children grew up they became susceptible to the infection as a result of sexual transmission. Endemic syphilis was probably widespread in Europe prior to the 15th century.

Whichever theory is favoured it is fact that an epidemic of syphilis swept through Europe in the late 15th and early 16th centuries. By the 18th century it was widely known that syphilis and gonorrhoea were transmitted by sexual intercourse but they had not been recognized as separate entities: many thought that gonorrhoea was the early symptom of syphilis. This view was maintained by the outstanding pioneer of scientific surgery, John Hunter (1728–1795) in his 'Treatise on the Venereal Disease', published in 1786 in which he said

> It has been supposed by many that the gonorrhoea and the chancre arise from two distinct poisons; . . . . . . yet, if we take up this question upon other grounds, and also have recourse to experiments, the result of which we can absolutely depend upon, we shall find this notion to be erroneous . . . . . the matter of a gonorrhoea will produce either a gonorrhoea, a chancre or the lues venera; and the matter of a chancre will also produce either a gonorrhoea, a chancre or the lues venera.

His erroneous opinion on the common identity of gonorrhoea and syphilis appears to have been due to misinterpretation of the results of his experiments rather than an inaccuracy of his observations of which many recorded by him would seem to be strongly in favour of a separate aetiology of the two diseases. John Hunter's records of experimental inoculations of patients with 'venereal matter' and the lack of evidence of a self-inoculation experiment, a story so often repeated in medical literature, are detailed more fully in George Qvist's scholarly appraisal of the genius of this remarkable man (Qvist 1981). In 1793, Benjamin Bell in Edinburgh, however, maintained that syphilis and gonorrhoea were different diseases. This view was later confirmed in 1837 by Philip Ricord of France who is usually credited with the separation of gonorrhoea and syphilis: the causal organisms were finally identified in 1879 (Albert Neisser) and 1905 (Schaudinn & Hoffmann) respectively.

TRANSMISSION OF INFECTION

Sexual

T. pallidum is so feebly viable outside its host that syphilis is ordinarily acquired by sexual intercourse. The organism has little intrinsic invasiveness and usually gains entry to its new host through minute abrasions in the epithelial surfaces which come into contact with the moist mucocutaneous lesions of an infected partner. An infected person usually ceases to be sexually infectious 2–4 years after acquiring the disease. Some individuals appear resistant to infection since not everyone exposed to early syphilis acquires the disease.

Accidental

Acquisition by means other than sexual intercourse usually involves direct contact. In such cases the organisms may gain entry through a small skin abrasion. Accidental inoculation has occurred under the following circumstances: in doctors and nurses who have examined a syphilitic lesion without wearing gloves; in laboratory workers by needle prick when inoculating pathogenic *T. pallidum* into rabbits or when handling large numbers of treponemes during isolation and purification procedures; in patients being transfused with blood from a donor suffering from early syphilis (Chambers et al 1969).

Many cases of transfusion acquired syphilis were reported prior to the 1950s. During the last few decades the number of cases reported has been very low. The decline is partly due to the lower incidence of syphilis and to more thorough screening of blood donors. More important, however, is that nowadays fresh blood is rarely used. In usual practice, when infected blood is stored at 4 °C in citrate anticoagulant, infectivity is lost between 96 and 120 h. The actual survival time may depend on the number of treponemes initially present in donor blood (van der Sluis et al 1982). Treponemes are not viable after storage for a few days to a few weeks at −10 °C to −20 °C. Treponemes are, however, viable when stored for extended periods at −45 °C and infectious for an indefinite period when stored at −78 °C. Freezing followed by desiccation kills the organism (Chambers et al 1969).

The risk of accidental infection by infected blood is highest when fresh heparinized blood is used. Such blood is favoured for exchange transfusion in neonates because it practically guarantees normal pH, electrolyte composition, and concentration of glucose and ionized calcium. An infant girl acquired syphilis in this way in Rotterdam in 1977 (Risseeuw-Appel & Kothe 1983). She showed typical features of early infectious syphilis three and a half months after the transfusion. Although the blood donor had negative serological tests for syphilis 5 days before giving the blood, later tests were positive indicating that he must have become infected shortly before donation of the blood. Although exceedingly rare, similar cases have been reported in adults. Soendjojo et al (1982) reporting from Indonesia described such a case in a 58-year-old Chinese woman who developed syphilis 7 weeks after receiving 2 units fresh whole blood from 4 different donors.

Congenital

Although it has previously been considered that *T. pallidum* was not transmitted to the fetus before the fourth month of gestation, possibly through the protective effect of the cytotrophoblastic (Langhan's) layer, recent studies have clearly demonstrated that infection of the fetus can occur before the tenth week (Harter & Benirschke 1976). A woman can transmit syphilis to her fetus long after she has ceased to be sexually infective, although the longer she has had syphilis the less likely this is to occur; transmission to the fetus is almost inevitable in the early stage.

Non-venereal

Endemic treponematosis is transmitted by direct or indirect non-venereal contact in early childhood, e.g. in playing, in sharing eating or drinking utensils and in close skin contact. It usually occurs in communities living in overcrowded and unhygienic conditions. Once common in parts of Europe, e.g. Yugoslavia, it is seen mainly in Africa as yaws, and in the Middle East as bejel and in certain parts of Central and South America as pinta (Ch. 13). There is no certain evidence of transmission from an infected mother to the fetus in utero.

COURSE OF UNTREATED SYPHILIS

The natural course of infection may span many decades and present a variety of clinical forms. The classification shown in Figure 7.1 represents the main stages of the disease.

ACQUIRED INFECTION

Clinical features are dealt with in detail in the following chapters but the infection, if untreated, may run courses outlined diagrammatically in Figure 7.1.

The clinical horizon in this figure separates the stages when clinical features are absent from those when these are present. The period before the disease shows itself (prepatent or incubation period) is usually about 25 days (range 9–90 days).

T. pallidum breaches the intact skin, probably through minute abrasions, or penetrates mucous membrane surfaces. The organisms quickly disseminate to the draining lymph nodes and within hours make their way via the blood and lymphatics to different tissues. Although treponemes rapidly disseminate they preferentially multiply at the site of entry, resulting in an inflammatory response as evidenced by the influx of mononuclear cells. As multiplication of treponemes continues the characteristic primary lesion or chancre

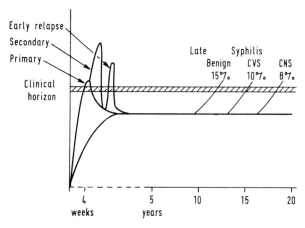

Fig. 7.1 Simplified diagrammatic representation of the course of untreated syphilis from the time of infection. The early stages, whether primary, secondary, early relapse of latent syphilis, are indicated together with the subsequent development of late-stage effects, whether late benign or gummatous, cardiovascular, central nervous system or late-stage latent syphilis. The percentage of effects may vary in different populations (modified from Kampmeier 1964).

seriously, cardiovascular or neurological disorders, bringing very serious disability and sometimes death.

The data in Figure 7.1 pertaining to late stage syphilis are based on the famous Oslo study of untreated syphilis (Gjestland 1955). During the period 1891–1910 approximately 2000 patients with primary and secondary syphilis were isolated in hospital when infectious, but otherwise they were not treated. The patients were those of Professor Boeck, who, convinced about the inadequacies of current therapy, withheld treatment. Later a study group analysed case histories of 1404 of Professor Boeck's original admissions to hospital.

As shown in Figure 7.1, infection may not run the 'typical' course and remains below the clinical horizon. Patients are diagnosed with latent infection who are completely unaware of having experienced primary or secondary symptoms. Symptoms are often suppressed during pregnancy. Antibiotics prescribed for other conditions may abort or delay early stage infection, minimizing or abolishing early symptoms.

tends to appear at the site of entry: treponemes are present in the fluid that can be expressed from the depth of the chancre. The time taken for a chancre to appear depends to some extent on the number of treponemes in the initial inoculum. In men the chancre is usually penile and noticeable, but in women a chancre on the cervix uteri could pass unnoticed in the same way as anal chancres in homosexual men. Chancres in other sites occur uncommonly (less than 1%). These primary lesions are painless and tend to heal spontaneously in 3 to 8 weeks, falsely reassuring the individual that all is well.

If the disease is not detected and treated in the primary stage, it progresses to the secondary stage, usually 6 to 12 weeks after contact, but occasionally this process may take up to 12 months. Secondary syphilis, characterized by a variety of macular, papular, papulosquamous, and other skin lesions, results from the generalized spread and multiplication of *T. pallidum* throughout the body; the treponemes may be carried to virtually every organ and tissue.

After the primary or secondary stage and probably also *ab initio* the infection becomes latent but mucocutaneous relapses may recur over a two-year period and render the infected person infectious again. Once the early infectious stage of the disease has run its course it enters the late non-infectious stage about two years after the initial contact. There may be no clinical evidence of this disease and latency, when disease is hidden, may persist for several decades, and even for life, but a proportion of patients (30–40%) will unpredictably develop either gummatous lesions or, more

CONGENITAL INFECTION (SEE ALSO CH. 12)

In congenital syphilis resulting from blood-borne infection of the fetus via the placenta there is no stage analogous to primary acquired syphilis. Clinically congenital infection is divided into the early stage, the late stage and the late latent stage with or without stigmata: the division between early and late stage is an arbitrary one.

Early stage pertains to the first two years of life and produces infectious lesions similar to those in the secondary stage of acquired syphilis. Lesions of late-stage congenital infection generally occur from two to three years of age and include gummata identical with those of benign tertiary acquired syphilis. The stigmata are scars and deformities of early or late lesions which are no longer active: these include the saddle-shaped nose, interstitial keratitis, Hutchinson's teeth and eighth nerve deafness. These differences in early and late-stage congenital syphilis may reflect the stage of infection of the mother and child during the pregnancy.

PATHOGENESIS AND IMMUNOLOGY

Attachment
Attachment to host tissues is an important initial step in syphilis (Fitzgerald 1981). Two receptors are involved: the surface receptor within tissue to which *T. pallidum* attaches and the surface receptor on *T. pallidum* that interacts with the host tissue receptor. Although *T. pallidum* attaches to a wide variety of cell types it attaches significantly better to some cells than

to others (Wong et al 1983). Cell surface receptors on cultured cells are uniformly distributed over the cell surface, probably as an intact layer. According to Fitzgerald et al (1979) the cell receptor that mediates treponemal attachment is the outer surface layer of mucopolysaccharide material. Acid mucopolysaccharides complexed with proteins form the ground substance or gel-like matrix between cells in almost every tissue of the body including nerve tissue. Thus the potential receptors for treponemal attachment are generally distributed throughout the body. The ability of *T. pallidum* to infect so many different tissues could reflect the presence of ground substance mucopolysaccharides within these tissues. Attachment may result from the enzymatic reaction of treponemal mucopolysaccharidase with its mucopolysaccharide substrate at the cell surface (Fitzgerald & Johnson 1979).

Dissemination

Syphilis can be described as a generalized infection of vascular tissues. Within lesions in each stage of syphilis treponemes localize primarily in vascular areas. After entering the host *T. pallidum* immediately disseminates to other tissues. Because of its rapid nature, dissemination must occur through the bloodstream, either by direct penetration of blood vessels or by penetration of lymphatic channels which subsequently empty into the blood. Electron micrographs suggest that *T. pallidum* penetrates between the junctions of endothelial cells to gain access to other tissues (Ovčinnikov & Delektorskij 1972).

Quist et al (1983) studied the interaction of *T. pallidum* with isolated rabbit capillary tissues. They considered that the mechanism of penetration may be partially attributed to treponemal hyaluronidase. Capillary endothelial cells are joined together by ground substance comprised of glycosaminoglycans (primarily hyaluronic acid), glycoproteins and proteins. *T. pallidum* may degrade the hyaluronic acid enzymatically thereby splitting the endothelial cell junctions. In support of the potential pathological role of hyaluronidase, *T. pertenue* possesses the enzyme and attaches to capillaries whereas the non-pathogenic treponemes lack the enzyme and do not attach. Treponemal hyaluronidase may also play a role in capillary destruction. Ground substance provides structural support for capillaries. With extensive perivascular multiplication of organisms degradation of the hyaluronic acid would damage capillary structural support. In turn collapsed vessels would result in the inhibited blood supply, necrosis, and ulceration that are characteristic of syphilitic histopathology.

With the exception of the gumma, clinical manifestations of syphilis result from multiplication of *T. pallidum* within tissues. Fitzgerald (1981) proposed a model for pathogenesis of syphilis in which treponemal multiplication is dependent on ground substance polysaccharide. This model helps explain the following: the primary stage involving dermal tissue which contains relatively high concentrations of mucopolysaccharides; the secondary stage involving most tissues, all of which contain varying amounts of ground substance; and the late stage, involving the aorta which also contains relatively high levels of mucopolysaccharides and nerve tissue which is composed of nerve fibres separated by ground substance. At least some of the birth defects of congenital syphilis may result from treponemal interference with ground substance mucopolysaccharide production during the very active fetal growth period.

Host response

It has been known for some time that humans exert some degree of natural resistance to *T. pallidum*. Shober et al (1983) have shown that approximately only 50% of at-risk sexual contacts of primary and secondary syphilis develop infection. The proportion reported is similar to that in the pre-antibiotic era.

Normal human serum contains a heat-stable cross-reactive treponemicidal antibody elicited by the non-pathogenic, host-indigenous *T. phagedenis* biotype Reiter. This antibody and the extent of the treponemal challenge dose may account in part for the relatively low infection rate (Bishop & Miller 1983).

Acquired immunity is slow to evolve and requires relatively prolonged periods of antigenic stimulation. In the Sing Sing study (Magnusson et al 1956) 62 patients with syphilis were experimentally challenged with Nichols strain of *T. pallidum*. The immunity of these patients was related to the duration of the initial infection; as the duration of untreated syphilis increased, lesions following challenge occurred less frequently. Also, as shown in the Oslo study (Gjestland 1955) 65% of untreated patients did not progress beyond the primary stage, implying a certain degree of immunity.

Humoral and cellular factors

Although early replication is primarily extracellular at least some treponemes become intracellular following attachment and penetration (Bishop and Miller 1983). The inflammatory response to primary infection in both the human and experimental rabbit disease consists essentially of infiltration by lymphocytes, plasma cells, and macrophages with a distribution depending upon the stage of lesion development versus healing. Healing may occur as a result of inactivation of *T. pallidum* by specific antibodies, with resultant enhanced phagocytosis and destruction by macrophages.

Phagocytosis

In infections such as listeriosis, toxoplasmosis and

tuberculosis destruction of the infecting organism is mediated by macrophages which have been activated by soluble products of specifically sensitized T-lymphocytes. Activated macrophages appear to play an important role in resistance to syphilis. Sensitized T-lymphocytes which arise early in infection produce migration inhibition factor as well as macrophage activation factor (Lukehart 1983). Living *T. pallidum* can be phagocytosed by macrophages in vitro in the presence of specific antibody. Macrophages play a major role in the clearance of organisms from the local site of infection. Immunofluorescence staining and electron microscopic studies reveal the presence of *T. pallidum* within macrophages in healing lesions.

Although degradation of ingested organisms within phagocytic vacuoles has been described, the direct killing of *T. pallidum* by macrophages has not yet been demonstrated.

Electron microscopic studies have documented the rapid uptake of *T. pallidum* into membrane-bound vacuoles in human polymorphonuclear leucocytes (PMNLs) in vitro after incubation for as little as five minutes. Leucocyte degranulation and loss of treponemal integrity was observed within a few hours. Intradermal injection of *T. pallidum* into rabbits caused a rapid accumulation of PMNLs. Thus, although PMNLs are attracted to, and appear to ingest *T. pallidum* they fail to eradicate the organisms following inoculation (Musher et al 1983).

Humoral response

In the naturally infected host, antibodies to *T.pallidum* are detected first by the fluorescent treponemal antibody absorbed (FTA-ABS) test followed by antibodies to cardiolipin (Ch. 5). The host responds first with the production of IgM and then IgG and IgA. Anti-treponemal IgE appears simultaneously with the IgG and IgA antibodies and is found in early as well as latent and late active syphilis (Bos et al 1980).

Recently, Hanff et al (1982) characterized the humoral immune response in human syphilis to polypeptides of *T. pallidum*. Serum IgG from uninfected individuals reacted weakly with three polypeptides of molecular weight (mol. wt.) 45 000, 33 000 and 30 000. All patients with syphilis have IgG antibody to at least four polypeptides of mol. wt. 45 000, 33 000, 30 000 and 15 000. Antibody to polypeptides of 42 000 and 16 500 mol. wt. appeared to be markers of non-primary syphilis. These six polypeptides have been termed the major antigenic proteins (MAP) of *T. pallidum*. Patients with secondary and early latent syphilis acquire antibodies to a set of 16 additional polypeptide antigens, whereas patients with latent and late syphilis have antibody to only four or five antigens in addition to MAP. One of the main antigens recognized early in infection

is the major axial filament polypeptide of mol. wt. 37 000 (Penn et al 1986). Thus there would appear to be an acquisition of antibodies to specific treponemal antigens as the disease progresses from primary to secondary and early latent or late syphilis. It is conceivable, therefore, that the development of antibody to particular antigens may explain the acquisition and retention of immunity and progression of the disease.

Antibodies may be important in healing of primary and secondary lesions as a result of inactivation of *T. pallidum* by treponemal antibody in concert with complement. Opsonins may also attach to *T. pallidum* resulting in enhanced phagocytosis and destruction by macrophages.

Antibodies are also important in the formation of immune complexes in the sera of patients with secondary syphilis. These complexes are thought to be present in the sera of most if not all patients with secondary disease (Solling et al 1978). Deposition of immune complexes is responsible for the nephropathy of secondary syphilis.

Cell-mediated immunity

Considerable controversy exists concerning the possible role of cell-mediated immunity (CMI) in host defence against treponemes. There are numerous reports involving the in vitro cell-mediated immune response in syphilis as shown by the phenomenon of blast transformation and macrophage migration inhibition (Fitzgerald 1981). Results of leucocyte migration inhibition suggest that CMI may be delayed in developing during the early stage of experimental *T. pallidum* infection in rabbits. These results are consistent with findings from delayed hypersensitivity skin testing and in vitro lymphocyte transformation studies. Changes such as depletion of lymphocytes in the paracortical areas of the lymph nodes and the areas surrounding the central arteriole of the spleen, associated with defective CMI, have been reported in patients with either congenital or secondary syphilis. Immune complexes may also prevent early activation of T-lymphocytes and CMI. In addition treponemes may possess a slime layer which helps protect them from host defences thus preventing activation of lymphocytes (Folds 1983).

In conclusion, although immunity develops following infection with *T. pallidum* it is slow to evolve and requires relatively prolonged periods of antigenic stimulation. Effective immunity most probably depends upon the co-operative action of both humoral and cell-mediated mechanisms. The reason(s) for survival of a limited number of treponemes following the healing process remains an enigma. However, it seems likely that protection from host immune mechanisms by virtue of an intracellular location may account for treponemal survival.

NOTE TO CHAPTER 7

Note 7.1

The name syphilis was not generally used until about 1850, some three centuries after Frascatorius of Verona wrote his famous poem 'Syphilis sive Morbus Gallicus'. This poem tells of one 'Syphilus' a shepherd who was afflicted by the disease because he had uttered blasphemy against the sun (Glendening 1942).

REFERENCES

Bishop N H, Miller J N 1983 Humoral immune mechanisms in acquired syphilis. In: Schell R F, Musher D F (eds) Pathogenesis and immunology of treponemal infection. Marcel Dekker, New York, ch 14, p 241–270

Bos J D, Hamerlinck F, Cormane R H 1980 Antitreponemal IgE in early syphilis. British Journal of Venereal Diseases 56: 20–25

Chambers R W, Foley H T, Schmidt P J 1969 Transmission of syphilis by fresh blood products. Transfusion 9: 32–34

Fieldsteel A H, Cox D L, Moeckli R A 1981 Cultivation of virulent Treponema pallidum in tissue culture. Infection and Immunity 32: 908–915

Fieldsteel A H, Cox D L, Moeckli R A 1982 Further studies on replication of virulent Treponema pallidum in tissue cultures of Sf1Ep cells. Infection and Immunity 32: 449–455

Fitzgerald T J 1981 Pathogenesis and immunology of Treponema pallidum. Annual Review of Microbiology 35: 29–54

Fitzgerald T J, Johnson R C 1979 Mucopolysaccharidase of Treponema pallidum. Infection and Immunity 24: 261–268

Fitzgerald T J, Johnson R C, Ritzi D M 1979 Relationship of Treponema pallidum to acidic mucopolysaccharides. Infection and Immunity 24: 252–260

Folds J D 1983 Cell-mediated immunity. In: Schell R F, Musher D F (eds) Pathogenesis and immunology of treponemal infection. Marcel Dekker, New York, ch 16, p 315–330

Gjestland T 1955 The Oslo study of untreated syphilis — an epidemiologic investigation of the natural course of untreated syphilis based on a study of the Boeck-Bruusgard material. Acta Dermato Venereologica 35: Suppl 34

Glendening G L 1942 Source book of medical history. Hoebner, London, p 120–121

Hackett C J 1963 On the origin of the human treponematoses (pinta, yaws, endemic syphilis and venereal syphilis). Bulletin of the World Health Organization 29: 7–41

Hanff P A, Fehniger T E, Miller J N, Lovett M A 1982 Humoral immune response in human syphilis to polypeptides of Treponema pallidum. Journal of Immunology 129: 1278–1291

Harter C A, Benirschke K 1976 Fetal syphilis in the first trimester. American Journal of Obstetrics and Gynecology 124: 705–711

Hovind-Hougan K 1976 Determination by means of electron microscopy of morphological criteria of value for classification of some spirochaetes, in particular treponemes. Acta Pathologica et Microbiologica Scandinavica Sect B Suppl 225: 1–41

Kampmeier R H 1964 The late manifestations of syphilis: skeletal, visceral cardiovascular. The Medical Clinics of North America, 48, 667–697

Lukehart S A 1983 Macrophages and host resistance. In: Schell R F, Musher D F (eds) Pathogenesis and immunology of treponemal infection. Marcel Dekker, New York, ch 18, p 349–364

Magnusson H J, Thomas E W, Olansky S, Kaplan B I, De Mello L, Cutler J C 1956 Inoculation of syphilis in human volunteers. Medicine 35: 33–82

Miao R, Fieldsteel A H 1980 Genetic relationship between Treponema pallidum and Treponema pertenue, two noncultivable human pathogens. Journal of Bacteriology 141: 427–429

Musher D M, Hague-park M, Gyorkey F, Anderson D C, Baughn R E 1983 The interaction between Treponema pallidum and human polymorphonuclear leucocytes. Journal of Infectious Diseases 147: 77–86

Norris S J 1982 In vitro cultivation of Treponema pallidum: independent confirmation. Infection and Immunity 36: 437–439

Ovčinnikov N J, Delektorskij V V 1972 Electron microscopy of phagocytosis in syphilis and yaws. British Journal of Venereal Diseases 48: 227–248

Penn C W, Bailey M J, Cockayne A 1986 Molecular and immunochemical analysis of Treponema pallidum. FEMS Microbiology Reviews 32: 139–148

Quist E E, Repesh L A, Zeleznikar R, Fitzgerald T J 1983 Interaction of Treponema pallidum with isolated rabbit capillary tissues. British Journal of Venereal Diseases 59: 11–20

Qvist G 1981 John Hunter, 1728–1793. William Heinemann Medical Books, London, p 42–53, 157–161

Risseeuw-Appel I M, Kothe F C 1983 Transfusion syphilis: a case report. Sexually Transmitted Diseases 10: 200–201

Schaudinn F, Hoffmann E 1905 A preliminary note upon the occurrence of spirochaetes in syphilitic lesions and in papillomata. In: Russell A E (ed) 1906. Selected essays on syphilis and small-pox. Translations etc. The New Sydenham Society, London, p 3–15

Schober P C, Gabriel G, White P, Felton W F 1983 How infectious is syphilis? British Journal of Venereal Diseases 59: 217–219

Smibert R M 1984 Genus III Treponema. In: Kreig N R, Holt J G (eds) Bergey's Manual of systematic bacteriology, vol 1. Williams and Wilkins, Baltimore/London, p 290–296

Soendjojo A, Boedisantoso M, Ilias M I, Rahardjo D 1982 Syphilis d'emblée due to blood transfusion. Case report. British Journal of Venereal Diseases 58: 149–150

Solling J, Solling K, Jacobsen K, From E 1978 Circulating immune complexes in syphilis. Acta Dermato Venereologica 58: 263–267

Thorburn A L 1971 Fritz Richard Schaudinn, 1871–1906 protozoologist of syphilis. British Journal of Venereal Diseases 47: 459–461

van der Sluis J J, Menke H E, Kothe F C 1982 Transfusion syphilis: survival of *Treponema pallidum* in donor blood. Antonie van Leeuwenhoek 48: 487–488

Willcox R R 1974 Changing patterns of treponemal disease. British Journal of Venereal Diseases 50: 169–178

Wong G H W, Steiner B, Faine S, Graves S 1983 Factors affecting the attachment of *Treponema pallidum* to mammalian cells *in vitro*. British Journal of Venereal Diseases 59: 21–29

8

Diagnosis of syphilis

In syphilis the social and medical implications are so serious that a clinical diagnosis must be confirmed in the laboratory either by:

1. demonstrating *Treponema pallidum* in the serous exudate obtained from the depth of early lesions and/or
2. demonstrating antibodies in the serum.

1. DEMONSTRATION OF *T.PALLIDUM* IN PRIMARY AND SECONDARY LESIONS

DARK GROUND MICROSCOPY

After cleansing the surfaces of the primary or secondary lesions with a swab soaked in physiological saline, serum is obtained from the depth of the lesion as described in Chapter 6 and examined by dark ground microscopy using the oil-immersion objective. *T. pallidum* is recognized by its slender structure, characteristic slow movements and angulation.

It must be carefully distinguished from the many other treponemes that may occur in genital ulcers (see Spirochaetaeceae in Ch. 2), but these tend to be surface organisms and are not found in the depth of lesions. If the initial test is negative the procedure should be repeated daily for at least three days: antibiotics should be withheld during this period although co-trimoxazole (sulphamethoxazole 5 parts, trimethoprim 1 part) in an oral dose of 960 mg every 12 hours for 5 days and local saline lavage may be used to reduce local sepsis. Many commensal treponemes occur in the mouth and therefore dark ground illumination is not suitable for examining oral lesions. Organisms are not easily found in skin lesions of secondary syphilis except those in moist skin areas.

Identification of *T. pallidum* requires a microscope with dark ground illumination and an experienced observer.

FLUORESCENCE MICROSCOPY

A smear of the material to be tested is made on a glass slide, dried, fixed in acetone and sent to the laboratory. In remote areas the specimen can be posted. On receipt in the laboratory the smear is stained with fluorescein-labelled antibody specific for *T. pallidum* and examined by fluorescence microscopy (Daniels & Ferneyhaugh 1977). This technique has not yet been properly evaluated and according to Luger (1981) immunofluorescence staining may give rise to non-specific results and is less reliable than dark ground microscopy.

The reliability of the method should be improved with the advent of monoclonal antibodies. Hook et al (1985) used a pathogen-specific fluorescein-conjugated monoclonal antibody to examine lesion exudates from 61 patients. Staining with the monoclonal antibody demonstrated *T. pallidum* in all 30 patients with early syphilis (22 primary, 8 secondary); 29 of the patients were positive by dark ground microscopy. Although 7 of 31 patients without syphilis had spiral organisms seen on dark ground microscopy, staining with monoclonal antibody was negative for all 31. Non-pathogenic spirochaetes were shown to be present in 5 of these patients by using a second monoclonal antibody reactive with non-pathogenic, as well as pathogenic, treponemes and related spirochaetes.

OTHER STAINING METHODS

Methods such as indian ink-staining and silver-staining are now obsolete. Silver-staining does not give a clear differentiation between *T. pallidum* and treponema-like shaped tissue fibres.

2. DEMONSTRATION OF ANTIBODIES IN THE SERUM

During treponemal infection, whether in syphilis or in the endemic treponemal diseases such as yaws or pinta, a variety of antibodies are produced. As shown in Table 8.1 these can be classified into non-specific anti-treponemal antibodies and antibodies specific for pathogenic treponemes: the main tests which are, or have been, used routinely in clinical practice are also shown along with their year of introduction.

The tests depicted in Table 8.1 all show reactivity with IgM as well as with IgG antibodies. The time course for the appearance and elimination of these antibodies is discussed on page 123 under the heading 'Detection of IgM antibodies against *T. pallidum*'.

Table 8.1 Tests to detect antibodies produced during treponemal infection. The year of introduction of each test is given in brackets.

Non-specific anti-treponemal antibodies	Antibodies specific for pathogenic treponemes
Antibodies to cardiolipin	
Wassermann reaction (1906)	TPI *Treponema pallidum* immobilization test (1949)
Kahn test (1928)	FTA-ABS Fluorescent treponemal antibody absorbed test (1964)
Venereal Disease Research Laboratory (VDRL) test (1946)	
	TPHA *Treponema pallidum* haemagglutination assay (1967)
Rapid plasma reagin test (1957)	
Automated reagin test (1968)	
Antibodies to group treponemal antigen	
Reiter protein complement fixation test (1953)	

In the following section the nature of the main serological tests is discussed and modifications for detecting specific anti-treponemal IgM described as a background to the rational application of these tests in clinical practice.

TESTS TO DETECT NON-SPECIFIC TREPONEMAL ANTIBODIES

Cardiolipin antigen tests

These tests are suitable for routine screening and usually become positive 10 to 14 days after the appearance of the chancre, the titre gradually increasing. The titre tends to diminish and the test tends to become negative after treatment. In late or latent syphilis the cardiolipin antigen tests are often negative.

1. Wassermann reaction (WR)

The complement fixation test introduced by Wassermann in 1906 was the first serological test for the diagnosis of syphilis: the historical background to this work can be found in a brief biography of August von Wassermann (Editorial 1968). The antigen in the original WR consisted of a saline extract of syphilitic tissues obtained from still-born fetuses with congenital infec-

tion. It was assumed that *T. pallidum* present in the infected tissue was responsible for the positive reactions obtained in patients with syphilis. Later it was shown that the same results were obtained with an alcoholic extract of heart muscle. In 1941 the diphospholipid cardiolipin was identified as the active component in beef heart extract (Pangborn 1941) and this led to new chemically defined lipoidal antigens being produced in the form of pure cardiolipin supplemented with lecithin and cholesterol.

The Wassermann complement fixation test has decreased markedly in popularity as it offers no advantage over the modern flocculation tests such as the Venereal Disease Research Laboratory (VDRL) test. The World Health Organization (1982) now recommends that complement fixation tests should be discontinued; the VDRL test is simpler, quicker and cheaper to perform and should be adopted as standard. Early flocculation tests such as the Kahn test are only of historical interest.

2. Venereal Disease Research Laboratory (VDRL) test

Because it is easy to standardize, simple and reproducible, the VDRL test (Harris et al 1946), introduced in 1946, is the preferred cardiolipin antigen test in most laboratories.

The test may be performed as a slide test in which the patient's serum, previously heated to inactivate complement, is mixed with a freshly prepared suspension of cardiolipin-lecithin-cholesterol antigen on a glass slide. The mixture is rotated, usually mechanically, and after a few minutes flocculation (aggregation of antigen-antibody complexes in suspension) is detected microscopically using a low power objective. Quantitative tests with serial dilutions of patient's serum are easily carried out.

The VDRL test is versatile and can be modified for testing unheated serum or plasma either by automated or manual techniques.

3. Rapid plasma reagin (RPR) test

(Reagin is an obsolete and confusing term and should no longer be used: unfortunately the term was used in naming certain currently used tests and reagin tests are widely referred to in the literature and in clinical practice. The preferred terms are cardiolipin antigen, or lipoidal antigen tests.)

VDRL test antigen suspended in choline chloride can be used to test plasma or unheated serum. By adding a chelating agent to remove metallic impurities the antigen remains stable for up to 6 months when stored at 4–10°C. In the RPR test (Portnoy et al 1957) finely divided carbon particles are added to the above antigen: results can be read with the naked eye instead of microscopically. The test can be performed with disposable equipment and plastic cards marked in circular areas. This makes the RPR test particularly suitable for use in field studies in developing countries. Unfortunately, the reagents are more expensive than simple VDRL slide test antigen. A form of this test known as the VDRL carbon antigen test, however, is now the preferred cardiolipin antigen test in most laboratories.

4. Automated reagin test (ART)
This test (McGrew et al 1968) uses the same antigen as the RPR test. Unheated serum or plasma are sampled automatically using auto-analyser equipment and passed through mixing and settling coils. The resultant mixture is deposited on a moving strip of filter paper. Positive reactions show clumping of the carbon particles while negative sera give a uniform grey suspension. The ART is particularly useful in laboratories serving blood transfusion centres.

Cardiolipin is widespread in nature and can be isolated from many mammalian tissues: it is a component of the inner membrane of the mammalian mitochondrion which accounts for the success of beef heart, which is rich in mitochondria, as a source of antigen. Historically the type of antibody reacting in the Wassermann reaction was termed reagin at a time when little was known of the nature of the reactions involved. The antibody is now generally considered to be directed against cardiolipin present in treponemes, i.e. it is antibody against a non-specific antigen shared by treponemes and mammalian tissues. Previously, it was considered that these antibodies were produced against host tissue cardiolipin released during treponemal infection.

Due to the widespread nature of cardiolipin, antibodies reacting with it are occasionally found in the sera of healthy individuals (less than 1% of the population) or patients without any clinical evidence of syphilis. These reactions are termed biological false-positive (BFP). BFP reactions are classified as acute if they disappear spontaneously within 6 months and chronic if they persist longer (p. 131). Acute BFP reactions are usually associated with acute febrile infectious diseases while chronic BFP reactors show a high incidence of auto-immune and related disorders. Other tests are required to distinguish between positive cardiolipin antigen tests resulting from BFP reactions and those resulting from treponemal infection.

TEST TO DETECT GROUP-SPECIFIC TREPONEMAL ANTIBODIES

Reiter protein complement fixation (RPCF) test
The RPCF test (D'Alessandro & Dardenoni 1953) detects antibodies against a group-specific treponemal antigen shared by pathogenic and commensal treponemes. The Reiter treponeme was isolated in 1920 at the Kaiser Wilhelm Institute in Berlin from a case of primary syphilis in man. For many years the Reiter treponeme was reputed to be an adapted strain of *T. pallidum* but it is now classified as a biovar of *T. phagedenis*. *T. phagedenis* biovar *Reiter* is avirulent for man and can be grown in relatively simple media accounting for its previous popularity as a source of antigen.

Although false-positive reactions occur with the RPCF test, the antibody detected by the RPCF test is distinct from that detected by cardiolipin antigen tests and differs from that causing false-positive reactions with the latter tests. The RPCF test can be used for screening purposes and a positive reaction in both this test and a cardiolipin test is strongly suggestive of treponemal infection. Unfortunately, the RPCF test is often negative in cases of late syphilis. The RPCF test has now been superseded by *T. pallidum* antigen tests.

TESTS TO DETECT ANTIBODIES SPECIFIC FOR PATHOGENIC TREPONEMES

The antigen used in these tests is derived from Nichols strain of *T. pallidum*. This strain, isolated in 1913 from the cerebrospinal fluid of a patient with neurosyphilis, is still virulent for man and is maintained in rabbits by intratesticular inoculation and weekly passage. Tests using pathogenic *T. pallidum* as antigen tend to remain positive following treatment. These tests have been used as verification tests to confirm the treponemal nature of a positive cardiolipin antigen test.

The *T. pallidum* immobilization (TPI) test
In this test (Nelson & Mayer 1949) live treponemes are incubated with heat-inactivated serum in the presence of complement and the number of organisms immobilized is determined by dark ground microscopy; if 50% or more treponemes are immobilized the result of the test is positive. The antibody detected by the TPI test is slow to develop and the test is often negative in untreated primary syphilis but usually positive in all other stages of the disease. The specificity of the TPI test has been accepted as absolute although it may rarely give false-positive results.

Following its introduction in 1949, the TPI test served for many years as the only reliable verification test for treponemal infection available to the clinician. The test, which is complicated, technically difficult to perform, expensive in animals and reagents, was restricted to a few reference laboratories. The development of microtechniques facilitated the introduction of new specific tests using immunofluorescence or haemagglutination techniques for the detection of antibody.

These newer tests have superseded the TPI test which is seldom used nowadays in clinical practice (Rein et al 1980, Sprott et al 1982). A few reference laboratories still perform the TPI test on selected sera and for research purposes.

Immunofluorescence staining

The fluorescent treponemal antibody absorbed (FTA-ABS) test

In the FTA-ABS test (Hunter et al 1964) the patient's serum is absorbed with a sonicate of Reiter's treponemes in order to remove group-specific antibody. Binding to *T. pallidum* of antibody specific for pathogenic treponemes is then demonstrated by the indirect immunofluorescence technique (Fig. 8.1). The indirect immunofluorescence technique is carried out in two stages. In the first stage a smear of *T. pallidum* is incubated with patient's serum: any anti-treponemal antibody in the patient's serum reacts with the treponemes on the slide. In the second stage fluorescein-labelled anti-human immunoglobulin is added to reveal any antibody which was bound in the first stage. Treponemes are located by dark ground microscopy and then examined by ultra-violet illumination. If the serum is positive the treponemes give bright apple-green fluorescence. The FTA-ABS test is an accepted reference test and is highly specific and sensitive at all stages of syphilitic infection although a small percentage of false-positive reactions occur.

False-positive results have been reported in patients with systemic lupus erythematosus and other connective tissue diseases (McKenna et al 1973). These false-positive results can be differentiated from positive FTA-ABS tests due to treponemal infection since the sera from patients with collagen disorders also give fluorescence with *Trypanosoma cruzi* and *Toxoplasma gondii* — absence of fluorescence with organisms pretreated with deoxyribonuclease demonstrates that cross-reaction is probably due to anti-DNA antibodies in patients with collagen disease (Wright 1973).

Excessive growth of commensal treponemes in the oral lesions of patients with ulcerative stomatitis produces high levels of group anti-treponemal antibody which may give a false-positive FTA-ABS test. Transitory false-positive results were reported in some cases of genital herpes infection (Wright et al 1975) although this was not confirmed by others (Chapel et al 1978). These false-positive results might arise due to the incomplete removal of group anti-treponemal antibody which is known to occur sometimes when 'Sorbent' comprising a heated and concentrated culture filtrate of Reiter treponemes is used instead of sonicate to remove group antibody (Wilkinson & Johnston 1975).

The FTA-ABS test is not suitable for screening large numbers of sera and is used as a confirmatory test when one of the screening tests is positive. It is also useful in suspected cases of primary syphilis.

Fluorescent treponemal antibody absorbed double staining procedure (FTA-ABS DS)

This modified procedure was introduced to update the FTA-ABS test for new microscopes equipped with incident illumination. The procedure incorporates a rhodamine-labelled class-specific anti-human immuno-

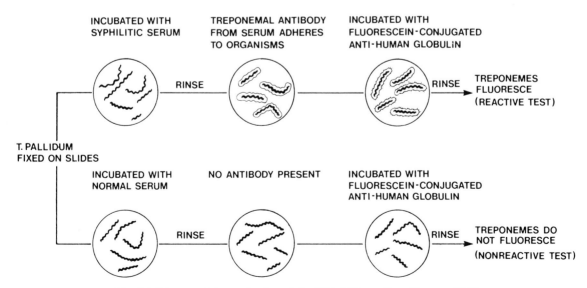

Fig. 8.1 Diagram of the mechanism of the FTA-ABS test (from Newman 1974).

globulin G primary stain and fluorescein-labelled anti-treponemal globulin as counterstain (Farshy et al 1983). The double staining method should overcome the difficulty of demonstrating the presence of antigen on non-reactive slides. It is considered to be less time-consuming and easier on the eyes than the conventional FTA-ABS test method and to result in fewer borderline reactions.

Solid-phase fluorimmunoassay

Unlike the FTA-ABS test, large numbers of sera could be screened by this immunofluorescence method. The entire test, which could be readily automated, yields an objective quantitative result. A lysate of virulent *T. pallidum* absorbed on a cellulose acetate disk is reacted with a serum dilution, rinsed and reacted with fluorescein-isothiocyanate-conjugated goat anti-human IgG followed by a second buffer rinse. Fluorescence signal units are measured with a fluorimeter. When fluorescence values were corrected with reference to appropriate controls, 62 sera reactive in the FTA-ABS test gave values of 64 to 178, whereas the values of 66 sera non-reactive in the FTA-ABS ranged from 20 to 46 (Stevens & Schell 1982). This test obviously merits further study.

Passive agglutination

The T. pallidum haemagglutination assay (TPHA)

In the TPHA (Rathlev 1967, Tomizawa and Kasamatsu 1966) sheep erythrocytes coated with an extract of *T. pallidum* are agglutinated by antibody from serum of patients with syphilis. Components of Reiter treponemes, rabbit testis and erythrocyte membranes are used to absorb test sera in order to eliminate haemagglutination due to antibody against any of these agents. Any serum giving a positive reaction is tested against control erythrocytes (i.e. not coated with *T. pallidum* antigen) to check the specificity of the agglutination. In spite of the absorption procedure about 0.1% of specimens agglutinate erythrocytes in the absence of antigen: this non-specific agglutination makes the individual test result invalid. The use of fowl erythrocytes in the TPHA test (Sequeira & Eldridge 1973) may decrease the number of non-specific agglutination reactions. The TPHA is simple to perform and as reagents based on sheep and fowl erythrocytes are available commercially, it has become the first of the specific tests suitable for routine screening.

Microhaemagglutination assay with T. pallidum antigen (MHA-TP)

Because of the expense of reagents the TPHA is almost always performed in microtitre plates. Although the micromethod is sometimes referred to as the MHA-TP

the two terms (TPHA and MHA-TP) are used synonymously in this text.

The TPHA is often negative in untreated primary syphilis but otherwise has a sensitivity and specificity comparable with the FTA-ABS test. The sensitivity of the test in early infections depends on the IgM binding capacity of the reagents which may vary between different kits from the same manufacturer. Such variations probably account for the discrepancies in the reported sensitivity of the TPHA test in primary syphilis. Whereas most workers (Young et al 1974, Larsen et al 1981, Huber et al 1983, Sequeira, 1983) find that antibodies detected by the TPHA appeared later or were of relatively lower titre than those detected by cardiolipin antigen tests, Dyckman et al (1980) reported that the TPHA generally became reactive earlier than the VDRL test.

Occasionally false-positive haemagglutination may result from heterophile antibody in the serum of patients with infectious mononucleosis; this only occurs if the control cells fail to agglutinate, otherwise a non-specific agglutination reaction would be recorded. In certain tropical countries a small percentage of BFP reactors have given apparent false-positive results: these positive results, due to the sensitivity of the TPHA test, could represent the residue of previous infection by endemic treponematosis (Manikowska-Lesinska et al 1978). According to Luger (1981) reactivity in the TPHA is almost always indicative of treponemal infection.

Automated microhaemagglutination assay with T. pallidum antigen (AMHA-TP)

In this modification filling of test plates and dilution steps are automated making the test less expensive and even more suitable for mass screening.

Microcapsule agglutination test for Treponema pallidum antibodies (MCA-TP)

The MCA-TP is similar to the TPHA apart from the replacement of erythrocytes by polyurea microcapsules (7 μm diameter) as the carrier for treponemal antigen (Kobayashi et al 1983). The addition of a red dye to the interior of the microcapsule improved the contrast, simplifying reading of the agglutination pattern. Microcapsules are chemically stable and are antigenically inert thus avoiding the problems associated with deterioration of erythrocytes and non-specific agglutination due to heterophile antibodies. Other advantages include the production of uniform quality microcapsules with the possibility of modifying certain particle characteristics such as size, specific gravity and surface properties according to the purpose of the test.

Preliminary studies with the MCA-TP test (Kobayashi et al 1983) allowed discrimination between sera from 65 patients with syphilis (titre of at least 160) and sera from 100 patients without syphilis (titre 10 to 40). The MCA-TP was markedly superior to the TPHA for detecting cases of primary syphilis; this difference may be partially attributable to improved binding of insoluble antigens to microcapsules as opposed to erythrocytes.

Enzyme-linked immunosorbent assay (ELISA)
ELISA is a relatively simple and fairly new serological technique. Patients' serum is allowed to react with antigen coated on the surface of small plastic beads or on the inside surface of plastic tubes or wells in a microhaemagglutination plate. Specific antibodies binding to the antigen are then quantitated by means of anti-immunoglobulin conjugated to an enzyme such as alkaline phosphatase or horseradish peroxidase. By use of appropriate enzyme substrates colour changes can be measured spectophotometrically allowing objective interpretation of the results. Another advantage of ELISA is the potential for automation.

Veldkamp & Visser (1975) using an ultrasonicate of *T. pallidum* as antigen concluded that ELISA was simple, reliable, and relatively quick and that its sensitivity in all stages of syphilis was equal to that of the FTA-ABS test.

Pope et al (1982), also using an ultrasonicate of *T. pallidum* as antigen, found ELISA to be less sensitive than the VDRL and FTA-ABS tests but more sensitive than the TPHA. In spite of using an anti-human IgG (gamma chain) conjugate the ELISA was considerably more sensitive than the TPHA in primary syphilis. ELISA obviously merits further study as a front-line screening procedure. However, among other factors, the widespread adoption of the technique will depend on commercial availability of suitable reagents.

Treponema pallidum immune adherence (TPIA) test
The immune adherence phenomenon, i.e. the adherence of specific antigen-antibody and complement-complex to primate erythrocytes or to non-primate platelets, was first described by Nelson (1953). In the TPIA test, *T. pallidum* antigen, test serum, and complement are incubated and group O human erythrocytes are added. After further incubation the mixture is centrifuged at low speed and the number of treponemes remaining in the supernatant counted. Because of their adherence to erythrocytes a decreased number of organisms is found with positive sera but not with negative sera. Although Tanaka et al (1978) described an improved method for the TPIA test the technique remains more time-consuming and technically demanding than other tests such as the TPHA or ELISA. The TPIA is unlikely to be used for other than research purposes.

DETECTION OF IgM ANTIBODIES AGAINST *T. PALLIDUM*

Tests such as the VDRL, TPHA and FTA-ABS described above, all show reactivity with IgM as well as with IgG antibodies. After infection the first humoral immune response is the production of antibodies of the IgM type. Specific anti-*T. pallidum* IgM is detectable during the second week of infection but disappears soon after elimination of the antigen; that is usually within 3–6 months of the beginning of treatment in cases of early syphilis or within 1–1.5 years of the beginning of therapy in late disease.

Production of specific anti-treponemal IgG begins around the fourth week after infection and usually reaches much higher titres than those for IgM. IgG secretion may be continued by memory cell clones long after elimination of the antigen thus accounting for the persistence of reactivity in sensitive tests such as the TPHA or FTA-ABS.

IgM-FTA-ABS test
This test is similar to the standard FTA-ABS test (p. 121) but uses a fluorescein-labelled mono-specific anti-human globulin, viz. anti-IgM, in place of the broad spectrum anti-human globulin conjugate. Although this was the first of the tests to detect anti-treponemal IgM, the extent of false-positive and false-negative results severely limits its clinical value. False-positive reactions may result due to rheumatoid factor (IgM antibody) in the serum reacting with treponemes already coated with anti-treponemal IgG (Wilkinson 1976). False-negative reactions are prone to arise when there are very high levels of IgG as at the beginning of the secondary stage and after reinfection: the smaller IgG molecules react with the receptors on the surface of *T. pallidum* before the larger IgM molecules can attach.

19S (IgM)-FTA-ABS test
This test was devised to overcome the erroneous reactions of the IgM-FTA-ABS test. The test is performed not with whole serum but with the 19S IgM fraction after separation by gel filtration or by high pressure chromatography. Müller & Lindenschmidt (1982) considered the 19S (IgM)-FTA-ABS test to be an infallible method for detecting patients with untreated syphilis. However, as expensive technical equipment and highly skilled personnel are required, this test can only be applied to a few problem sera.

19S (IgM)-TPHA test
In this test, serum is fractionated as for the 19S (IgM)-FTA-ABS test. After gel filtration eight fractions starting with the peak of the first elution maximum are tested quantitatively with commercially available TPHA

reagents. To obtain the titre of 19S (IgM) antibodies the highest titre estimated in the range of the 19S (IgM) elution is multiplied by the dilution factor produced by gel filtration. Titres for the 19S (I9M)-FTA-ABS test are calculated in a similar way. Because the test also relies on fractionation of serum its use is limited. According to Muller & Lindenschmidt (1982) the 19S (IgM)-TPHA test is not suitable for demonstrating anti-treponemal IgM; the reading of the titre in the test is difficult in some cases and impossible in others.

Solid-phase haemadsorption (IgM-SPHA)
This was one of the first specific anti-treponemal IgM tests which was simple and cheap enough to be applied on a large scale (Schmidt 1980). Wells in a polystyrene microtitre plate are coated with rabbit anti-human IgM (μ-chain specific) and are then filled with a mixture of patient's serum and absorbing diluent. After incubation for 2 h the plate is washed and TPHA antigen added. Specific anti-treponemal IgM antibody in sera from untreated patients becomes linked to the TPHA antigen and prevents the erythrocytes from sinking to the bottom of the well. A preliminary reading is possible after 3–4 h but the final result is best read after 18 h.

Negative results in the IgM-SPHA correlate well with treated infection (Luger 1981, Muller & Lindenschmidt 1982). However, Muller & Lindenschmidt (1982) reported false-negative results in more than half of patients with untreated primary syphilis and in just over one-quarter of patients with untreated secondary and late syphilis. These false-negative results may be attributable to the mechanism of the test. To obtain a reactive IgM-SPHA the percentage of treponemal-specific 19S (IgM) antibodies of the total 19S (IgM) in a serum sample must be very high otherwise the specific anti-treponemal IgM is blocked by non-specific IgM. The indirect haemadsorption which forms the second step of the test is insensitive and fails to detect levels of specific anti-treponemal IgM detectable by more sensitive techniques such as ELISA. Although Schmidt (1980) found a higher sensitivity in early syphilis he excluded sera that showed competitive inhibition.

Treponema pallidum specific IgM enzyme immunoassay (TP-IgM-EIA)
Polystyrene beads coated with a purified ultrasonicate of T.pallidum are incubated with dilutions of patient's serum for 2 h at 37°C. After washing, beads are incubated for 1 h with anti-human IgM (μ chain specific) labelled horseradish peroxidase. After further careful washing, enzyme activity is determined by incubation with the appropriate enzyme substrate (hydrogen peroxide and 2, 2'-azino-diethyl-benzothiazoline). The extent of the enzyme reaction which is related to the

amount of anti-treponemal IgM can be measured accurately with a spectrophotometer.

The overall specificity of the test was 97% when tested against sera from 1192 patients with adequately treated syphilis (Muller & Moskophidis 1984). As the test is performed with unfractionated serum rheumatoid factor can give false positive reactions. Therefore specimens giving positive results should be re-tested after absorption with latex particles coated with IgG. False negative results may arise from competition between high IgG and lower IgM antibody concentrations for binding sites on the T. pallidum coated beads. This may account for the lower sensitivity (about 93%) on latent syphilis and reinfection compared with 97.3% and 98% for primary and secondary syphilis respectively.

CAPTIA Syphilis-M monoclonal antibody enzyme-linked immunosorbent assay
This test which is available commercially (Mercia Diagnostics) depends upon IgM capture and is not subject to interference by rheumatoid factor or by competition from anti-treponemal I.G.

Rabbit antibodies against human IgM (μ chain-specific) are coated on the inner surface of microtitre wells. When test sera, diluted 1 in 50, are incubated in the wells a portion of the total IgM is captured. Washing removes unbound antibodies and other serum proteins. Specific anti-treponemal IgM within the total bound IgM is then detected by adding a tracers system prepared by mixing T. pallidum antigen, biotinylated monoclonal antibody reactive with an epitope on the 37 000 (mol. wt.) axial filament, and streptavidin-horse radish peroxidase conjugate. After further washing, bound horse radish peroxidase is detected by adding tetramethylbenzidine substrate. Because the horse radish peroxidase is indirectly bound to the specific anti-treponemal IgM through the streptavidin-biotinylated monoclonal antibody-T. pallidum antigen, the intensity of the coloured reaction product is directly proportional to the amount of anti-T. pallidum IgM in the original serum.

This test is potentially a highly sensitive and specific method for detecting anti-treponemal IgM, particularly in early infection (Luger 1987).

Treponema pallidum specific IgM haemagglutination (TP-IgM-HA)
IgM in unfractionated serum is captured by erythrocytes sensitized with rabbit anti-human IgM (μ chain specific). Prior to IgM capture the serum is usually absorbed with a sonicate of T. phagedenis to remove group specific antibody. Specific anti-treponemal IgM is detected by adding a second reagent comprising erythrocytes sensitized with sonicated T. pallidum. As

the entire test is carried out in a microtitre plate it can easily be applied to a large number of specimens.

Sato et al (1984) in a study involving 37 patients with untreated primary syphilis, 45 patients with untreated secondary syphilis and 1872 patients without syphilis (including 69 with rheumatoid arthritis) found the TP-IgM-HA test had a sensitivity and specificity of 97.6% and 99.7% respectively. If further studies including significant numbers of patients with untreated and adequately treated late active and late latent syphilis corroborate these findings, and provided that reliable reagents can be manufactured commercially, this test has considerable potential.

SEROLOGICAL TESTS IN CLINICAL PRACTICE

RATIONALE OF SEROLOGICAL SCREENING AND CLINICAL INTERPRETATION OF TEST RESULTS

The demand for serological tests parallels the recent overall increase in STD and far exceeds the present incidence of the disease. Since syphilis can be acquired concomitantly with any other STD all patients attending the clinic should be screened to exclude syphilis. As syphilis may mimic a variety of dermatological, medical and surgical conditions serological tests are of value in excluding this disease. Serological screening of all antenatal patients and blood donors is carried out to prevent congenital and transfusion-acquired infection respectively (Ch. 7).

The large number of specimens to examine and the long duration of the infection dictate that a suitable serological test should be: sensitive at all stages of infection; specific for syphilis and not react with sera from patients with other conditions; reproducible; simple and rapid to perform; and preferably inexpensive. Unfortunately no single serological test meets these requirements and, as outlined in Table 8.1, many tests have been developed over the years.

Screening with a combination of VDRL and TPHA tests

When used together, the VDRL and TPHA tests provide a highly efficient screen for the detection or exclusion of treponemal infection; their activity is complementary, both are simple to perform and can be readily quantitated. The VDRL test is more sensitive than the TPHA in the detection of very early syphilis while the TPHA is more sensitive than the VDRL in the detection of latent and late infection (Young et al 1974).

Any of the cardiolipin antigen tests can be used for routine screening and all behave in a similar manner with respect to stage of infection, effect of treatment, etc. Because it is easy to standardize, simple and reproducible, the VDRL test (VDRL carbon antigen or rapid plasma reagin test) is the recommended cardiolipin antigen test. This view is endorsed by the World Health Organization (1982) who also consider that complement fixation tests should be discontinued.

Although the VDRL carbon antigen and TPHA tests can be performed without inactivation, heating patient's serum at 56° for 30 minutes is recommended: this not only decreases the incidence of non-specific agglutination but also destroys the Acquired Immune Deficiency Syndrome (AIDS) associated virus, HIV (Ch. 31).

The VDRL carbon antigen test (or rapid plasma reagin test)

Patient's serum is tested undiluted. If any agglutination of the antigen is noted the test is repeated with a series of two-fold dilutions of patient's serum and the reciprocal of the final dilution of serum causing unequivocal agglutination is termed the titre, e.g. if agglutination occurred only with undiluted serum the result would be reported as 'positive-undiluted serum' whereas if 1 in 16 was the last dilution showing agglutination the test would be reported as 'positive-16'. It is important to test all specimens showing any degree of agglutination quantitatively in order to detect a prozone reaction (i.e. inhibition of agglutination due to excess antibody in the serum).

The VDRL test usually becomes positive 10 to 14 days after the appearance of the chancre or approximately 3 to 5 weeks after acquiring the infection. It is positive in approximately 75% of cases of primary syphilis. After the secondary stage the VDRL titre declines and eventually becomes negative in approximately 30% of untreated latent and late cases. The VDRL test also tends to become negative after treatment, particularly in early syphilis.

The TPHA test

Patient's serum is screened at a final dilution of 1 in 80: if any haemagglutination is noted the test is repeated with a series of two-fold dilutions from 1 in 80 to 1 in 5120. The reciprocal of the final serum dilution resulting in marked haemagglutination is termed the titre. TPHA titres are reported as positive-80, positive-160, etc. Each specimen is also tested against control cells (no antigen) at a serum dilution of 1 in 80: if the control cells agglutinate the serum is reported as 'non-specific agglutination — test invalid'.

The TPHA is usually negative in early primary syphilis but may become positive at low titre (80 to 320) towards the end of the primary stage. The TPHA titre may give some indication of the duration of the infection. Titres rise sharply during the secondary stage and commonly reach 5120 or greater. The TPHA titre declines during the latent stage but invariably remains positive at low titre (80 to 640).

The only stage of syphilis likely to escape detection by screening with a combination of VDRL and TPHA tests is early primary syphilis, although repeated tests over a three month period will detect such an infection. Most such cases of seronegative primary syphilis should be detected by a careful clinical examination and dark ground investigation. Since the FTA-ABS is normally the first test to become positive following infection it is a useful aid in the diagnosis of primary syphilis. Although it cannot be applied to all specimens the test can be carried out, and should be requested, in cases of suspected primary syphilis.

Table 8.2 Commonly observed pattern of results of serological tests in different stages of acquired syphilis. (In endemic treponemal diseases, such as yaws, bejel or pinta, patterns are similar to syphilis — see text for fuller details.)

VDRL	TPHA	FTA-ABS	Likely diagnosis
+	−	−	(False-positive reaction. (Repeat to exclude primary
+	− or +	+	(Primary. Dark field (investigation of lesion may be positive.
+	+	+	(Untreated (or recently (treated). Probably beyond primary stage.
−	+	+	(Treated or partially (treated at any stage. Untreated latent or late.
−	+	−	History of treated syphilis.

+ = positive; ∓ = weakly reactive; − = negative

CONFIRMATION OF DIAGNOSIS AND QUANTITATIVE TESTS

The FTA-ABS test should be used as a verification test in the case of specimens showing reactivity in the VDRL and/or TPHA tests during screening. Quantitative VDRL and TPHA tests should be carried out at the same time as the confirmatory FTA-ABS test. In order to minimize the risk of transfer or transposition errors which may have occurred during mass screening,

these tests should be performed with a further specimen of serum removed from the original blood tube.

When such a system is employed the pattern of results obtained (Table 8.2) may give valuable information as to the stage of infection. This figure is only a guide: each case must be interpreted individually in the light of available clinical and epidemiological data.

PATTERNS OF SEROLOGICAL RESULTS

Biological false-positive reaction
Sera positive only in the VDRL test are most likely to be biological false-positive reactions. A further specimen of blood should be taken and the test repeated to exclude technical error or an atypical primary pattern. In screening for early syphilis, tests should be repeated over a period of at least three months. If the VDRL test remains the only test positive for longer than six months then investigations should be instigated to exclude the various conditions often associated with a chronic biological false-positive reaction.

Primary syphilis
A typical pattern of primary syphilis is VDRL and FTA-ABS positive but TPHA negative or weakly reactive. During the primary stage the VDRL titre may rise to 8 or 16 whereas the TPHA may become positive at low titre (80–320) towards the end of the primary stage. Very early in the infection the FTA-ABS may be the only test positive. Dark ground examination of serum obtained from the depth of mucocutaneous lesions may also be positive for *T. pallidum* at this stage.

Secondary syphilis
VDRL titres of 16–128 are commonly found in secondary syphilis. TPHA titres also rise sharply during the secondary stage and usually reach 5120 or greater. Titres tend to decline after the secondary stage. Therefore when quantitative VDRL and TPHA tests are positive to high titre and the FTA-ABS is also positive the most likely diagnosis is secondary syphilis or early latent syphilis. The same pattern of results can be obtained in late syphilis or in recently treated secondary syphilis so it is clear that interpretation of syphilis serology is dependent on the history and clinical findings.

Late-stage syphilis
The VDRL titre declines after the secondary stage and eventually becomes negative in approximately 30% of untreated latent and late infections. However, titres may be high (16–128) in active cardiovascular and neuro-syphilis and in those with gummatous lesions. The TPHA titre declines during the latent stage but unlike the

VDRL test it invariably remains positive at low titre (80–640). High titres (5120 or greater) can be expected in active late syphilis. Therefore, when quantitative VDRL and TPHA tests are positive regularly over a period of time at low titre in patients without signs then the infection is likely to be beyond the early latent stage and may have been modified by coincidental curative or subcurative antibiotic treatment.

When the TPHA is the only positive test it is usually of low titre, and a history of syphilis, treated as many as 20 to 40 years previously, may be obtained. Sometimes there is merely a hint of some half-forgotten incident. Luger (1981) also considered that a positive haemagglutination assay is strongly suggestive of previous syphilis which has either cured itself spontaneously or been cured by antibiotic treatment.

ACTIVITY OF INFECTION AND RESPONSE TO TREATMENT

Quantitative VDRL test

All cardiolipin antigen tests tend to become negative after treatment, particularly in early syphilis. Serial quantitative tests should be carried out for up to two years following treatment for early acquired syphilis and for up to five years in late-stage infection. In interpreting a fall or rise in titre in early-stage syphilis a four-fold change is considered significant but a two-fold change is not. Fluctuating antibody levels are sometimes found in treated late and congenital syphilis. These do not necessarily indicate a need for further treatment.

As a general guide the VDRL titre should become negative within one to two years of effective treatment for early syphilis. After adequate treatment of late infection the VDRL test may remain reactive (titre $\leqslant 8$) for many years. VDRL titres of > 16 rarely persist in adequately treated infections.

A negative VDRL test can be expected in up to 30% of patients with *untreated* late syphilis.

Quantitative TPHA

In many instances quantitative tests when interpreted in the light of clinical signs and symptoms, and with a knowledge of the patient's history, will support a diagnosis of untreated early syphilis. However, the TPHA titre is of little help in assessing treatment status in cases of late syphilis.

The TPHA test remains positive for life even in those who have been fully treated with adequate doses of penicillin. In such cases, the detection of a positive TPHA, perhaps later in life, is not an indication for further treatment and investigation, provided the patient has been adequately treated in the past and

provided he has not been at risk since. The TPHA test presents the clinician with the problem of differentiating between treated and untreated or partially treated infection. The reliable detection of latent and late syphilis by the TPHA test is, however, very important since, if untreated, a proportion of these patients will unpredictably develop the clinical manifestations of late infection. The widespread use of antibiotics for many other conditions, often trivial, has produced a situation where untreated infections are now a rarity. The clinical and pathological features of partially treated or suppressed infection require further study and screening by the TPHA test is of value in this respect.

DETECTION OF ANTI-TREPONEMAL IgM

The presence of anti-treponemal IgM in the sera of neonates and adults is an indication of the persistence of treponemal antigen within the body. Very occasionally false-negative reactions may result from suppression of the specific IgM antibody response by high levels of circulating IgG (Uhr & Moller 1968, Araujo & Remington 1975, Muller & Moskophidis 1984).

Of the various methods of detecting anti-treponemal IgM described earlier, reactivity in the 19S (IgM)-FTA-ABS provides the most reliable correlation with treatment status in all stages of infection (Muller & Lindenschmidt 1982). Effective treatment is indicated by a negative 19S (IgM-FTA-ABS test: within three months of the beginning of treatment in cases of early syphilis; within one year of the beginning of treatment in cases of late disease. Unfortunately experience with the 19S (IgM)-FTA-ABS test is restricted to a very few laboratories.

For the near future, simple tests such as the TP-IgM-HA or the Captia Syphilis-M monoclonal antibody ELISA test (Luger 1987) may bring reliable anti-treponemal IgM detection within the scope of most laboratories serving genito-urinary medicine clinics. Whenever an investigation for specific anti-treponemal IgM is to be undertaken, the lability of the large IgM molecule must be borne in mind: blood samples should preferably be transported under refrigeration and, once separated, the serum should be tested without heat inactivation (Luger 1987).

CONGENITAL SYPHILIS

The diagnosis of congenital syphilis can present a considerable problem since it depends mainly on the results of serological tests and also because most neonates so affected are asymptomatic at birth. Early-stage congenital syphilis is a rarity in the United Kingdom and there are few up-to-date serological data available.

As the standard serological tests for syphilis depend on responses involving IgG and IgM antibodies their interpretation is extremely difficult; the IgG found in the serum of neonates is largely passively acquired through the placenta and does not represent the infant's own response. Whereas a rising or higher titre in the neonate than in the mother is suggestive of infection, the 19S (IgM)-FTA-ABS test is currently the most reliable test for confirming a diagnosis of congenital infection. Whilst fractionation of serum will overcome the problem of false-negative reactions resulting from competition between IgG and IgM for treponemal binding sites during the test it cannot overcome the theoretical possibility of suppression of IgM synthesis in the neonate due to high levels of circulating maternal anti-treponemal IgG (Johnston 1972).

There was no suppression of IgM synthesis in the 9 cases of congenital syphilis reported from Seville, Spain, where the mean number of cases of congenital syphilis over a 3-year period was 0.81 per 1000 live births (Borobio et al 1980). In addition to the demonstration of specific treponemal IgM, Borobio et al (1980) found that all infected infants had raised total IgM, usually in the range of 1 to 4 g/l. After treatment, total IgM returned to normal, specific anti-treponemal IgM and other antibody test titres decreased and tended to become negative. In 3 cases considered to have passively transferred antibody, anti-treponemal IgM was absent and total IgM levels were near normal ($\leqslant$ 0.7 g/l). Lower titres in neonates when compared to their mothers are also suggestive of passively transferred antibody. In the absence of infection passively transferred antibody detected by the VDRL will decrease and the tests will become negative in approximately 3 months. In the case of the TPHA, the titre will become low and the test negative in 6 to 12 months.

In late-stage infection, either treated or untreated, test results tend to fluctuate over a period of months or years. The VDRL test often remains positive at low titre in association with a low TPHA titre and positive FTA-ABS test. Data on specific anti-treponemal IgM in late-stage congenital infection are inadequate.

DIAGNOSIS OF NEUROSYPHILIS

The use of cerebrospinal fluid (CSF) for routine screening tests in patients in whom there is no clinical suspicion of syphilis is unjustified; a negative TPHA test on the blood will virtually exclude active neuro-syphilis and is a better screen for the detection of all forms of late syphilis (Leading Article 1977).

In cases selected on clinical grounds and backed by a positive TPHA result on blood, however, investigations should be carried out on the CSF to detect early invasion of the central nervous system (CNS). Because invasion of the CNS can be detected before symptoms develop, and also because the (early) effects of syphilis on the CNS can often be reversed by penicillin treatment, CSF examinations are important in the assessment of patients with the disease.

In the case of early syphilis it is traditional policy to carry out a lumbar puncture 12 months after treatment as part of the test of cure. In the case of patients with syphilis of uncertain duration or in the late symptomatic or late latent stage, CSF examination is an essential part of the investigation necessary before treatment. When there is evidence of clinical relapse or a four-fold rise is noted in the titre of the serological tests in the follow-up of a patient, CSF examination is necessary (Catterall 1977).

In cerebrospinal and ocular fluids treponemes indistinguishable from T. pallidum may be found sometimes after treatment, in late syphilis. The presence of these treponemes is of uncertain clinical significance and they are not necessarily associated with progression of the disease nor are they indicators that the patient can transmit his disease at that stage (Collart et al 1962). The search for such treponemes in the centrifuged deposit of the CSF and by inoculation of experimental rabbits with CSF are research procedures rather than routines required in day-to-day clinical practice.

Examination of the cerebrospinal fluid (CSF)
A total volume of 8–10 ml is usually sufficient for the tests required, which should be carried out as soon as possible after collection; note that contamination of the CSF specimen with even a small amount of blood can give misleading results. Investigation of the CSF should include: (1) serological tests; (2) a cell count; (3) estimation of total protein, IgG, IgM and albumin. Serological tests and estimation of IgG and albumin should be performed in parallel on serum.

1. Serological tests
A negative result in either the TPHA or the FTA-ABS test on CSF excludes neurosyphilis. A negative VDRL test is not reliable for excluding neurosyphilis since the VDRL test is non-reactive in approximately 30–60% of patients with active neurosyphilis.

A positive TPHA or FTA-ABS test on CSF does not necessarily indicate active disease since reactivity may be caused by transudation of immunoglobulins from the serum into the CSF. Although CSF TPHA titres of $\geqslant$ 2560 are suggestive of active neurosyphilis, results can be misleading where there is a severe breakdown of the blood/CSF barrier function. Calculation of the TPHA index (see below) allows for such impaired barrier function.

2. Cell count

Cell counts are carried out in a Fuchs-Rosenthal haemocytometer. The total and differential white blood cell counts are performed. Normally there are less than 3 leucocytes per mm^3 (3×10^6 per litre) and the first indication of involvement of the CNS by syphilis may be a count of 10 lymphocytes or more per mm^3 (10×10^6 per litre).

After treatment with penicillin in cases of neurosyphilis or asymptomatic neurosyphilis, the leucocyte count in the CSF reverts rapidly towards normal; with tetracycline and erythromycin, given to those who are allergic to penicillin, more careful CSF follow-up with re-treatment is advised as confidence and experience with these antibiotics in the treatment of neurosyphilis is less than with penicillin.

3. Total protein and immunoglobulins

The total protein is normally 10–40 mg per 100 ml (100–400 mg per litre) and in neurosyphilis the increase may be only slight or may reach levels of 100–200 per 100 ml (1000–2000 mg per litre). Total protein tends to revert towards normal after treatment more rapidly than more complex qualitative changes such as those detected by electrophoresis. In the absence of virus disease, an increase in immunoglobulin (IgG) above 13% of total protein is supportive evidence of neurosyphilis or multiple sclerosis (Millar 1975). In such cases CSF protein should be submitted, where possible and practicable, to polyacrylamide gel electrophoresis at pH 8.8 as a quantitative analysis of these immunoglobulins may help in the assessment of CSF activity. In neurosyphilis IgM may be elevated in the CSF and it tends to fall rapidly after treatment (Oxelius et al 1969).

The Lange colloidal gold test is a traditional test used over many years to indicate alteration in the albumin/globulin ratio. Colloidal gold activity resides in the gamma globulin fraction; gamma globulins are more positively charged in solution and have a greater tendency to precipitate the negatively charged gold sol. Because the results of this test are not always precise or reproducible the method has now been discarded. A more modern approach is to examine oligoprotein banding patterns on gel electrophoresis.

Oligoproteins

Proteins in CSF are derived partly by filtration of serum, partly from interstitial fluid which includes proteins from brain cells, and partly from cells of the CSF itself. If polyacrylamide is used as the support medium in the electrophoresis of CSF the migration of proteins is retarded according to their size, since the polyacrylamide has an internal structure like that of a molecular sieve and as a result some 30 bands may be seen. The technique requires only a small amount (1.0 ml) of fresh unconcentrated fluid, free from red cells, and diluted serum from the same patient should be run alongside the CSF. A densitometer can be used to scan the stained gel.

This form of electrophoresis can detect protein abnormalities, particularly in the gamma region; these consist predominantly of immunoglobulins. When the immunoglobulins, as in neurosyphilis, are locally produced they are more basic and tend to run near the cathode in the slow part of the gamma region. Instead of being diffusely stained, as would be expected with polyclonal immunoglobulins of varying size and charge, the locally synthesized immunoglobulins run in 'bands' visible against a diffuse background (Fishman 1980). Such immunoglobulins are the product of a small (oligo) number of B-cell clones and when the oligoclonal pattern is more prominent in the CSF than in the serum from the same patient then this is strong evidence for local synthesis of IgG within the CNS. In neurosyphilis such an oligoclonal pattern may be seen and may alter following treatment (Thompson & Johnson 1982).

Blood/CSF barrier function and the TPHA index

Conventional criteria such as raised CSF cell count and increased total protein may give evidence of an inflammatory response in the CNS, but these examinations are not specific for neurosyphilis. In addition normal cell counts and total protein values do not exclude absolutely involvement of the CNS. Luger et al (1981) have investigated the following parameters as aids to the accurate diagnosis of neurosyphilis.

Albumin quotient

$$\text{The albumin quotient} = \frac{\text{CSF albumin (mg/dl)} \times 10^3}{\text{serum albumin (mg/dl)}}$$

This quotient provides a means of defining the normality or degree of impairment of the blood/CSF barrier. Normal values range from 3.0 to 8.0 depending on the age of the patient.

TPHA index

$$\text{The TPHA index} = \frac{\text{CSF TPHA titre}}{\text{albumin quotient}}$$

The TPHA index relates the CSF TPHA titre to the

albumin quotient and thereby attempts to exclude errors from disturbed function of the blood/brain barrier. The normal range is below 100 provided that the albumin quotient is not extremely high (e.g. above 20–30).

Luger et al (1981) found all but 1 sample from 11 patients with active neurosyphilis had TPHA indices above 100 (range 160 to greater than 12 000); 1 patient with a marked breakdown of the blood/CSF barrier as evidenced by an albumin quotient of 380 had a CSF TPHA titre of 10 240, giving a TPHA index of 27.

IgG index

$$\text{The IgG index} = \frac{\text{IgG quotient}}{\text{albumin quotient}}$$

The IgG quotient is analogous to the albumin quotient described above and is calculated as follows:

$$\text{IgG quotient} = \frac{\text{CSF IgG (mg/l)} \times 10^3}{\text{serum IgG (mg/dl)}}$$

The IgG index estimates whether the IgG antibody concentration in the CSF is greater than could be accounted for by mere transudation from the serum to the CSF. Because of their different molecular weights, two molecules of albumin will cross the barrier for every one molecule of globulin, giving a normal IgG index of 0.5. An IgG index of ≥ 0.85 is usually taken to indicate that the IgG concentration in the CSF is greater than can be accounted for by mere transudation from the serum. A raised IgG index is no more than a sign of a specific perivascular inflammation in the close vicinity of the CSF and does not necessarily indicate neurosyphilis. Nevertheless, all but one of the patients with active neurosyphilis studied by Luger et al (1981) had pathological IgG indices.

Although the above parameters have been suggested as useful indices of neurosyphilis, they require more detailed study in other centres involving larger numbers of patients with all forms of late syphilis. Other indicators which also require further study include the detection of specific anti- treponemal immunoglobulins such as IgM and IgA. Gschnait et al (1981) found *T.pallidum* specific IgA in the CSF of patients with neurosyphilis but not those with late latent syphilis. It was suggested that *T.pallidum* specific IgA may play a role in the pathogenesis of neurosyphilis by competing with IgG molecules for receptor sites on the treponeme: since binding of IgA does not activate the classical complement pathway it blocks the complement-dependent IgG bactericidal activity.

SCREENING BY OTHER THAN A COMBINATION OF VDRL AND TPHA TESTS

The continuous serological screening of pregnant women, blood donors, and 'at-risk' groups should be maintained as part of the overall effort to detect and control syphilis. The combination of the VDRL (or RPR or ART tests) and TPHA tests is now accepted as giving the best coverage for detection or exclusion of all forms of treponemal infection (WHO 1982). In conditions of high prevalence and limited resources, either the VDRL or RPR alone should be used for screening.

In the UK in 1983 as shown in Table 8.3, the vast majority (86%) of laboratories employ a screening schedule comprising a 'reagin' flocculation or agglutination test in combination with the TPHA. It is clear that the Reiter protein complement fixation test and the Wassermann complement fixation reaction performed in only 3% and 2% of laboratories respectively have been superseded by the TPHA in combination with one of the newer 'reagin' tests.

Table 8.3 Combination of serological tests for syphilis used by laboratories participating in a nationwide quality control survey. (Reproduced from Summary of Distribution No. 253, June 1983, by kind permission of the Organizer of the National External Quality Assessment Scheme; for full details, see Acknowledgements.)

Test combination	Number of laboratories using stated combination of tests
Reagin/TPHA/FTA	87
Reagin/TPHA	76
Reagin	11
Reagin/TPHA/FTA/Reiter	3
Reagin/TPHA/FTA/WR	3
Reagin/FTA	2
Reagin/TPHA/Reiter	2
Reagin/TPHA/FTA/TPI	1
Reagin/WR	1
TPHA	1
Reagin/Reiter	1
Reagin/TPHA/TPI	1

It has been suggested (Diggory 1983) that the VDRL test should be withdrawn from initial testing for syphilis except where primary disease is suspected. However, until TPHA reagents with improved and reliable IgM binding capacity become widely available the VDRL test should remain as a cover for primary infection. As the VDRL is both cheap and simple to perform it is probably just as cost-effective to screen all specimens by both tests as it is to initiate a reliable system of test selection in the case of suspected primary syphilis.

Traditionally, in areas such as blood transfusion, cardiolipin antigen tests have been used to detect donations from patients with early syphilis. Although a cardiolipin antigen test alone will provide an adequate screen for early infection, sera from patients with secondary syphilis may give false negative reactions resulting from the 'prozone' phenomenon. The TPHA test performed in combination is not only useful in detecting sera with very high levels of antibody likely to give a prozone reaction in the cardiolipin antigen test, but will also identify virtually all patients with late syphilis, whether treated or not. Puckett & Pratt (1982) described a modified, miniaturized version of the TPHA for use in blood transfusion centres but cautioned that neither the TPHA nor cardiolipin tests should be relied upon alone in screening.

ELISA is a more sensitive test system than agglutination and, in spite of using anti-human IgG (gamma chain) conjugate, an ELISA test was more sensitive than the TPHA in primary syphilis (Pope et al 1982). Results of screening with a new commercially avilable ELISA for anti-treponemal IgG (CAPTIA Syphilis-G, Mercia Diagnostics) were comparable to screening with a combination of VDRL and TPHA tests (Young et al 1987). The potential for automation and computerized data analysis will in the near future make such a test attractive for rapid screening of large numbers of specimens for current or past infection.

Whichever screening system is used, human and technical errors may result and *a diagnosis of syphilis should never be made on the results of a single blood specimen.*

BIOLOGICAL FALSE-POSITIVE (BFP) REACTORS

BFP reactors are those patients whose serum gives a positive cardiolipin antigen test result but negative specific treponemal antigen tests in the absence of past or present treponemal infection (Catterall 1972). There are several possible reasons for obtaining a BFP reaction. It may be the result of tissue destruction and liberation of cardiolipin from mitochondria. Infection with microorganisms containing cardiolipin, or serum protein disturbances may also result in BFP reactions. Anticardiolipin antibody is present in small quantities in the sera of healthy individuals, where it is normally inhibited by a globulin known as the inhibitor. If the amount of inhibitor is reduced a cardiolipin antigen test can give a positive result (Kiraly 1973).

The frequency of BFP reactions depends upon the test used and appears to be lower with the VDRL test than with the Wassermann reaction. The lower the incidence of treponemal infection within the community, the higher the relative frequency of BFP reactors among positive cardiolipin screening tests. Chronic BFP reactors are seen more frequently in the female and in the elderly as a result of tissue wear and tear. A high frequency of BFP reactions also occurs among drug addicts although the significance of this is not clear at present. The BFP reaction may sometimes have a genetic basis.

The acute or transient BFP may occur shortly after an acute febrile infectious disease (e.g. infectious mononucleosis, infective hepatitis, measles, upper respiratory tract infection) or be provoked by strong immunological stimuli such as vaccination and pregnancy. The acute BFP disappears within a few weeks or months after the acute illness has subsided. Approximately 60% of acute BFP reactors are under 30 years of age.

In contrast, the chronic BFP reaction persists longer than six months, and approximately 60% of reactors are over 30 years of age. Chronic BFP reactions are also more common in women than men. They may be associated with auto-immune and related diseases, e.g. rheumatoid arthritis, systemic lupus erythematosus (SLE), Sjögren's disease, auto-immune thyroiditis and auto-immune haemolytic anaemia.

The sera of approximately 10% of patients with SLE contain a non-specific circulating anticoagulant called 'lupus anticoagulant' which is directed against the prothrombin converting complex. BFP reactions are found in approximately 70% of SLE patients with lupus anticoagulant compared with only 10% of patients lacking the anticoagulant (Shoenfeld et al 1980). It was also noted that thrombocytopenia is found more frequently in SLE patients who give BFP reactions. The association between circulating anticoagulant, the BFP reaction and thrombocytopenia is due to an immunological cross-reaction resulting from antibody directed against the phospholipid component of the different antigens such as the prothrombin converting complex, cardiolipin and phospholipid sites on the platelet membrane.

Antibody of class IgG giving rise to a BFP reaction may cross the placenta and be detected in the neonate. On serial testing the antibody should disappear and the tests become negative in two to three months.

Repeated serological tests are necessary in order to differentiate between acute and chronic BFP reactors and cases of treponemal infection: great care should be exercised in the interpretation of results to prevent misdiagnosis. By mechanisms quite distinct from the BFP reaction patients with SLE may give a false-positive result in the FTA-ABS test. Similarly, a proportion of patients with infectious mononucleosis may give a false-positive TPHA test due to high levels of heterophile antibody. Very occasionally, both treponemal tests may be falsely reactive. Russell Jones et al (1983) described a patient with essential mixed cryoglobulinaemia whose serum gave false-positive reactions in the FTA-ABS and TPHA tests; and an anti-complementary TPI test. After removal of antiglobulin activity by immunoabsorption with heat-aggregated gamma globulin, all serological test results for treponemal infection became negative.

The TPI test is less sensitive than either the FTA-ABS or TPHA tests in late syphilis and, if relied upon, patients with treponemal infection could be falsely classified as BFP reactors. Since the chronic BFP reaction may precede the clinical manifestations of systemic lupus erythematosus or other auto-immune disease, the diagnosis of chronic BFP reactor may eventually have serious implications for the patient. About 20% of women and 5% of men who are chronic BFP reactors may give a history of hypersensitivity to penicillin, underlining the importance of accurate diagnosis of this group (Catterall 1972).

REINFECTION

The natural course of syphilis indicates that immune mechanisms are involved in the host-treponeme relationship. An initial attack does not give complete immunity but the majority of patients maintain a level of immunity sufficient to limit the disease to such an extent as to remain latent, i.e. a balance is struck between the infecting organisms and the specific cellular immune process. Humoral mechanisms of immunity do exist in syphilis but appear to be relatively inefficient and of uncertain protective value. It is a well-known clinical finding that patients with early acquired syphilis may have high levels of circulating antibody yet become reinfected after treatment.

Fiumara (1980) studied 36 patients who became reinfected with primary, secondary or latent syphilis. The titres of antibody to cardiolipin were consistently higher during reinfection than during the first infection, and the serological responses to treatment were always slower. These findings and the series of serological test results (Fig. 8.2) for one of our patients who became reinfected after treatment for secondary syphilis demonstrate the importance of *quantitative* serological tests in detecting reinfection.

CASE HISTORY

The patient, a homosexual male, attended the clinic in late October 1974. Although there was no history of syphilis the FTA-ABS test was positive, the VDRL titre was 8 and the TPHA titre 1280. The rise in VDRL titre from 8 to 32 in the next 7 days suggested an early secondary infection.

Following a course of penicillin treatment the VDRL titre decreased and became negative by February 1975, again indicating an early infection. Although the TPHA titre decreased to 80 by mid-November, characteristically it did not become negative. In mid-December the VDRL had risen to 4 and the TPHA titre to 2560, suggesting reinfection. By mid-January the VDRL titre was 64 and the TPHA 5120. On clinical examination the patient had a maculopapular rash and an anal chancre abounding with treponemes. Following the second course of penicillin therapy titres again declined.

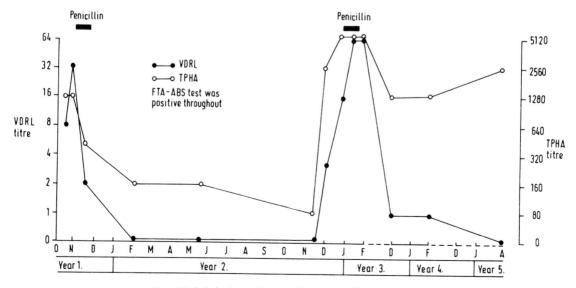

Fig. 8.2 Reinfection with syphilis: see case history in text.

NEW TECHNOLOGICAL APPROACHES TO DIAGNOSIS AND CONTROL

MONOCLONAL ANTIBODIES

Murine anti-*T. pallidum* (Nichols strain) lymphocyte hybridoma cell lines secreting monoclonal antibodies against a variety of treponemal antigens have been generated (Robertson et al 1982). When certain of these antibodies were used as primary antibody source in a solid-phase immunoblot assay system they were able to detect approximately 1 to 2×10^3 treponemes (Norgard et al 1984). The antibodies were directed against an abundant 47 000 dalton surface-exposed antigen. Most of the monoclonal antibodies reacted specifically with *T. pallidum*, either purified or within primary chancre lesions of experimental rabbits and not with *T. phagedenis* biotype *Reiter*, *Haemophilus ducreyi*, *Neisseria gonorrhoeae*, herpes simplex virus type 2, or normal rabbit testicular tissue. Such monoclonal antibodies should facilitate the development of diagnostic tests designed to detect low numbers of pathogenic treponemes in lesion exudates or other body fluids such as CSF (Lukehart & Baker-Zander 1987). Therapeutic use of monoclonal antibodies remains another possibility.

GENE CLONING

The technology provided by molecular biology is currently being applied to the study and manipulation of *T. pallidum* genes and surface antigens. Van Embden et al (1983) cloned *T. pallidum* DNA in *Escherichia coli* K12 and demonstrated that the *T. pallidum* genes were able to direct the synthesis of *T. pallidum* protein antigens in the recombinant *E. coli* strain. Treponemal antigens which have now been cloned in *E. coli* include the major 47 000 mol. wt. surface immunogen (Norgard et al 1986) as well as a 39 000 mol. wt. basic membrane protein (Dallas et al 1987).

Whilst cloned treponemal antigens almost certainly have great potential in the serodiagnosis of syphilis, seroreactivities of the various antigens require extensive characterization with respect to the human humoral immune response to *T. pallidum*. By careful selection, it may be possible to obtain antigens with a bias towards detection of specific stages of infection and to use combined antigens to detect infection at any stage. Several groups have already started to characterize the immune response to cloned antigens (Coates et al 1986, Hindersson et al 1986, Radolf et al 1986).

The combined technologies of gene cloning and monoclonal antibodies may aid the selection and testing of candidate vaccine antigens. Highly specific monoclonal antibodies and suitably selected antigens may allow the differentiation between vaccinated and infected individuals, thus overcoming a major diagnostic difficulty which would be associated with the introduction of a conventional vaccination programme. However, as a proportion of patients may develop syphilis in a latent form only, the assessment of the effectiveness of any vaccine would be very difficult.

REFERENCES

Araujo F G, Remington J S 1975 IgG antibody suppression of the IgM antibody response to *Toxoplasma gondii* in newborn rabbits. Immunology 115: 335–338

Borobio M V, Nogales M C, Palomares J C 1980 Value of serological diagnosis in congenital syphilis: report of nine cases. British Journal of Venereal Diseases 56: 377–380

Catterall R D 1972 Systemic disease and the biological false positive reaction. British Journal of Venereal Diseases 48: 1–12

Catterall R D 1977 Neurosyphilis. British Journal of Hospital Medicine 17: 585–604

Chapel T, Jeffries C D, Brown W J, Stewart J A 1978 Influence of genital herpes on results of the FTA-ABS test. British Journal of Venereal Diseases .54: 299–302

Coates S R, Sheridan P J, Hansen D S, Laird W J, Erlich H A 1986 Serospecificity of a cloned protease-resistant *Treponema pallidum* specific antigen expressed in *Escherichia coli*. Journal of Clinical Microbiology 23: 460–464

Collart P, Borel L J, Durel P 1962 Étude de l'action de la pénicilline dans la syphilis tardive. Persistance du tréponème role après traitement. Annales de l'Institut Pasteur 102: 596–615

D'Alessandro G, Dordanoni L 1953 Isolation and purification of the protein antigen of the Reiter treponeme. American Journal of Syphilis, Gonorrhea and Venereal Diseases 37: 137–150

Dallas W S, Ray P H, Leong J, Benedict C D, Stamm L V, Bassford P J 1987 Identification and pirification of a recombinant *Treponema pallidum* basic membrane protein antigen expressed in *Escherichia coli*. Infection and Immunity 55: 1106–1115

Daniels K C, Ferneyhaugh H S 1977 Specific direct fluorescent antibody detection of *Treponema pallidum*. Health Laboratory Science 14: 164–171

Diggory P 1983 Role of the Venereal Disease Research Laboratory test in the detection of syphilis. British Journal of Venereal Diseases 59: 8–10

Dyckman J D, Storms S, Huber T W 1980 Reactivity of microhaemagglutination fluorescent treponemal antibody absorption and Venereal Disease Research Laboratory tests in primary syphilis. Journal of Clinical Microbiology 12: 629–630

Editorial 1968 August von Wassermann (1866–1925) Wassermann reaction. Journal of the American Medical Association 204: 1000–1001

Farshy C E, Kennedy E J, Hunter E F, Larsen S A 1983 Fluorescent treponemal antibody absorption double-staining test evaluation. Journal of Clinical Microbiology 17: 245–248

Fishman R A 1980 Cerebrospinal fluid in diseases of the nervous system. W B Saunders Philadelphia, p 180

Fiumara N J 1980 Reinfection primary, secondary and latent syphilis: the serologic response after treatment. Sexually Transmitted Diseases 7: 111–115

Gschnait F, Schmidt B L, Luger A 1981 Cerebrospinal fluid immunoglobulins in neurosyphilis. British Journal of Venereal Diseases 57: 238–240

Harris A, Rosenberg A A, Riedel L M 1946 A microflocculation test for syphilis using cardiolipin antigen. Journal of Venereal Disease Information 27: 169–175

Hindersson P, Cockayne A, Schouls L M, van Embden J D A 1986 Immunochemical characterization and purification of *Treponema pallidum* antigen TpD expressed by *Escherichia coli* K12. Sexually Transmitted Diseases 13: 237–244

Hook E W, Roddy R E, Lukehart S A, Hom J, Holmes K K, Tam M R 1985 Detection of *Treponema pallidum* in lesion exudate with a pathogen-specific monoclonal antibody. Journal of Clinical Microbiology 22: 241–244

Huber T W et al 1983 Reactivity of microhaemagglutination fluorescent treponemal antibody absorption Venereal Disease Research Laboratory and rapid plasma reagin tests in primary syphilis. Journal of Clinical Microbiology 17: 405–409

Hunter E F, Deacon W E, Meyer P E 1964 An improved FTA test for syphilis, the absorption procedure (FTA-ABS). Public Health Report, Washington 79: 410–412

Johnston N A 1972 Neonatal congenital syphilis. Diagnosis by the absorbed fluorescent treponemal antibody (IgM) test. British Journal of Venereal Disease 48: 465–469

Kiraly K 1973 Immunoallergologic aspects of syphilis. WHO/VDT/RES Document 73.304

Kobayashi S, Yamaya S-I, Sugahara T, Matuhsi T 1983 Microcapsule agglutination test for Treponema pallidum antibodies: a new serodiagnostic test for syphilis. British Journal of Venereal Diseases 59: 1–7

Larsen S A, Hambie E A, Pettit D E, Perryman M W, Kraus S J 1981 Specificity, sensitivity and reproducibility among the fluorescent treponemal antibody-absorption test, the microhaemagglutination assay for *Treponema pallidum* antibodies, and the haemagglutination treponemal test for syphilis. Journal of Clinical Microbiology 14: 441–445

Leading Article 1977 Routine tests for syphilis on cerebrospinal fluid. Lancet ii: 595

Luger A 1981 Diagnosis of syphilis. Bulletin of the World Health Organization 59: 647–655

Luger A 1987 Serological diagnosis of syphilis: current methods. In: Young H, McMillan A (eds) Immunological diagnosis of sexually transmitted diseases. Marcel Dekker, New York p 249–274

Luger A, Schmidt B L, Steyrer K, Schonuald E 1981 Diagnosis of neurosyphilis by examination of the cerebrospinal fluid. British Journal of Venereal Diseases 57: 232–237

Lukehart S A, Baker-Zander S A 1987 The diagnostic potential of monoclonal antibodies against *Treponema pallidum*. In: Young H, McMillan A (eds) Immunological

diagnosis of sexually transmitted diseases. Marcel Dekker, New York p 213–247

McGrew B E, Ducros M J F, Stout G W, Falcone V H 1968 Automation of a flocculation test for syphilis. American Journal of Clinical Pathology 50: 52–59

McKenna C H, Schroeter A L, Kierland R R, Stilwell G C, Pien F D 1973 The fluorescent treponemal antibody absorbed (FTA-ABS) test beading phenomenon in connective tissue diseases. Mayo Clinical Proceedings 48: 545–548

Manikowska-Lesinska W, Linda B, Zajac W 1978 Specificity of the FTA-ABS and TPHA tests during pregnancy. British Journal of Venereal Diseases 54: 295–298

Millar J H D 1975 The demyelinating diseases. In: Mathews W B (ed) Present advances in clinical neurology. Churchill Livingstone, Edinburgh, p 218–233

Müller F, Lindenschmidt E-G 1982 Demonstration of specific 19S (IgM) antibodies in untreated and treated syphilis: comparative studies of the 19S (IgM)-TPHA test and the solid-phase haemabsorption assay. British Journal of Venereal Diseases 58: 12–17

Müller F, Moskophidis M 1984 Evaluation of an enzyme-linked immunoassay for IgM antibodies to *Treponema pallidum* in syphilis in man. British Journal of Venereal Diseases 60: 288–292

Nelson R A 1953 The immune-adherence phenomenon. An immunologically specific reaction between microorganisms and erythrocytes leading to enhanced phagocytosis. Science 118: 733–737

Nelson R A, Mayer M M 1949 Immobilization of *Treponema pallidum in vitro* by antibody produced by syphilitic infection. Journal of Experimental Medicine 89: 369–393

Newman R B 1974 Laboratory diagnosis of syphilis CRC Critical Reviews in Clinical Laboratory Sciences 5: 1–28

Norgard M V, Selland C K, Kettman J R, Miller J N 1984 Sensitivity and specificity of monoclonal antibodies directed against antigenic determinants of *Treponema pallidum* Nichols in the diagnosis of syphilis. Journal of Clinical Microbiology 20: 711–717

Norgard M V, Chamberlain N R, Swancutt M A, Goldberg M S 1986 Cloning and expression of the major 47-Kilodalton surface immunogen of *Treponema pallidum* in *Escherichia coli*. Infection and Immunity 54: 500–506

Oxelius V-A, Rorsman H, Laurell A-B 1969 Immunoglobulins of cerebrospinal fluid in syphilis. British Journal of Venereal Diseases 45: 121–125

Panghorn M C 1941 A new serologically active phospholipid from beef heart. Proceedings of the Society for Experimental Biology and Medicine 48: 484–486

Pope V, Hunter E F, Feeley J C 1982 Evaluation of the micro-enzyme linked immunosorbent assay with *Treponema pallidum* antigen. Journal of Clinical Microbiology 15: 630–634

Portnoy J, Garson W, Smith C A 1957 Rapid plasma reagin test for syphilis. Public Health Report, Washington 72: 761–766

Puckett A, Pratt G 1982 Modification of the system of screening for antisyphilis antibodies in a blood transfusion centre featuring a miniaturisation of the *Treponema pallidum* haemagglutination assay. Journal of Clinical Pathology 35: 1349–1352

Radolf J D, Lernhardt E B, Fehniger T E, Lovett M A 1986 Serodiagnosis of syphilis by enzyme-linked immunosorbent assay with purified recombinant *Treponema pallidum* antigen 4D. Journal of Infectious Diseases 153: 1023–1027

Rathlev J 1967 Haemagglutination test utilizing pathogenic

Treponema pallidum for the sero-diagnosis of syphilis. British Journal of Venereal Diseases 43: 181–185

Rein M F, Banks G W, Logan L C et al 1980 Failure of the *Treponema pallidum* immobilization test to provide additional diagnostic information about contemporary problem sera. Sexually Transmitted Diseases 7: 101–105

Robertson S M, Kettman J R, Miller J N, Norgard M V 1982 Murine monoclonal antibodies specific for virulent *Treponema pallidum* (Nichols). Infection and Immunity 36: 1076–1085

Russell Jones R, Pusey C, Schifferli J, Johnston N A 1983 Essential mixed cryoglobulinaemia with false-positive serological tests for syphilis. British Journal of Venereal Diseases 59: 33–36

Sato T, Kubo E, Yokota M, Kayashina T, Tomigawa T 1984 *Treponema pallidum* specific IgM haemagglutination test for serodiagnosis of syphilis. British Journal of Venereal Diseases 60: 364–370

Schmidt B L 1980 Solid phase hemadsorption: a method for rapid detection of *Treponema pallidum*-specific IgM. Sexually Transmitted Diseases 7: 53–58

Sequeira P J L 1983 Serological diagnosis of untreated early syphilis. Importance of the differences in THA, TPHA, and VDRL test titres. British Journal of Venereal Diseases 59: 145–150

Sequeira P J L, Eldridge A E 1973 Treponemal haemagglutination test. British Journal of Venereal Diseases 49: 242–248

Shoenfeld Y, Shaulion E, Shaklai M, Kniglack J, Fenerman E, Pukhas J 1980 Circulating anticoagulant and serological tests for syphilis. Acta Dermato Venereologica 60: 365–367

Sprott M S, Selkon J B, Turner R H 1982 Evaluation of the role of the *Treponema pallidum* immobilisation test in Britain. British Journal of Venereal Diseases 58: 147–148

Stevens R W, Schell R F 1982 Solid-phase fluorimmunoassay for treponemal antibody. Journal of Clinical Microbiology 15: 191–195

Tanaka S, Suzuki T, Numata T 1978 *Treponema pallidum* immune adherence test for serodiagnosis of syphilis 1: An improved method of the TPIA test. British Journal of Venereal Diseases 54: 369–373

Thompson E J, Johnson M H 1982 Electrophoresis of CSF proteins. British Journal of Hospital Medicine 28: 600–608

Tomizawa T, Kasamatsu S 1966 Haemagglutination tests for diagnosis of syphilis: a preliminary report. Japanese Journal of Medical Science and Biology 19: 305–308

Uhr J W, Moller G 1968 Regulatory effect of antibody on the immune response. Advances in Immunochemistry 8: 81–127

Van Embden J D, van der Donk H J, van Eijk R V, van der Heide H G, de Jong J A, van Olderen M F 1983 Molecular cloning and expression of *Treponema pallidum* DNA in *Escherichia coli* K-12. Infection and Immunity 42: 187–196

Veldkamp J, Visser A M 1975 Application of the enzyme-linked immunosorbent assay (ELISA) in the serodiagnosis of syphilis. British Journal of Venereal Diseases 51: 227–231

Wilkinson A E 1976 Some aspects of research on syphilis: serological evidence of activity of the disease. In: Catterall R D, Nicol C E (eds) Sexually transmitted diseases. Academic Press, London, p 214–218

Wilkinson A E, Johnston N A 1975 Comparison between sorbent and Reiter sonicate in the absorbed fluorescent treponemal antibody test. Annals of the New York Academy of Sciences 254: 395–399

World Health Organization 1982 Treponemal infections. Technical report series 674. World Health Organization, Geneva

Wright D J M 1973 The significance of the fluorescent treponemal antibody (FTA-ABS) test in collagen disorders and leprosy. Journal of Clinical Pathology 26: 968–972

Wright J T, Cremer A W, Ridgway G L 1975 False positive FTA-ABS results in patients with genital herpes. British Journal of Venereal Diseases 51: 329–330

Young H, Henrichsen C, Robertson D H H 1974 *Treponema pallidum* haemagglutination test as a screening procedure for the diagnosis of syphilis. British Journal of Venereal Diseases 50: 341–346

Young H, Moyes A, McMillan A, Robertson D H H 1988 Screening for treponemal infection by a new enzyme immunoassay. Genitourinary Medicine, (in press).

TREATMENT OF EARLY SYPHILIS (primary, secondary, latent syphilis of less than one year's duration)

Benzathine penicillin 1.836 g (approximately equivalent to 1.44 g or 2.4 million i.u. of benzylpenicillin) given intramuscularly once (CDC 1985), *or*, procaine penicillin 900 mg (approximately equivalent to 545 mg or 908 174 i.u. benzylpenicillin) or up to 1.2 g (approximately equivalent to 727 mg or 1 210 898 i.u. benzylpenicillin) for heavier patients should be given daily for 10 days in seronegative primary syphilis; and for seropositive primary and secondary syphilis for 14 days. In the authors' practice, in early syphilis, treatment with procaine penicillin is preferred to benzathine penicillin and given daily as described above. Benzathine penicillin in a single dose is not routine, although approved in the 1985 CDC guidelines and clearly a useful alternative for patients intending to travel.

In early latent syphilis it is difficult to obtain direct information regarding the duration of the disease and it is advisable in cases of doubt to examine the cerebrospinal fluid (CSF), because when it is abnormal a diagnosis of asymptomatic neurosyphilis can be made, and treatment with procaine penicillin can be given daily over a 21-day period. Kern (1971) in Berlin set the desirable duration of the long-acting penicillin course at 15 days in the case of all forms of early-stage syphilis and at 30 days for later stages.

In patients with secondary syphilis, admission to hospital is advisable for the first one or two days of treatment at least. The patient can then receive care during the Jarisch-Herxheimer reaction (Leading Article (Lancet) 1977) and the opportunity can be taken to give explanations, to help with social problems, and to interview closely regarding possible sexual contacts.

TREATMENT IN PATIENTS WHO ARE HYPERSENSITIVE TO PENICILLIN

Tetracycline hydrochloride, 500 mg four times a day by mouth for 15 days, (CDC 1985). Oxytetracycline may be used similarly as an alternative. Doxycycline 100 mg 12-hourly by mouth for 28 days has given promising results (Onoda 1979).

Those who give a history of hypersensitivity to penicillin and who cannot tolerate tetracycline should have their allergy confirmed, and if compliance in treatment and follow-up can be assured, then erythromycin can be given as follows: erythromycin (stearate, ethylsuccinate or base), 500 mg four times a day by mouth for 15 days (CDC 1985).

These antibiotics appear to be effective, but results have been evaluated less fully than in the case of penicillin therapy. Clinical and serological follow-up are therefore very important.

TREATMENT OF SYPHILIS OF MORE THAN ONE YEAR'S DURATION (latent syphilis of indeterminate or more than one year's duration, cardiovascular or late benign syphilis) except neurosyphilis

Benzathine penicillin 1.836 g (approximately equivalent to 1.44 g or 2.4 million i.u. of benzylpenicillin) given intramuscularly weekly for 3 successive weeks (CDC 1985), *or*, procaine penicillin 900 mg (approximately equivalent to 545 mg or 908 174 i.u. benzylpenicillin) or up to 1.2 g (approximately equivalent to 727 mg or 1 210 898 units benzylpenicillin) for heavier patients, should be given daily for 14 days.

Optimal treatment schedules for syphilis of greater than one year's duration are less well established than those for early syphilis. Cerebrospinal fluid (CSF) examinations are mandatory in suspected symptomatic neurosyphilis and desirable in other patients with syphilis of greater than one year's duration.

In the circumstances of out-patient clinics for sexually transmitted disease it is wise to avoid penicillin injections, particularly in those with a history of penicillin hypersensitivity, asthma, eczema or other illnesses due to hypersensitivity. In neurosyphilis penicillin should be given wherever possible. Alternative antibiotics recommended by the Center for Disease Control, USA (CDC 1985) are as follows.

1. Tetracycline hydrochloride, 500 mg four times daily by mouth for 30 days. (Oxytetracycline in the same dose may be used as an alternative to tetracycline.) Compliance may be difficult to ensure with this regimen — re-attendance and successive issue of one week's treatment may assist in this regard. In patients who are allergic to penicillin and who cannot tolerate tetracycline, erythromycin may be given as follows:

2. Erythromycin stearate, ethylsuccinate or base, 500 mg four times daily by mouth for 30 days.

CSF examinations and follow-up are important in patients being treated with these regimens as their efficacy in the long term is not yet clear.

NEUROSYPHILIS

Early diagnosis and the rapid institution of treatment are of prime importance in neurosyphilis. Results of treatment depend to a very great extent upon how much irreversible damage to the central nervous system has occurred before treatment has begun, and it is clear that any patient should be seen as a matter of urgency. For a long time it seemed that in neurosyphilis there was little evidence that more clinical benefit could be obtained by using doses higher than those recommended (Kelly 1964) or by giving benzylpenicillin rather than long-acting forms such as benzathine penicillin or procaine penicillin. Furthermore, Wilner & Brodie (1968) found that in 40% of cases of general paresis treated with penicillin new neurological signs would develop subsequently after months or years. Such progression of disease occurred in the absence of deterioration in the CSF findings and was thought to be due to irreversible cerebrovascular damage before treatment, with further loss of neurones as a result of ageing. Currently this explanation is under challenge, as is the practice of using long-acting or repository forms of penicillin in the treatment of neurosyphilis.

Some clinicians have never wholly relied upon long-acting forms of penicillin for treating neurosyphilis and now there is a strong movement in clinical practice in the United States and elsewhere to use specifically benzylpenicillin and, furthermore, to give it intravenously rather than intramuscularly. It is known that, although blood levels may be adequate and treponemicidal, penetration of penicillin into the cerebrospinal fluid is poor. In normal circumstances about 0.2–2.0% of the blood concentration of penicillin is achieved, whereas in the presence of inflammation, as in the case of purulent meningitis, the ratio is higher viz. 2.0–6.0% (Barling & Selkon 1978). Mohr et al (1976) treated 13 patients with neurosyphilis with 2.754 g of benzathine penicillin (equivalent to 2.160 g or 3.6 million units of benzylpenicillin) once-weekly for four weeks. In 12 patients there was no detectable penicillin in the CSF; in 1 there was 0.1 mg/l CSF. Encouraging CSF values in 2 patients were obtained after giving 5 and 10 million units (respectively 3.0 g and 6.0 g) benzylpenicillin daily intravenously. Ethical and practical difficulties surround the problem of conducting trials of treatment, and arguments for using intravenous penicillin tend to be based on pharmacological and bacteriological rather than clinical criteria for determining effectiveness. Benzylpenicillin given intramuscularly fails to achieve a steady penicillin level, but when given in large doses by continuous intravenous (vena cava) infusion maintained by an automatic injection unit it was possible to do so (Ritter et al 1975). By this means a serum level of 30–42 mg (50 000–70 000 i.u.)/l was sufficient to maintain CSF levels of 1.8–3.0 mg (3 000–5 000 i.u.)/l. Ritter et al thought that the giving of benzylpenicillin in doses of 12 g (20 million i.u.)/4 hours — with an infusion time of 30 minutes each and a total dosage of 72 g (120 million i.u.) per day — over a period of several treponemal generation cycles (say 3–5 days) might prevent the high failure rates seen with 'insufficient' dosage of depot or long-acting forms of penicillin.

Tramont (1976) reported the isolation of *Treponema pallidum* in rabbits inoculated with CSF from a patient who had been treated intramuscularly with 918 mg benzathine penicillin (approximately equivalent to 720 mg or 1.2 million i.u. benzylpenicillin) three times weekly for three weeks. After intravenous penicillin, however, subsequent attempts at isolation by the inoculation of CSF into rabbits were unsuccessful. Again, in a case of neurosyphilis (Greene et al 1980), progressive deterioration occurred despite treatment with benzathine penicillin, but subsequently after intravenous therapy with high doses of benzylpenicillin both subjective and objective improvement occurred. In their study in Montreal, Ducas & Robson (1981) found that in patients with latent syphilis — none of whom had evidence of neurosyphilis — none of the 18 treated weekly for three weeks with 1.836 g benzathine penicillin (approximately equivalent to 1.44 g or 2.4 million i.u. of benzylpenicillin) intramuscularly and only 2 of 15 given 3.672 g (approximately equivalent to 2.88 g or 4.8 million i.u. of benzydpenicillin) had adequate penicillin levels in the CSF. Probenecid 500 mg by mouth four times daily gave rise to problems in patient compliance and did not regularly produce CSF levels greater than 0.018 mg (30 i.u.)/l CSF. As a result it was considered that benzathine penicillin should not be employed as a first-line agent in the treatment of neurosyphilis. Their policy is to admit patients to hospital for a 14-day course of intravenous benzylpenicillin 14.4 g (24 million i.u.) daily. CSF concentrations of benzylpenicillin are determined after 3 days therapy to establish that adequate levels have been achieved.

Unwanted effects of high dosage of penicillin

A cautionary note is needed. A number of individuals have received benzylpenicillin intravenously in doses of 24–48 g (40–80 million units) daily for as long as four weeks without untoward effects, but parenteral administration of benzylpenicillin in daily doses of more than 12 g (20 million i.u.), or less in the case of those patients with renal insufficiency, may produce confusion, twitching. multifocal myoclonus or generalized epileptiform seizures. These are most apt to occur in the presence of localized central nervous system lesions, hyponatraemia or renal insufficiency. When concentration of benzylpenicillin in the CSF exceeds 10 mg/l significant dysfunction of the central nervous system is frequent. The injection of 12 g (20 million i.u.) of benzylpenicillin potassium which contains 34 mEg of potassium may lead to severe or even fatal hyperkalaemia in persons with renal dysfunction (Gilman et al 1985). Risks, also, of haemolytic anaemia developing in those given benzylpenicillin intravenously in doses of about 6 g or more should be considered (Ries et al 1975, Reynolds 1982).

Probenecid

The proposition that probenecid may be used in neurosyphilis requires consideration. Fishman's data from experiments in dogs (Fishman 1966) supported the theory of the existence of a transport system close to the CSF, presumably in the choroid plexus, which actively transports organic acids, such as penicillin, from the CSF. Probenecid achieves higher CSF levels of penicillin by: 1. raising the blood level; 2. inhibiting the active transport of penicillin from CSF; and 3. increasing the diffusible penicillin in plasma by competition for binding to serum protein. Probenecid may actually interfere with the accumulation of penicillin in the brain tissue; in Fishman's experiments in rats there was evidence of competition between penicillin and probenecid for entry into the brain. The suggestion is that probenecid may achieve higher CSF and blood levels but may not necessarily be a useful adjunct in the treatment of bacterial infection of the nervous system. The special permeability characteristics of the brain depend upon the net transfer characteristics of multiple complex membranes which constitute the cerebral capillaries, glia and neurons, and on brain metabolism which serves also to stabilize neuronal enviroments (Fishman 1966).

Penicillin therapy in neurosyphilis: recommendations in current practice

The CDC (1985) guidelines refer to the fact that 3.6–5.4 g (6–9 million i.u.) of benzylpenicillin over a 3–4 week period is satisfactory in about 90% of patients with neurosyphilis, but suggest a number of potentially effective regimens in answer to a criticism that failures in treatment(s) have been recorded for regimens relying on long-acting forms of penicillin when treponemicidal levels in the CSF may not be consistently reached. The CDC (1985) guidelines give three potentially effective regimens, none of which has been adequately studied, as follows:

Benzylpenicillin 1.2–2.4 g (2–4 million i.u.) intravenously every 4 hours for 10 days, followed by a course of one or more of the long-acting penicillins:
1. Benzathine penicillin 1.836 g (approximately equivalent to 1.44 g or 2.4 million i.u. benzylpenicillin) intramuscularly once weekly for 3 doses, or
2. Procaine penicillin 2.378 g (approximately equivalent to 1.44 g or 2.4 million units benzylpenicillin) intramuscularly once-daily plus probenecid 500 mg by mouth 4 times daily, both for 10 days and followed by benzathine penicillin 1.836 g (approximately equivalent to 1.44 g or 2.4 million i.u. benzylpenicillin) intramuscularly weekly for 3 doses, or
3. Benzathine penicillin 1.836 g (approximately equiv-

alent to 1.44 g or 2.4 million i.u. benzylpenicillin) intramuscularly weekly for 3 doses.

The authors consider that in (1) the dose of procaine penicillin should be less, viz. between 900 mg (approximately equivalent to 545 mg or 908 174 i.u. benzylpenicillin) or up to 1.2 g (approximately equivalent to 727 mg or 1 210 898 units benzylpenicillin) for heavier patients daily for 10 days.

Intravenous administration of benzylpenicillin in neurosyphilis

It is certain that early diagnosis and rapid initiation of penicillin treatment is of prime importance. With benzylpenicillin given intravenously there may be problems with the unwanted effects of very large doses discussed above. With probenecid there are theoretical objections to its use in bacterial infections of the brain, and clearly long-acting forms of penicillin, viz. benzathine penicillin and procaine penicillin, may not always be successful in the treatment of neurosyphilis. The position with regard to the optimum management of neurosyphilis is still very uncertain but the disease is probably best treated with high-dose intravenously administered benzylpenicillin (Rein 1981), taking into consideration known hazards in this form of treatment.

Benzylpenicillin for Injection BP (either as benzylpenicillin sodium or benzylpenicillin potassium) is prepared by dissolving the sterile contents of the sealed container in the required amount of water for injections. Intravenous doses above 1.2 g (2 million i.u.) should be administered slowly at a rate of not more than 300 mg per minute to avoid irritation of the central nervous system (Reynolds 1982). A slow intravenous infusion technique with very high doses over the 3–5 day period described by Ritter et al (1975) is an approach which requires further study.

Oral amoxycillin plus probenecid

An oral therapeutic antibiotic (amoxycillin plus probenecid) regimen may be effective (Morrison et al 1985) in the dosage given (amoxycillin 2 g by mouth three times a day plus probenecid 500 mg by mouth twice a day for 14 days) since CSF amoxycillin concentrations greater than 0.3 μg/ml are consistently attained, although theoretical objections to the use of probenecid are not yet possible to discount.

SYPHILIS IN PREGNANCY

In localities where the number of reported cases of transplacental (congenital) syphilis are more than very rare the antenatal care, with regular serological testing, of pregnant women is a matter of major importance and will enable the eradication of congenital syphilis.

Penicillin is recommended for pregnant women in dosage appropriate for the stage of syphilis. The authors prefer to use benzylpenicillin 600 mg (1 million i.u.) 8-hourly intramuscularly for the first 5 days in the case of early syphilis, followed by daily intramuscular procaine penicillin 900 mg (approximately equivalent to 545 mg or 908 174 i.u. benzylpenicillin) or up to 1.2 g (approximately equivalent to 727 mg or 1 210 898 units benzylpenicillin) for heavier patients, for 9 days (a 14-day dosage altogether). Procaine penicillin 900 mg daily for 14 days may be used in late or latent stages in pregnancy.

Pregnant women should be followed up carefully clinically and have monthly quantitative cardiolipin antigen serological tests, preferably the VDRL, for the remainder of the current pregnancy. A four-fold rise in titre is an indication for re-treatment.

It is the authors' practice to give a single 10-day course of procaine penicillin during early pregnancy in any patient who has had syphilis, even if adequately treated in the past. This 'insurance course' is justified on the grounds that treponemes appear to persist in the host in spite of treatment and might be transmitted transplacentally. It is difficult, however, not only to test the validity of this argument but also doubtful whether it is ethical to do so if it brings a risk of transmission to the fetus.

Alternative antibiotic therapy in pregnant women with a history of hypersensitivity to penicillin

In those gravid women allergic to penicillin, tetracyclines should not be used. Erythromycin has been offered as a suitable alternative to penicillin and may be given in an oral dose of 500 mg four times daily for 20 days (Spence 1977); the CDC (1985) guidelines suggest the same dosage and approach as that recommended for the treatment of non-pregnant patients. If gastrointestinal symptoms preclude its use, admission to hospital for desensitization before giving penicillin treatment is suggested. With oral erythromycin serum levels may be unsatisfactory and even after multiple maternal doses the average fetal blood level may only be 0.06 μg/ml. As placental transfer is unpredictable and the problem of patient compliance very serious, the evidence suggests that oral erythromycin is not a good agent in the treatment of in utero syphilis (Fenton & Light 1976). In the case reported by these authors a 24-year-old gravid woman with syphilis was treated with erythromycin stearate 750 mg four times daily for 12 days; during her pregnancy her serum VDRL titre declined from 16 to 2. Notwithstanding this apparently satisfactory response in the mother the female infant, apparently normal on physical examination at birth, developed an ill-defined rash on the face at 7 weeks and florid effects of early congenital syphilis (papulosquamous skin lesions, stuffy nose, adenopathy and osteochondritis of the right index finger) at 11 weeks. The VDRL at birth, 7 weeks and 11 weeks showed titres of 2, 1 and 256 respectively.

South et al (1964) first recorded this problem in a pregnant woman who was treated for secondary syphilis with erythromycin estolate in an oral dose of 500 mg thrice-daily for 10 days; her syphilis was apparently controlled but the infant had severe congenital syphilis.

In view of the unpredictable placental transfer of erythromycin during treatment of the pregnant woman for syphilis with this antibiotic full treatment of the infant with penicillin, beginning at birth, is an essential precaution (Fenton & Light 1976, CDC 1985) and it is clear that admission to hospital is desirable to ensure that the prescribed dosage is in fact taken at the required intervals. Estimations of serum erythromycin levels (Ryden 1978) are desirable.

Fenton & Light (1976) suggest that in cases of suspected hypersensitivity to penicillin in maternal syphilis the use of intravenous erythromycin should be investigated and that the history of allergy to penicillin, often vague, should be closely scrutinized and practical methods should be applied to predicting penicillin reactions.

Cephaloridine crosses the placenta to achieve levels in the cord or fetal blood approximately 60% of that in the maternal circulation. Holder & Knox (1972) recommended for this reason, and on the basis of reports of its effectiveness, intramuscular cephaloridine as a reasonable alternative and refer to doses of 0.5 g daily for 10 days as a possible course; more data are required on dosage and possible teratogenic effects.

There is, of course, a calculated risk, which these authors recognized, as there is a cross-allergenicity between penicillins and cephalosporins. The incidence of allergic reactions to cephalosporins in patients not allergic to penicillin is given as 1.7% and in those who are so allergic 8.2% (Petz 1971). From a wide study of the literature, Dash (1975) concluded that 91–94% of patients with a history of penicillin allergy have not reacted to a cephalosporin. Cephalosporins are nevertheless *not* recommended for patients with an *authentic* history of penicillin hypersensitivity (Garrod et al 1981).

In the case of syphilis in the pregnant woman who gives a history of hypersensitivity to penicillin, treatment is problematic. Treatment with erythromycin may control the infection in the gravid patient but it may fail to prevent or cure the infection in her fetus.

Green (1975) has discussed the problem in relation to optimal antibiotic therapy for patients with a history of penicillin allergy who have a life-threatening infection such as bacterial endocarditis. About 60% (34/56) of Green's patients with bacterial endocarditis who gave a history of hypersensitivity to penicillin were treated with this antibiotic without incident. 4 patients reacted severely enough to discontinue treatment and 1 had a severe, although not fatal, anaphylactic type reaction. It is through the fear of the latter reaction that physicians tend to avoid giving penicillin to all who give a history of penicillin allergy.

Type 1 hypersensitivity reactions (Roitt 1988) (anaphylactic sensitivity) are very rare indeed and occur in about 3 in every 100 000 cases, and fatalities in less than 2 in every 100 000. The rare and fatal reactions occur mainly in those known to have had a prior reaction to penicillin or an allergic diathesis (Green 1975). Predictive tests for penicillin allergy cannot yet be widely applied in general practice (Garrod et al 1981) and the serious and feared Type 1 hypersensitivity reaction, and indeed fatal anaphylactic reactions, have been reported in patients with a negative skin test to penicillin.

As a general rule patients giving a history of allergy to penicillin should be treated with an antibiotic of a different type. In unusual instances where treatment with penicillin is essential, skin tests may be of some help (Solley et al 1982). Lack of response to benzyl-penicilloyl-polylysine (PRE-PEN) makes it unlikely that a patient will develop an immediate or accelerated reaction to penicillin. Those with a positive response to PRE-PEN are at significant risk of developing a severe reaction, and two-thirds of those will develop some form of allergic reaction. In order further to reduce the likelihood of an immediate severe reaction sensitivity to minor antigenic determinants should also be tested. Unfortunately mixtures of the minor determinants are not commercially available (Gilman et al 1985) and scratch tests with penicillin have the disadvantages already emphasized.

It appears therefore that penicillin is withheld from many individuals who could tolerate it because of the fear that they may develop the rare anaphylactic Type 1 reaction.

It is wholly justifiable in a life-threatening condition such as bacterial endocarditis to give penicillin, when it is considered to be the best antibiotic, to patients who give a history of allergy to this antibiotic, although its administration should be in hospital under the guidance of a physician knowledgeable in the handling of acute allergic states (Green 1975) and skilled in intensive medical care.

Although the scheme may be justified in life-threatening bacterial endocarditis, is it justified to put the life of a pregnant woman at risk, even if remote, to protect or cure with certainty a fetal infection in utero? The infection in the fetus might or might not be seriously damaging and would be treatable effectively with penicillin at birth, although damage already sustained would not necessarily be reversed.

The problem is not wholly solved. The clinician requires a test to recognize liability to systemic anaphylactic sensitivity (Type 1 hypersensitivity) and a means of preventing it. These questions, of an immunological nature, have not yet been fully answered. In a small series of cases, however, a satisfactory outcome to the treatment of syphilis in pregnant women who were allergic to penicillin has been reported using a protocol of skin testing; desensitization with oral phenoxymethylpenicillin; and subsequent treatment with benzathine penicillin.

Skin testing has been reported as a means of predicting in those positive to the test a 41–67% chance that a clinically detectable reaction will occur, with up to half of reactions involving respiratory obstruction or hypotension. In those negative to the test there is a 1–4% risk of a cutaneous reaction, and no life-threatening reactions have been reported. Desensitization and a state of unresponsiveness by host cells to specific antigen may be induced with increasing doses of antigen. Using phenoxymethylpenicillin (penicillin V) by the oral route, a safer desensitization procedure than with parenteral benzylpenicillin, Wendel et al (1985) have followed a protocol which was effective therapeutically in pregnant women with syphilis. In this procedure an elixir of phenoxymethylpenicillin was given orally in doses of initially 0.059 mg (approximately equivalent to 0.06 mg or 100 i.u. of benzylpenicillin) and increasing by approximately doubling the oral dose every 15 minutes for 14 doses. During the desensitization procedure in hospital intravenous lines were established and close personal medical supervision was maintained for 24 hours. Mild cutaneous reactions were allowed to resolve spontaneously or were. treated with diphenhydramine 25 mg intravenously. After the desensitization process patients were able to tolerate intramuscular benzathine penicillin treatment in doses appropriate to their infection although close observation was given on re-admission for an oral test dose of 236 mg phenoxymethylpenicillin (equivalent to 240 mg or 400 000 i. u. of benzyl penicillin) followed by observation for 1 hour. The injection of benzathine penicillin was then given and the patients monitored overnight.

CONGENITAL SYPHILIS

Congenital syphilis is considered more fully in Chapter 12. The discovery of congenital syphilis is an indication of defective antenatal care or failure of antibiotic treatment, e.g. as with erythromycin.

The Centers for Disease Control, US Public Health Service (1985) advise that the CSF should be examined before treatment in infants with congenital syphilis to provide a baseline for follow-up. Regardless of the CSF results, children should be treated with a regimen effective for neurosyphilis. The regimens recommended are as follows.

1. Benzylpenicillin 30 mg (50 000 i.u.) per kg body weight intramuscularly or intraveously daily in two divided doses for a minimum of 10 days, *or*

2. Procaine penicillin 49.55 mg (approximately equivalent to 30 mg or 50 000 i.u. benzylpenicillin) per kg body weight intramuscularly daily for a minimum of 10 days.

After the neonatal period the dose should be the same dosage used for neonatal congenital syphilis. For larger children the total dose need not exceed the dosage advised in adult syphilis for more than one year's duration. If hypersensitive to penicillin, erythromycin may be used. Tetracycline or oxytetracycline should not be used in children under 8 years of age.

FOLLOW-UP AFTER TREATMENT

The CDC (1985) guidelines advise that quantitative non-treponemal tests (e.g. VDRL) should be taken 3, 6 and 12 months after treatment. If disease is of more than one year's duration, serological tests for syphilis should be repeated 24 months afterwards. Follow-up is especially important in patients treated with antibiotics other than penicillin. CSF is examined at the last follow-up after treatment with alternative antibiotics. In patients with neurosyphilis a follow-up after treatment is advised with periodic quantitative cardiolipin tests (e.g. VDRL), clinical evaluation and repeat CSF examinations, for at least 3 years (CDC 1985). A lifetime follow-up is, however, generally recommended.

In the authors' practice case holding tends to continue for longer than outlined in the preceding paragraph. In the case of early syphilis a 2–3-year follow-up is maintained when possible.

In the case of cardiovascular syphilis follow-up by a cardiologist is advisable. In neurosyphilis a lifetime follow-up is best. Liaison with the general practitioner responsible for primary care is essential, particularly in late-stage cases where re-investigation may be started unnecessarily if the patient is admitted to hospital for investigation of some possibly unrelated complaint.

RE-TREATMENT

Reinfection with syphilis is a possibility, particularly in the promiscuous who have casual relationships and where contacts, as in the case of some homosexual men particularly, may fear or neglect to surface for medical help. A CSF examination should be carried out before re-treatment unless reinfection and a diagnosis of early syphilis is clearly established.

Re-treatment should be considered under the following circumstances (CDC 1985):

1. If clinical signs or symptoms persist or recur.
2. If there is a four-fold increase in the titre of a non-treponemal test.
3. If an initially high titre non-treponemal test fails to show a four-fold decrease in titre within a year.

When a patient is re-treated one treatment course is indicated and the course used will be that recommended for syphilis of more than one year's duration.

TREATMENT ON EPIDEMIOLOGICAL GROUNDS

Patients who have clearly been exposed to infectious syphilis and who are not likely to cease sexual intercourse for three months, or to attend for surveillance, should be considered on epidemiological grounds for treatment and followed up; the regimen advised is that for early syphilis. It is our practice to treat couples such as husband and wife simultaneously if possible, if one partner develops early syphilis. Every effort is made, however, to establish a diagnosis beforehand in such cases.

In the case of early-stage syphilis immediate treatment for the infected person or 'epidemiologic' treatment for potentially infected contacts will interrupt a possible chain of infection. Although about one-third of recently exposed persons will develop syphilis and two-thirds will not, the United States Public Health Service has advocated 'epidemiologic' treatment (preventive) of all contacts because of the inability to identify quickly those who will develop the disease (Kaufman et al 1974). In the authors' practice this is not generally applied as early syphilis is currently not common in this city and is sporadic in appearance. In favour of the concept of 'epidemiologic' treatment it must be said that on occasions contacts of early syphilis, particularly in those who are homosexual and promiscuous, have been lost to follow-up. They have not infrequently defaulted from the prolonged serological testing necessary for the exclusion of syphilis. The CDC (1985) guidelines recommend that those exposed to infectious syphilis within the preceding three months and those who, on epidemiological grounds are at high risk for early syphilis should be treated as for early.

RESPONSE TO TREATMENT AND ASSESSMENT OF CURE

1. Response to treatment: early-stage syphilis

Penicillin in sufficient dosage causes disappearance of *T.pallidum* from early surface lesions within 6–26 hours (Idsoe et al 1972). Infectivity appears to be lost very soon and lesions heal often within a few days. Obvious induration, depth, size and number of lesions will vary in relation to the duration of the disease and healing may be correspondingly longer. The infection can no longer be transmitted by sexual contact and relapse after adequate treatment is exceedingly rare, recurrences being usually due to reinfection.

In addition to careful clinical assessment of the patient, serological tests (cardiolipin tests e.g. VDRL) must be performed serially over a period of time to ensure that treatment has been satisfactory. These tests should be carried out immediately after completion of treatment, monthly for the first three months and there-after three-monthly in the first year and twice in the second year.

Following satisfactory treatment, quantitative tests for cardiolipin antibody (e.g. VDRL) gradually become negative, usually within three to six months, unless the initial titre was high, in which case positive results may be obtained, at lower titres, for a much longer period (e.g. Fig. 8.2 which shows the changes in titres of serological tests taken after treatment of a patient who is later reinfected).

The now obsolete Reiter's protein complement fix-ation test (RPCFT), like tests for cardiolipin antibody, usually becomes negative within six months of treat-ment of early syphilis.

The TPHA, which detects mainly IgG antibody, remains positive for years after treatment, unless this was given very early in the course of the disease when the titre in the serum was low (e.g. 1 in 80). Unlike the cardiolipin antibody tests, the TPHA is therefore of very little value in assessing efficacy of treatment and like the *T. pallidum* immobilization test remains positive often for years, or even for life. The FTA-ABS test and probably the ELISA also remain positive for many years after treatment. More experience is required in the use of the FTA-IgM test before it can be used routinely.

To ensure that treatment of secondary syphilis has been adequate it is generally considered good practice, even after penicillin therapy, to examine the CSF fluid (cell count, total protein content, IgG content, VDRL,

TPHA and FTA-ABS test) about a year after treatment. Such examinations are essential after treatments with antibiotics other than penicillin.

Abstinence from sexual intercourse is advised in a patient being treated for early syphilis until the disease cannot be transmitted. This is usually achieved within a few days, but it is wise for the patient to abstain until after the course of antibiotic when all lesions will be healed, and possibly for one month after treatment if resumption of intercourse with an uninfected partner is to take place. If one partner is infected and has put the other at risk simultaneous treatment of both is advisable as reinfection of the treated by the untreated can occur. Such treatment on epidemiological grounds in a person at very high risk will call for the same follow-up and assessment of cure as in the patient in whom a diagnosis is established.

2. Response to treatment; late-stage syphilis

Response to treatment is discussed in Chapter 11 with respect to gummatous syphilis, neurosyphilis and cardiovascular syphilis. Titres of cardiolipin antigen tests tend to diminish over the years in some patients but persistence of a high titre does not necessarily indicate a need for further treatment If penicillin has been given in an adequate dosage further courses are not necessarily indicated. In cases of neurosyphilis the advisability of higher penicillin dosage requires consider-ation as levels in the cerebrospinal fluid after doses of long-acting penicillin preparations may be very low.

JARISCH-HERXHEIMER REACTION (JHR)

This reaction is a complication that usually follows within a day of the initial treatment of a number of organismal diseases, including syphilis, and it is charac-terized by fever and an aggravation of existing lesions together with their attendant symptoms and signs (Warrell et al 1971, Bryceson 1976, Leading Article 1977).

In 1895 Jarisch recorded the fact that the spots of roseolar syphilis became clearer and more numerous after treatment with mercury. Later, in 1902, Herx-heimer and Krause pointed out that the reaction followed soon after an adequate dose of mercury and was accompanied by a rise in temperature. The reaction is generally confined to the first day of treatment and it occurs also after treatment with antibiotics such as penicillin; it can be evoked twice in the same patient if the first injection of penicillin is only 10 20 i.u. per kg body weight (Gudjonsson & Skog 1968). The JHR develops in about 55% of cases of VDRL negative primary syphilis, also in 95% of patients with general paralysis of the insane — in those with high CSF cell counts, the JHR may be expected to occur after treatment when there may be exacerbation of mental signs or symptoms. Generally no reaction is noted following treatment of very early and late-stage latent syphilis. The JHR may occur in early-stage congenital syphilis, most frequently in children under the age of 6 months, but is rare after treatment of late-stage congenital syphilis.

The salient features of the JHR are as follows (Bryceson et al 1972)

1. A rise and then a fall in body temperature: the rise is accompanied by a chill and the fall by sweating.

2. Aggravation of pre-existing lesions and their attendant symptoms and signs, e.g. flaring of the rash in syphilis and acute myocarditis in louse-borne relapsing fever.

3. Characteristic physiological changes, which include early vasoconstriction, hyperventilation and a rise in blood pressure and cardiac output, and later a fall in blood pressure associated with a low peripheral resistance.

In 1895 Jarisch postulated that the cause of the reaction was a toxin liberated from degenerating treponemes, but it was not until 1961 that endotoxin-like activity was detected in a spirochaete, *Borrelia vincentii* (Leading Article 1977), and only in 1973 was a lipopolysaccharide, resembling that of Gram-negative organisms, identified in *T. pallidum* (Jackson & Zey 1973). In louse-borne relapsing fever, due to *Borrelia recurrentis*, the JHR is much more severe than in syphilis and Bryceson et al (1972) found that in 1 case out of the 4 examined, the plasma taken from a patient during the JHR induced fever 60 minutes after transfusion into that patient on the following day. In addition endotoxin has been detected by the limulus amoebocyte lysate assay in the plasma of patients at the time they were undergoing the JHR and this was accompanied by depression of the third component of complement (Gelfand et al 1976). Findings of Fulford et al (1976) suggested activation of the classical pathway resulting from antigen-antibody interaction, rather than the alternative pathway, although some alternative pathway antibody by treponemal endotoxin could not be excluded. Polymorphonuclear activation may lead to pyrogen release and resulting fever. These authors also found that levels of IgM fluorescent treponemal antibodies (FTA) were higher in patients who developed reactions than in those who did not. Combination of these antibodies with newly available antigenic sites could lead to complement binding. They suggested that antigenic determinants, particularly those corresponding to FTA antibody, placed deeply within the treponemes, may be released after death and breakdown of treponemes by treatment.

In neurosyphilis exacerbation of signs may occur in patients treated with penicillin (Tucker & Robinson 1946, Hoekenga & Farmer 1948) and this may resemble, but be less severe than, the reactive encephalopathy seen in patients with *Trypanosoma brucei rhodesiense* or *T.b.gambiense* meningoencephalitis treated with melarsoprol (Robertson 1963). In neither general paralysis of the insane nor in secondary syphilis, however, are these JHR as severe as in louse-borne relapsing fever. In a number of instances a possible flare-up of local lesions is feared, as for example in acute labyrinthitis of early syphilis when irreversible deafness is a threat (Vercoe 1976). In the now rare gummata of the brain and larynx, which contain numerous treponemes, treatment has proved on occasions fatal (Moore et al 1948). In local lesions of the aorta involving the coronary ostia (Leading Article 1977) a JHR may have serious consequences.

The late lesions of syphilis described are now rare in western countries. The use of prednisolone in high initial dosage is advised on rather limited evidence in acute labyrinthitis and may be considered, again on limited evidence of its efficacy, in late forms of disease where exacerbation of local inflammation is feared. In the louse-borne relapsing fever model of the JHR, high-dose hydrocortisone infused before and during the JHR reduced the patient's baseline temperature but did not mitigate the febrile, physiological or local inflammatory features of the JHR in any way (Warrell et al 1970). The clinical value of steroids remains unproven, although prednisone may reduce pyrexia (Gudjonsson & Skog 1968).

In relapsing fever administration of meptazinol, a partial opioid agonist, has been shown to diminish the JHR, and the hypothesis made is that there is endogenous opioid withdrawal in the JHR; the administration of the opioid agonist is therefore beneficial (Wright 1983). This approach would be worth consideration in the treatment of syphilis when reduction of the intensity of the JHR would be beneficial.

Clinical phases of the Jarisch-Herxheimer reaction (JHR)

There are four clinical phases, and the effects are greatest in secondary syphilis and in general paralysis of the insane. In primary syphilis the effects are usually mild. The reaction develops within four hours of starting treatment, becomes most intense at six to eight hours and resolves within 24 hours.

The clinical phases are:

1. *Prodromal phase* with aches and pains.
2. *Rigor* or *chill*. Temperature rises by an average 1°C. (Range 0.2 °–2.7 °C) four to eight hours after treatment.

3. *Flush*. Temperature reaches a peak, usually at about eight hours after the first injection, and is associated with hypotension.

4. *Defervescence*, which lasts up to 12 hours.

Other clinical and physiological observations

The patient may feel discomfort in the local lesions, which become more pronounced and show an acute transient inflammatory reaction. Histologically it is found that neutrophil and mononuclear cells appear and migrate through the swollen vascular endothelium into the surrounding oedematous tissue.

There is a leucocytosis and a fall in the lymphocyte count. The metabolic rate is increased and peaks with the rigor. Pulmonary ventilation and cardiac output exceed metabolic requirements and pulmonary oxygen uptake is impaired.

During the rigor phase there is early hyperventilation; the systemic arterial blood pressure rises due to vaso-constriction, but falls in the flush phase due to decrease in vascular resistance as a result of vasodilatation.

The reaction to specific treatment, whether antibiotic or not, is seen in diseases other than syphilis, namely in louse-borne relapsing fever, rat-bite fever, lepto-spirosis, yaws, brucellosis, tularaemia, glanders, anthrax and in African trypanosomiasis, particularly in that due to *T.b.rhodesiense*. In relapsing fever and leptospirosis the reaction is much more severe than in syphilis, and it can be fatal.

ADVERSE EFFECTS OF PENICILLIN

Penicillins are virtually non-toxic in the doses discussed, but by far the most serious reactions are due to hyper-sensitivity — Type 1 anaphylactic sensitivity — (Note 10.1) and penicillin is one of the most common causes of this and other forms of hypersensitivity. Anaphylactic reactions may occur at any age. Their incidence is thought to be 0.04–0.2% of patients treated with penicillins, and about 0.001% of patients treated may die from anaphylaxis, most often following *injection* of penicillin. Anaphylaxis has also been observed after oral ingestion of drug and has even resulted from the intra-dermal instillation of a very small quantity for the purpose of testing for the presence of hypersensitivity (Gilman et al 1985). There appears to be no completely safe and reliable practical method of detecting sensi-tivity to penicillin, but inquiry concerning reactions to previous treatment should always be made. Patients who suffer from sensitivities to other agents are more liable to react adversely to penicillin, and sensitivity induced by one penicillin may lead to similar reactions to others. Reactions include skin rashes of all types, fever, arthralgia, lymphadenopathy, stomatitis and gloss-

itis, but Type 1 hypersensitivity (anaphylactic reaction) with severe hypotension and rapid death is the most dramatic and sudden. Bronchospasm with severe asthma, or abdominal pain, nausea and vomiting, or extreme weakness and fall in blood pressure, or diar-rhoea and purpuric skin eruptions have characterized anaphylactic episodes in other instances (Gilman et al 1985).

Occasionally very serious reactions and even death, occurring during or shortly after an injection of peni-cillin, may result from accidental intravenous injection with subsequent pulmonary embolism. Some of these reactions may simulate anaphylaxis. Injection of procaine penicillin may result in an immediate reaction, characterized by dizziness, tinnitus, headache, halluci-nations and sometimes seizures. This is due to the rapid liberation of toxic concentrations of procaine (Green et al 1974). It has been reported to occur in 1 of 200 patients receiving 4.757 g procaine penicillin (approxi-mately equivalent to 2.88 mg or 4.8 million units benzylpenicillin) for a sexually transmitted disease (Gilman et al 1985).

In syphilis the Jarisch-Herxheimer reaction occurs within the first 24 hours of treatment and it is particu-larly prominent in secondary syphilis.

ADVERSE EFFECTS OF TETRACYCLINES

As tetracyclines are selectively taken up by the growing teeth and bones of fetus or child the use of tetracyclines should be avoided in pregnancy or in childhood. Tetra-cyclines other than doxycycline should be avoided in patients with impaired renal function as acute renal failure may be precipitated. Doxycycline, in particular, commonly induces photosensitization, and patients should be warned regarding the risks of sun-bathing if receiving this treatment.

Gastrointestinal side effects of tetracycline therapy such as nausea, vomiting and mild diarrhoea, are common. Less commonly there is suppression of normal microbial flora leading to superinfection of skin and mucous membrane with organisms such as *Candida* spp, *Staphylococcus aureus*, *Proteus* spp. Rarely a fulminating staphylococcal enterocolitis results.

ERYTHROMYCIN

Erythromycin given orally, as the stearate, is well absorbed from the gastrointestinal tract, peak levels being obtained two to four hours after ingestion. Eryth-romycin estolate is hepatotoxic, and the stearate ester (ethylsuccinate or base) should be used in the treatment of syphilis. The dosage recommended is not toxic, nausea and vomiting are uncommon side effects, occurring in less than 5% of cases.

Erythromycin, although apparently safe to use in pregnancy, is unpredictable in its effects on the fetus in in utero syphilis.

APPENDIX: REACTIONS TO PENICILLIN

Hypersensitivity reactions (instructions for out-patient clinic)
Precautions

1. Avoid penicillin in those with a history of:
   - Previous penicillin reactions
   - Bronchial asthma
   - Tendency to allergic reactions, e.g. in biological false-positive reactors
2. The injections should be given to the patient in the lying down position, or a couch should be nearby.
3. The patient should have rested for 5 minutes before the injection and he/she should wait for 25 minutes afterwards.
4. Avoid unintentional intravenous injections by observing the following technique:
   a. Use one needle for drawing up the contents of the ampoule.
   b. Use another needle for the injection.
   c. Insert the needle into the upper and outer quadrant of the buttocks.
   d. Patient should be in the prone position.
   e. Leave the needle for 30 seconds after insertion and suck back before injection.
   f. If a vein is entered, withdraw the needle and reinsert.

Emergency kit
Adrenaline injection BP ampoule 1 ml   3
Disposable syringe (2 ml + needles)   3
Chlorpheniramine maleate (Piriton) ampoule 10 mg   3
Aminophylline injection BP (250 mg in 10 ml)   3
Disposable syringes (10 ml)   3
Hydrocortisone sodium phosphate (Efcortesol, Glaxo 100 mg) ampoules   3
Oxygen and means of administration
Sphygmomanometer

Procedure
1. On appearance of signs of reaction patient should lie down — (head down and feet up position). Call the doctor.
2. Take blood pressure.
3. If BP is low give 0.5–1.0 ml adrenaline intramuscularly into upper arm.
4. If no response give 100 mg of hydrocortisone sodium phosphate i.m. or i.v.
5. If angioneurotic oedema give i.m. or i.v. chlorpheniramine (Piriton).
6. If cough, dyspnoea, respiratory distress give aminophylline i.v.

Type 1 hypersensitivity reactions (anaphylactic-type reactions)
After a penicillin injection patients should be observed for 30 minutes, particularly after the first injection. The serious and life-threatening complication of penicillin which is feared is a Type 1 hypersensitivity reaction (anaphylactic-type reaction) and this calls for an immediate intramuscular injection of adrenaline (see above).

The signs and symptoms of a Type 1 hypersensitivity reaction (anaphylactic-type) include generalized pruritus, particularly of the palms of the hands and soles of the feet. Hyperaemia develops with facial flushing, bronchospasm, laryngeal oedema, hypotension, tachycardia and shock (Drusin 1972). Early intramuscular adrenaline BP 0.5–1.0 ml is the most important form of therapy.

Additional facilities which may be required in hypersensitivity reactions (see Green 1975 for fuller details).
Equipment for intravenous infusion and tracheostomy, including tourniquet, venous cutdown equipment and 5% glucose; oxygen supply with means of administering it, and endotracheal tube.

NOTE TO CHAPTER 10

Note 10.1: Expressions of dosage of benzylpenicillin and long-acting forms of penicillin.

UNITS

Both the BP and USP used a biological method of assay when monographs for penicillin were first introduced. As soon as chemical assay, became available, however, both pharmacopoeias switched to the chemical assay, and the less accurate biological assay, where potency was expressed in units, was abandoned. Units therefore became redundant and were abandoned by the BP, and dosage was expressed on the basis of weight. The USP does the assay in terms of weight but calculates into units (British Pharmacopoeia 1980, United States Pharmacopoeia XXI).

UNITS PER MG

A mass of approximately 60 mg was chosen to express a potency of 100 000 units (it may be that the particular mass chosen (60 mg) may reflect the influence of the Apothecary System (62.5 mg — 1 grain).

EQUIVALENTS

Various approximate equivalents to units or mg of benzylpenicillin are given for various long-acting forms of penicillin in Martindale (28th edition, i.e. Reynolds 1985) and in manufacturers' data on commercial products, but a more 'scientific' approach to the determination of equivalents (on the basis of weight) is to use calculations based on molecular weights (mol. wt.) (Table 10.1).

In order to determine the weight of, say, procaine penicillin equivalent to 600 mg of benzylpenicillin sodium the following relationship may be used:

$$\text{Weight of procaine penicillin} = \frac{\text{mol.wt. of procaine penicillin} \times 600 \text{ mg}}{\text{mol.wt. of benzylpenicillin sodium}}$$

N.B. the unit is defined in terms of benzylpenicillin sodium (mol. wt. = 356.4) not benzylpenicillin (mol. wt. = 334.4).

The above approach bypasses the intermediate stage of having to convert weight to units and then back to the weight of a different salt.

REFERENCES

Barling R W A, Selkon J B 1978 The penetration of antibiotics into cerebrospinal fluid and brain tissue. Journal of Antimicrobial Chemotherapy 4: 203–227

Bryceson A D M 1976 Clinical pathology of the Jarisch-Herxheimer Reaction. Journal of Infectious Diseases 133: 696–704

Bryceson A D M, Cooper K E, Warrell D A, Perine P L, Parry E H O 1972 Studies of the mechanism of the Jarisch-Herxheimer reaction in louse-borne relapsing fever: evidence for the presence of circulating Borrelia endotoxin. Clinical Science 43: 343–354

Centers for Disease Control US Public Health Service 1985 STD Treatment guidelines. Morbidity and Mortality Weekly Report, Supplement 34: 94S–99S

Collart P. Borel L-J, Durel P 1962a Étude de l'action de la pénicilline dans la syphilis tardive: Persistance du tréponème pale. Premiere partie. La syphilis tardive experimentale après traitement Annales de l'Institut Pasteur de Lille 102: 596–615

Collart P, Borel L-J, Durel P 1962b Étude de l'action de la pénicilline dans la syphilis tardive: Persistance du tréponème pale. Seconde partie. La syphilis tardive humaine après traitement. Annales de l'Institut Pasteur de Lille 102: 693–704

Collart P, Borel L-J, Durel P 1964 Significance of spiral organisms found after treatment in late human and experimental syphilis. British Journal of Venereal Diseases 40: 81–89

Dash C H 1975 Penicillin allergy and the cephalosporins. Journal of Antimicrobial Chemotherapy 1(3) (Suppl): 107–118

Drusin L M 1972 The diagnosis and treatment of infectious and latent syphilis. Medical Clinics of North America 56(5): 1161–1173

Ducas J, Robson H G 1981 Cerebrospinal fluid penicillin levels during therapy for latent syphilis. Journal of the American Medical Association 246(22): 2583–2584

Dunlop E M C 1972 Persistence of treponemes after treatment. British Medical Journal 2: 577–580

Fenton L J, Light I J 1976 Syphilis after maternal treatment with erythromycin. Obstetrics and Gynecology 47: 492–494

Fishman R A 1966 Blood-brain and CSF barriers to penicillin and related organic acids. Archives of Neurology 15: 113–124

Fulford K W M, Johnson N, Loveday C, Storey J, Tedder R S 1976 Changes in intravascular complement and antitreponemal antibody titres preceding the Jarisch-Herxheimer reaction in secondary syphilis. Clinical and Experimental Immunology 24: 483–491

Garrod L P, Lambert H P, O'Grady F, Waterworth P M 1981 Penicillins. Antibiotic and chemotherapy, 5th edn. Livingstone, Edinburgh, ch 3, p 58–90; ch 24, p 61

Gelfand J A, Elin R J, Berry F W, Frank M M 1976 Endotoxemia associated with the Jarisch-Herxheimer reaction. New England Journal of Medicine 295: 211–213

Giles A J H, Lawrence A G 1979 Treatment failure with penicillin in early syphilis. British Journal of Venereal Diseases 55: 62–64

Gilman A C, Goodman L S, Rall T W, Murad F (eds) 1985 Goodman and Gilman's, the pharmacological basis of therapeutics. McMillan, New York, p 1115–1137

Green G R 1975 In: Stewart G T, McGovern J P (eds) Penicillin allergy: Clinical and immunological aspects. C C Thomas, Springfield, Illinois, USA, p 162

Greene B M, Miller N R, T E Bynum 1980 Failure of penicillin G benzathine in the treatment of neurosyphilis. Archives of Internal Medicine 140: 1117–1118

Green R L, Lewis J E, Kraus S J, Frederickson E L 1974 Elevated plasma procaine concentrations after administration of procaine penicillin G. New England Journal of Medicine 291: 223–226

Gudjonsson H, Skog E 1968 The effect of prednisolone on the Jarisch-Herxheimer reaction. Acta Dermato-venereologica 48: 15–18

Hare R 1970 The birth of penicillin and the disarming of microbes. Allen and Unwin Ltd

Hoekenga M T, Farmer T W 1948 Jarisch-Herxheimer reaction in neurosyphilis treated with penicillin. Archives of Internal Medicine 82: 611–622

Holder W R, Knox J M 1972 Syphilis in pregnancy. Medical Clinics of North America 56: 1151–1160

Idsoe O, Guthe E, Willcox R R 1972 Penicillin in the treatment of syphilis: the experience of three decades. Bulletin of the World Health Organization vol 47 Supplement. World Health Organization, Geneva

Jackson S W, Zey P N 1973 Ultrastructure of lipopolysaccharide isolated from *Treponema pallidum*. Journal of Bacteriology 114: 838–844

Kaufman R E, Blount J H, Jones O G 1974 Epidemiologic treatment in early syphilis. Public Health Reviews 3: 175–198

Kelly R 1964 The Treatment of neurosyphilis. Symposium on Neuropharmacology. The Practitioner 192: 90–95

Kern A 1971 Grundlagen und gestaltung der penicillin-therapie der syphilis. Medicamentum, Berlin 12: 194

Lamanna C, Mallette M F, Zimmerman L 1973 Limits of mutation. In: Basic bacteriology, its biological and chemical background. Williams and Wilkins, Baltimore, p 626

Leading Article 1977 The Jarisch-Herxheimer reaction. Lancet i: 340–341

Mohr J A, Griffiths W, Jackson R, Saadah H, Bird P, Riddle J 1976 Neurosyphilis and penicillin levels in cerebrospinal fluid. Journal of the American Medical Association 236: 2208–2209

Moore J E, Mohr C F 1952 Biologically false positive serologic tests for syphilis. Type, incidence and cause. Journal of the American Medical Association 150: 467–473

Moore J E, Farmer T W, Hoekenga M T 1948 Penicillin and the Jarisch-Herxheimer reaction in early, cardiovascular and neurosyphilis. Transactions of the Association of American Physicians 61: 176–183

Morrison R E, Harrison S M, Tramont E C 1985 Oral amoxicillin an alternative treatment for neurosyphilis. British Journal of Genitourinary Medicine 61: 359–362

Onoda Y 1979 Therapeutic effect of oral doxycycline on syphilis. British Journal of Venereal Diseases 55: 110–115

Petz L D 1971 Immunologic reactions of humans to cephalosporins. Postgraduate Medical Journal 47 Supplement: 64–67

Rein M F 1981 Treatment of neurosyphilis. Editorial. Journal of the American Medical Association 246: 2613

Reynolds F E F (ed) 1982 Martindale, the extra pharmacopoeia, 28th edn. The Pharmaceutical Press, London, p 1101–1110; 1206

Ries C A, Rosenbaum J J, Garatty G, Petz L D, Fudenberg H 1975 Penicillin-induced hemolytic anaemia. Journal of the American Medical Association 233: 432–435

Ritter G, Volles E, Müller F, Nabert-Bock G 1975 Blut-liquor-kinetik von penicillin-G bei neurosyphilis. Munchenen Medizinische Wochenschrift 117(35): 1383–1386

Robertson D H H 1963 The treatment of sleeping sickness (mainly due to *Trypanosoma rhodesiense*) with melarsoprol. I. Reactions observed during treatment. Transactions of the Royal Society of Tropical Medicine and Hygiene 57: 122–133

Roitt I 1988 Essential immunology. Blackwell Scientific Publications, Oxford, p 193–200

Ryden E 1978 Erythromycin. In: Reeves D S, Phillips I, Williams J D, Wise R (eds) Laboratory methods in antimicrobial chemotherapy. Churchill Livingstone, Edinburgh, p 208

Solley G O, Gleich G J, van Dellen R G 1982 Penicillin allergy: clinical experience with a battery of skin-test reagents. Journal of Allergy and Clinical Immunology 69: 238–244

South M A, Short D H, Knox J M 1964 Failure of erythromycin estolate therapy in in utero syphilis. Journal of the American Medical Association 190: 70–72

Spence M R 1977 Genital infections in pregnancy. Medical Clinics of North America 61(1): 139–151

Tramont E C 1976 Persistance of *Treponema pallidum* following penicillin G therapy: Report of two cases. Journal of the American Medical Association 236(19): 2206–2207

Tucker H A, Robinson R C V 1946 Neurosyphilitic patients treated with penicillin. Probable Herxheimer reaction. Journal of the American Medical Association 132: 281–283

Turner T B, Hollander D H 1957 Biology of the treponematoses. World Health Organization, Monograph Series 35: 43

Vercoe G S 1976 The effect of early syphilis on the inner ear and auditory nerves. Journal of Laryngology and Otology 90: 853–861

Warrell D A, Pope H M, Parry E H O, Perine P L, Bryceson A D M 1970 Cardiorespiratory disturbances associated with infective fever in man: studies of Ethiopian louse-borne relapsing fever. Clinical Science 39: 123–145

Warrell D A, Perine P L, Bryceson A D M, Parry E H O, Pope H M 1971 Physiologic changes during the Jarisch-Herxheimer reaction in early syphilis. American Journal of Medicine 51: 176–185

Wendel G D Jr, Stark B J, Jamison R B, Molina R D, Sullivan T J 1985 Penicillin allergy and desensitization in serious infections during pregnancy. The New England Journal of Medicine 312(19): 1229–1232

Willcox R R 1953 Progress in venereology. Heinemann, London, p 97

Willcox R R 1979 The management of sexually transmitted diseases. Regional Office for Europe, World Health Organization, Copenhagen

Wilner E, Brodie J A 1968 Prognosis of general paresis after treatment. Lancet ii: 1370–1371

Wright D J M 1983 Endogenous opioid withdrawal in the Jarisch-Herxheimer reaction; hypothesis. Lancet i: 1135–1136

Wright J T 1975 Single dose penicillin therapy. Correspondence, British Journal of Venereal Diseases 51: 410

11

Acquired syphilis: late-stage

In the early years of a syphilis infection the lesions already described (chancre, mucous patch, condyloma latum) are infectious and there is evidence of a recurrent spirochaetaemia and recurring mucocutaneous lesions. In pregnant women, also, infection of the fetus in utero is inevitable in untreated early-stage syphilis. Syphilis then enters a subclinical stage of latency, in which the only readily detectable evidence of infection is serological, and this latency may persist for years or even for life. Transmission of the disease by sexual intercourse does not occur although in the case of pregnancy the woman can infect her fetus long after she has ceased to be infectious sexually. Further activity of the disease may, at any time during latency, cause profound effects (Kampmeier 1964) and lead to death as long as three decades or more after infection. The main forms of late-stage syphilis are described below although the protean manifestations call for the consideration of syphilis in the differential diagnoses of many diseases involving particularly the cardiovascular or central nervous system.

The decline in the incidence of late-stage syphilis (Martin 1972) and of neurosyphilis and cardiovascular syphilis in particular has been discussed in Chapter 3. By 1969, for example, deaths in England and Wales from these two main causes declined further to 73 and 148 respectively and in 1973 to 38 and 85.

LATE-STAGE LATENT SYPHILIS

The diagnosis rests on the finding of positive specific serological tests for syphilis (Ch. 8), and the absence of other evidence of disease. Before reaching this diagnosis the cerebrospinal fluid (Ch. 8) should be examined and the heart and aorta screened by fluoroscopy to exclude changes due to involvement of the aortic valve and the first part of the aorta particularly. In the absence of obvious stigmata of congenital syphilis, corneal microscopy should be carried out in patients with latent syphilis, as the finding of traces of a healed interstitial keratitis will assist in differentiating a congenital infection from an acquired. Latent syphilis is the commonest manifestation of late syphilis, probably made more common because the patient will have had courses of antibiotics for other conditions which will have prevented the emergence of the late effects such as neurosyphilis.

In syphilis of longer than two years' duration longer courses and sometimes higher doses of penicillin are considered necessary (Ch. 10). Clear-cut demonstration of the value of treatment is not always so apparent as in early syphilis except perhaps in gummatous skin lesions and in some cases of neurosyphilis. In late-stage latent syphilis the prognosis with treatment is good. The differentiation between early-stage latent and late-stage latent is an arbitrary distinction, but treatment prevents the emergence of late effects although it cannot reverse damage already sustained. This general rule appears to be sound clinically although it should be noted that only careful examinations will detect the cardiovascular changes, and the methods currently used to detect involvement of the central nervous system, e.g. cerebrospinal fluid, may not be entirely sensitive.

There are problems too in the diagnosis of reinfection, and present serological tests may not give clear answers. Clinical judgement must be used therefore in deciding whether to re-treat a patient whose life style brings him into continuous risk of reinfection.

LATE-STAGE GUMMATOUS SYPHILIS

This is now very rare. It is characterized by gumma formation (syphilitic granulation tissue) which may develop because there is reactivation of residual treponemes in sensitized persons who have been untreated or inadequately treated. Possibly re-exposure may induce gumma formation in sensitized persons who have been adequately treated (Olansky 1964).

Serological tests for syphilis give positive results (Ch. 8). Gummatous lesions tend to be solitary or few in number. They are asymmetrical, indurated and indolent. On the skin late-stage lesions tend to be arcuate in outline because without treatment they tend to heal partially in the centre and extend peripherally. Atrophic or hyperpigmented scars form. Gummatous lesions respond rapidly to treatment. A gumma may form a nodule in the subcutaneous tissue which increases in size, breaks down and may produce a gummatous ulcer, often described as 'punched out' as it tends to have vertical walls. The granular floor of such an ulcer may have a 'wash leather' appearance due to slough. The sites commonly involved are the upper part of the leg below the knee, the scalp, face, sternoclavicular region or the buttocks.

The mouth and throat are much less frequently involved by a gummatous lesion than the skin and bones. The submucosa is involved first but either the soft or hard palate may be affected, leading to perforation. A gumma of the tongue can develop but a diffuse lesion with infiltration and a chronic superficial glossitis is more common. In such a case the patchy epithelial necrosis and the leukoplakia which develops, produce white areas of adherent epithelium on the tongue (Fig. 11.1). Mouth lesion should always be biopsied as malignant change is not uncommon and a careful life-long follow-up is necessary. Infiltration of the laryngeal mucosa may occur with or without ulceration.

Two main types of late syphilis of bone are recognized. Gummatous periostitis without destruction but with bony proliferation may lead to the development of

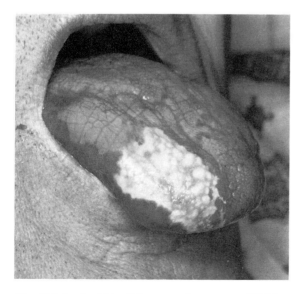

Fig. 11.1 Leukoplakia of the tongue (late-stage syphilis) in a 70-year-old male. Mouth lesions should be biopsied as malignant change is not uncommon. Careful life-long follow-up is also necessary.

'sabre tibia'. Gummatous osteitis may cause a destructive lesion. Clinically, in late syphilis of the bone, the patient may have boring pain and localized redness or swelling.

In congenital syphilis of the acute form, many treponemes are found in the liver, and a pericellular fibrosis results. Gummata of the liver may occur in late syphilis. A gumma of the testis produces a smooth painless swelling; the testis must be removed surgically to exclude malignant neoplasm (Ch. 18). Lesions of the oesophagus, stomach and intestine have been reported. An opacity, however, detected in a chest X-ray of a patient with syphilis is nearly always due to a carcinoma as a gumma is very rare in this site (Morgan et al 1952).

Gummatous lesions generally respond rapidly to treatment although when fibrosis is marked resolution will be slow. Reference has already been made to the importance of biopsy and a careful follow-up in cases of mouth lesions where malignant change is a recognized hazard.

NEUROSYPHILIS

Although *Treponema pallidum* may invade the central nervous system and involve particularly the meninges during early syphilis, causing minor changes in the cerebrospinal fluid (CSF), overt manifestations may occur only in about 5% of cases. In those cases, meningeal symptoms or signs may appear abruptly (headache or drowsiness, amaurosis with papilloedema, cranial nerve palsies or hemiplegia). Neurological abnormalities in early syphilis have been referred to in Chapter 9.

Neurosyphilis of the late stage is uncommon, but its sporadic appearance and often very good response to antibiotic therapy make it vitally important to make a diagnosis as early as possible. It may appear in a form with more localized and less striking clinical effects (Heathfield 1968, Joffe et al 1968) than were seen in the classical forms of parenchymatous neurosyphilis which were so much commoner in times before antibiotic and chemotherapy, when the wards of every mental hospital were crowded with cases in various stages of mental and physical deterioration. Although late-stage neurosyphilis can be classified into various forms there may be considerable overlap.

It is clearly important in all hospital departments to consider syphilis in diagnosis and to use treponemal serological tests (e.g. TPHA, FTA-ABS) as non-treponemal serological tests (e.g. VDRL) are sometimes negative in late syphilis (see Ch. 8). In recent years early infectious syphilis has been commoner in homosexual males, and in a series of 17 cases of neurosyphilis, 1 occurred in a woman and 16 in men, of whom 7 were homosexual (Joffe et al 1968).

PATHOLOGY OF NEUROSYPHILIS

In all forms of meningovascular syphilis there is a widespread, often diffuse, thickening of the pia-arachnoid and infiltration with lymphocytes and plasma cells. The basal meningitis of the secondary stage may be carried into the late stage with increased fibrosis and the formation of small miliary gummata. This can lead to hydrocephalus and papilloedema. The basal meningitis may be continued over the upper cervical segments of the spinal cord, or a diffuse spinal arachnoiditis may reveal its presence by root signs and symptoms. Meningeal gummata are very rare.

Lesions of the cerebral vessels may accompany any form of neurosyphilis but syphilitic vascular disease is not a common cause of cerebral vascular accidents. The classical lesion is endarteritis obliterans with fibroblasts and eventually collagenous thickening of the intima.

In tabes dorsalis the lesions are concentrated on the dorsal roots and columns, most often at the lumbosacral and lower thoracic levels. In classical paretic dementia (general paralysis of the insane), in a patient who dies demented after several years of illness, the brain is shrunken and covered with opaque thickened arachnoid. Microscopical examination at any stage shows the lesions to be concentrated in the cerebral cortex, corpus striatum and hypothalamus. In the cerebral cortex, particularly in the prefrontal cortex, all cellular elements are involved with a striking loss of cortical architecture. The meningeal and perivascular infiltrations, microglial and astrocytic hyperplasia and the degeneration and disappearance of nerve cells are similar to those found in other forms of subacute or chronic encephalitis such as African trypanosomiasis (due to *Trypanosoma brucei rhodesiense* or, more particularly, in that due to *T.b.gambiense*) and subacute sclerosing panencephalitis.

Although neurosyphilis is classified as parenchymatous or meningovascular, overlapping processes are found. The classification of tabes dorsalis among the parenchymatous forms of neurosyphilis is justified by the concentration of the lesions in the dorsal roots and columns. In most cases of tabes dorsalis in which cerebral symptoms appear and which are diagnosed clinically as taboparesis the cerebral lesions are those of meningovascular syphilis. Again, primary optic atrophy is commonly associated with tabes dorsalis and sometimes with meningovascular syphilis, but rarely with general paralysis of the insane (Harriman 1976).

CLINICAL FORMS OF ACQUIRED LATE-STAGE NEUROSYPHILIS

Asymptomatic neurosyphilis
The diagnosis rests on CSF findings, indicative of syphilis of the CNS in the absence of clinical symptoms or signs. It is reasonable to conclude that the inflammatory process is more restricted than in those forms of the disease with overt signs and symptoms. The investigation in such a case should not be restricted to serological tests for syphilis and CSF examination but should include a full clinical examination and fluoroscopic chest examination to exclude signs of syphilis in other systems.

Meningovascular syphilis
Symptoms and signs of meningovascular involvement may develop even during the secondary stage when the effect is predominantly meningeal with signs discussed already.

Meningovascular syphilis of the late stage may produce headache associated with cranial nerve palsies, particularly of the third and sixth; the auditory or vestibular nerves may also be affected. The optic nerves or chiasma may be involved in a basal meningitis. If cerebral vessels are affected mental deterioration and focal signs such as aphasia or hemiplegia will occur. If the gummatous infiltration involves the spinal cord progressive paraplegia can develop and occasionally there is a transverse myelitis due to occlusion of the anterior spinal artery. In meningovascular and, indeed, all forms of late-stage neurosyphilis pupillary abnormalities are common and the fully developed sign is the Argyll Robertson pupil.

Argyll Robertson pupil
In December 1868, at a meeting of the Edinburgh Medico-Chirurgical Society (Robertson 1869). Douglas Argyll Robertson described reflex pupillary paralysis to light in a case of spinal disease and later he defined the sign now known by his name:

> Although the retina is quite sensitive, and the pupil contracts during the act of accommodation for near objects, yet an alteration of the amount of light admitted into the eye does not influence the size of the pupil.

In all forms of late neurosyphilis, overt or latent, pupillary abnormalities in the presence of good vision are common. In more than 80% of cases and in tabes in particular, pupil abnormalities develop in the course of time. The fully developed condition already described and known as the Argyll Robertson pupil is a valuable sign although not pathognomonic of neurosyphilis, as it has been described as a curiosity in conditions such as diabetes, alcoholic neuropathy, hypertrophic polyneuropathy and tumours of the pineal region when there is also, as a rule, a defect of upward conjugate gaze (Walton 1985).

Earlier manifestations of reflex iridoplegia (failure to react to light) may be found in neurosyphilis, and during neurological examination the eye should be examined carefully to discover whether:

1. Reaction to light is reduced in amplitude.
2. Reaction to light is not sustained.
3. Latent period is longer than usual.
4. Reaction may be brisker in one eye.
5. Consensual reflex may be brisker than the direct.
6. Rarely a dilatation may occur in response to light.

In addition, oculosympathetic paralysis may be seen with no dilatation of the pupil in response to a scratch on the neck. Ptosis with compensatory wrinkling of the brow may also occur. Patchy depigmentation of the iris may give it a watery blue colour. Both pupils are usually affected, but unequally.

The fully developed Argyll Robertson pupil may best be described as 'small, constant in size and unaltered by light or shade; it contracts promptly and fully on convergence and dilates again promptly when the effort to converge is relaxed; it dilates slowly and imperfectly to mydriatics.'

The method of testing is important.

The light reflex
1. Ask the patient to look at a distant object.
2. Cover the other eye to eliminate the consensual reaction.
3. Test by shining light into the eye and look for contraction of the pupil.

Accommodation reflex
1. Ask the patient to look at distant object.
2. Then, ask him to look at examiner's finger which is brought gradually to within 2 inches of the eyes. The reaction consists of contraction of the medial recti muscles and contraction of the pupil.

The site of the lesion continues to excite controversy and is not entirely settled. The reflex paths in the midbrain are the most popular site for the causal injury, although a peripheral lesion in the iris has been suggested. The location of a lesion in the periaqueductal region of the midbrain by magnetic resonance imaging in a patient with Argyll Robertson pupils due to neuro-ophthalmic complications of acute sarcoidosis (Poole 1984) was in keeping with the midbrain theory. The suggestion is that the Argyll Robertson syndrome is caused by interruption of the light reflex pathway and inhibitory supranuclear pathways to the Edinger-West-phal nucleus at a point dorso-rostral to the oculomotor complex, while fibres controlling accommodation, being placed more ventrally, are left unaffected.

General paresis (dementia paralytica, general paralysis of the insane or GPI)

This can develop 7–15 years after a primary infection. The clinical syndrome now encountered is often one of simple mental deterioration, sometimes with depression, not distinguishable from the commoner and less specific presenile dementia. In the classical form of GPI the disease is insidious in its development and is characterized by episodes of strange behaviour at variance with the previous good character of the individual. Comprehension and aesthetic feelings are dulled and the alterations in the patient's personality distress his friends and relatives. Grandiose delusions and euphoria used to be commonly seen but are rare now. Writing may be tremulous and tremors of the tongue, hands and facial muscles may develop. Pronunciation difficulties may distort words beyond recognition. Epileptic fits and transient attacks of hemiplegia and aphasia are frequent. Tremor of the hands and a slow slurred speech are characteristic as the disease progresses. Spastic weakness of the legs develops and the final stage is that of paralysis and dementia (Matthews & Willer 1972).

Neurosyphilitic psychosis most commonly presents now as a depressive illness or a simple dementia, and patients presenting with grandiose delusions are very rare (Dewhurst 1969).

Tendon reflex abnormalities are common and degrees of iridoplegia, irregularity and inequality of the pupils are valuable signs. The fully developed Argyll Robertson pupil may be found in 25% of cases.

Tabes dorsalis

The lesions in tabes dorsalis are concentrated on the dorsal spinal roots and dorsal columns of the spinal cord, most often at the lumbosacral and lower thoracic levels. The dorsal roots are thin and grey and contrast with the thick white ventral roots. The dorsal columns show shrinkage although the dorsal root ganglia show less definite atrophy. The reasons for this selective degeneration are not understood.

Among the subjective manifestations are lightning pains, so called from their sudden brief stabbing quality. A brief jab of severe pain striking a localized point of one leg may make the patient wince. Such pains can be felt as girdle pains around the trunk or in the area supplied by the trigeminal nerve. The patient may complain of paraesthesiae, saying that he feels as if he is walking on cotton wool. He may have defects in his sensation of the need to defaecate or to empty his bladder.

Various paroxysmal painful disorders of the viscera

known as tabetic crises, probably reflecting irritation of the dorsal roots, may occur as a result of spasm of.smooth muscle. In gastric crises attacks of epigastric pain and ceaseless vomiting may mimic the 'acute abdomen' and last for several days. Laryngeal crises present with dyspnoea, cough and stridor. Tenesmus and bladder and penis pain occur in rectal and vesical crises respectively.

Other symptoms and signs are explained in terms of loss of sensory function. The patient is ataxic as there is loss of position sense, he tends to walk on a broad base, staggering and lifting his feet with a stamping gait. In Romberg's sign the patient demonstrates his inability to keep his balance with his eyes closed and his feet together. Muscles are hypotonic, the tendon reflexes diminished or absent. Vibration sense, deep pain sense and position sense are all diminished or absent.

Trophic changes may be seen. In the neuropathic joint (Charcot's joint) affecting a knee (Fig. 11.2), a wrist, or other joints, there is bone destruction with osteophyte formation. The joint is swollen and deformed with marked crepitus but quite painless. Collapse of the lumbar spine can cause nerve root compression. Perforating trophic ulcers may develop on the soles of the feet.

Charcot's joints are not pathognomonic of syphilis, being found in other neurological conditions such as syringomyelia, subacute combined degeneration of the spinal cord, diabetic neuropathy, or following intra-articular injections of corticosteroids (Boyle & Buchanan 1971).

Optic atrophy and a bilateral ptosis with compensatory wrinkling of the brow is common in tabes.

Optic atrophy
Optic atrophy as an isolated condition occurs as blindness in a third form of late-stage neurosyphilis. The discs are small and pale. The atrophy may progress to cause complete blindness in about one-third of patients, even with penicillin treatment. Atrophic fibres cannot regenerate whatever treatment is given. Recognition of syphilis at an early stage and penicillin therapy are vital in the prevention of these serious late-stage effects.

Modified late-stage forms of neurosyphilis
In countries of the West since the introduction and widespread use of antibiotics the classical clinical picture of late-stage neurosyphilis is seldom seen, but the disease may appear as modified neurosyphilis (Hooshmand et al 1972) with more isolated, localized and less striking signs. The diagnosis is backed by the sensitive and highly specific serological tests such as the FTA-ABS and/or TPHA tests (Ch. 8). In such modified forms the differential diagnosis needs careful thought.

1. Ophthalmological signs indicative of neurosyphilis
Argyll Robertson pupil or an irregular, unequal fixed pupil sometimes with synechiae of the iris and with positive serological tests for syphilis is indicative of neurosyphilis.

2. Ophthalmological signs in which positive serum treponemal antibody tests may be coincidental
Such findings (Duke-Elder 1971) should not be attributed automatically to syphilis, although full treatment for late-stage syphilis is nevertheless mandatory.

a. Choroido-retinitis. This is a manifestation of posterior uveitis and is now more commonly due to *Toxocara* or *Toxoplasma* infestation than to syphilis.

b. Secondary pigmentary degeneration of the retina. This may be a sequel to syphilitic neuroretinitis and resemble retinitis pigmentosa, an entity where there is a family history of the condition, and the patient will complain of night blindness. There is concentric constriction of the visual fields and pigmentation obscures the choroidal blood vessels, which are narrowed.

c. Ptosis. In bilateral ptosis consider also myasthenia gravis or a rare localized ocular myopathy. If the ptosis

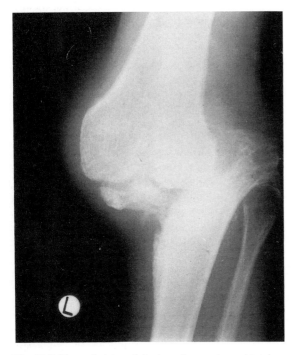

Fig. 11.2 Charcot's joint of the knee in a patient with tabes dorsalis.

is unilateral a neoplasm or aneurysm in the chest or neck, or diabetes are possibilities as well as syphilis.

d. Optic atrophy. This may be associated with an insidious glaucoma, multiple sclerosis or the result of injury or retro-orbital neoplasm or inflammation. In cases of optic atrophy associated with temporal arteritis the patient is ill, has continuous headache and a high erythrocyte sedimentation rate.

3. Neurological features attributable to localized inflammatory lesions of syphilis
In this group patients may present with epileptiform fits or as incomplete tabes with tendon reflex changes such as absent ankle jerks or a Babinski sign. Some may have a sensory abnormality and in some the signs of cervical spondylosis are due to syphilitic pachymeningitis rather than arthropathy.

4. Psychiatric disorders
Here it may be difficult to attribute depression, mania, personality disorder or dementia, to syphilis unless there are definite CSF changes.

TREATMENT OF NEUROSYPHILIS

The question of dosage of penicillin is considered in Chapter 10. There is little evidence that more clinical benefit is obtained by using doses higher than those recommended or by giving more than one course. There does not appear to be any correlation between the size of the penicillin dosage and the likelihood of developing new symptoms and it has been found that in 40% of cases of general paresis new neurological signs may develop. Such progression of the disease occurs in the absence of a deterioration in the CSF and it may be due to irreversible cerebrovascular disease before treatment (Wilner & Brodie 1968).

The first principle of effective treatment of neurosyphilis is early diagnosis. This is a matter of great importance as the effectiveness of treatment will depend upon how much irreversible damage to the central nervous system has occurred before treatment has begun. The appearance of neurosyphilis is the result of a failure to detect syphilis at the early stage when treatment will prevent the emergence of late-stage disease. In those forms of neurosyphilis modified by previous courses of antibiotics given for other reasons, both the recognition of the disease and the detection of objective signs of improvement after treatment will be difficult.

Any case thought to be neurosyphilis should be regarded as one of medical urgency and the patient should be assessed within 24 hours. A careful examination of the patient will include an examination of the CSF, an investigation which is essential in every case of late-stage syphilis except in those over 60 years of age, when its omission in the absence of neurological signs may be justified. Having established the diagnosis, treatment with penicillin should be started immediately.

A Jarisch-Herxheimer reaction with pyrexia occurs in over 90% of patients with general paresis with grossly abnormal cerebrospinal fluids but in other forms of neurosyphilis it is much less frequent (less than 40%). Clinical reactions are of special importance in general paresis when 10% of patients may be expected to develop a sudden intensification of somatic or psychotic symptoms (convulsions, coma, focal vascular accidents, excitement, confusion, mania, hallucinations or paranoid delusions) (Moore et al 1948).

TREATMENT, FOLLOW-UP AND PROGNOSIS OF NEUROSYPHILIS

The prognosis and follow up after treatment depend upon the type of neurosyphilis (Kelly 1964) and the amount of permanent damage caused before treatment is started.

Syphilitic meningitis
With the predominantly meningeal involvement, which occurs in early-stage syphilis beyond the primary stage, treatment is very effective. When there is an acute labyrinthitis with eighth cranial nerve dysfunction recovery may be slow and deafness can persist. Where there is a labyrinthitis, prednisolone in a high initial dosage together with penicillin is justified as an attempt to reduce the chance of an irreversible deafness (Vercoe 1976). Recovery from other meningitic effects is usual.

Meningovascular neurosyphilis
In late-stage meningovascular neurosyphilis the effects are due to foci of ischaemia due to the syphilitic arteritis, and although there is often considerable recovery after penicillin and an arrest of the disease process, ischaemic effects will persist and together with gliosis will cause persistent focal neurological effects such as aphasia, hemiplegia and cranial nerve involvement. In patients with predominantly psychiatric disorders differentiation from other psychosis is most important. Early treatment produces often remarkable improvement, but complete recovery is not to be expected.

General paresis (dementia paralytica, general paralysis of the insane)
Early diagnosis and the rapid institution of treatment are vital. In patients who have an acute onset of symptoms and are seen within weeks treatment can be spectacular in its effect. Patients have been able to resume

the practice of a profession within weeks of treatment and have remained efficient subsequently.

In those with a greater degree of damage recovery is often remarkable and the patients will feel much better, wishing to return to work as soon as possible. Sometimes their enthusiasm is not matched by the return of their intellectual ability, and psychological assessment is a necessary prelude to retraining for an occupation requiring less intellectual effort and less responsibility.

In patients who have become demented over a few years, and in whom the disease has presented with a more insidious course, there is often a serious loss of cortical neurones. Although treatment will arrest part of the disease process new signs of neurological disease may develop in a third of patients (Wilner & Brodie 1968) and these signs of progression do not seem to be limited by further courses of penicillin or by larger amounts of this antibiotic. The new signs described include grand-mal epilepsy, hand paraplegia, hemiparesis, amyotrophy, tabes dorsalis, optic atrophy or oculomotor palsy. Case reports (Greene et al 1980, Tramont 1976) of good response to high dose intravenous treatment with benzyl penicillin (e.g. 20 million units daily for 20 days) following progression in spite of benzathine penicillin (e.g. 2.4 million units weekly for 3 weeks) are among those quoted, together with observations that benzathine penicillin regimens do not secure adequate treponemicidal levels in the CSF, in favour of using the high-dose regimens in neurosyphilis.

Tabes dorsalis

This condition is rare and may present in an incomplete form. In some patients the disease is recognized as a result of a chance medical examination or because they seek advice for ataxia or lightning pains. Treatment with penicillin sometimes appears to halt the progress but deterioration often occurs in spite of treatment. Lightning pains, tabetic crises, bladder dysfunction, Charcot's arthropathy, and optic atrophy, may progress after treatment. In the follow-up of a case of tabes dorsalis there are particular points to consider.

The paroxysmal painful disorders of visceral function known as crises can be cut short by an injection of pethidine hydrochloride, 100 mg but this and other potentially addictive drugs should be avoided unless absolutely essential. In the case of a gastric crisis the patient should have a barium meal as the failure to diagnose a gastric ulcer in a tabetic may be more disastrous for the patient than to mistake an organic lesion of the stomach for a gastric crisis. In severe recurrent cases benefit has followed section of lower thoracic spinal dorsal roots, and very rarely upper thoracic chordotomy may be necessary (Walton 1985).

The loss of circulatory reflexes and orthostatic hypotension may result from interruption on the afferent side of the reflex arc from baroreceptors as part of the deep sensory loss characteristic of tabes. Such patients learn that they can rise to their feet only slowly if they are to avoid fainting but few have more than an occasional loss of consciousness (Spalding 1974).

Tabetic pains can be controlled sometimes by analgesics although the assessment of the value of individual drugs in the relief of the characteristic lightning pains is notoriously difficult in this now rare condition. In some cases analgesics are effective and their use should follow the principles of analgesic medication (Mehta 1973). If the antipyretic analgesic, acetyl salicylic acid (as aspirin soluble tablets BP) in a dose of 0.6 g (up to 0.9 g) every four to six hours is ineffective or unsuitable because of gastrointestinal side effects, paracetamol 0.5 g repeated every four to six hours may be tried. Mefenamic acid in a total daily dose of 1.0 g (each capsule contains 250 mg) may be used as an alternative; repeated changes within this group will delay tolerance and minimize side effects. If the pains are very intense, one of the weak narcotics, dihydrocodeine tablets BP in an oral dose of 30 mg can be tried, or alternatively the narcotic antagonist with analgesic activity, pentazocine (as tablets BP) in the oral dose of 25–50 mg may be given after food.

The pains of tabes are paroxysmal, brief and often very intense and this similarity to the pains of trigeminal neuralgia suggested the use of carbamazepine. It appeared to be effective when given as an initial dose of 200 mg twice daily, increasing to a maximum maintenance dose of 400–800 mg daily (Ekbom 1972).

In tabes the bladder becomes atonic and distended because there is damage to the posterior roots and ganglia which give loss of both deep pain and deep postural sensation including that of the bladder (Spalding 1974). If there is no evidence of hydronephrosis the patient should be instructed to empty the bladder every three hours during the day by the clock, before retiring and again early in the morning. Precipitancy of micturition may be relieved by propanethiline 15 mg three times daily (Walton 1985). Attempts may be made to empty an atonic bladder by giving an anticholinesterase (e.g. distigmine bromide (Ubretid, Berk Pharmaceuticals), 5 mg by mouth half an hour before breakfast or by an intramuscular injection of 0.5 mg for the first few days), or by reducing the resistance at the bladder neck with a transurethral resection. Manual compression can be dangerous as more urine may pass up the ureter than is expelled. When renal function is impaired or there is urinary infection which has failed to respond to chemotherapy surgery may be necessary (Walton 1985). Permanent drainage with a urethral or suprapubic catheter may be advised or the urine can be diverted to the skin. Urine must not be diverted into the colon in tabes as it will leak from the anus which is supplied by the same nerve roots as the bladder (Newsam & Petrie 1981).

In Charcot's arthropathy attempts are made to reduce the weight carried by the joint and improve its stability. Various calipers are available for the patient to use while walking. Perforating ulcers should be prevented by wearing well-fitting socks and shoes and by careful treatment of corns on the feet. When ulcers do develop, rest, clean dressings and antibiotic treatment will aid healing (Catterall 1977).

Ataxia may be improved by careful exercises which give confidence, supervised by a physiotherapist.

Optic atrophy

Acute optic neuritis in secondary syphilis will respond well to penicillin and the visual prognosis is good when there is acute visual loss. In optic atrophy the prognosis is poor although prednisone 30–60 mg daily with penicillin therapy may be given in an attempt to halt its progress. The help of an ophthalmologist should be sought in all such cases.

CARDIOVASCULAR SYPHILIS

Reference has already been made to the decline in the numbers of deaths from cardiovascular syphilis in England and Wales, a decline shared by all forms of late-stage syphilis, although the improvement in incidence has been much more apparent in its neurological than in its cardiovascular forms.

Gummata tend to occur in the interatrial septum or in the upper portion of the interventricular septum. Because of their proximity to the atrioventricular node, they may disturb the conducting system of the heart and provide one of the rare causes of the Stokes-Adams syndrome (complete heart block).

The second category of cardiac lesions in acquired syphilis are those which lead to aortic valve insufficiency. In all stages of syphilis arteritis is a constant feature. There is an endarteritis obliterans with a cellular reaction which radiates at some distance round the lesion in the form of a cuff within the periarterial tissues. This form of arteritis is important in two situations — the aorta and the brain. Involvement of the aorta is the commonest manifestation of late-stage syphilis. The severest lesions are usually in the aortic ring and the ascending part of the aorta, possibly because the vasa vasorum with their circumvascular lymphatics are most numerous in these portions of the vessel. The elastic tissue and muscle of the tunica media are destroyed and hence there is weakening of the aortic wall and loss of its elastic recoil. As the vessel becomes unable to withstand the force of the blood pressure it dilates. The dilatation often affects the root of the aorta

and hence widens the ring of the aortic valve. This is not the only cause of incompetence, for the cusps suffer damaging changes of a distinctive kind. There is an ingrowth of fibroblasts from the intima of the aorta along the free margin of the valve, which is given a cord-like or 'rolled edge' deformity.

Granulomatous lesions often involve the openings of the coronary arteries particularly in those patients in whom, as a developmental anomaly, the vessels arise above the level of the aortic sinus and are consequently nearer to the region of the greatest damage to the aorta.

Weakening of the media in syphilis often leads to general dilatation of the aorta, and in addition localized dilatation may occur, almost always in the ascending thoracic aorta. Such an aneurysm may press on neighbouring structures including the vertebrae, sternum and ribs which can be eroded by continuing pressure. The recurrent laryngeal nerve may be stretched and the oesophagus compressed. Rupture of the aueurysm is a common cause of death.

The coronary ostial stenosis, coupled with the low diastolic pressure accompanying the valvular insufficiency, gravely lessens the blood supply to the myocardium. The ischaemia may cause angina and sudden death due to infarction.

Aortic lesions in syphilis are maximal in the first part of the aorta and the arch; they are absent below the diaphragm. In contrast, in atheroma the lesions increase progressively from the arch to the bifurcation. In syphilis an aneurysm is usually thoracic and the aortic valve incompetent; in atheroma, the aneurysm is usually abdominal and if the aortic valve is involved it is stenosed (Symmers 1976).

CLINICAL FEATURES

Compensation for aortic regurgitation is so efficient that patients may live for many years with minimal symptoms. They may be aware of the heaving cardiac impulse in bed and may notice transient dizziness following changes in posture. The compensation is achieved because the refluxing blood augments that which enters the left ventricle through the mitral valve to produce increased stretching and hence more powerful contraction of the ventricle. Gross hypertrophy and dilatation of the left ventricle has produced some of the largest hearts to be found at autopsy.

The symptoms and signs depend upon the site and the anatomical nature of the lesion. Coronary ostial stenosis will cause angina. Dilatation of the aorta may cause an aortic systolic murmur and a characteristic loud aortic component of the second sound. Aortic regurgitation is responsible for an early diastolic murmur, often best heard in the second right intercostal space with the patient leaning forward and holding his breath.

An aortic aneurysm may cause pulsation of the anterior chest wall or occasionally obstruction of the superior vena cava, causing facial oedema. Pressure of the aneurysm on the bronchi can cause a tracheal tug felt by the examiner as a downward pull on the thyroid cartilage. Hoarseness, dysphagia and bone pain are other symptoms.

Electrocardiogram changes may show evidence of myocardial ischaemia or signs of left ventricular hypertrophy. The radiograph of the chest shows dilatation of the aorta, and linear calcification of the surrounding portion is a useful early sign. The most useful diagnostic measure is an injection of radio-opaque dye into the ascending aorta by catheterization which demonstrates the degree of reflux into the ventricle in diastole. As long as compensation is maintained cardiac catheterization will show that the end diastolic pressure in the left ventricle and the left atrial pressures are normal.

DIAGNOSIS

In any case of aortic regurgitation or aneurysmal dilatation syphilis should be suspected. Syphilis seldom causes ischaemic heart disease alone without producing aortic regurgitation. In any form of late-stage syphilis the chest should be examined by fluoroscopy as when the aorta is involved there is a loss of parallelism of its walls and often calcification of the first part before aneurysmal changes are pronounced (McCann & Porter 1956). Serological tests for syphilis will indicate the aetiology (Ch. 8).

TREATMENT OF CARDIOVASCULAR SYPHILIS

Treatment with penicillin should take the form advised for late-stage syphilis other than neurosyphilis (Ch. 10)

although objective evidence of cardiovascular improvement can seldom be obtained (Macfarlane et al 1956). Nonetheless, such a course of treatment should be given and it should be remembered that neurosyphilis may co-exist with cardiovascular syphilis, when a longer course is advised.

In uncomplicated syphilitic aortitis, diagnosed on the basis of fluoroscopic detection of dilatation of the aorta in the absence of aortic incompetence, there is no appreciable threat to life during the first seven years after the discovery. Progression to aortic incompetence occurs in about a third of patients within four years, and the quantity of penicillin treatment given does not appear to influence these changes (Irvine 1956).

The progression of uncomplicated aortitis to aortic incompetence is not certainly halted by antibiotic treatment. Compensation for aortic regurgitation is so efficient that patients may live for many years with minimal symptoms such as an awareness of the heaving cardiac impulse in bed or transient dizziness following sudden changes in posture. Failure of compensation is indicated by angina and shortness of breath. As life expectancy is so good and the long-term effects of valve replacement are still unpredictable, physicians may be reluctant to refer patients for surgery until they develop symptoms. This excessive conservatism has its disadvantages as the results of surgery will be adversely affected if the operation is deferred until the ventricle has become irreparably damaged.

In surgery of aneurysm of the ascending aorta a mortality as high as 40% may be expected. Resection of an aneurysm of the aortic arch is the most demanding operation in surgery and carries a very high mortality (Collis et al 1976).

In coronary ostial stenosis surgical intervention can produce dramatic relief and although antibiotic treatment is given, as in other forms of cardiovascular syphilis, a decision about the advisability of surgery will require a cardiological assessment including a coronary arteriogram.

REFERENCES

Boyle J A, Buchanan W W 1971 In: Clinical rheumatology. Blackwell Scientific Publications, Oxford, p 359–360

Catterall R D 1977 Neurosyphilis. British Journal of Hospital Medicine 17: 585–605

Collis J L, Clarke D B, Smith R A 1976 In: d'Abreu's Practice of cardiothoracic surgery, 4th edn. Edward Arnold, London, p 431–435, 516–518

Dewhurst K 1969 The neurosyphilitic psychoses today. A survey of 91 cases. British Journal of Psychiatry 115: 31–38

Duke-Elder Sir Stewart 1971 In: System of ophthalmology, neuro-ophthalmology, vol XII. Kimpton, London, p 660

Ekbom K 1972 Carbamazepine in the treatment of tabetic lightning pains. Archives of Neurology (Chicago) 26: 374–378

Greene B M, Miller N R, Bynum T E 1980 Failure of penicillin G benzathine in the treatment of neurosyphilis. Archives of Internal Medicine 140: 1117–1118

Harriman D G F 1976 In: Blackwood W, Corsellis J A N (eds) Greenfield's Neuropathology, bacterial infections of the central nervous system. Arnold, London, p 238–268

Heathfield K W G 1968 Neurosyphilis. Correspondence. British Medical Journal 1: 765–766

Hooshmand H, Escobar M R, Koff S W 1972 Neurosyphilis: A study of 241 patients. Journal of the American Medical Association 219 : 729

Irvine R E 1956 Outcome of uncomplicated syphilitic aortitis. British Medical Journal 1: 832–834

Jaffe R, Black M M, Floyd M 1968 Changing clinical picture of neurosyphilis: Report of seven unusual cases. British Medical Journal 1: 211–212

Kampmeier R J 1964 Late manifestations of syphilis: skeletal, visceral and cardiovascular. The Medical Clinics of North America. Syphilis and other venereal diseases 48: 667–697

Kelly R 1964 The treatment of neurosyphilis. The Practitioner 192: 90–95

Macfarlane W V, Swan W C A, Irvine R E 1956 Cardiovascular disease in syphilis. A review of 1330 patients. British Medical Journal 1: 827–832

McCann J S, Porter D C 1956 Calcification of the aorta as an aid to the diagnosis of syphilis. British Medical Journal 1: 826–827

Martin J M 1972 Conquest of general paralysis. British Medical Journal 2: 159–160

Mehta M 1973 In: Intractable pain: treatment. Saunders, London, p 61–88

Moore J E, Farmer T W, Hockenga M T 1948 Penicillin and the Jarisch-Herxheimer reaction in early, cardiovascular, and neurosyphilis. Transactions of the Association of American Physicians 61: 176–183

Morgan A D, Lloyd W E, Price-Thomas Sir Clement 1952 Tertiary syphilis of the lung and its diagnosis. Thorax 7: 125–133

Newsam J E, Petrie J J B 1981 Urology and renal medicine, 3rd edn. Churchill Livingstone, Edinburgh, p 259–260

Olansky S 1964 Late benign syphilis (gumma). The Medical Clinics of North America. Syphilis and other venereal diseases 48: 653–665

Poole C J M 1984 Argyll Robertson pupils due to neurosarcoidosis: evidence for site of lesion. British Medical Journal 289 : 356

Robertson D M C L Argyll 1869 (a) On an interesting series of eye-symptoms in a case of spinal disease, etc. Edinburgh Medical Journal 14: 696–708. (b) Four cases of spinal myosis, etc. Edinburgh Medical Journal 15: 487–493

Spalding J M K 1974 In: Disorders of the autonomic nervous system. Blackwell Scientific Publications, Oxford, p 96, 235

Symmers W St C 1976 In: Symmers W St C (ed) Systemic pathology, vol 1. Churchill Livingstone, Edinburgh, p 39, 136

Tramont E C 1976 Persistence of *Treponema pallidum* following penicillin G therapy: Report of two cases. Journal of the American Medical Association 236(19): 2206–2207

Vercoe G S 1976 The effect of early syphilis on the inner ear and auditory systems. Journal of Laryngology and Otology 90: 853–861

Walton Sir John 1985 Brain's Diseases of the nervous system. 9th edn Oxford University Press, Oxford, p 104, 271–272

Wilner E, Brodie J A 1968 Prognosis of general paresis after treatment. Lancet ii: 1370–1371

12

Congenital syphilis

INTRODUCTION

Congenital syphilis is an uncommon disease in the United Kingdom. In England during the 12 months ending in December 1982 there were 126 cases reported and a case rate of 0.27 per 100 000 population for that year (Department of Health and Social Security 1983). Antenatal examination routinely includes serological tests for syphilis and this screening, together with adequate treatment of infected mothers, accounts for the low incidence of the disease in this country. In Africa and South America congenital syphilis is still common, although where yaws is endemic an immune effect may modify the consequences of syphilis in the adult female and its transmissibility to the fetus. It can be prevented in utero by treatment of the infected woman with penicillin during early pregnancy or cured later in pregnancy; its occurrence in a community is an indicator of defective antenatal care and the result of insufficient primary medical care.

TRANSMISSION OF INFECTION

Although it had long been considered that involvement of the fetus did not occur before the fourth month of gestation, studies have now clearly demonstrated that infection may occur within 10 weeks of conception (Harter & Benirschke 1976). Any infection before 20 weeks gestation will not stimulate immune mechanisms because the fetal immune system is not as yet well developed and thus no histological evidence of fetal reaction to infection will be seen (Silverstein 1962). The theory that the cytotrophoblastic layer (Langhan's layer) of the early placenta protects — until its disappearance at 18–20 weeks gestation — against transmission of the organism from the maternal to the fetal circulation (Curtis & Philpott 1964), has now been discounted. Electron microscopic studies have shown that this layer of cells does not completely atrophy (Benirschke 1974).

Infection of the fetus is more likely to occur when the mother's infection is in the early stage, as at this time considerable numbers of organisms are present in the circulation. During the first year of infection in an untreated woman there is an 80 to 90% chance that the infection will be transmitted to the fetus. The probability of fetal infection declines rapidly after the second year of infection in the mother and becomes rare after the fourth year. In general, the greater the duration of syphilis in the mother, the less chance there is of the fetus being affected.

In pre-antibiotic days it was common for a mother of a child with congenital syphilis to give a history of previous miscarriages succeeded by a premature stillbirth, then a stillbirth at term, and later an apparently healthy child at birth. The widespread use of antibiotics for concomitant infection has completely altered this pattern of events, and such an obstetrical record is now virtually unknown.

Although uncommon, a woman with late syphilis, however, may give birth to a child with syphilis, although the child of a previous pregnancy had been apparently healthy. This may be explained by the speculation that there is an intermittent release of treponemes from lymphoid tissue into the circulation in late syphilis. Should such an event occur the fetus may become infected.

If a mother with early-stage syphilis is not treated, 25 to 30% of fetuses die in utero; 25 to 30% die after birth; and of the infected survivors 40% develop late symptomatic syphilis (Thomas 1949).

CLINICAL FEATURES

The manifestations of congenital syphilis may conveniently be divided into two stages, early and late; the end of the second year of life is the arbitrary point of division between the two stages. Fuller details of the clinical features of congenital syphilis may be found in Nabarro's book (Nabarro 1954) and in a review by Robinson (1969) as well as by reference to individual papers quoted.

Early congenital syphilis

When congenital syphilis was common it was rare to find acute signs of syphilis in the newborn and in cases that occurred, death usually followed within a few days. Infants were often born prematurely or, if full-term, were often of low birth weight. The skin was wrinkled and there was a bullous skin rash (syphilitic pemphigus). particularly on the soles and palms. The clear or purulent fluid from the bullae contained large numbers of *T. pallidum* and was highly infectious. Other skin lesions, most often maculopapules, were usually present and were found around the body orifices. Rhinitis produced a mucoid or mucopurulent nasal discharge, and a hoarse cry resulted from laryngitis.

Abdominal distension was common, and hepatic and splenic enlargement almost invariably found. Haemorrhagic manifestations occasionally occurred. This has been shown to have been due to thrombocytopenia and macroglobulinaemia (Marchi et al 1966). The majority of infants infected with syphilis appear healthy at birth, as the characteristic clinical features do not develop until between 2 and 12 weeks. After a period of normal development, the child fails to thrive and the clinical picture of congenital syphilis becomes apparent.

It is convenient to describe the manifestations according to the particular part of the body affected.

Cutaneous manifestations

Skin rashes of varied character are found in 70 to 90% of infants with congenital syphilis. The rash is symmetrical in distribution and erythematous macular, papular and papulosquamous lesions may exist together in different parts of the body. On the face the eruption is particularly prominent around the mouth. Where the skin is moist, for example on the buttocks and external genitalia, the rash appears eczematous. In these sites hypertrophic lesions resembling condylomata lata may appear, usually as a manifestation of a recurrence following resolution of the initial rash. Deep fissures develop round the body orifices, and healing of these lesions leaves characteristic scars (rhagades).

The skin of the palms and soles may show peeling. In severe cases, the hair becomes scanty and brittle and involvement of the nails leads to shedding, and replacement by narrow, atrophic nails.

In addition to the eruptions described, the skin may show wrinkling from weight loss and there is café-au-lait pigmentation.

If an infant is not treated, or is inadequately treated, the skin lesions usually heal within a year, but there may be recurrences during the second year. Recurrent lesions usually differ from those seen in the original rash and include condylomata lata.

Mucosal lesions

Clinical evidence of rhinitis is found in 70 to 80% of infected infants. There is nasal obstruction and a mucoid nasal discharge which becomes mucopurulent and occasionally blood-stained (syphilitic snuffles). Numerous treponemes may be demonstrated in the discharge, which is highly infectious. Arrested development of nasal structures, and continued pressure changes within the nose as a result of obstruction lead to deformities of the nose (saddle nose).

Mucous patches resembling those seen in secondary acquired syphilis may occur in the mouth and pharynx. Laryngitis produces a hoarse or aphonic cry.

Lymphadenitis and splenic enlargement

Although not a constant accompaniment of early congenital syphilis, moderate generalized enlargement of the lymph nodes is common. The spleen is enlarged in at least 60% of infected infants.

Bone and joint manifestations

Bone disease, diagnosed by clinical or radiological examination, or both, occurs in at least 85% of infected infants under the age of 1 year (Nabarro 1954). In only about 40% of cases is there clinical evidence of bone involvement. Bones are usually affected symmetrically, but one side may be more involved than the other. The child cries when adjacent joints are passively moved and he rarely moves affected limbs (Parrot's pseudoparalysis).

Radiological examination of infected infants under the age of 12 months, who have no clinical evidence of bone involvement, demonstrates abnormalities in at least 75% of cases. Multiple long-bone involvement is most commonly found, the metaphyses being particularly affected. Variable degrees of calcification at the growing ends of the bone result in a variety of radiological changes (Hira et al 1985). Most commonly there is an irregular (saw tooth) dense zone of calcification overlying an osteoporotic area at the metaphysis. Peripheral osteoporosis of the metaphysis is less often observed, as is the appearance of dense bands sandwiching such zones.

Irregular patchy areas of loss of bone density are commonly found in both metaphyses and diaphyses. A characteristic sign is loss of density of the upper medial aspect of the tibiae (Wimberger's sign). In severe cases there may be a fracture at the site of bone destruction in the metaphysis, with impaction or displacement of the epiphysis.

Periostitis appears radiologically either as a single layer or as multiple layers of new-bone formation along the cortex of the shaft of the bone; it is common in early congenital syphilis, particularly amongst children aged four weeks and over (Hira et al 1985). Although any long bone may be affected, the distal femur and radius and the proximal tibia and humerus are the most often involved. The changes described are not specific for syphilis, similar radiological findings being encountered in rubella, cytomegalovirus infection, rickets and haemolytic disease of the newborn (Cremin & Fisher 1970). Occasionally in early congenital syphilis lens-shaped areas known as Parrot's nodes appear around the anterior fontanelle on the frontal and parietal bones. These nodes are probably due to periostitis. Usually the changes described resolve within the second 6 months of life, but periostitis persists and may become more pronounced.

During the later stages of early congenital syphilis, dactylitis, manifest clinically as painless, spindle-shaped swelling of the fingers, may occur in a small number of cases (less than 5%). Radiographic examination shows that up to 25% of all infected children under the age of two years have dactylitis.

Hepatic and pancreatic involvement

The liver is almost invariably enlarged, usually in association with the spleen, in congenital syphilis appearing in the neonatal period, and in at least 60% of older infants. Jaundice is an uncommon feature, but its presence in the neonate should alert the physician practising in areas where syphilis is common, to the possibility that syphilis may be the cause of the jaundice.

Although not clinically apparent, pancreatitis is a common finding at autopsy of infants dying of congenital syphilis in the neonatal period (Oppenheimer & Hardy 1971).

Renal involvement

The nephrotic syndrome may rarely be associated with early congenital syphilis, and is thought to be the result of deposition of soluble complexes of treponemal antigen and anti-treponemal antibody in the glomeruli (Yuceoglu et al 1974). Acute nephritis is a rarity (Taitz et al 1961).

Broncho-pulmonary involvement

In the aborted fetus and stillborn infant, the lungs are always affected, as bronchi and lung parenchyma have developed abnormally.

Neurological involvement

Although meningitis is common in early congenital syphilis, particularly during the exanthem stage, clinical signs relating to the nervous system are uncommon. Epileptiform seizures, irritability and bulging of the anterior fontanelle may occur. There may be focal changes in the cerebral tissue due to thrombotic occlusion of blood vessels affected by a panarteritis. These cerebral lesions may produce hemiplegia, monoplegia and cranial nerve palsies.

In about a third of infants under the age of 12 months, the cerebrospinal fluid is abnormal with respect to cell content and protein levels, and gives positive results when examined by the serological tests for syphilis.

Ocular manifestations

Iritis is rare in early congenital syphilis. Choroido-retinitis is considerably more common during the first year of life. Examination with ophthalmoscope shows small spots of pigment surrounded by yellow areas (salt and pepper fundus). If untreated the inflammatory process progresses, and if the macular or optic disc regions are involved, blindness may result.

Haematological abnormalities

Anaemia of varying severity occurs in at least 20% of infants with congenital syphilis. Normocytic, normochromic anaemia reflects depression of haematopoiesis in the bone marrow as a result of the chronic infection. Increased haemolysis probably plays a small part in the development of the anaemia. Secondary iron deficiency produces a microcytic, hypochromic anaemia. Occasionally a leuco-erythroblastic anaemia occurs.

Thrombocytopenia, associated with a bleeding disorder during the first few weeks of life, has been described (Freiman & Super 1966). Macroglobulinaemia may be associated with the bleeding diathesis (Marchi et al 1966).

In early congenital syphilis, the white cell count is usually elevated, with lymphocytosis.

LATE CONGENITAL SYPHILIS

Infected and untreated children are said to have entered the late stage of syphilis after their second birthday. In at least 60% of affected children there are no clinical signs of the disease, the only abnormal finding being positive serological tests, that is latent congenital syphilis.

Interstitial keratitis

This is the most common clinical manifestation of late congenital syphilis, occurring in about 40% of affected children. Interstitial keratitis appears to be the result of immunological reaction in the cornea to the treponeme, penicillin treatment having no influence on the course of this manifestation. In most cases this develops between the ages of 6 and 14 years, but it may occur earlier or very much later (even over the age of 30 years). Although commencing in one eye, both become involved in more than 90% of cases; the second eye shows features of the condition a few days to several months after the first. The patient complains of pain in the affected eye, photophobia with excessive lacrimation and dimness of vision. A diffuse haziness near the centre of the cornea of one eye is the earliest clinical sign, but within a few weeks the whole cornea becomes opaque. This is usually associated with circumcorneal sclerotic congestion.

Examination by slit-lamp microscopy shows that these corneal changes are attributable to blood vessels extending into the cornea from the sclera, and to exudation of cells from these vessels.

The condition gradually improves over a period of 12 to 18 months, leaving a variable degree of corneal damage which may lead to blindness or be only detectable by slit-lamp examination. This latter investigation may show empty blood vessels (ghost vessels) within the cornea of patients who have had interstitial keratitis earlier in life, but have had no apparent residual scarring (Dunlop & Zwink 1954).

After resolution of the initial episode of interstitial keratitis, 20 to 30% of patients suffer a relapse of this condition.

Bone lesions

The essential bone lesion in late congenital syphilis is hyperplastic osteoperiostitis, a process which may be diffuse, resulting in sclerosis of bone, or localized (periosteal node or gumma). Gumma formation may lead to necrosis of underlying cortex with softening of the bone. The tibiae are most commonly affected by these changes.

Usually bone lesions develop between the 5th and 20th year of life, when the patient complains of pain in the affected bone. Palpation may reveal nodules on the anterior surface of the bone, and rarely ulceration may be observed where a gumma has involved skin and bone. In older children, thickening of the anterior surface of the tibia may result in forward bowing of that bone (sabre tibia).

Painless gummatous lesions may be found on the hard and soft palates or in the pharynx. These are often extensive, with considerable necrosis of tissue. Perforation of the palate, absence of the uvula and scarring about the oropharynx may be the result.

Destructive gummatous lesions of the nasal septum may cause perforation of the septum with or without deformity of the lower part of the nose.

Joint lesions

The commonest type of joint lesion (Clutton's joints), seen in about 20% of untreated children, is bilateral effusion into the knee joints (Scott Gray & Philp 1963). This condition, like interstitial keratitis, is unaffected by antibiotic treatment, and appears to be an immuno-

logical reaction to *T. pallidum*. Less commonly, other joints are similarly affected. Although most frequently occurring in children between the ages of five and ten years, joint involvement may be seen at any age from three years to the mid-twenties.

The onset of the arthritis is acute, often with a history of antecedent trauma. Although most commonly painless, the affected joints may be acutely painful, particularly at the onset. Radiological examination reveals no specific changes in the joint.

There is gradual resolution of the arthritis over many months, with recovery of full function.

Neurosyphilis

In about 20% of infected children over the age of one year neurosyphilis is latent or hidden and diagnosis depends upon the detection of abnormalities in the cerebrospinal fluid.

As a late result of the meningitis of early-stage congenital syphilis, epileptiform seizures, mental deficiency and cranial nerve palsies may be found in children over the age of two years. Parenchymatous involvement produces two main clinical conditions, juvenile general paralysis of the insane and tabes dorsalis.

Juvenile general paralysis (juvenile GPI)

This occurs in about 1% of affected children, appearing about the age of 10 years, but occasionally much earlier or much later, as in middle age. The sexes are affected equally (in contrast to the GPI of acquired syphilis in which males are more often affected than females). There is usually a gradual onset of symptoms, the child becoming dull, irritable, apathetic and forgetful. Later, delusions, usually paranoid in type, occur and speech becomes disturbed. The voice is monotonous, articulation becomes stumbling and tremulous, and speech is eventually lost. There is generally tremor of the lips, hands and legs. Handwriting becomes indistinct. Epileptiform seizures are common at a late stage of the disease.

Pupillary abnormalities are seen in over 90% of cases; the pupils are of the Argyll Robertson type or immobile and dilated. Optic atrophy occurs in between 10 and 35% of cases.

Other physical findings resemble those found in general paralysis of acquired syphilis.

Juvenile tabes

This is much rarer than general paralysis. The onset of the condition is generally between the ages of 10 and 17 years. Failing vision and paraesthesiae are the most common symptoms; lightning pains and ataxia are rare. Later in the course of the disease headaches, photophobia and diplopia occur frequently. Sphincter disturbances are uncommon although enuresis may be found. Clinical examination may detect nystagmus, pupillary abnormalities, optic atrophy, and absent or diminished tendon reflexes. Trophic disturbances are rare and it is unusual to find evidence of loss of cutaneous sensation.

Ear disease

The middle ear may be affected by a painless otolabyrinthitis, showing as a slight purulent aural discharge. Conduction deafness may result without treatment. The deafness of congenital syphilis, however, is predominantly sensory.

In sections of the temporal bone of individuals with long-standing sensorineural deafness which has resulted from congenital syphilis, there is patchy osteitis with inflammation of all three layers of the otic capsule. Hydrops of the cochlear duct, saccule and utricle occurs and there is degeneration of the organ of Corti with loss of cochlear neurones. Similar changes may affect the sensory epithelium or neurones of the vestibular system (Karmody & Schuknecht 1966).

Even after what has been considered adequate penicillin treatment, treponemes have been demonstrated in endochondral bone, a dense structure into which antibiotics do not readily diffuse.

Subjective hearing impairment is commonly a late manifestation, often not occurring until adult life, although it can occur in childhood. In addition the patient may not be seen first till middle age, when the diagnosis of congenital syphilis may not come readily to mind unless there are other stigmata of the disease.

Vestibular disease is frequent in patients with congenital syphilis. The symptoms, which include dizziness, unsteadiness of gait and paroxysmal vertigo, usually begin with the onset of deafness (Morrison 1975).

Audiograms show a variety of patterns. The most common (35%) is high-tone loss, followed by a flat audiogram (25% of cases) and low-tone loss (15% of cases) (Morrison 1975). There is progressive deterioration of deafness although spontaneous fluctuation may occur. The most severe difficulty is in discrimination of speech. It is usually an isolated finding, bilateral, although one side is often more severely affected than the other. There are usually no abnormalities in the cerebrospinal fluid (Hahn et al 1961).

Skin lesions

Gummata similar to those occurring in late acquired syphilis may be found.

Cardiovascular lesions

Myocarditis may be found in children dying of congenital syphilis, but aortitis is exceedingly rare.

Liver disease

Gummata of the liver are rarely found.

Paroxysmal cold haemoglobinuria

This rare condition, occurring in less than 1% of patients with late congenital syphilis, may be seen also in acquired syphilis. Large quantities of haemoglobin are excreted in the urine after exposure to cold.

Shivering or a rigor heralds the attack and this is rapidly followed by fever, headache and pains in the back or limbs. A generalized urticarial rash may also develop. Within the next few hours the urine becomes dark brown in colour and contains haemoglobin, methaemoglobin, but few red blood cells. In most cases, the clinical features described resolve within several hours, but occasionally mild jaundice may develop and persist for some days. This condition is liable to recur periodically when the patient is exposed to cold of varying severity.

Cold haemolysins are found in the blood, and demonstrated by the Donath Landsteiner test. The basis of this test is the ability of the haemolysin to unite with red cells when the blood is chilled; when the blood is then warmed to 37°C, these sensitized cells are lysed in the presence of complement.

STIGMATA OF CONGENITAL SYPHILIS

Lesions of early and late congenital syphilis may heal leaving scars and deformities characteristic of the disease. Such scarring and deformities constitute the stigmata of congenital syphilis, but only in some 40% of patients do they occur.

Stigmata of early lesions

1. Facial appearance

The 'saddle-nose' deformity may result from rhinitis. The palate may appear high-arched as a result of underdevelopment of the maxilla.

2. Teeth

The tooth germs of deciduous teeth are fully differentiated by the 10th week of gestation before tissue reaction to treponemes appears to occur; hence these teeth are usually unaffected. Teeth which develop later may, however, be affected. Two groups of teeth bear the brunt, the upper central incisors and the 1st molars.

Typically the affected upper incisor is smaller than normal, and darker in colour and peg-like, instead of being flat, with the sides converging to the cutting edge which classically has a notched centre (Fig. 12.1), the

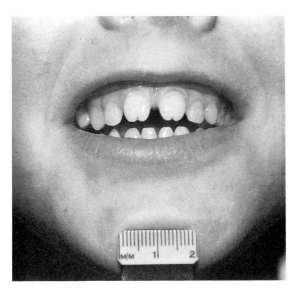

Fig. 12.1 Hutchinson's incisors, one of the classical stigmata of congenital syphilis. Note the peg-like appearance with convergence towards the cutting edge, which classically has a notched centre. Affected incisors do not always have this typical appearance (see text.)

so-called Hutchinson's incisor (Hutchinson 1858). Affected incisors do not always show this typical appearance but may often be thickened anteroposteriorly, with rounding of the incisal angles; they may have a shallow depression on the incisal edge rather than a notch.

The typically affected molar, Moon's molar, shows a constricted occlusal surface and rounded angles. The cuspules of the molar are poorly developed and appear crowded together. Such teeth are prone to dental caries and as a result are lost early.

In one series (Putkonen 1962), in 45% of patients with congenital syphilis the upper central incisors were affected, and in about 20% the first molars were involved. The incidence of dental changes is high in patients who also develop interstitial keratitis.

3. Rhagades
The deep cutaneous lesions around the orifices of the body heal, producing scars radiating from the orifice known as rhagades.

4. Nails
Atrophy and deformity of the nails may be seen in adult life as a result of nail-bed inflammation in infancy.

5. Choroidal scarring
Healing of choroido-retinitis produces white scarred areas surrounded by pigmentation on the retina.

Stigmata of late lesions

1. Corneal lesions
Opacities of the cornea and ghost vessels observed on slit-lamp examination are the result of interstitial keratitis (Dunlop & Zwink 1954).

2. Bone lesions
Sabre tibia resulting from osteoperiostitis may be observed, as may the scars of destructive lesions of the oropharyngeal and nasal regions. Broadening of the skull may result from osteoperiostitis of the frontal and parietal bones.

3. Optic atrophy
This may occur as a single entity without iridoplegia (e.g. Argyll Robertson pupils) (Robinson 1969).

4. Nerve deafness

DIAGNOSIS

It is important to ascertain that a child born to a mother who has been apparently adequately treated for syphilis is not infected. An infected infant may appear healthy at birth. Blood from the neonate should be examined at birth, using VDRL and TPHA tests. As a result of transplacental passage of maternal antibody, those tests which are positive in the mother are also likely to be positive in the infant, and at a similar titre. Within 6 months, however, these maternal antibodies will have disappeared from the infant's serum and, if the child is not infected, the tests will have become negative. Persistently positive serological tests, or a rising titre, suggest congenital infection and the need for treatment.

The use of the FTA-ABS test, using monospecific antisera to detect specific IgM antibodies in the infant's blood has been described. It is important to remember that this test may be negative at birth in a child with active infection and may not become positive until the age of 3 months. Serial serological tests up to 6 months are therefore required in apparently healthy babies born to mothers with positive serological tests for syphilis, particularly if untreated or suspected to be so.

In western industrialized countries, the discovery of positive serological tests in an otherwise healthy person often raises the question as to whether syphilis has been acquired before birth or later. This problem is difficult as stigmata appear to be rare now. A family history may be misleading. Patients should, however, be carefully examined for the presence of obvious stigmata, and slit-lamp microscopy of the cornea should be included in the investigation to search for ghost vessels, as a trace of previous interstitial keratitis (Dunlop & Zwink 1954). Nerve deafness may be obvious or, if mild, demonstrable by audiography. In doubtful cases, serological examination of parents or brothers and sisters may be helpful, and to avoid serious social upset consultation and collaboration with the general practitioner is advised.

TREATMENT OF CONGENITAL SYPHILIS

Early congenital syphilis
Although infants with massive infection may still die in the neonatal period, the majority will be cured by adequate penicillin treatment. Stigmata, particularly dental, will, however, be detectable.

Prior to instituting treatment, the CSF should be examined to detect neurological involvement. Benzylpenicillin in an intramuscular dose of 30 mg (50 000 i.u.) per kg should be given daily in two divided doses.

Alternatively, procaine penicillin 49.55 mg (approximately equivalent to 30 mg or 50 000 i.u. benzylpenicillin) per kg per day may be used (Hager 1978). Treatment should be continued for at least 10 days, and preferably longer if the CSF is abnormal. Further details on prevention, treatment and the problem when erythromycin has been used for treatment of the pregnant woman with syphilis are discussed in Chapter 10.

Late congenital syphilis
The dosage of procaine penicillin required for the treatment of late congenital syphilis is similar to that used in the therapy of late acquired syphilis. Treatment, however, does not prevent the development or course of interstitial keratitis, hydrarthrosis and neural deafness.

a. Management of interstitial keratitis
Patients with interstitial keratitis should be managed in hospital, in consultation with an ophthalmologist.

Topically-applied corticosteroids rapidly suppress the inflammatory reaction in the cornea and anterior uveal tract, and their use, until spontaneous cure occurs, has revolutionized the management of this condition. Although the infiltration of the cornea by inflammatory cells resolves, scarring from previous episodes of keratitis is not affected.

Betamethasone eye drops, BPC 0.1%, instilled into the affected eye(s) every 1 to 2 hours, is a useful preparation. Treatment should be continued until the corneal inflammatory infiltrate has cleared, and visual acuity restored to the patient's normal level. Slit-lamp examination is essential before steroid treatment is discontinued, as mild degrees of keratitis may not be apparent otherwise. Regular examination is required after cessation of treatment, as corneal scarring may result from continuing mild inflammation.

During steroid treatment, mydriatics such as atropine eye drops BPC 1%, may be useful adjuvants by reducing ciliary muscle tension.

Corneal grafting may be required in patients with corneal scarring acquired during attacks of interstitial keratitis.

b. Hydrarthrosis (Clutton's joints)
This is a self-limiting disorder, and does not require any specific therapy.

c. Nerve deafness
Despite previous treatment of congenital syphilis with what have been regarded as adequate doses of penicillin, progressive neural deafness may develop at any age, but most commonly in the adult of middle age. This may be the result of failure of the drug to reach adequate concentrations in the perilymph or endolymph.

Morrison (1975) advocated the use of benzylpenicillin in a dosage of 300 mg (500 000 i.u.) given by intramuscular injection every six hours for 17 days, together with probenecid in a dose of 1 g six hourly by mouth. During the first week of treatment, 30 mg of prednisone is given orally, the dose thereafter being reduced to 25 mg daily for three weeks. As a response to treatment is seen within the first month, treatment may be discontinued if there has been no improvement at that time. When the response has been satisfactory, steroids may be continued for three to six months in gradually diminishing doses. A further course of penicillin is then given. Occasionally patients have required maintenance treatment with low doses of steroids to abolish vertigo and maintain hearing.

In advanced cases where there has been considerable tissue damage, however, no response to medical treatment occurs.

Ampicillin in a dosage of 1.5 g six-hourly for four weeks, together with prednisolone 30 mg daily for 10 days, tailing off over the succeeding 10 days has been used in the management of this condition (Kerr et al 1973).

Audiometry may give useful information regarding response to treatment.

The value of treatment has not been fully assessed. In some cases the disease process may be arrested, but in others improvement in hearing may only be temporary.

REFERENCES

Benirschke K 1974 Syphilis in the placenta and the fetus. American Journal of Diseases of Children 128: 142–143

Cremin B J, Fisher R M 1970 The lesions of congenital syphilis. British Journal of Radiology 43: 333–341

Curtis A C, Philpott O S 1964 Prenatal syphilis. Medical Clinics of North America 48: 707–719

Department of Health and Social Security 1983 Sexually transmitted diseases: Extract from the annual report of the Chief Medical Officer of the Department of Health and Social Security for the year 1983. Genitourinary Medicine 61: 204–207

Dunlop E M C, Zwink F B 1954 Incidence of corneal changes in congenital syphilis. British Journal of Venereal Diseases 30: 201–209

Freiman I, Super M 1966 Thrombocytopenia and congenital syphilis in South African Bantu infants. Archives of Diseases of Childhood 41: 87–90

Hager W D 1978 Transplacental transmission of spirochetes in congenital syphilis: a new perspective. Sexually Transmitted Diseases 5: 122–123

Hahn R D, Rodin P, Haskins H L 1961 Treatment of neural deafness with prednisone. Journal of Chronic Diseases 15: 395–410

Harter C A, Benirschke K 1976 Fetal syphilis in the first trimester. American Journal of Obstetrics and Gynecology 124: 705–711

Hira S K, Bhat G J, Patel J B et al 1985 Early congenital syphilis: clinico-radiologic features in 202 patients. Sexually Transmitted Diseases 12: 177–183

Hutchinson J 1858 On the influence of hereditary syphilis on the teeth. Transactions of the Odontological Society 2 : 95

Karmody C S, Schuknecht H F, 1966 Deafness in congenital syphilis. Archives of Otolaryngology (Chicago) 83: 18–27

Kerr A G, Smyth G D L, Cinnamond M J 1973 Congenital syphilitic deafness. Journal of Laryngology and Otology 87: 1–12

Marchi A G, Tambussi A M, Famularo L 1966 Un insolito guadro della disprotidemia luetica connatale: la crioglobulinemia. Present azrione di un caso. Minerva Pediatrica 18: 1155–1157

Morrison A W 1975 Management of sensorineural deafness. Butterworths, London. ch 4, p 109–144

Nabarro D 1954 Congenital syphilis. Edward Arnold, London

Oppenheimer E H, Hardy J B 1971 Congenital syphilis in the newborn infant: Clinical and pathological observations in recent cases. Johns Hopkins Medical Journal 129: 63–82

Putkonen T 1962 Dental changes in congenital syphilis. Relationship to other stigmata. Acta Dermato-venereologica (Stockholm) 42: 44–62

Robinson R C V 1969 Congenital syphilis. Review article. Archives of Dermatology 99: 599–610

Scott Gray M, Philp T 1963 Syphilitic arthritis. Annals of the Rheumatic Diseases 22: 19–25

Silverstein A M 1962 Congenital syphilis and the timing of immunogenesis in the human foetus. Nature 194: 196–197

Taitz L S, Isaacson C, Stein H 1961 Acute nephritis associated with congenital syphilis. British Medical Journal 2: 152–153

Thomas E W 1949 Syphilis: its course and management. Macmillan, New York

Yuceoglu A M, Sagel I, Tresser G, Wasserman E, Lange K 1974 The glomerulopathy of congenital syphilis. Journal of the American Medical Association 229: 1085–1089

13

Endemic treponematoses

In 1905, Castellani, working in Ceylon, discovered the causative organism of yaws, and Schaudinn discovered and characterized *Spirochaeta pallida* (translated 'pale spiral hair'; later the name was changed to *Treponema pallidum*) in syphilis, and confirmed that the causative organisms of yaws and syphilis were morphologically identical (Castellani 1905, Castellani 1906, Schaudinn & Hoffman 1906). Since the very time of this discovery the biological and epidemiological relationships of the treponemes of venereal syphilis and the non-venereal treponemal diseases, such as yaws and pinta, have continued to fascinate — for there are clinical, epidemio-

logical and immunological similarities which continue to defy attempts to separate and distinguish the organisms. The various biological differences appear, rather, to illustrate the remarkable adaptability of the treponeme and its ingenuity for survival. A number of other morphologically identical treponemes are known in mammals also and cannot yet be clearly distinguished from *Treponema pallidum* in the laboratory. These include *T. luiscuniculi* which causes a venereal disease in rabbits, and a treponeme found in the popliteal lymph nodes of the feral *Cynocephalus* (dog-headed ape) or baboon of Guinea. It is better to regard these trepo-

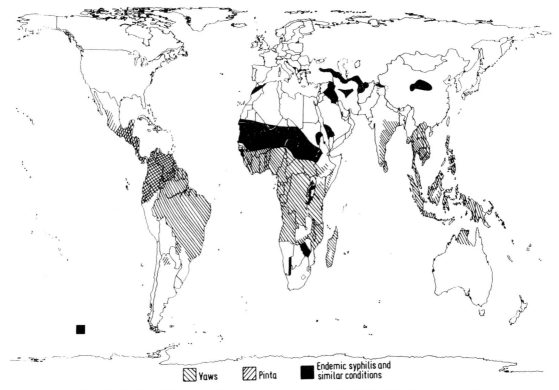

Fig. 13.1 Geographical distribution of the endemic treponematoses in the early 1950s. World map, Arno Peters projection; data from WHO Scientific Group 1982.

nemes as varieties or adaptations to secure survival than as distinct species.

The treponematoses of man have developed in differing geographical and epidemiological situations as parasite and host and have evolved a modus vivendi. The non-venereal diseases tend to exist among primitive peoples in rural communities, where transmission occurs by skin contact in childhood with other younger or older children who, themselves, have relapsing crops of infective skin lesions. If infected in childhood, susceptibility to venereal syphilis later as adults is diminished.

In the world maps provided, the geographical distribution of the endemic treponematoses in the early 1950s (Fig. 13.1) is contrasted with that of the 1980s (Fig. 13.2).

Syphilis, on the other hand, probably evolved as a venereal disease as a result of social and climatic change, as in populations who began to wear clothes and, apart from sexual contact, tended to live more separate existences. The survival and transmission of the treponeme under these circumstances became possible only when susceptible adults, escaping yaws in childhood, became infected by contact with genital lesions at sexual intercourse.

PINTA (synonyms: in Mexico *mal de pinto*, in Colombia and Venezuela *carate*, and in Chile and Peru *azul*)

This is a disease of remote rural communities affecting the skin (blue-stain disease) and it is the least damaging of the human treponematoses. The causative organism is *Treponema carateum*, the most attenuated of the pathogenic treponemes. Pinta used to be prevalent in semi-arid regions of Brazil, Colombia, Cuba, southern Mexico and Venezuela, with scattered foci in Central and South American countries and the Caribbean islands; today only scattered foci remain in northern South America and Mexico (Perine et al 1984). It differs from yaws and endemic syphilis in that it affects children and adults of all ages. Throughout its course the disease is confined to the skin, where pigmented and achromic lesions may remain infective for years, permitting spread by direct skin to skin contact.

Clinical features
The primary or initial lesion develops usually after two to three weeks, often on an uncovered part of the body, as a lenticular and slightly scaly papule which enlarges to form a plaque; mostly the initial lesion is to be found

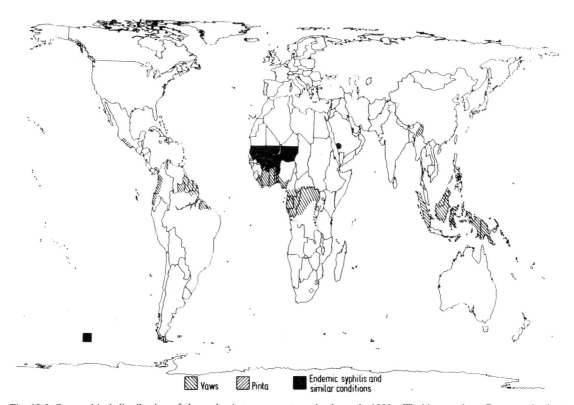

Fig. 13.2 Geographical distribution of the endemic treponematoses in the early 1980s. World map, Arno Peters projection; data from WHO Scientific Group 1982.

on the legs, the dorsum of the foot, the forearm or the back of the hands. At first pink in colour in fair skins it becomes pigmented or hypochromic to a variable degree as it enlarges; lymph nodes draining the area enlarge. After two months or up to a year later, secondary lesions develop, some on occasions appearing on the same site as the initial lesion. At first erythematous and afterwards copper coloured, these 'pintids' become pigmented to a varying degree, changing slowly from a copper colour to lead-grey and slate-blue as a result of photosensitization, and areas of erythema, hypopigmentation and leucoderma develop. The polychromic lesions become keratotic.

In late-stage pinta, residual areas of hyperchromia and achromia develop in isolated patches to form multicoloured lesions; the depigmentation process occurs at different rates even within the same lesion. No disability or complication other than leucoderma occurs (Perine et al 1984).

The causative organism, *T. carateum*, is detected by dark ground illumination microscopy in serum obtained from the base of a lesion after abrading the surface; although numerous in early-stage lesions, treponemes persist through to the late dyschromic stage (Marquez 1975).

YAWS (synonyms: *pian* — French; *framboesia* — German, Dutch; *bouba* — Portuguese: *buba* — Kiswahili).

Yaws has shown the greatest changes in regional prevalence since the mass treatment campaigns of the 1950s. In South America, only scattered foci of active yaws persist; Brazil and Surinam are almost yaws free and in Colombia, Ecuador, French Guiana and Guyana only a few dozen or a hundred cases are reported annually. In south east Asia yaws still exist in Indonesia and Papua New Guinea.

Africa remains the part of the world most affected, although where there is improved rural medical care and improved standards of living, as in the Ivory Coast and

Table 13.1 Classification of yaws lesions (Hackett 1951, 1957, Perine 1984).

Yaws lesions	Examples	'Infectiousness' + to +++
Early-stage cutaneous (often pruritic; tendency to cropping; often polymorphous; modified by climate; if lesions moist then infectious)		
Initial lesion	Papule, papilloma	+++
Papillomata	papilloma; some serpiginous; some ulcerated	+++
Macules		++
Micropapules, papules		+++
Squamous macules		+
Squamous micropapules, papules		++
Polymorphous or mixed		++
Plaques		+
Nodules	e.g. front of knees	+
Hyperkeratosis	palmar, plantar (as in cráb yaws — painful)	−
Early-stage bone		
Osteoperiostitis	polydactylitis	−
	tibia	−
	goundou (osteitis of nasal processes of maxilla)	
Early-stage joint	ganglion, hydrarthrosis	−
Late-stage cutaneous		
Hyperkeratosis	palmar, plantar	−
Ulcer with characteristic tissue destruction (gummatous)		−
Late-stage bone		
Gummatous osteoperiostitis	sabre tibia; monodactylitis	−
	gangosa	−
Late-stage joint		
	ganglion	−
	hydrarthrosis	−
	bursitis	−
	juxta-articular nodes	−

Nigeria, the numbers of clinical cases are declining (WHO Scientific Group 1982). In Ghana, however, resurgence of yaws occurred following cessation of active yaws surveillance; the numbers of reported cases of infectious yaws increased 21-fold between 1969 and 1976 (Agadzi et al 1983).

In a WHO survey in the Central African Republic, Congo and Gabon, clinical yaws was detected in over 20% of the pygmy population and positive serological tests in 80% (WHO Scientific Group 1982). Out of a total pygmy population of 100 000–200 000, two major groups have undergone less assimilation than the others — the Binga of the tropical rain forests to the west of the Ubangi River, and the Mbuti, several hundred miles to the east in the Ituri Forest (Anonymous 1978). In a survey (486 examined) of the former group in 1978/79, in the dry season, a time when these nomadic forest people were accessible, it was found that there were clinical signs of yaws in 50% and serological tests (VDRL and TPHA) were positive in 86% of the children and 95% of the adults. In the case of neighbouring non-pygmy peasant-cultivators clinical evidence of yaws was also common (30%) and 78% of the children and 98% of the adults had positive serological tests (Widy-Wirski et al 1980). Eradication campaigns had clearly not reached such isolated populations, and total mass treatment (see antibiotics in treatment and control in endemic treponematoses) would be the appropriate medical strategy. To achieve success, however, anthropological understanding would be an essential, as the forest pygmies have no formal social structure and organization and small bands constantly change in size and composition throughout the year (Turnbull 1963, Anonymous 1978).

Clinical features

Yaws is a contact disease of childhood, caused by *Treponema pertenue* (Chambers 1938), and is characterized by crops of highly infectious and relapsing skin lesions in the first five or six years of the natural course of the infection. The classification and nomenclature for the lesions of yaws were established in an illustrated monograph of the World Health Organization (Hackett 1957) and the bone lesions were discussed more fully by Hackett (1951). A classification of lesions and the degrees of infectiousness of such lesions, based on Perine et al (1984), are summarized in Table 13.1.

The most characteristic lesion in early yaws is the papilloma, and in the exudate of all early lesions, which may be macular, maculopapular or papular (Fig. 13.3), treponemes are numerous. The early papule enlarges to form a papillomatous lesion bearing some resemblance to a raspberry (a synonym is framboesia). There may also be adenitis. After two to six months the initial lesion heals, often without scarring. Further papil-

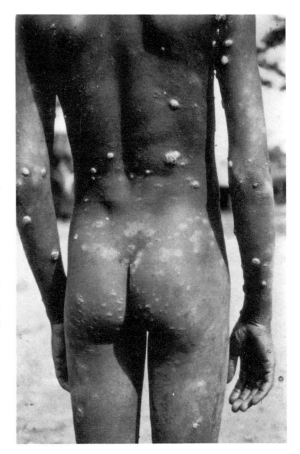

Fig. 13.3 Back of patient showing papillomata and papules. Over the inner surface of the buttocks are papular lesions and on the posterior surface of the upper limbs are macular lesions. On the back are acuminate micropapules. The association of macular and maculopapular lesions with papillomata is frequent in the early stages of the disease.

lomata, often in crops, develop most often around the body orifices, near the nose, mouth, anus and vulva. A change in climate may influence the number and morphology of yaws lesions: in the dry season lesions tend to be fewer in number and macular in form, and papillomata tend to be more concentrated in moist areas of the skin such as the axilla (Fig. 13.4) and anal cleft. Hyperkeratotic lesions occur on the soles of the feet and palms of the hands. On the feet plaques develop, which are painful, and walking becomes difficult (crab yaws).

A periostitis may affect long bones or cause a polydactylitis affecting the phalanges and metacarpals (Fig. 13.5). An osteitis of the nasal processes of the maxilla produces paranasal swellings (goundou) and is common in Africa. The tibia may become sabre-shaped. Nocturnal bone pain and tenderness of the tibial shaft are common in early yaws.

Ganglions, particularly at the wrist, and hydrarthrosis

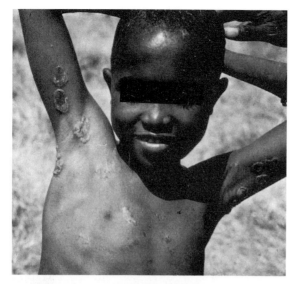

Fig. 13.4 Circinate early papules in yaws.

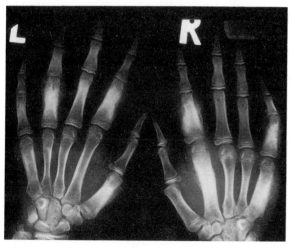

Fig. 13.5 X-ray showing oesteoperiostitis of early yaws in a boy aged 12 years with polydactylitis and circinate early stage lesions in the axilla.

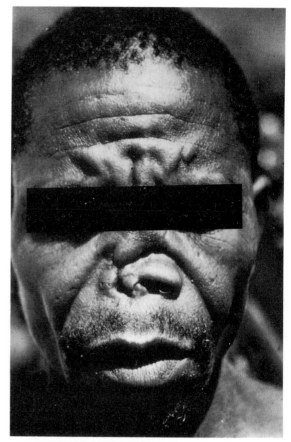

Fig. 13.6 Gangosa in late-stage yaws (effect due to gummatous lesions of late yaws).

that there is no bone lesion that occurs in yaws that does not also occur in syphilis (Hackett 1951).

There is no certain evidence of transplacental or congenital infection in yaws. Serologically it cannot be distinguished from syphilis.

ENDEMIC SYPHILIS (synonyms: *bejel* — Arabic; in Zimbabwe *njovera*, *dichuchwa*; endemic syphilis, in Bosnia. Extinct forms of disease: *sibbens* in Scotland, *radesyge* in Norway and *skerljevo*, of the Croatian coast, Yugoslavia)

Endemic syphilis is prevalent today primarily among the semi-nomads in the Arabian peninsula and along the southern border of the Sahara desert. A recent survey found thousands of cases of early endemic syphilis in Mali, Mauretania, Niger and Upper Volta; in sub-Saharan Africa the disease may be a greater problem today than it was formerly (WHO Scientific group 1982). It used to be found also in scattered foci in

can also occur in early yaws. There is also an early latent stage which may be interrupted by relapses of active early lesions.

Late-stage lesions (Table 13.1) develop five or more years after the infection, and the characteristic late lesion is a destructive ulcer, which may involve skin, subcutaneous tissue, the mucosae and the bones and joints. Deep destructive lesions are typified by the hideous mutilation of the central part of the face (rhinopharyngitis mutilans) called gangosa (Fig. 13.6), in which there is destruction of cartilage and bone structures of the septum, palate and posterior part of the pharynx (Kerdel-Vegas 1986). It is probable, however,

Central Asia, Australia and India but these have been eliminated by the mass penicillin treatment campaigns of the 1950s (Perine et al 1984).

The infection may be spread in the early stage through the use of recently contaminated drinking vessels (Grin 1953); by direct skin to skin contact; or by the fingers contaminated with saliva and mucus from infective lesions containing treponemes (Perine et al 1984).

In Arabia endemic syphilis, known as bejel, presents in its early stage and generally in children aged 2–15 years, with a mucocutaneous eruption and exuberant papules, predominantly around the genitalia and anus. Mucous papules or shallow ulcerations (mucous patches) appear on the lips, in the mouth and in the fauces. Symptoms such as hoarseness, dysphagia or dyspnoea have been attributed to extension of the mucous patches to the larynx. Condylomata may be seen in the moist areas of the skin. Periostitis also occurs (Hudson 1958).

Late lesions are granulomatous and destructive, and the nose and its bony structure, the oral cavity and the hard palate and larynx are favourite sites. Hudson (1958) remarks that in his time 'cleft palate voices were common in the market place'. Destructive skin ulcers, plantar keratosis, juxta-articular nodes and depigmented lesions are common late manifestations.

CONTROL OF ENDEMIC TREPONEMATOSES

Although the treatment of whole communities with long-acting penicillin preparations for the control of endemic treponematosis of childhood was followed initially by a remarkable regression of the community disease, early clinical yaws has not been eliminated in large endemic areas where transmission continues and periodic focal outbreaks tend to occur (Guthe et al 1972, WHO Scientific Group 1982). Without renewed control programmes, gains made by mass treatment campaigns of the 1950s and afterwards may be lost, particularly for yaws in some African countries (Perine et al 1984).

In the 1950s, on the basis of pilot studies in yaws in Haiti, endemic syphilis in Yugoslavia and pinta in Mexico, mass treatment campaigns with penicillin were undertaken in 46 countries in the context of the World Health Organization Treponematoses Campaign. Up till 1970 some 160 million people had been examined and in 50 million clinical cases, latent cases and contacts, treatment had been given. In Western Samoa, for example, the prevalence of clinically active yaws was about 11% in 1955, with about 3% with infectious lesions. On re-survey of the population after mass treatment a year later clinically active yaws was found in only 0.06% and infectious cases in 0.02%. In Bosnia,

Yugoslavia, the prevalence of endemic syphilis varied from district to district and was highest in north-eastern Bosnia, where about 14% of the population were infected. Of all those found during the campaign to have the treponemal disease, about 10% had early infectious lesions, 0.2% congenital, 85% latent and 5% late (Grin 1953). During the follow-up period after mass treatment it soon became evident that the chief risk of perpetuating the disease lay, not in treatment failures, but rather in infected persons escaping examination, in migrants from other districts with early lesions, in those with latent infections or those incubating the disease at the time of examination. In Yugoslavia the careful campaign, follow-up and progressive environmental changes reduced the rate of endemic syphilis to nil. In Haiti, more than 1.3 million clinical cases, latent cases and contacts were treated, and surveys showed steady progress to low infectious levels of 0.01% in 1961.

Clinical surveys for active yaws may be conducted without any sophisticated laboratory test, but surveys for latent disease require serological tests (WHO Scientific Group 1970a). The original indices were clinical, and the detection of cases of active yaws is likely to continue to be the mainstay of surveillance and most appropriate for economic and logistic reasons. Age-specific seroreactor rates are, however, useful to define areas as hyperendemic, mesoendemic and hypoendemic, and in surveys after mass treatment such profiles demonstrate the age at which infections are occurring. In areas where very well conducted campaigns have been carried out, an occasional seroreactive child is discovered with no evidence of past or present clinical disease, so there is a possibility of persisting subclinical infection. If the proportion of the population examined and treated is too low then seroreactors will be common in early age groups of a sample and a further mass campaign will be necessary.

False seroreactions in cardiolipin tests (biological false-positives) become relatively important when the seroreactor rates are declining, and particularly so in childhood. Special techniques of storing serum in liquid nitrogen (WHO Scientific Group 1970b) and other facilities have been developed to ensure that reliable specific antibody tests (TPHA or FTA tests) can be carried out for those working in the field.

The socio-economic status of a large segment of the populations in the rural areas of West Africa has either not improved or has actually regressed in the last decade. In these areas, patients with reported yaws infection now number tens of thousands, but epidemiological estimates place the true incidence as four times higher. In areas of increasing prevalence, atypical early yaws lesions may be underdiagnosed owing to the inexperience of clinicians unfamiliar with the manifestations of the disease (WHO Scientific Group 1982).

Antibiotics in treatment and control in endemic treponematoses

Benzathine benzylpenicillin has been recommended by a recent WHO Expert Committee on Venereal Diseases and is preferred to other forms of penicillin for the treatment of treponemal diseases. Since a single deep intramuscular injection of benzathine benzylpenicillin 1.836 g (approximately equivalent to 1.44 g or 2.4×10^6 i.u. benzylpenicillin) (Penidural L-A) in a healthy ambulant adult produces a penicillinaemia above the treponemicidal level for more than three weeks, this dose is effective not only for curing treponemal diseases but also for providing protection against reinfection during this period. Currently schedules for the endemic treponematoses (not including venereal syphilis) are: a single intramuscular injection of 459 mg benzathine benzylpenicillin (approximately equivalent to 360 mg or 600 000 i.u. of benzylpenicillin) for patients and contacts aged under 10 years; and 918 mg benzathine benzylpenicillin (approximately equivalent to 720 mg or 1.2×10^6 i.u. benzylpenicillin) for those over 10 years (Perine et al 1984).

The extent of treatment given to a community, village or other group living close to one another, is based on the prevalence of clinically active yaws in the community. World Health Organization treatment policies recommend for hyperendemic areas (approximate prevalence of clinically active yaws in the community of over 10%) benzathine benzylpenicillin treatment to the entire population viz. total mass treatment (TMT); for mesoendemic areas (approximate prevalence of clinically active yaws in the community of 5–10%) treatment with benzathine benzylpenicillin in all active cases, all children under 15 years of age, and obvious contacts of infectious patients viz. juvenile mass treatment (JMT); and for hypoendemic areas (approximate prevalence of clinically active yaws in the community under 5%) treatment with benzathine benzylpenicillin in all active cases and all household or other obvious contacts. In isolated and remote villages TMT may be appropriate even if the prevalence of active yaws is less than 10% (Perine et al 1984).

Penicillin treatment always carries the risk of serious side effects including fatal anaphylaxis. During the initial mass treatment campaigns, when almost all those treated were receiving penicillin for the first time, risks were very low. Those undertaking such campaigns should be prepared to treat such drug reactions. Alternatives have been suggested (e.g. tetracycline or erythromycin 500 mg orally four times daily for 15 days is probably effective). Children between eight and 15 years of age may be given half doses of either drug, and those under eight years of age only erythromycin in doses appropriate to their body weight. Tetracycline is not recommended in pregnancy (Perine et al 1984).

Adults who may have acquired yaws in childhood may be seen in the clinics of western countries, when the results of serological tests will not differentiate from syphilis; in such cases, treatment appropriate for syphilis is advised.

REFERENCES

Agadzi V K, Aboagye-Atta Y, Nelson J W, Perine P L, Hopkins D R 1983 Resurgence of yaws in Ghana. Lancet ii. 389–390

Anonymous 1978 Peoples of Africa. Pygmies. Marshall Cavendish, London, p 154–157

Castellani A 1905 On the presence of spirochaetes in two cases of ulcerated parangi (yaws). British Medical Journal 2: 1280

Castellani A 1906 On the prevalence of spirochaetes in yaws. In: Russell A E (ed) Selected essays on syphilis and smallpox. New Sydenham Society, London, p 80–83

Chambers H D 1938 Yaws (framboesia tropica). Churchill, London.

Grin E I 1953 Epidemiology and control of endemic syphilis. WHO, Monograph Series No. 11, Geneva

Guthe T, Ridet J, Vorst F, D'Costa J, Grab B 1972 Methods for surveillance of endemic treponematoses and sero-immunological investigations of 'disappearing' disease. Bulletin of the World Health Organization 46: 1–14

Hackett C J 1951 Bone lesions of yaws in Uganda. Blackwell Scientific Publications, Oxford

Hackett C J 1957 An international nomenclature of yaws lesions. World Health Organization, Geneva

Hudson E H 1958 Non-venereal syphilis. Livingstone, Edinburgh

Kerdel-Vegas F 1986 Yaws. In: Rook A, Wilkinson D S, Ebling F J G, Champion R H, Burton J L Textbook of Dermatology, 4th edn. Blackwell, London, vol. 1, p 871–878

Marquez F 1975 Pinta. In: Canizares O (ed) Clinical tropical dermatology. Blackwell, London, p 86

Perine P L, Hopkins D R, Niemel P L A. St John R K, Causse G, Antal G M 1984 Handbook of endemic treponematoses. World Health Organization, Geneva

Schaudinn F, Hoffman E 1906 A preliminary note upon the occurrence of spirochaetes in syphilitic lesions and in papillomata (English translation of 1905 paper) In: Russell A E (ed) Selected essays on syphilis and smallpox. New Sydenham Society, London, p 2–15

Turnbull C M 1963 The forest people. Reprint Society, London

WHO Scientific Group 1970a Multipurpose serological surveys and WHO Serum Reference Banks. WHO Technical Report Series, No 454

WHO Scientific Group 1970b Treponematoses research. WHO Technical Report Series, No 455, p 61

WHO Scientific Group 1982 Endemic treponematoses making a comeback. WHO Chronicle 36(2): 77–78

Widy-Wirski R, D'Costa J, Meheus J 1980 Prévalence du pian chez les pygmées en Centrafique. Annales de la societé Belge de médecine tropicale (Bruxelles) 60: 61–67

14

Gonorrhoea: aetiology and pathogenesis

Gonorrhoea, an infection of the mucosal surfaces of the genito-urinary tract with the bacterium *Neisseria gonorrhoeae*, is mainly transmitted by sexual intercourse. In men the infection is associated with an acute purulent urethritis in approximately 90% of cases, but the organisms may spread also to the epididymis and the prostate. In women the urethra and cervix are infected in 65–75% and 85–90% of cases respectively, and the rectal mucosa in 25–50%. Occasionally (about 10%) infection extends from the cervix to the endometrium and Fallopian tubes. Infection of the fauces may occur in both sexes (5–15%); eye infections are seen rarely in adults. In homosexual men, who act as passive partners in anal intercourse, rectal infections also occur. In a small percentage of untreated cases, systemic spread gives rise to an entity known as disseminated gonococcal infection, characterized clinically by arthritis with or without skin lesions.

The causative organism, *Neisseria gonorrhoeae*, commonly referred to as the gonococcus, derives its generic name from Albert Neisser who described it in 1879. The bacteria are small Gram-negative cocci, kidney-shaped and arranged in pairs (diplococci) with the long axes in parallel and the opposed surfaces slightly concave; the organisms are typically intracellular.

By microscopy it is impossible to differentiate the gonococcus from *N. meningitidis* or from other non-pathogenic or potentially pathogenic neisseriae, or *Branhamella catarrhalis* (synonymous with *Moraxella b. catarrhalis* see Ch. 2, p. 29), commonly found in the upper respiratory tract. *N. meningitidis* and commensal neisseriae can also be found on the mucous surfaces of the genito-urinary tract and anal canal, particularly in women and homosexual men respectively. The differentiation of the gonococcus from other neisseriae and *B. catarrhalis* is discussed in Chapter 15.

The gonococcus is a delicate organism with exacting nutritional and environmental requirements. Media containing blood or serum, a temperature of 36°C to 37°C and a moist atmosphere, enriched with 10% carbon dioxide, must be provided to ensure growth. The organism is liable to die if separated from its host and is also readily killed by drying, soap and water, and many other cleansing or antiseptic agents.

In nature, *N. gonorrhoeae* is a strictly human pathogen although infections have been induced experimentally in the urethra of the chimpanzee (Lucas et al 1971, Brown et al 1972).

TRANSMISSION OF INFECTION

Owing to the poor viability of the gonococcus away from the mucosal surfaces of the host, gonorrhoea is ordinarily acquired by sexual intercourse with an infected person. There are so many variable factors that it is difficult to assess the risk of acquiring an infection from a single exposure. Gonorrhoea is regarded, however, as being of high infectivity, the risk for a female having intercourse with an infected male being higher, 60–90% (Barlow et al 1976, Chipperfield & Catterall 1976, Evans 1976), than that for a male with an infected female, 20–50% (Holmes et al 1970, Hooper et al 1978). The risk of transmission per exposure with an infected partner was 0.19 for white American men and 0.53 for black American men. The higher risk of infection among black Americans may be related to the increased susceptibility to neisserial infection of patients with blood group B (Blackwell et al 1985). On repeated exposure with a single infected partner the majority of men are susceptible to gonococcal infection.

Human volunteer studies associated with vaccine trials in men suggest that inoculum size is important in establishing infection. In challenge studies, increasing the challenge dose from 10^3 to 10^5 piliated gonococcal colony forming units (cfu) overcame the efficacy of a parenteral gonococcal pilus vaccine (Tramont et al 1985). Similar numbers of organisms are readily acquired during sexual intercourse, as the number of gonococci recovered from cervical aspirates ranges from 5×10^3 to 8×10^6 cfu/ml (mean 1.0×10^6 cfu/ml): the corresponding figures for vaginal aspirates are 1.0×10^2 to 1.0×10^6 (mean 8.4×10^4) (Young H et al 1983).

Studies on the inocula required to cause endocervical infection have not been done because of the risk of salpingitis and subsequent infertility. The observation, however, that the first 20–30 ml of urine from infected men contains 4.0×10^3 to 1.0×10^6 cfu/ml (mean 1.1×10^5 cfu/ml) (Young, unpublished observations) gives some idea of the numbers of gonococci likely to be transmitted.

The incubation period in the male tends to be about 3–5 days (range 2–10 days). In the female a precise incubation period is difficult to determine since approximately 70% or more of infections may cause no symptoms. Such asymptomatic infections make it possible for individuals to remain as sources of infection within the community whilst at risk themselves of developing pelvic inflammatory disease or disseminated infection: the risk of developing these sequelae is generally given as 10% and 1% respectively. Patients infected with certain strains of gonococci are at greater risk of developing disseminated infection.

The gonococcus can be transmitted to the pharynx by orogenital contact. Infection is usually without symptoms. During 1985 the prevalence of pharyngeal infection in patients with gonorrhoea in Edinburgh was 9% for heterosexual men, 15% for women, and 28% for homosexual men (Young, unpublished observations). Pharyngeal transfer of gonococci by kissing is a rare occurrence (Tice & Rodriguez 1981). Oral to genital transmission is rare although it has been reported in relation to subsets of prostitutes in South East Asia who specialize in oral sex (Soendjojo 1983).

In males, rectal infection results from anal intercourse. Particular strains of gonococci are associated with rectal infection in men. Colonization of the rectal mucosa in the female is common (25–50%) (Bhattacharyya & Jephcott 1974) and ordinarily results from backward extension of the infection due to contamination by infected vaginal secretions.

Vulvo-vaginitis in young children under the age of puberty is caused more commonly by organisms other than *N. gonorrhoeae*, but such infections can result from accidental contamination of the child with discharge when sleeping with an infected parent. On occasions, it may be the result of a sexual assault, which is often difficult to prove.

During birth, a baby passing through an infected cervix may acquire gonococcal conjunctivitis of the newborn (ophthalmia neonatorum): this condition is uncommon nowadays in this locality due to general improvements in antenatal care and the detection and treatment of gonococcal infection. Gonococcal conjunctivitis in older children and in adults is usually acquired by contact with fingers and/or moist towels contaminated with fresh pus.

PATHOGENESIS

Primary infection commonly occurs in the columnar epithelium of the urethra and para-urethral ducts and glands of both sexes; the greater vestibular glands (Bartholin's); the cervix; the conjunctiva; and the rectum. Primary infection may also occur in the soft stratified squamous epithelium of the vagina of young girls: involvement of this type of epithelium in other parts of the body such as the skin of the glans penis, cornea and mouth is extremely rare.

During acute gonococcal urethritis, by the third day of infection, gonococci have penetrated the mucosal lining of the urethra and have become established in the subepithelial connective tissue (Harkness 1948). The capillaries are dilated, and there is an exudation of cells and serum. Dense cellular infiltrations, consisting of polymorphonuclear leucocytes, plasma cells and mast cells, soon make their appearance beneath the columnar epithelium, being particularly numerous in the region of Littré's glands and ducts. The inflammatory reaction involves the deep tissue of the corpus spongiosum and may extend into the corpora cavernosa. Gonococci are thought to penetrate the intact mucosal surface by invasion through the cells rather than by passing between cell junctions; the intracellular penetration of gonococci into mucosal cells desquamated from the cervix and urethra of infected patients has been demonstrated (Watt et al 1978).

Electronmicroscopy of human Fallopian tubes challenged with gonococci in vitro has suggested the following sequence of events (Watt et al 1978). Gonococci first adhere to non-ciliated columnar epithelial cells of the genital tract, thus allowing the bacteria to become established despite the flow of mucus and other secretions. The ciliated cells are then damaged and slough. This may be due to gonococcal lipopolysaccharide (LPS) as the cell damage can be reproduced by purified gonococcal LPS. Next the gonococci enter the non-ciliated cells: microvilli of the host cell make initial contact with the gonococci which then become engulfed by the cell membrane and lie within a phagocytic vacuole inside the cell. Intracellular multiplication then occurs and very large numbers of gonococci can be present in a cell. Gonococci damage the epithelial cells, resulting in cell lysis with the release of gonococci into the submucosal spaces. This process normally gives rise to the local inflammatory response that is responsible for the typical symptoms of gonorrhoea. Host responses usually localize the infection, but occasionally gonococci evade host defences resulting in disseminated infection.

According to one concept, gonococcal pathogenicity may be based primarily on internal disorganization of human macrophages (Novotny et al 1977). Gonococci in pus appear in specific clusters in which they are surrounded by organelles and granules derived from the host cells in which they multiplied. These clusters are called infectious units because:

1. the cocci multiply within them,
2. the whole complex makes contact with epithelial cells,
3. the cocci in units are not recognized by polymorphs as long as the coating of granules is dense enough, and
4. the cocci are probably protected against humoral defence mechanisms.

Gonococci phagocytosed by polymorphonuclear leucocytes are killed. Those phagocytosed by macrophages, however, interfere with the cells' regulatory processes, survive and form a cluster of multiplying gonococci surrounded by granules and remnants of macrophages, i.e. the infectious units; the host cell remnants are utilized, the gonococci become less and less coated and are re-phagocytosed, and the cycle is repeated. Depending on the nature of the phagocytic cells involved, an abortive infection or a self-cure of gonorrhoea may occur.

GONOCOCCAL SURFACE STRUCTURES AND PATHOGENICITY

The ability to attach to, and subsequently invade, the mucosal surface of the genital tract distinguishes gonococci from non-invasive commensal neisseriae. As the outer membrane of the gonococcal cell envelope interacts with the host mucosal surfaces and with the immune system, gonococcal surface components are important in gonococcal virulence and pathogenicity.

The cell envelope of Gram-negative bacteria including *N. gonorrhoeae* is composed of three macromolecular components, the outer membrane, the cytoplasmic membrane and the rigid peptidoglycan layer. The outer membrane is composed of lipopolysaccharide, phospholipids and proteins. Pili, also called fimbriae, are filamentous protein appendages that extend several μm from the gonococcal cell surface. Although several investigators have concluded that gonococci have a capsule, the putative capsular material has never been isolated and characterized chemically.

Certain of these surface components are discussed in the following sections. For a more detailed discussion of gonococcal virulence and pathogenicity see the reviews by Blake & Gotschlich (1983) and Britigan et al (1985).

Pili

In 1963 Kellogg et al described four distinct colony types of gonococci referred to as T1 to T4. Later an additional colony type (T5) was recognized (Jephcott & Reyn 1971). Bacteria from colony types 1 and 2 are virulent for human volunteers and possess pili, whereas colony types 3 and 4 are essentially avirulent and lack pili (Kellogg et al 1963, Jephcott et al 1971). Freshly isolated strains from clinical specimens are predominantly colony type 1, but on non-selective subculture in the laboratory the avirulent colony types become established.

Attachment

Piliated gonococci attach more successfully than non-piliated variants to a variety of human cells including spermatozoa, erythrocytes, vaginal epithelial cells, Fallopian tube epithelium and buccal cell epithelium (Buchanan 1977). Cells from tissue sites of natural gonococcal infection bind more pili per square micron than cells from sites not usually infected.

Pili promote attachment by non-specific as well as specific interactions; the pilus receptor, however, has not yet been fully characterized. The hydrophobic nature of the pilus protein helps overcome the electrostatic repulsive barrier which exists between the negatively charged surfaces of bacterium and host cell (Heckels et al 1976). Once the bacterium and host cell are more closely aligned, pili can attach to specific receptors on the epithelial cell surface. Other gonococcal outer membrane proteins such as protein II are important in the final adhesion involving direct contact of the gonococcal outer envelope and host cell surfaces.

Structure and function

Pili are made up of a series of apparently identical repeating protein subunits termed pilin proteins, which have molecular weights of 18 000 to 22 000 daltons. Each pilin molecule contains about 175–180 amino acids.

The 53 or so amino acids at the amino terminus of the polypeptide are conserved in all pili from *N. gonorrhoeae*. A semi-variable region extends between amino acids 54 and 114 and contains many different amino acid substitutions depending on the pilin examined. Finally there is a hypervariable region extending from amino acid 115 to the carboxy terminus. This contains deletions as well as insertions of 1–4 amino acids in different pili variants.

The constant region common to all gonococcal pili is only weakly immunogenic. The highly variable amino acid sequences of the carboxy terminal end are immunodominant and account for the antigenic heterogeneity of gonococcal pili: there is approximately 10% shared antigenicity with rabbit antisera and 50% shared antigenicity with human sera (Brinton et al 1978, Buchanan 1978). Both the conserved and variable regions are involved in binding to cell receptors (Schoolnik et al 1982, Virji & Heckels 1983).

There is an epithelium and erythrocyte binding domain in the conserved region. A region spanning the conserved and variable domains has been shown to bind to cervical cells but not to HeLa or buccal epithelial cells. The variable domain, apart from conferring antigenic specificity, may also have specific cell-binding functions. Pili are associated with virulence properties other than adhesion. In comparison to non-piliated variants, piliated gonococci are more resistant to phagocytosis, bind iron more avidly and are more efficient in the uptake of transforming DNA.

Phase and antigenic variation

In pilus phase variation, pilin genes are reversibly switched on (to produce piliated or P^+ cells) at a high rate.

Antigenic variation involves the generation of biochemical and antigenic diversity in pilus type and results from the expression of alternative pilin genes. These two processes are probably closely linked, as the transition between P^+ and P^- is accompanied by genome rearrangements; P^- derivatives that switch back to P^+ frequently express pili that are antigenically distinct from those produced by the initial P^+ strain (Hagblom et al 1985, Segal et al 1985).

Frequent changes in the antigenic structure of pili may assist in avoiding host immune responses. Gonococcal isolates from the urethra of men and from the cervix and urethra of their female partners often differ in pilus type (Zak et al, 1984). Variations in pili may also be associated with differential attachment to, and virulence for, host cells suggesting that one role of antigenic variation is to allow sequential adhesion to different cell types during natural infection (Virji and Heckels, 1984).

The genetic control of phase variation (P^+ to P^- to P^+ etc.) and antigenic variation is complex but can be explained by chromosomal rearrangements that result from intragenic recombination between a repertoire of casettes of different pilin genes (Hagblom et al, 1985; Segal et al, 1985).

Outer membrane proteins

There are three major clones of protein in the outer membrane of *N. gonorrhoeae* and they account for over 60% of the total protein of the membrane. The three proteins are termed protein I, protein II and protein III (Johnston & Gotschlich 1974).

Protein I

Protein I has previously been called by a variety of names, such as principal outer membrane protein

(POMP) and major outer membrane protein (MOMP). Protein I accounts for 50–60% of the total membrane protein and has a subunit molecular weight which ranges from 32 000 to 39 000 daltons. Protein I is always present in the same subunit molecular weight in any one strain.

Protein I can be subdivided into two subgroups termed IA and IB. The protein IA subgroup contains the protein I molecules with a lower molecular weight, whereas the IB subgroup contains those protein I molecules with a higher molecular weight. These can be considered mutually exclusive forms of protein I, an individual strain possessing either protein IA or IB. Differences in protein I form the basis of a serogrouping and a serotyping system.

Protein I is primarily a protein which forms channels or pores in the outer membrane through which hydrophilic molecules and ions can enter the cell (Douglas et al 1981). Three protein I molecules may be complexed with a protein III molecule to form the pore. JDE Young et al (1983) estimated the diameter of the pore was 11 Å. Pores formed by proteins IA and IB may have different sizes (Blake, personal communication, cited by Barrera & Swanson 1984).

Interactions between protein I and the host cell membrane may be important in gonococcal pathogenesis. Protein I on whole gonococci can insert into artificial lipid bilayers and into the membranes of red blood cells. It is possible that the insertion of gonococcal protein I into epithelial cell membranes may alter the membrane potential of the epithelial cells and possibly trigger phagocytosis and internalization of gonococci (Blake & Gotschlich 1983). Protein IA molecules are more efficient at inserting into lipid bilayers than protein IB molecules. This is of interest as gonococcal strains with protein IA cause disseminated infection much more frequently than do gonococci with protein IB (Cannon et al 1983). Protein I also interacts with natural IgG and complement in the bactericidal reaction observed with normal serum.

Protein II

The molecular weight of protein II molecules ranges from 24 000 to 30 000 daltons (Swanson 1980). There are a number of different protein II species, and gonococcal strains may express one or more of these, depending on growth conditions and the anatomical site from which the organism was isolated. Protein II has also been referred to as heat modifiable protein (protein II changes its molecular weight on boiling), leucocyte association protein and opacity associated protein. Opaque and transparent colonies of gonococci can be differentiated on translucent media: gonococci from opaque colonies invariably have one or more protein II, whereas gonococci from transparent colonies are generally considered to lack protein II, or if they do have protein II it is of a different molecular weight from that found in opaque colonies. Gonococcal isogenic opacity variants of a single strain have been shown to contain protein IIs of different molecular weights (Lambden et al 1979): these proteins have been termed IIa–f.

Function The major function of protein II is in the attachment of gonococci to each other and to surface receptors on various cell types. Greater numbers of gonococci from opaque colonies attach to eukaryotic cells than do gonococci from transparent colonies (James et al 1983). Lambden et al (1979) found that all strains which produced extra protein IIs showed decreased binding to erythrocytes, compared with the parent strain not producing protein II. Strains producing protein IIa showed increased association with polymorphonuclear leucocytes (PMNs) whereas another variant producing protein IIb showed decreased association with PMNs. Protein IIa, which has a molecular weight of 28 500 daltons, is probably the same as the previously reported leucocyte association factor with a molecular weight of 28×10^3 to 29×10^3 daltons (Swanson & King 1978).

Protein II has conserved and variable domains, with the variation occurring on the surface exposed part of the molecule (Heckels 1981, Judd 1985). Changes in non-exposed parts of the molecule, however, might cause conformational changes in the protein II, resulting in new domains being exposed on the surface.

Variations in expression of protein II almost certainly occur in vivo since different types have been reported from different sites of infection in male and female sex partners (Zak et al 1984). Gonococci that form opaque colonies tend to be isolated from patients with symptomatic genital infections, but are rarely associated with invasive disease. Gonococci forming transparent colonies predominate in the cervix at the time of menstruation, and are usually isolated from men with asymptomatic genital infections who are also consorts of women with salpingitis or disseminated infection. The proportions of transparent and opaque colonies vary in apparent association with environmental change associated with the menstrual cycle (James & Swanson 1978).

As in pilus expression, the ability of the gonococcus to alter protein II expression rapidly may allow the bacteria to adapt efficiently to particular microenvironments.

Protein III
Protein III (molecular weight 30×10^3 to 31×10^3 daltons) is a species-specific protein and is virtually identical in all strains of gonococci examined. The majority of protein III is buried deeply within the membrane (Blake & Gotschlich 1983). Surface labelling and monoclonal antibody studies, however, have shown that the same portion of the protein III molecule is exposed at the surface in all gonococcal strains examined (Judd 1982, Swanson et al 1982).

Lipopolysaccharide (LPS)
LPS is composed of three parts: the 'O' or somatic antigen (a polysaccharide chain which contains a series of monosaccharides); the reducing end of the O-somatic antigen is linked to a core oligosaccharide composed of different monosaccharides such as heptose, glucose, mannose, glucosamine, and an eight carbon sugar acid, 3-deoxy-D-manno-octulosonic acid (KDO); and lipid A which is bound to the core, usually by the KDO residue. LPS which is composed of all three components is called smooth LPS (S-LPS). LPS lacking the O-antigen is termed rough LPS (R-LPS). Most gonococci growing under normal conditions produce LPS which is largely, if not entirely, of the R-type. Chemical analysis has produced conflicting evidence for and against the presence of O antigens and about the detailed composition of gonococcal LPS (Perry et al 1975, Stead et al 1975, Wiseman & Caird 1977).

LPS is found on the outermost part of the Gram-negative outer membrane and can be lost spontaneously. In the neisseriae the loss of LPS has been visualized as a process of outer membrane 'blebbing'. Studies on human Fallopian tube organ cultures challenged with gonococci suggest that while bacteria bind to non-ciliated columnar epithelium cells the released LPS is responsible for the sloughing off and death of ciliated epithelial cells (Melly et al 1981). Although the contribution of LPS to virulence in the natural infection is unclear, anti-LPS antibodies are protective in a number of animal models. Antibodies directed against LPS are bactericidal for the gonococcus. The bactericidal activity of normal human serum is largely due to the presence of antibodies cross-reactive with LPS. Serum resistance of gonococci associated with disseminated infection may be due, in part, to lack of an LPS determinant (Schneider et al 1982, Winstanley et al 1983).

IgA protease
IgA protease has been found in *N. gonorrhoeae*, *N. meningitidis*, *Haemophilus influenzae* and certain oral streptococci (Kornfield & Plaut 1981). It splits antibodies of the IgA_1 subclass of IgA at specific amino acid sites in the hinge region of the molecule. Once split, the IgA loses its antibody activity. The role of IgA protease in gonococcal pathogenesis is not clear. Although the enzyme presumably inactivates secretory IgA_1 on the mucosal surface, antibody of the IgA_2 subclass is unaffected.

HOST RESPONSE

Invasion of the genital tract mucosal surfaces early in infection brings the gonococcus into contact with plasma. IgG and complement components are also found in cervical secretions, and may contribute a primary defence system. Activation of the early components of complement aids opsonization of bacteria, while the sequential action of the terminal components results in the formation of the membrane attack system C5b-9 which will kill bacteria. Complement can be activated by the classical pathway (including antibody antigen complexes and Cl, C4 and C2) and/or by the alternate pathway. The alternate pathway misses out the C1, C4 and C2 components and starts at the C3 step. The mechanism of activation does not depend upon the same part of the immunoglobulin molecule as the classical pathway and can be activated by aggregated immunoglobulins and various polysaccharides, including bacterial endotoxin.

The acute inflammatory response induced in localized gonococcal infection is in part mediated by the interaction of invading gonococci with natural antibody and complement (Watt & Medlen 1978). These interactions generate chematoxins which attract phagocytes to the site of infection.

OPSONIZATION, PHAGOCYTOSIS AND KILLING

Examination of urethral exudates suggests that antibody-complement-mediated opsonization and PMN phagocytosis with intracellular killing of the gonococci is important in the host's defence against gonococcal infection.

The opsonization, phagocytosis and subsequent killing systems are not as important in protection from disseminated gonococcal (and meningococcal) infections as is the antibody-complement-mediated bactericidal system.

The role of complement in serum bactericidal activity has been shown to be important in preventing systemic neisserial infections (Lim et al 1976, Peterson et al 1976, Lee et al 1978). Patients with hereditary deficiencies in the complement system, resulting in the lack of the terminal components C6, C7 and C8, are susceptible to repeated attacks of bacteraemic neisserial infections. These patients have normal opsonization and PMN chemotaxis but lack serum bactericidal function produced by the terminal complement membrane attack complex (Lee et al 1978).

Individuals with normal antibody and complement systems do not become bacteraemic with serum-sensitive gonococci because of the antibody-complement-mediated killing of the bacteria. Gonococci from patients with disseminated gonococcal infection are commonly resistant to the bactericidal action of antibody and complement (Brooks et al 1976, Schoolnik et al 1976). A natural antibody may block receptors for bactericidal antibody on the gonococcal surface, thus protecting gonococci from killing.

NATURAL ANTIBODY AND IMMUNE RESPONSES

Natural gonococcal bactericidal antibody is present in the serum of most normal adults and arises without obvious immunization or specific infection (Schoolnik et al 1976). These antibodies may arise due to pharyngeal carriage of non-gonococcal neisseriae. Natural antibody of IgG, IgM and IgA classes were detected by an indirect immunofluorescence test (Cohen 1967).

Natural IgM

Natural IgM in conjunction with complement is responsible for the bactericidal activity of normal human serum (NHS) (Schoolnik et al 1979). The development of natural antibody is age-dependent, attaining adult levels at approximately two years of age. Rice & Kasper (1977) showed that the bactericidal activity of NHS could be inhibited by gonococcal endotoxin but not by gonococcal protein. This is in keeping with the suggestion that natural IgM reacts with LPS (Schoolnik et al 1979).

Natural IgG

McCutchan et al (1978) examined the mechanisms by which N. gonorrhoeae isolated from cases of DGI resisted the bactericidal activity of normal human serum (NHS). They concluded that natural IgG-blocking antibody binds to gonococci possessing the appropriate receptor and protects them from killing by bactericidal antibody and complement by preventing bactericidal antibody binding to the gonococcal cells.

Mechanisms by which different gonococci resist the bactericidal activity may be different and depend upon the type of LPS they produce (Shafer et al 1984): there may be differences in the conformation of LPS or an increase in the number of receptor sites made available to blocking IgG. This may result in a greater degree of IgG-blocking antibody binding to serum resistant strains, inhibiting the binding of natural IgM by steric hindrance. It has also been proposed that serum resistance may be due to conformational changes in LPS, rendering the complement membrane attack complex C5b-9 ineffectual (Harriman et al 1982). Although the C5b-9 complex bound to the surface of both serum-sensitive and serum-resistant gonococci it was unable to penetrate the membrane and kill serum resistant gonococci.

IgG-blocking antibodies in NHS may be effective against convalescent bactericidal antibody as well as against the natural IgM responsible for the bactericidal activity of NHS. Recent evidence suggests that protein III is a major antigenic determinant for these IgG-blocking antibodies (Rice et al 1985). IgG-blocking antibody was purified by affinity chromatography using a mixture of gonococcal outer membrane proteins free from LPS contamination. The immuno-adsorbed IgG showed a 40-fold increased blocking activity per mg of IgG compared with unabsorbed IgG in assays using a disseminated gonococcal infection strain and convalescent bactericidal antibody. Using an ELISA test, the purified IgG-blocking antibody showed a 57-fold increase in titre against protein III.

The intimate relationship of protein III with protein I, which in turn appears to be tightly bound to LPS, suggests that binding sites for bactericidal and blocking antibodies are located in close proximity of the outer membrane.

Natural IgG can also function as a heat-stable opsonin promoting phagocytosis of gonococci by human PMNs. In this way it may constitute a part of the host's early defence mechanisms prior to the development of a specific antibody response. Studies with monoclonal antibodies suggest that the natural IgG in NHS acting as an opsonin attaches to protein I (Sarafian et al 1983).

Humoral antibody response

Serum antibody to gonococci can be detected within a few days of infection but such antibodies are not protective with regard to mucosal reinfection.

Following gonococcal infection, the majority of patients develop increased levels of serum IgG, IgM and IgA reactive with the gonococcus.

The serum IgA is secretory, implying absorption from the mucosal surface (Glynn & Ison 1978). Humoral antibody responses may vary in different gonococcal syndromes and the antibodies produced detect different gonococcal antigens. Infected patients develop increased IgG and IgM against gonococcal LPS. These antibodies are important in the antibody-complement-mediated bactericidal action of serum and may be protective against bacteraemia caused by serum sensitive strains. Pili and protein II are important surface antigens in the serum IgG and IgA response. Antigenic variation mitigates against effective immunity resulting from antibody responses to these surface antigens.

Although infected patients and immunized volunteers make antibody against protein I, this antigen is not very immunogenic for humans in terms of the serum antibody response (Buchanan et al 1982). Nevertheless, antibody against protein I can be protective against the recurrence of complicated gonococcal infection. Women with pelvic inflammatory disease (PID) who produced an antibody response to protein I were protected from subsequent attacks of PID with gonococci of the same protein I serotype. These antibodies were, however, unable to protect women from repeated local genital infection by strains with homologous protein I serotype (Buchanan et al 1980).

Mucosal antibody response

Using whole cell gonococcal antigen in an immuno fluorescence test, anti-gonococcal antibody could be demonstrated in cervical exudate from 97% of women with gonorrhoea (McMillan et al 1979b). The antibodies were predominantly of the IgG and IgA class. IgM was detected in approximately 40% of women and was associated with infections of less than 15 days duration. IgA appeared to be mainly secretory IgA. Similar findings were reported for men with gonococcal urethritis (McMillan et al 1979a). Of 132 men with gonorrhoea, 129 had antibodies to the gonococcus in their urethral secretions. IgA was found in all 129, IgG in 119 and IgM in 64. Successful treatment resulted in the rapid decline of IgA and more gradual decline of IgG.

Tramont et al (1980) reported antibodies in vaginal secretions were reactive with pili, outer membrane complexes and LPS. Vaginal secretions from infected patients inhibited attachment of the infecting strain of gonococcus to epithelial cells (Tramont 1977). A pilus vaccine also induced antibodies capable of inhibiting the pilus-mediated attachment of the strain of N. gonorrhoeae used to make the vaccine (McChesney et al 1982). The finding of anti-gonococcal IgA and IgG in the secretions of 12 women who had no evidence of gonococcal infection but who were contacts of men with gonorrhoea (McMillan et al 1979b) suggests that a mucosal antibody response may be involved in limiting or eradicating infection in some individuals. The significance of gonococcal IgA protease in relation to gonococcal-IgA interactions at the mucosal surface is not known.

Cell-mediated immunity

There is little evidence that cell-mediated immunity is important in protection from infection. A wide range in degree of lymphocyte response in both men and women has been noted. Cell-mediated responses are found more frequently in patients with a history of multiple infections, with greater blastogenic transformation in those with three or more gonococcal infections. Cell-mediated immunity in gonococcal infection has been reviewed by Watson (1978).

Non-specific immunity

A degree of non-specific immunity to gonococcal infection probably exists, since not everyone exposed to an infection acquires the disease. The effectors of this immunity are poorly understood but are likely to include urine pH, osmolarity and urea concentration as well as the influence of hormones and genital pH in women (Braude 1982). Certain components of the normal endocervical flora are antagonistic towards gonococci and prevent the establishment of gonococcal infection (Saigh et al 1978).

In spite of non-specific defence mechanisms and the ability to mount an antibody response, the vast majority of individuals who are exposed to the gonococcus become infected. From the number of patients with well-documented, repeated infections, it is obvious that immunity to the gonococcus sufficient to be protective does not result from an earlier infection. Failure to develop effective immunity is probably not due to the rapid elimination of infection with antibiotics, since repeated infections were common before these were available. Many infections in female patients are also asymptomatic for a long time.

The host response is directed against a bewildering array of gonococcal antigens and varies from patient to patient. The gonococcus in turn appears to have a formidable battery of virulence determinants which enable it to evade the host immune response, and is thus a very successful host specific pathogen. The variable immune response, lack of protection against reinfection and the very large numbers of gonococcal antigens make the selection of antigen(s) for a gonococcal vaccine to prevent mucosal infection very difficult. In the infectious unit, too, the cocci are probably protected against humoral defence mechanisms, and phagocytic cells will not recognize the cocci as long as the coating of granules is sufficiently dense. The protection from complicated infection observed when patients are reinfected with the same protein I serotype lends more optimism to the development of vaccines to prevent complicated infection.

EPIDEMIOLOGY

Since man is the only natural host for *N. gonorrhoeae*, the epidemiological factors that are important in gonococcal infection relate to human behavioural factors as well as to properties of the organism. Behavioural factors have been dealt with in Chapter 1, whilst data on gonococcal epidemiology in relation to the epidemiology of sexually transmitted diseases can be found in Chapter 5. The remainder of this section is concerned with properties of the organism and will deal with the epidemiology of antibiotic resistance, epidemiological markers, and the application of gonococcal typing methods.

Gonorrhoea is common in developed as well as devel-

oping countries. On a global scale there are in the region of 200 million cases per year. Differences and inadequacies in reporting systems make absolute comparisons of data between countries difficult. Nevertheless the data do give a reasonable guide as to trends.

In many countries, including the United Kingdom and the United States, the sharp increase in the incidence of gonorrhoea noted in the 1960s and mid-1970s stabilized and decreased slightly during the late 1970s and early 1980s. For some areas, including Edinburgh, there has been a marked decrease in the incidence of homosexually acquired gonorrhoea, most probably resulting from concern over AIDS.

In the United Kingdom statistics for Scotland are recorded separately from those of England and Wales. In Scotland, 5528 (106.39 per 100 000 population and a male:female ratio of 1.7 : 1) new cases of gonorrhoea were reported in 1977. In 1979, although the male:female ratio remained the same the number of new cases had decreased to 4938, a rate of 95.96 per 100 000 population (Communicable Diseases Scotland, Summary of Sexually Transmitted Diseases 1972–79). In England there were 55 156 cases of gonorrhoea reported in 1982 giving an incidence rate of 111.39 per 100 000 population and a male:female ratio of 1.7 : 1 (Extract from the report of the Chief Medical Officer 1985).

In the United States in 1981 a total of 990 864 cases were reported (435 per 100 000 population): 92% of cases occurred in those under 35. The male:female ratio decreased from 2.4 : 1 in 1960 to 1.4 : 1 in 1981 (US Department of Health and Human Services 1982). The decrease in the male:female ratio is due in part to Public Health Service programmes of more culture screening to detect infected women who are often without symptoms. As it has been estimated that the cost of pelvic inflammatory disease in the United States is 700 million dollars per year, there is a strong economic incentive to control gonorrhoea (US Department of Health and Human Services 1981).

The incidence of gonorrhoea in developing countries in Asia, Africa, Central and South America is not known because of inadequacies in the reporting systems. The World Health Organization considers that gonorrhoea is a major cause for the high prevalence of infertility in parts of Africa (World Health Organization Scientific Group 1978). Insofar as the data from the few studies carried out in those regions represent the true picture, the incidence is very high. For example, in Nairobi 17.5% of women attending a family planning clinic had gonorrhoea (Hopcraft et al 1973); in rural Uganda gonorrhoea was found in 9% of men and 18% of women randomly selected for testing (Arya et al 1973); and in Salisbury, Zimbabwe, 35% of men and 23% of women attending an STD clinic were infected (Latif 1981).

Prostitution probably plays an important part in the spread of infection in developing countries. According to the World Health Organization prostitution is relatively unimportant in the transmission of disease in developed countries (World Health Organization Scientific Group 1978).

EPIDEMIOLOGY OF ANTIBIOTIC RESISTANCE

Antibiotic resistance in the gonococcus results from mutations in chromosomal genes and/or from plasmid mediated β-lactamase production.

Chromosomally mediated resistance

Fully sensitive wild strains of gonococci have penicillin minimum inhibitory concentrations (MICs) of less than 0.06 mg/l. Mutations at a series of loci on the chromosome result in small additive increases in penicillin resistance, resulting in isolates with penicillin MICs of 1 mg/l or greater, levels at which currently recommended doses of penicillin become ineffective. These levels of resistance are over 100 times greater than those which prevailed when penicillin therapy was introduced in the 1960s.

The main genetic loci involved in chromosomal resistance are *pen*A, *pen*B and *mtr* (Sarubbi et al 1974, Sparling et al 1975). Mutation at the *pen* A locus results in an eight-fold increase in resistance to penicillin alone. Mutation at the *mtr* locus results in a two- to four-fold increase in resistance to penicillin and to other antibiotics, dyes and detergents. Mutation at a locus termed *pen* B_2 results in a four-fold increase in resistance to penicillin and tetracycline: *pen* B_2 is only expressed phenotypically when a mutation at *mtr* is present within the same cell. For the laboratory the accumulative effect of these three mutations is a 128-fold increase in penicillin resistance, a situation similar to that observed with clinical isolates over the last 40 years. As these mutations exert their effect by altering the permeability of the gonococcal cell envelope, isolates with clinically significant levels of resistance to penicillin are likely to be relatively resistant to a range of antibiotics such as erythromycin, tetracycline and chloramphenicol. Resistance to tetracycline and chloramphenicol is controlled by specific loci (*tet* and *cam*) as well as the non-specific loci *pen* B and *mtr*.

There is considerable geographical variation in the proportion of strains showing significant levels (MIC $\geq$ 0.5 mg/l) of resistance to penicillin. Strains from countries in South East Asia tend to be most resistant. In Singapore 64% of strains have MICs of $\geq$ 0.5 mg/l, resulting from chromosomally mediated resistance (Sng et al 1984). Similar levels of resistance are common in parts of Africa (Sparling 1977). Presumably the lack of antibiotic control in these areas leads to indiscriminate prophylactic use, and treatment with suboptimal dosages of penicillin and contributes to the selection of resistant strains. In this context, it is of interest that the first strains of gonococci totally resistant to penicillin, due to the production of a plasmid-coded β-lactamase, were linked epidemiologically with South East Asia and West Africa.

With the speed and extent of modern travel there is a continual influx of resistant strains. Whether such strains persist and become endemic amongst the indigenous gonococcal population depends on the ability of such strains to survive and compete successfully. If drug resistance has an adverse effect on virulence, such strains will be unsuccessful in surviving.

There is another set of gonococcal mutations termed *env*. Strains carrying these mutations are much more sensitive (hypersensitive) to antibiotics, dyes and detergents (Maness & Sparling 1973, Sarubbi et al 1975).

The *env* mutation suppresses the phenotypic expression of the *mtr* mutation if the two occur within the same strain (Sarubbi et al 1975). The phenotypic expression of the *env* mutation is an alteration in the cell envelope so that it becomes more permeable to inhibitory substances. As *env* mutations are selected and maintained it has been speculated that the increased membrane permeability aids uptake of nutrients and gives a growth advantage in vivo: in contrast *mtr* mutations decrease permeability and may limit uptake of nutrients. Gonococcal strains carrying the *env* mutation account for 15% of clinical isolates in North Carolina (Eisenstein & Sparling 1978). These strains help to offset the effects of stable chromosomal antibiotic-resistance mutations.

Plasmid-mediated penicillin resistance

Plasmids are small circular pieces of DNA that can replicate within a bacterial cell independent of the chromosome. Gonococci totally resistant to penicillin due to a plasmid coding for a β-lactamase (penicillinase) enzyme were first reported in 1976 (Ashford et al 1976, Phillips 1976). Before considering the advent of what would appear to be exogenously acquired penicillin resistance in 1976, it is worth considering the naturally occurring or endogenous plasmids of gonococci (Riou & Courvalin 1985).

Endogenous gonococcal plasmids

The following plasmids are considered endogenous because their GC ratio of 0.5 (the ratio of the nucleotide bases guanine + cytosine to guanine + cytosine + adenine + thymine) is indistinguishable from that of the chromosomal DNA of the gonococcus.

2.6 Mdalton (Mdal) plasmid. This was the first plasmid discovered in the gonococcus. It occurs in almost all gonococcal strains and there are usually 24–32 copies per cell (Mayer et al 1974). No phenotypic character has been attributed to this plasmid and it is therefore termed 'cryptic'. This plasmid has been used in the non-cultural detection of gonorrhoea. Particular strains of gonococci lacking this plasmid may cause a diagnostic problem in certain geographical areas.

7.8 Mdalton plasmid. This plasmid, which was described by Johnson et al (1983), also appears to be cryptic. Restriction enzyme analysis suggests that it is a trimer of the 2–6 Mdal plasmid.

24.5 Mdalton plasmid. This plasmid co-exists with the 2.6 Mdal plasmid but is not found in all strains (Stiffler et al 1975). It has conjugative properties and is able to mobilize other plasmids such as resistance (R) plasmids between gonococci (Roberts & Falkow 1979). The 24.5 Mdal plasmid occurs in about 7–8% of gonococcal strains, although it may be as high as 40% in strains originating in South East Asia.

Tetracycline resistant strains of *N. gonorrhoeae* (TRNG) were recognised recently in the United States (Morse et al, 1986). These isolates are highly resistant due to the insertion of the resistance determinant *tetM*, initially found in the genus *Streptococcus* into the 24.5 Mdal plasmid. This results in a plasmid of 25.2 Mdal.

Exogenous gonococcal plasmids
Penicillinase-producing *Neisseria gonorrhoeae* (PPNG) were reported simultaneously in the United Kingdom (Phillips 1976) and the United States (Ashford et al 1976); the respective isolates were linked epidemiologically with West Africa and South East Asia. The production of β-lactamase was shown to be due to the presence of a 3.2 Mdal plasmid in strains from Africa and Europe and a 4.4 Mdal plasmid in strains from Asia and the United States. The 24.5 Mdal plasmid,

although absent from the original PPNG isolates, was shown to be present in up to 40% of the 'Asian' strains carrying the 4.4 Mdal plasmid. PPNG spread rapidly throughout the world (Table 14.1): strains from South East Asia tended to include other parts of Asia and the American continent while the African strains predominated in Europe. Within a few years the 24.5 Mdal plasmid was found in strains carrying the 3.2 Mdal plasmid (Ansink-Schipper et al 1982, Johnston & Kolator 1982). As a result the terms 'African' and 'Asian' can only be used to describe the plasmid type and not the geographical origin of the isolate.

An apparently new plasmid of 2.9 Mdal was described by van Embden et al (1985). This plasmid, which also codes for β-lactamase production, appears to be closely related to the other β-lactamase-producing plasmids. The 3.2 and 2.9 Mdal plasmids are identical to parts of the 4.4 Mdal plasmid with deletions of between 2.0 and 2.5 kilo bases in the smaller plasmids.

Irrespective of the plasmid size, the β-lactamase enzyme produced is identical and of the TEM-1 type. It has been shown by DNA homology studies that strains containing either the 4.4 or 3.2 Mdal plasmid contain approximately 40% of the transposable DNA sequence TnA. This sequence contains the gene Tn2 encoding for TEM β-lactamase production (Elwell et al 1977). The TnA sequence is commonly found in the R plasmids of enteric bacteria such as *E. coli*, and the TEM-1 enzyme often found in these bacteria is identical to the enzyme of *Haemophilus influenzae* and *H. ducreyi* (Heffron et al 1975, 1979).

These observations suggest a common origin for the resistance (R) plasmids in the gonococcus and *Haemophilus spp*. Plasmid-mediated resistance in *H. influenzae* and *H. parainfluenzae* appeared in 1974 (Khan et al 1974) before that in *N. gonorrhoeae*. If the gonococcal R plasmids had arisen as a result of a transposition of TnA to an indigenous gonococcal plasmid, it would have been expected that the R plasmids would have had a GC ratio of 0.5 similar to the chromosome. The gonococcal R plasmids, however, show a much lower

Table 14.1 Geographical areas reporting β-lactamase-producing *Neisseria gonorrhoeae* by May 1981 (Centers for Disease Control 1982).

Africa	East Asia	South East Asia	Europe	Americas
Morocco	Philippines	Indonesia	France	Canada
Ghana	Hong Kong	Singapore	Belgium	United States
Mali	Taiwan	Malaysia	Netherlands	Mexico
Nigeria	Guam	Thailand	United Kingdom	Panama
Central African Republic	Japan	India	West Germany	Argentina
Gabon	Republic of Korea	Sri Lanka	Denmark	Colombia
Zaire	New Zealand		Poland	
Madagascar	New Hebrides		Switzerland	
Zambia	Australia		Sweden	
Senegal			Norway	
			Finland	

GC ratio, in the range 0.4 to 0.41. It is open to speculation whether or not gonococci and *Haemophilus spp* acquired their R plasmids coincidentally from another species, for example one of the Gram-negative enteric bacteria. Alternatively, *Haemophilus spp* could have acted as an intermediary in the spread of the R plasmid to the gonococcus.

The worldwide occurrence of PPNG is evident from Table 14.1. Although the first infections with PPNG strains in the United Kingdom were acquired overseas, PPNG soon became endemic, albeit at a low level. The incidence of PPNG increased exponentially between 1977 and 1982. In 1977 there were 15 reported cases of PPNG, compared with 443 in 1981. Between 1978 and 1980, 62–68% of the isolates were acquired abroad and 20–26% were acquired within the United Kingdom (McCutchan et al 1982).

In St Mary's Hospital, London, where a significant proportion of PPNG seen in the United Kingdom are isolated, the prevalence of PPNG infection rose from less than 1% in 1980 to 6.5% in 1982. In 1983 there was a further increase to 8.7%, but this was a far smaller rise than in the previous two years. In 1984 the prevalence of PPNG decreased to 6.5% (Easmon 1985).

A similar trend was seen in Edinburgh where the prevalence of PPNG increased from 0.1% in 1977 to 1.7% in 1984, but decreased to 1.1% during 1985.

The prevalence of PPNG infections also fell in the United States during 1983, suggesting that the phenomenon is not a local one.

Early diagnosis, effective therapy and intensive contact-tracing have undoubtedly contributed to the decrease in PPNG infections. It may also be, however, that in the absence of selective pressure, such as that provided by uncontrolled penicillin usage, PPNG isolates may have a diminished capacity to compete with non-PPNG.

EPIDEMIOLOGICAL MARKERS (TYPING OF GONOCOCCI)

Typing of gonococci is important in epidemiological studies. The ability to divide the gonococcus into groups and subgroups allows the variety of organism types to be determined, as well as their distribution and prevalence in specific geographical areas. The main methods of typing are outlined before discussing their application in epidemiological studies.

Auxotyping

Auxotyping was developed in 1973 by Catlin (Carifo & Catlin 1973, Catlin 1973). It is based upon the nutritional profile of gonococcal isolates growing on chemically defined media containing amino acids, nucleic acid

bases and certain vitamins. By the exclusion of single or multiple components, such media can be used for the so-called auxotyping of gonococci. 35 auxotypes have been identified (Catlin 1977). These range from gonococci that are prototrophic (Proto) or wild type and are thus able to grow on media lacking one or more nutrients, to those strains which require the addition of up to six nutrients.

Auxotypes are most often distinguished according to the requirement of the tested strains for proline (Pro-), arginine (Arg-), hypoxanthine (Hyx-), uracil (Ura-) and methionine (Met-). Strains that require arginine can be subdivided by testing with media lacking arginine but containing one or other of the arginine precursors ornithine and citrulline. The auxotype of a strain is stable during subculture.

Although auxotyping has provided valuable information about *N. gonorrhoeae*, it is a laborious and expensive method. Its use has been largely restricted to reference laboratories and specialised research centres. For a more detailed discussion of auxotyping see Knapp (1985).

Serogrouping and serotyping

The only serological classification scheme which is simple enough for routine use is the coagglutination (CoA) system described by Sandstrom & Danielsson (1980). The CoA system is based upon the attachment of anti-gonococcal IgG, by its Fc portion, to protein A on whole killed cells of *Staphylococcus aureus*. The addition of gonococci which have determinants that react with the antibody binding site on the specific IgG attached to the staphylococci results in agglutination which is visible to the naked eye. The method is used in the identification of cultured gonococci (Ch. 15).

The development of the CoA serogrouping system stems from the work of Johnston et al (1976) who, using immunoprecipitation of the purified outer membrane, recognized 16 serotypes of gonococci on the basis of differences in the molecular weight of protein I (then termed major outer membrane protein or MOMP) and a covariant minor protein. Strains representative of these various serotypes have become known as the MOMP reference strains. By careful selection of MOMP reference strains for immunization and absorption, Sandstrom & Danielsson (1980) produced a panel of CoA reagents which allowed gonococci to be classified into three serogroups, WI, WII and WIII. Serogrouping of clinical isolates can be performed in a few minutes by testing a boiled suspension of cells of the test strain with the appropriate CoA reagents. Reactions with CoA reagents are stable and reproducible and are not altered by changes in colonial morphology or on subculture.

Unfortunately, subdivision within serogroups WI, WII and WIII was not possible with polyclonal antibody reagents. This problem was overcome as a result of the following detailed serological analysis which provided the background to the successful development of a serotyping system based on monoclonal antibodies.

Buchanan and Hildebrandt (1981), using purified protein I in an ELISA inhibition assay, demonstrated that there were nine different protein I serotypes within the 16 serotypes described by Johnston et al (1976). Strains of CoA serogroup WI corresponded to protein I serotypes 1, 2 and 3; CoA serogroups WII strains usually corresponded to serotypes 4, 5, 6, while WIII strains corresponded to serotype 9. Some of the WII and WIII strains gave reactions representative of both serotypes 8 and 9 and were termed WII/III strains (Sandstrom et al 1982b). Strains belonging to the WI serogroup possessed the type of protein I molecules designated IA, whereas strains belonging to serogroup WII or WIII possessed a distinctly different protein I designated protein IB (Sandstrom et al 1982a).

Two commercial groups have produced monoclonal antibodies specific for epitopes (antigen sites) on protein IA and protein IB: CoA reagents prepared with these monoclonal antibodies tend to give stronger reactions than reagents prepared with absorbed polyclonal antisera (Bygdeman 1987). Separate panels of monoclonal antibodies have been developed by the two groups, and these are termed GS-antibodies (Genetic Systems Corporation, Seattle) and Ph-antibodies (Pharmacia, Uppsala, Sweden).

On the basis of the pattern of reaction of a gonococcal strain to the panel of reagents, particular serovars (serovariants) can be recognized. Using CoA reagents prepared with monoclonal antibodies against protein IA, 21 different serovars within serogroup WI could be recognized with a panel of nine GS-antibodies, compared with 12 WI serovars recognized with a panel of five Ph-antibodies. Using reagents prepared with monoclonals against protein IB, 62 WII serovars could be defined with a panel of nine GS-antibodies, compared with 38 WII serovars with a panel of nine Ph-antibodies. By combining the two sets of antibodies, a total of 27 WI serovars and 93 WII/III serovars could be recognized (Sandstrom et al 1985).

Unfortunately, two different systems of serovar nomenclature have been proposed (Knapp et al 1985). Both systems of nomenclature use the prefix IA or IB to denote whether a strain possesses protein IA or IB as determined by the reaction with IA-specific or IB-specific monoclonal antibody reagents. Knapp et al (1984) then use a numerical designation according to the frequency with which strains of a particular reaction pattern (serovar) were encountered in a worldwide survey of gonococci. For example, serovar IB-1 was the most frequently occurring serovar, while serovar IB-28 was uncommon. This nomenclature lacks flexibility and would become less meaningful if rare serovars became more prevalent. In addition, the relationships between the reaction patterns are not evident from the single numerical designation.

The system proposed by Bygdeman et al (1985), although superficially more cumbersome, is also more flexible. Individual serovars are named by listing letters that denote the monoclonal antibodies with which the strain reacts. For example, serovar IB-1 of Knapp et al (1984) reacts with antibodies a, b, c and k and is termed serovar Babck, while serovar IB-28 reacts with c, h and k and becomes Bchk. This system allows differences in the reaction patterns to be observed and gives an insight into the relatedness of different serovars. New monoclonal antibodies could be readily incorporated into the system.

Monoclonal antibody serotyping, although still essentially in the developmental stage is likely to become the most widely used method of strain differentiation. The most appropriate panel of monoclonal antibodies remains to be decided. For a detailed review of serotyping with monoclonal antibodies see Bygdeman (1987).

Restriction endonuclease analysis

Restriction endonucleases are enzymes that recognize specific nucleotide sequences and cleave both strands of DNA at sites internal to the molecule. After endonuclease digestion the separation of the DNA fragments by electrophoresis produces patterns of band 'fingerprints' in the gel. These 'fingerprints' have been used to characterize individual isolates of gonococci (Falk et al 1985). This method is suitable for research and reference laboratories only.

APPLICATION OF EPIDEMIOLOGICAL MARKERS

Auxotyping

Extensive studies on auxotyping of isolates from different parts of the world have shown that the gonococcus is heterogeneous and the distribution and prevalence of auxotypes is varied (Knapp 1985). The AHU$^-$ strains have received most attention, as this auxotype predominates in patients with disseminated gonoccocal infection (DGI). Strains with the AHU$^-$ auxotype are usually hypersensitive to penicillin and resistant to the bactericidal action of normal human serum. AHU$^-$ strains predominate in men with asymptomatic gonococcal infection, thus allowing the strains a greater opportunity to disseminate.

No association has been found between auxotype and PID, although non-AHU$^-$ auxotypes are more prevalent. The prevalence of AHU$^-$ strains varies widely among different geographical areas. For example,

AHU⁻ strains have not been isolated in the Philippines but account for up to 40% of isolates in Stockholm, while within cities in the United States levels range from 8% to 57%. The wide variation in the prevalence of AHU⁻ in American cities may correlate with racial differences: the AHU⁻ auxotype is isolated more often from white patients than from black patients (Noble & Miller 1980). As AHU⁻ strains are often sensitive to vancomycin, the use of gonococcal selective media containing vancomycin (Ch. 15) may be a significant factor in the apparent prevalence of AHU⁻ strains in different areas.

Serogrouping

Studies with polyclonal antibody reagents have also shown differences in serogroup in relation to various geographical areas (Bygdeman 1987). The most comprehensive data are available from Sweden, where it has been noted that serogroup WII strains predominate, accounting for around 55% of isolates in the larger cities, whereas WI strains may account for almost 80% of isolates in smaller cities. The situation in Edinburgh is similar to that in the larger Swedish cities (Reid & Young 1984). Serogroup WIII is rare in Europe (0–7%) and is usually associated with infections acquired abroad. Serogroup WII strains predominate in South East Asia, while serogroup WI accounts for only 0–25% of strains (Bygdeman 1987).

There is also a correlation between serogroup and antibiotic susceptibility. Gonococci with decreased susceptibility, the so-called multi-resistant strains, belong to serogroups WII and WIII, whereas those with high sensitivity to β-lactamase antibiotics, tetracyclines and other antibiotics belong to serogroup WI (Bygdeman 1981). These findings are supported by experience in clinical practice, where treatment failures are most often associated with serogroup WII/III infections.

Bygdeman et al (1983) considered that greater antibiotic pressure in larger towns than in smaller ones might account for their observed higher incidence of WII strains in larger towns. Isolates from infections acquired in the Far East, where antibiotic pressure is very high owing to the lack of antibiotic control, show reduced sensitivity to a wide variety of antibiotics and are predominantly of serogroup WII or WIII (Bygdeman 1981).

Isolates from homosexual men

There is a strong correlation between serogroup WII and homosexually acquired infection (Reid & Young 1984). Whereas serogroups WI and WII are, in general, fairly evenly distributed amongst the heterosexual population, some 95–100% of homosexually acquired infections are with isolates of serogroup WII.

Mtr phenotype strains are also significantly more prevalent among isolates from homosexual men than among heterosexual men and women (Morse et al 1982, Reid et al 1985). Although the Mtr phenotype is associated with serogroup WII in isolates from homosexual men, there is no such association in the case of heterosexually acquired infections. Although this is true for Europe, serogrouping of a limited number of strains from heterosexual men who acquired their infection in the Far East are usually of serogroup WII and the Mtr phenotype. It has been proposed that the Mtr phenotype and serogroup WII are selected independently as a result of a general selective pressure such as antibiotic usage (Reid et al 1985). The characteristics of isolates from homosexual men could account for the high failure rate when single dose regimens are used to treat rectal gonorrhoea in men.

Clinical correlation

Serogroup WI is correlated with disseminated gonococcal infection (DGI). Sandstrom et al (1984) reporting from the United States found that 84% of 101 isolates from patients with DGI belonged to serogroup WI, compared with 40% of 168 isolates from patients with uncomplicated gonorrhoea. There was a better correlation between DGI and serogroup WI than between DGI and the AHU⁻ auxotype.

Although serogrouping with polyclonal antibodies has provided much useful information, the inability to resolve isolates into subgroups is a major limitation of the system. With the development of suitable panels of monoclonal antibody reagents, the fine subdivision of gonococcal strains is now possible.

Serovar determination with monoclonal antibodies

The epidemiological observations made with regard to serogrouping have been extended and confirmed by the serological classification into serovars. Bygdeman (1987) has found this to be a valuable tool in specific micro-epidemics caused by the introduction of new strains into the community. Recognition and monitoring of a newly introduced strain, which could be a PPNG for example, enables contact-tracing to be guided and used more effectively.

Serovar analysis can also be used in medico-legal cases. In one instance a two-year-old girl was infected with a serogroup WII strain of serovar combination Bcgjk/Bopys. Of the two adult men suspected to be the source of the infection, one was infected with a strain of the same serovar combination, whereas the other was infected with a totally different serogroup of serovar combination Aedgkih/Arost. As the serovar combination Bcgjk/Bopys was seen in only 2% of strains from the same city, there was a high probability that the girl had acquired her infection from the man with the identical strain (Bygdeman 1987). Serovar determination has also proved useful in recognizing multiple infection and differentiating between reinfection and treatment failure.

PPNG

A combination of serovar analysis, auxotyping and determination of plasmid profile has proved valuable in the epidemiology of PPNG. There has been a change from the early pattern observed among PPNG strains, where those originally described as African type were of the auxotype Arg⁻ and contained a 3.2 Mdal plasmid, while those of the Asian type were auxotype Proto or Pro⁻ and contained a 4.4 Mdal plasmid, usually in conjunction with a 24.5 Mdal transfer plasmid. PPNG strains of a diversity of different auxotypes and serovars have emerged, expressing the spread of the β-lactamase encoding plasmids between strains of different serovar/auxotype combinations. PPNG strains harbouring the 3.2 Mdal plasmid can now be Proto and Pro-, and the majority belong to serogroup WI. Studies carried out in Sweden showed that the most common serovar/auxotype combination of such strains associated with Africa was Ae/Proto, although a few were Aedgkih/Pro⁻ and some of these contained the 24.5 Mdal transfer plasmid (Bygdeman 1987). PPNG of serovars Ae and Aedgkih have not been isolated among strains from Asia. Aedgkih/Pro⁻ strains carrying the 4.4 Mdal plasmid and the 24.5 Mdal plasmid are, therefore, probably indigenous in Africa. Likewise, it seems probable that Aedgkih/Pro⁻ strains carrying both the 3.2 Mdal and the 24.5 Mdal plasmids are not the result of a deletion of the 4.4 Mdal plasmid in Asian type PPNG, but rather the result of a genetic exchange between locally existing strains. Serogroup WI PPNG isolated in Asia are usually serovar Aedih/Pro⁻ or Aedih/Proto.

In Asia most PPNG are serogroup WII and there is a greater number of different serovar/auxotype combi-

nations. In Bangkok, Singapore and Korea, PPNG strains of 9, 11 and 6 different serovars respectively, were identified with a total of 14 different serovars. The most common serovar/auxotype combinations were Bcgjk/Proto, Bcegk/Proto and Bacjk/Pro⁻. The spread of β-lactamase encoding plasmids to strains of new serovars with the capacity to survive seems to be more developed among strains of serogroup WII/III than among those of serogroup WI (Bygdeman 1987).

EPIDEMIOLOGICAL CHANGES

The pattern of gonococcal strains of different types may change owing to the importation of new strains or by genetic exchanges in locally existing strains. Both mechanisms are likely to operate most effectively in patients at high risk of repeated and double infections.

Studies involving serovar analysis should also be helpful in the development and assessment of gonococcal vaccines. Since repeated gonococcal infections are not unusual, if protective antibodies are produced against epitopes on the protein I, gonococcal strains of new serovars might have an advantage over those that are more common in a given area. The possibility of being re-exposed to a strain of the same serogroup, but antigenically different from that of an earlier infection, is greater for WII/III strains than for WI strains, since in each region a greater diversity of serovars has been found within the WII/III serogroup (Bygdeman et al 1983). This hypothesis might explain why WII/III strains are more common among homosexual men than among heterosexual patients and more frequent among heterosexual men than among women. Continual epidemiological surveillance is necessary to increase our understanding of the transmission between individuals and to direct the development of meaningful strategies to reduce the global problem.

REFERENCES

Ansink-Schipper M C, van Embden J D A, van Klingeren B, Woudstra R 1982 Further spread of plasmids among different auxotypes of penicillinase-producing gonococci. Lancet i: 445

Arya O P, Nsanzumuhire H, Taber S R 1973 Clinical, cultural and demographic aspects of gonorrhoea in a rural community in Uganda. Bulletin of the World Health Organization 49: 587–595

Ashford W A, Golash R G, Hemming V C 1976 Penicillinase-producing Neisseria gonorrhoeae. Lancet ii: 657–658

Barlow D, Nayyar K, Phillips I, Barrow J 1976 Diagnosis of

gonorrhoea in women. British Journal of Venereal Diseases 52: 326–328

Barrera O, Swanson J 1984 Proteins IA and IB exhibit different surface exposures and orientations in the outer membranes of Neisseria gonorrhoeae. Infection and Immunity 44: 565–568

Bhattacharyya M N, Jephcott A E 1974 Diagnosis of gonorrhoea in women. Role of the rectal sample. British Journal of Venereal Diseases 50: 109–112

Blackwell C C, Winstanley F P, Weir D M, Kinane D F 1985 Host-parasite interactions influencing susceptibility to diseases caused by the pathogenic Neisseria species. In:

Schoolnik G K, Brooks G F, Falkow S, Frasch E, Knapp J S, McCutchan J A, Morse S A (eds). The pathogenic Neisseriae. American Society for Microbiology, Washington DC, p 452–455

Blake M S, Gotschlich E C 1983 Gonococcal membrane proteins: speculation on their role in pathogenesis. Progress in Allergy 33: 298–313

Braude A I 1982 Resistance to infection with the gonococcus. Journal of Infectious Diseases 45: 623–634

Brinton C C, Bryan J, Dillon J-A et al 1978 Uses of pili in gonorrhoea control: Role of bacterial pili in disease, purification and properties of gonococcal pili, and progress in the development of a gonococcal pilus vaccine for gonorrhoea. In: Brooks G F, Gotschlich E C, Holmes K K, Sawyer W D, Young F E (eds) Immunobiology of Neisseria gonorrhoeae. American Society for Microbiology, Washington DC, p 155–178

Britigan B E, Cohen M S, Sparling P F 1985 Gonococcal infection: a model of molecular pathogenesis. The New England Journal of Medicine 312: 1683–1694

Brooks G F, Israel K S, Peterson B H 1976 Bactericidal and opsonic activity against Neisseria gonorrhoeae in sera from patients with disseminated gonococcal infection. Journal of Infectious Diseases 134: 450–462

Brown W J, Lucas C T, Kuhn U S G 1972 Gonorrhoea in the chimpanzee: infection with laboratory-passed gonococci and by natural transmission. British Journal of Venereal Diseases 48: 177–178

Buchanan T M 1977 Surface antigens: Pili In: Roberts R B (ed) The gonococcus, J Wily, New York, p 255–272

Buchanan T M 1978 Antigen-specific serotyping of Neisseria gonorrhoeae. I. Use of an enzyme-linked immunosorbent assay to quantitate pilus antigens on gonococci. The Journal of Infectious Diseases 138: 319–325

Buchanan T M, Hildebrandt J F 1981 Antigen-specific serotyping of Neisseria gonorrhoeae: Characterization based upon principal outer membrane protein. Infection and Immunity 32: 985–994

Buchanan T M, Eschenbach D A, Knapp J S, Holmes K K 1980 Gonococcal salpingitis is less likely to occur with Neisseria gonorrhoeae of the same principal outer membrane protein antigenic type. American Journal of Obstetrics and Gynecology 138: 978–980

Buchanan J M, Siegel M S, Chen K C S, Pearce W A 1982 Development of a vaccine to prevent gonorrhea. In: Weinstein L, Fields B N (eds) Seminars in infectious diseases. iv. Bacterial vaccines. Thieme-Stratton, New York, p 160–164

Bygdeman S 1981 Antibiotic susceptibility of Neisseria gonorrhoeae in relation to serogroups. Acta Pathologica et Microbiologica Scandinavica, Section B 89: 227–237

Bygdeman S M 1987 Polyclonal and monoclonal antibodies applied to the epidemiology of gonococcal infection. In: Young H, McMillan A (eds) Immunological diagnosis of sexually transmitted diseases. Marcel Dekker, New York, p 117–165

Bygdeman S, Danielsson D, Sandstrom E 1983 Gonococcal W serogroups in Scandinavia. A study with polyclonal and monoclonal antibodies. Acta Pathologica et Microbiologica Scandinavica, Section B 91: 293–305

Bygdeman S M, Gillenius E-C, Sandstrom E G 1985 Comparison of two different sets of monoclonal antibodies for the serological classification of Neisseria gonorrhoeae. In: Schoolnik G K, Brooks G F, Falkow S, Frasch C E. Knapp J S, McCutchan, J A, Morse S A (eds) The pathogenic Neisseriae. American Society for Microbiology, Washington DC, p 31–36

Cannon J G, Buchanan T M, Sparling P F 1983 Confirmation of association of protein I serotype of Neisseria gonorrhoeae with ability to cause disseminated infection. Infection and Immunity 40: 816–819

Carifo K, Catlin B W, 1973 Neisseria gonorrhoeae auxotyping: Differentiation of clinical isolates based on growth responses on chemically defined media. Applied Microbiology 26: 223–230

Catlin B W 1973 Nutritional profiles of Neisseria gonorrhoeae, Neisseria meningitidis and Neisseria lactamica in chemically defined media and the use of growth requirements for gonococcal typing. Journal of Infectious Diseases 128: 178–194

Catlin B W 1977 Nutritional requirements and auxotyping. In: Roberts R (ed) The gonococcus. John Wiley, New York, p 91–109

Centers for Disease Control 1982 Global distribution of Penicillinase-producing Neisseria gonorrhoeae (PPNG). Morbidity and Mortality Weekly Report, January 22nd 1982. U.S. Department of Health and Human Services, Public Health Service

Chipperfield E J, Catterall R D 1976 Reappraisal of Gram-staining and cultural techniques for the diagnosis of gonorrhoea in women. British Journal of Venereal Diseases 52: 36–39

Cohen I R 1967 Natural and immune human antibodies reactive with antigens of virulent Neisseria gonorrhoeae: Immunoglobulins G, M and A. Journal of Bacteriology 94: 141–148

Communicable Diseases Scotland (1982) Summary of Sexually Transmitted Diseases 1972–79. Communicable Diseases (Scotland) Unit, Ruchhill Hospital, Glasgow

Douglas J T, Lee M D, Nikaido H 1981 Protein I of Neisseria gonorrhoeae outer membrane is a porin. FEMS Microbiology Letters 12: 305–309

Easmon C S F 1985 Gonococcal resistance to antibiotics. Journal of Antimicrobial Chemotherapy 16: 409–417

Eisenstein B I, Sparling P F 1978 Mutations to increased antibiotic sensitivity in naturally-occurring gonococci. Nature 271: 242–244

Elwell L P, Roberts M, Mayer L W, Falkow S 1977 Plasmid-mediated beta-lactamase production in Neisseria gonorrhoeae. Antimicrobial Agents and Chemotherapy 11: 528–533

Evans B A 1976 Detection of gonorrhoea in women. British Journal of Venereal Diseases 52: 40–42

Extract from the report of the Chief Medical Officer 1985 Sexually transmitted diseases: extract from the annual report of the Chief Medical Officer of the Department of Health and Social Security for the year 1983. Genitourinary Medicine 61: 204–207

Falk E S, Danielsson D, Bjorvatn B, Melby K, Sorensen B, Kristiansen B-E 1985 Genomic fingerprinting in the epidemiology of gonorrhoea. Acta Dermato Venereologica 65: 235–239

Glynn A A, Ison C 1978 Antibodies to a gonococcal envelope protein in acute gonorrhy. In: Brooks G F, Gotschlich E C, Holmes K K, Sawyer W D, Young F E (ed) Immunobiology of Neisseria gonorrhoeae, American Society for Microbiology, Washington DC, p 387–388

Hagblom P, Segal E, Billyard E, So M 1985 Intragenic recombination leads to pilus antigenic variation in Neisseria gonorrhoeae. Nature 315: 156–158

Harkness A H 1948 The pathology of gonorrhoea. British Journal of Venereal Diseases 56: 227–229

Harriman G R, Podak E R, Braude A I, Corbeil L C, Essex A F, Curd J G 1982 Activation of complement by serum-resistant *Neisseria gonorrhoeae*. Journal of Experimental Medicine 156: 1235–1249

Heckels J E 1981 Structural comparison of Neisseria gonorrhoeae outer membrane proteins. Journal of Bacteriology 145: 736–742

Heckels J E, Blackett B, Everson J S, Ward M E 1976 The influence of surface charge on the attachment of *Neisseria gonorrhoeae* to human cells. Journal of General Microbiology 96: 359–364

Heffron F, Sublett R, Hedges R W, Jacob A, Falkow S 1975 Origin of the TEM beta-lactamase gene formed on plasmids. Journal of Bacteriology 122: 250–56

Heffron F, McCarthy B J, Ohtsubo H, Ohtsubo E 1979 DNA sequence analysis of the transposon Tn3: three genes and three sites involved in transposition of Tn3. Cell 18: 1153–1163

Holmes K K, Johnson D W, Trostle H J 1970 An estimate of the risk of men acquiring gonorrhea by sexual contact with infected females. American Journal of Epidemiology 91: 170–174

Hooper R R, Reynolds G H, Jones O G et al 1978 Cohort study of venereal disease. I. The risk of gonorrhea transmission from infected women to men. American Journal of Epidemiology 108: 136–144

Hopcraft M, Verhagen A R, Ngigi S, Hagu A C A 1973 Genital infections in developing countries: experience in a family planning clinic. Bulletin of the World Health Organization 48: 581–586

James J F, Swanson J 1978 Color/opacity colonial variants of *Neisseria gonorrhoeae* and their relationship to the menstrual cycle. In: Brooks G F, Gotschlich E C, Holmes K K, Sawyer W D, Young F E (eds) Immunobiology of *Neisseria gonorrhoeae*. American Society for Microbiology, Washington DC, p 388–343

James J F, Lammel C J, Draper D L, Brown D A, Sweet R L, Brooks G F 1983 Gonococcal attachment to eukaryotic cells. Sexually Transmitted Diseases 10: 173–179

Jephcott A E, Reyn A 1971 *Neisseria gonorrhoeae*. Colony variation I. Acta Pathologica et Microbiologica Scandinavica, Section B 79: 609–614

Jephcott A E, Reyn A, Birch-Anderson A 1971 Brief report. *Neisseria gonorrhoeae* III. Demonstration of presumed appendages to cells from different colony types. Acta Pathologica et Microbiologica Scandinavica, Section B 79: 437–439

Johnson S R, Anderson B E, Biddle J W, Perkins G H, DeWitt W E 1983 Characterization of concatameric plasmids of *Neisseria gonorrhoeae*. Infection and Immunity 40: 843–846

Johnston K H, Gotschlich E C 1974 Isolation and characterization of the outer membrane of *Neisseria gonorrhoeae*. Journal of Bacteriology 119: 250–257

Johnston K H, Holmes K K, Gotschlich E C 1976 The serological classification of *Neisseria gonorrhoeae*. I. Isolation of the outer membrane complex responsible for serotypic specificity. Journal of Experimental Medicine 143: 741–758

Johnston N A, Kolator B 1982 Emergence in Britain of beta-lactamase-producing gonococci with new plasmid combinations. Lancet i: 445–46

Judd R C 1982 ^{125}I-peptide mapping of protein III isolated from four strains of *Neisseria gonorrhoeae*. Infection and Immunity 37: 622–631

Judd R C 1985 Structure and surface exposure of protein IIs of *Neisseria gonorrhoeae* Infection and Immunity 48: 452–457

Kellogg D S Jr, Peacock W L Jr, Deacon W E, Brown L, Pirkle C I 1963 *Neisseria gonorrhoeae* I. Virulence linked to colonial variation. Journal of Bacteriology 85: 1274–1279

Khan W, Ross S, Rodriguez W, Controni G, Saz A K 1974 *Haemophilus influenzae* type B resistant to ampicillin. A report of two cases. Journal of the American Medical Association 229: 298–301

Knapp J S 1985 Typing of gonococci. In: Brooks G F, Donegan E A (eds) Gonococcal infection. Edward Arnold, London, p 159–167

Knapp J S, Tam M R, Nowinski R C, Holmes K K, Sandstrom E G 1984 Serological classification of *Neisseria gonorrhoeae* with use of monoclonal antibodies to gonococcal outer membrane protein I. Journal of Infectious Diseases 150: 44–48

Knapp J S, Bygdeman S, Sandstrom E, Holmes K K 1985 Nomenclature for the serological classification of *Neisseria gonorrhoeae*. In: Schoolnik G K, Brooks G F, Falkow S, Frasch C E, Knapp J S, McCutchan J A, Morse S A (eds) The pathogenic Neisseriae. American Society for Microbiology, Washington DC, p 4–5

Kornfield S I, Plaut A G 1981 Secretory immunity and the bacterial IgA proteases. Review of Infectious Diseases 3: 521–534

Lambden P R, Heckels J E, James L T, Watt P J 1979 Variations in surface protein composition associated with virulence properties in opacity types of *Neisseria gonorrhoeae*. Journal of General Microbiology 114: 305–312

Latif A S 1981 Sexually transmitted disease in clinic patients in Salisbury, Zimbabwe. British Journal of Venereal Diseases 57: 181–183

Lee T J, Schmoyer A, Synderman R, Yount W J, Sparling P F 1978 Familial deficiencies of the sixth and seventh components of complement associated with bacteremic *Neisseria* infections. In: Brooks G F, Gotschlich E C, Holmes K K, Sawyer W D, Young F E (eds) Immunobiology of *Neisseria gonorrhoeae*. American Society for Microbiology, Washington DC, p 204–206

Lim D, Gewurz A, Lint T F, Ghaze M, Sapheri B, Gewurz H 1976 Absence of the sixth component of complement in a patient with repeated episodes of meningococcal meningitis. Journal of Paediatrics 89: 42

Lucas C T, Chandler F, Martin J E, Schmale J D 1971 Transfer of gonococcal urethritis from man to chimpanzee. An animal model for gonorrhea. Journal of the American Medical Association 216: 1612–1614

McChesney D, Tramont E C, Boslego J W, Ciak J, Sadoff J, Brinton C C 1982 Genital antibody response to a parenteral gonococcal pilus vaccine. Infection and Immunity 36: 1006–1012

McCutchan J A, Katzenstein D, Norquist D, Chikami G, Wunderlich A, Braude A I 1978 Role of blocking antibody in disseminated gonococcal infection. Journal of Immunology 121: 1884–1888

McCutchan J, Adler M W, Berrie J R H 1982 Penicillinase-producing *Neisseria gonorrhoeae* in Great Britain, 1977–81; alarming increase in incidence and recent development of endemic transmission. British Medical Journal 285: 337–340

McMillan A, McNeillage G, Young H 1979a Antibodies to *Neisseria gonorrhoeae*: A study of the urethral exudates of 232 men. Journal of Infectious Diseases 140: 89–95

McMillan A, McNeillage G, Young H, Bain S S R 1979b Secretory antibody response of the cervix to infection with *Neisseria gonorrhoeae*. British Journal of Venereal Diseases 55: 265–270

Maness M J, Sparling P F 1973 Multiple antibiotic resistance due to a single mutation in *Neisseria gonorrhoeae*. Journal of Infectious Diseases 128: 321–330

Mayer L W, Holmes K K, Falkow S 1974 Characterization of plasmid deoxybonucleic acid from *Neisseria gonorrhoeae*. Infection and Immunity 10: 712–717

Melly M A, Gregg C R, McGee Z A 1981 Studies of toxicity of *Neisseria gonorrhoeae* for human fallopian tube mucosa. Journal of Infectious Diseases 143: 423–431

Morse S A, Lysko P G, McFarland L, Knapp J S, Sandstrom E, Critchlow C, Holmes K K 1982 Gonococcal strains from homosexual men have outer membranes with reduced permeability to hydrophobic molecules. Infection and Immunity 37: 432–438

Morse S A, Johnson S R, Biddle J W, Roberts M C 1986 High-level tetracycline resistance in *Neisseria gonorrhoeae* is result of acquisition of streptococcocal *tetM* determinant. Antimicrobial Agents and Chemotherapy 30: 664–670

Noble R C, Miller B R 1980 Auxotypes and antimicrobial susceptibilities of Neisseria gonorrhoeae in black and white patients. British Journal of Venereal Diseases 56: 26–30

Novotny P, Short J A, Hughes M et al 1977 Studies on the mechanism of pathogenicity of *Neisseria gonorrhoeae*. Journal of Medical Microbiology 10: 347–363

Perry M B, Daoust V, Diena B B, Ashton F E, Wallace R 1975 Lipopolysaccharides of *Neisseria gonorrhoeae* colony types 1 and 4. Canadian Journal of Biochemistry 53: 623–629

Peterson B H, Graham J A, Brooks G F 1976 Human deficiency of the eighth component of complement. Journal of Clinical Investigation 58: 1163–1173

Phillips I 1976 B-lactamase-producing penicillin resistant gonococcus. Lancet 2: 656–657

Reid K G, Young H 1984 Correlation of coagglutination serogroup WII with homosexually acquired infection. British Journal of Venereal Diseases 60: 302–305

Reid K G, Warbrick J, Young H 1985 Correlation of cell-envelope phenotypes of *Neisseria gonorrhoeae* with site of infection and serogroup. Journal of Medical Microbiology 20: 379–386

Rice P A, Kasper D K 1977 Characterisation of gonococcal antigens responsible for induction of bactericidal antibody in disseminated infection. Journal of Clinical Investigation 60: 1149–1158

Rice P A, Tam M R, Blake M S 1985 Immunoglobulin G antibodies in normal human serum directed against protein III block killing of serum-resistant *Neisseria gonorrhoeae* by immune human serum. In: Schoolnik G K, Brooks G F, Falkow S, Frasch C E, Knapp J S, McCutchan J A, Morse S A (eds) The pathogenic Neisseriae. American Society for Microbiology, Washington DC, p 427–430

Riou J Y, Courvalin P 1985 *Neisseria gonorrhoeae* plasmids: Theoretical study and practical consequences. WHO/VDT/RES/GON/85.146 World Health Organization, Geneva

Roberts M, Falkow S 1979 *In vitro* conjugal transfer of R plasmids in *Neisseria gonorrhoeae*. Infection and Immunity 24: 982–984

Saigh J H, Sanders C C, Saders W E 1978 Inhibition of *Neisseria gonorrhoeae* by aerobic and facultatively anaerobic components of the endocervical flora: evidence for a protective effect against infection. Infection and Immunity 19: 704–710

Sandstrom E, Danielsson D 1980 Serology of *Neisseria gonorrhoeae*. Classification by coagglutination. Acta Pathologica et Microbiologica Scandinavica Section B 88: 27–38

Sandstrom E G, Chen K C S, Buchanan T M 1982a Serology of *Neisseria gonorrhoeae*: coagglutination serogroups WI and WII/III correspond to different outer membrane protein I molecules. Infection and Immunity 38: 462–470

Sandstrom E G, Knapp J S, Buchanan T M 1982b Serology of *Neisseria gonorrhoeae*: W-antigen serogrouping by coagglutination and protein I serotyping by enzyme-linked immunosorbent assay both detect protein I antigens. Infection and Immunity 35: 229–239

Sandstrom E, Knapp J S, Reller B, Thompson S, Hook E W, Holmes K K 1984 Serogrouping of *Neisseria gonorrhoeae*: Correlation of serogroup with disseminated gonococcal infection. Sexually Transmitted Diseases 11: 77–80

Sandstrom E, Lindell P, Harfast B, Blomberg F, Ryden A-C, Bygdeman S 1985 Evaluation of a new set of *Neisseria gonorrhoeae* serogroup W-specific monoclonal antibodies for serovar determination. In: Schoolnik G K, Brooks G F, Falkow S, Frasch C E, Knapp J S, McCutchan J A, Morse S A (eds) The pathogenic Neisseriae. American Society for Microbiology, Washington DC, p 26–31

Sarafian S K, Tam M R, Morse S A 1983 Gonococcal protein I-specific opsonic IgG in normal human serum. Journal of Infectious Diseases 148: 1025–1032

Sarubbi F A, Blackman E, Sparling P F 1974 Genetic mapping of linked antibiotic resistance loci in *Neisseria gonorrhoeae*. Journal of Bacteriology 120: 1284–1292

Sarubbi F A, Sparling P F, Blackman E, Lewis E 1975 Loss of low-level antibiotic resistance in *Neisseria gonorrhoeae* due to *env* mutations. Journal of Bacteriology 124: 750–756

Schneider H, Griffis J M, Williams G D, Pier G B 1982 Immunological basis of serum resistance of *Neisseria gonorrhoeae*. Journal of General Microbiology 128: 13–22

Schoolnik G K, Buchanan T M, Holmes K K 1976 Gonococci causing disseminated infection are resistant to the bactericidal action of normal human sera. Journal of Clinical Investigation 58: 1163–1173

Schoolnik G K, Ochs H D, Buchanan T M 1979 Immunoglobulin class responsible for gonococcal bactericidal activity of normal human sera. Journal of Immunology 122: 1771–1779

Schoolnik G K, Tai J Y, Gotschlich E C 1982 Receptor binding and antigenic domains of gonococcal pili. In: Schlessinger D (ed) Microbiology — 1982. American Society for Microbiology, Washington DC, p 312–316

Segal E, Billyard E, So M, Storzbach S, Meyer T F 1985 Role of chromosomal rearrangement in *N. gonorrhoeae* pilus variation. Cell 40: 293–300

Shafer W M, Joiner K, Guymon L F, Cohen M S, Sparling P F 1984 Serum sensitivity of *Neisseria gonorrhoeae*: The role of lipopolysaccharide. Journal of Infectious Diseases 149: 175–183

Sng E H, Lim A L, Yeo K L 1984 Susceptibility to antimicrobials of *Neisseria gonorrhoeae* isolated in Singapore: implications on the need for more effective treatment regimens and control strategies. British Journal of Venereal Diseases 60: 374–379

Soendjojo A 1983 Gonococcal urethritis due to fellatio. Sexually Transmitted Diseases 10: 41–42

Sparling P F 1977 Antibiotic resistance in the gonococcus. In: Roberts R B (ed) The gonococcus. John Wiley, New York, p 111–135

Sparling P F, Sarubbi F A, Blackman E 1975 Inheritance of low-level resistance to penicillin, tetracycline and chloramphenicol in *Neisseria gonorrhoeae*. Journal of Bacteriology 124: 740–749

Stead A, Main J S, Ward M E, Watt P J 1975 Studies on lipopolysaccharides isolated from strains of *Neisseria gonorrhoeae*. Journal of General Microbiology 88: 123–131

Stiffler P N, Lerner S A, Bohnhoff M, Morello J A 1975 Plasmid deoxyribonucleic acid in clinical isolates of *Neisseria gonorrhoeae*. Journal of Bacteriology 122: 1293–1300

Swanson J 1980 ^{125}I-labelled peptide mapping of some heat-modifiable proteins of the gonococcal outer membrane. Infection and Immunity 37: 359–368

Swanson J, King G 1978 *Neisseria gonorrhoeae* — granulocyte interactions. In: Brooks G F, Gotschlich E C, Holmes K K, Sawyer W D, Young F E (ed) Immunobiology of *Neisseria gonorrhoeae*. American Society for Microbiology, Washington DC, p 221–226

Swanson J, Mayer L W, Tam M R 1982 Antigenicity of *Neisseria gonorrhoeae* outer membrane protein(s) III detected by immunoprecipitation and western blot transfer with a monoclonal antibody. Infection and Immunity 38: 668–672

Tice A W, Rodriguez V L 1981 Pharyngeal gonorrhea. Journal of the American Medical Association 246: 2717–2719

Tramont E C 1977 Inhibition of adherence of *Neisseria gonorrhoeae* by human genital secretions. Journal of Clinical Investigation 59: 117–124

Tramont E C, Ciak J, Boslego J, McChesney D G, Brinton C C, Zollinger W 1980 Antigenic specificity of antibodies in vaginal secretions during infection with *Neisseria gonorrhoeae*. Journal of Infectious Diseases 142: 23–31

Tramont E C, Boslego J W, Chung R et al 1985 Parenteral gonococcal pilus vaccine. In: Schoolnik G K, Brooks G F, Falkow S, Frasch C E, Knapp J S, McCutchan J A, Morse S A (eds) The pathogenic Neisseriae. American Society for Microbiology, Washington DC, p 316–322

US Department of Health and Human Services 1981 STD fact sheet 35. Basic statistics on the sexually transmitted disease problem in the United States. Public Health Service Centers for Disease Control. VD Control Division, Atlanta, Georgia, HHS Publication (CDC) 81-8195, p 1–35

US Department of Health and Human Services 1982 Sexually transmitted diseases (STD) statistical letter (formerly VD statistical letter), calendar year 1981. Public Health Service, Centers for Disease Control, VD Control Division, Atlanta, Georgia, p 1–55

van Embden J D A, Dessens-Kroom M, van Klingeren B 1985 A new B-lactamase plasmid in *Neisseria gonorrhoeae*. Journal of Antimicrobial Chemotherapy 15: 247–250

Virji M, Heckels J E 1983 Antigenic cross-reactivity of *Neisseria* pili: Investigations with type- and species-specific monoclonal antibodies. Journal of General Microbiology 129: 2761–2768

Virji M, Heckels J E 1984 The role of common and type-specific pilus antigenic domains in adhesion and virulence of gonococci for human epithelial cells. Journal of General Microbiology 130: 1089–1095

Watson R R 1978 Cell-mediated immune response to *Neisseria gonorrhoeae*. In: Brooks G F, Gotschlich E C, Holmes K K, Sawyer W D, Young F E (eds) Immunobiology of *Neisseria gonorrhoeae*. American Society for Microbiology, Washington DC, p 290–292

Watt P J, Medlen A R 1978 Generation of chemotaxins by gonococci. In: Brooks G F, Gotschlich E C, Holmes K K, Sawyer W D, Young F E (eds). Immunobiology of *Neisseria gonorrhoeae*. American Society for Microbiology, Washington DC, p 239–241

Watt P J, Ward M E, Heckels J E, Trust T S 1978 Surface properties of *Neisseria gonorrhoeae*: Attachment to and invasion of mucosal surfaces. In: Brooks G F, Gotschlich E C, Holmes K K, Sawyer W D, Young F E (eds) Immunobiology of *Neisseria gonorrhoeae*. American Society for Microbiology, Washington DC, p 253–257

Winstanley F P, Blackwell C C, Weir D M, Kinane D F 1983 ABO blood groups and susceptibility to gonococcal infection. II. The relationship of lipopolysaccharide type to gonococcal sensitivity to the bactericidal activity of normal serum. Journal of Clinical and Laboratory Immunology 11: 27–32

Wiseman G M, Caird J D 1977 Composition of the lipopolysaccharide of *Neisseria gonorrhoeae*. Infection and Immunity 16: 550–556

World Health Organization Scientific Group 1978 *Neisseria gonorrhoeae* and gonococcal infections. Technical Report Series 616. World Health Organization, Geneva

Young H, Sarafian S K, Harris A B, McMillan A 1983 Non-cultural detection of *Neisseria gonorrhoeae* in cervical and vaginal washings. Journal of Medical Microbiology 16: 183–191

Young J D E, Blake M, Mauro A, Cohn Z A 1983 Properties of the major outer membrane protein from *Neisseria gonorrhoeae* incorporated into model lipid membranes. Proceedings of the National Academy of Sciences USA 80: 3831–3835

Zak K, Diaz J-L, Jackson D, Heckels J E 1984 Antigenic variation during infection with *Neisseria gonorrhoeae*: detection of antibodies to surface proteins in sera of patients with gonorrhea. Journal of Infectious Diseases 149: 166–174

15

Diagnosis of gonorrhoea: laboratory and clinical procedures

Microbiological tests are mandatory in making a diagnosis of gonorrhoea. Because of the short incubation period and high infectivity, rapid diagnosis followed by immediate treatment and contact-tracing are important in the control of infection within the community.

Neisseria gonorrhoeae is a very fastidious organism and very careful techniques are necessary for the collection of specimens and their transport to the laboratory for culture and investigation. Ideally the patient is seen at a clinic with an adjacent or closely-sited laboratory. Under these conditions the majority of infected patients (about 90–95% of males and 50–60% of females) can receive appropriate effective treatment on the first attendance after examination of Gram-stained smears. Cultural diagnosis of additional cases and confirmation of smear-positive cases can be made within 24 to 72 hours.

SPECIMENS REQUIRED FOR BACTERIOLOGICAL EXAMINATION

Specimens from males

In males, material for examination is obtained by inserting a sterile bacteriological loop into the everted urethral meatus and gently scraping the walls of the terminal part of the urethra. A loopful or less of the exudate obtained may be examined by microscopy of a Gram-stained smear and by culture. If recent anal intercourse is acknowledged or suspected a cotton wool tipped applicator stick should be passed gently and blindly into the anal canal to a distance of 5 cm; a proctoscope should be passed, and if mucopus is seen it may be examined microscopically and by culture. Direct microscopy of rectal material is often unhelpful as there are large numbers of other organisms in this site, and interpretation of a Gram-stained smear may be difficult. If there has been orogenital contact with a person who may possibly have been infected, material should be obtained for culture from the tonsillar crypts or bed and pharynx. Ideally, in every case of gonorrhoea or in known contacts, it is wise to take this test without seeking details of sexual practice, which patients may be reluctant to discuss.

If the patient is known to have had sexual intercourse with an infected partner and he has no obvious signs of urethritis, it is often helpful to re-examine him when he has held his urine for several hours, preferably overnight. Any exudate which may have collected may then be massaged to the urethral orifice and examined by microscopy and culture. Even in the absence of an obvious discharge, specimens for culture should be obtained by gently scraping the urethral walls with a bacteriological loop. Occasionally examination of prostatic fluid may detect an asymptomatic infection.

Normally a single examination is sufficient to diagnose or exclude urethral gonorrhoea in men. If rectal or pharyngeal infection are suspected, however, cultures should be repeated if the first tests are negative.

Specimens from females

In female patients specimens for cultural investigation should be taken from the urethra (Ur) (traditionally specimens are taken from the urethra after massaging from above downwards to expel any discharge from the para-urethral glands), external cervical os and cervical canal (Cx), rectum (R) and throat (T). If pus is expressed from the orifice(s) of the ducts of the greater vestibular glands, this should be similarly examined. Smears should be taken from the urethra and endocervix for microscopic examination after Gram-staining.

If the first set of culture tests (Ur, Cx, R and possibly T) is negative the tests should be repeated one week later before reassuring the patient that she does not have gonorrhoea. A third set of tests is a justified additional precaution in the case of contacts of gonorrhoea who have given two negative cultures. The use of non-selective medium should be considered for second and third tests in gonorrhoea contacts.

Tests in disseminated gonococcal infection

When disseminated gonococcal infection (DGI) is suspected, the routine tests described and several blood cultures should be taken before commencing therapy. As procedures in routine blood culture may not be optimal for the gonococcus it is most important to inform the laboratory that DGI is a possible diagnosis. Although immunofluorescent techniques may reveal gonococcal antigen in skin lesions these procedures are of research interest and are not for routine diagnosis. Fluid obtained by aspiration of a joint effusion should be examined by culture. For these investigations a non-selective medium should be employed in parallel with a selective medium. Although patients with suspected DGI may have no genital symptoms it is important to take ano-genital (and pharyngeal) cultures as these are most likely to yield gonococci (Barr & Danielsson 1971).

Importance of culture site and number of diagnostic tests

Repeated testing of multiple sites is necessary since not all infections in women will be detected on first attendance. The proportion of infected women detected at their first attendance has been variously reported as 66% (Catterall 1970), 90% (Thin et al 1971) 91% (Chipperfield & Catterall 1976) and 98% (Young et al 1979). Provided that the microbiological service consistently reaches a high standard, only two sets of investigations need to be taken to diagnose or exclude gonorrhoea in women (Barlow et al 1976, Young et al 1979). It is prudent, however, to carry out a third set of tests in the case of gonorrhoea contacts.

The efficiency of detecting gonorrhoea varies depending on factors such as the culture medium used. For example, a single endocervical culture detected 90% of infections when Modified New York City (MNYC) medium was used but only 78% when conventional Thayer Martin (TM) medium was used (Young et al 1979). A figure as low as 40% has been reported (Norins 1974).

In terms of a screening schedule more infections are detected by testing additional sites at the first attendance than by re-screening by endocervical culture (Young et al 1979).

A 'high vaginal swab' is totally inadequate for diagnosing or excluding gonorrhoea and if this is the only specimen taken, one in three infected women is likely to be missed (Bhattacharyya et al 1973). The poor results with vaginal specimens are to be expected since this material detects only gonococci which may have contaminated the area, particularly from the cervix, a site of infection where gonococci are actively multiplying.

Rectal cultures are important in the female: approximately 25–50% of patients have ano-rectal involvement, and 5–10% may be positive only in this site (Bhattacharyya & Jephcott 1974). Since rectal infection is usually symptomless, and may be an important cause

of treatment failure, rectal cultures are essential in screening for infection and assessing effectiveness of treatment.

In males who may have acquired their infection through homosexual contact it is important to obtain screening cultures from all sites that might possibly be infected, regardless of the symptoms. For example, in a series of 278 homosexual men with gonorrhoea (McMillan & Young 1978) the urethra was infected in 169 (60.8%), the ano-rectum in 114 (41.0%) and the throat in 23 (8.3%). This study also stressed the importance of repeat testing in diagnosing rectal and pharyngeal infection: by relying on only one set of tests, 8 (7.0%) patients with rectal gonorrhoea and 6 (26.1%) patients with pharyngeal gonorrhoea would have been missed. Detection of rectal and pharyngeal gonorrhoea in homosexual men is particularly important. Because the biological properties of gonococci associated with homosexually acquired infection tend to make them more resistant (see Ch. 14), treatment of rectal and pharyngeal gonorrhoea in homosexual men requires higher penicillin dosage than does urethral infection or ano-genital infection in women.

Heterosexual men and women with pharyngeal gonorrhoea also require higher penicillin dosage than those with uncomplicated infection. The importance of detecting pharyngeal infection, which has increased in incidence in all patient groups in recent years (Table 15.1), has been emphasized by Young & Bain (1983). In the United Kingdom there seems to be little risk associated with pharyngeal gonorrhoea, either to the individual, in terms of developing disseminated gonococcal infection, or to their sexual partner(s). In general, the detection of endocervical infection, urethral infection in heterosexual men, and ano-rectal infection in homosexual men is much more important than the

Table 15.1 Pharyngeal gonorrhoea in patients attending the Department of Genitourinary Medicine, Edinburgh Royal Infirmary (1978–85).

Year	Number (and percentage) of infected patients* with pharyngeal gonorrhoea		
	Heterosexual	Homosexual	Female
	(n = 3488)	(n = 627)	(n = 2355)
1978	14 (2.5)	11 (12.6)	27 (6.9)
1979	18 (3.6)	5 (9.4)	25 (7.1)
1980	12 (2.7)	10 (15.4)	27 (8.1)
1981	19 (4.6)	4 (6.0)	27 (9.5)
1982	21 (5.2)	18 (16.1)	40 (15.3)
1983	35 (9.8)	15 (13.8)	45 (17.2)
1984	45 (11.5)	12 (15.0)	37 (17.5)
1985	37 (9.0)	15 (27.8)	38 (14.6)
Total	201 (5.2)	90 (13.8)	266 (9.3)

*Expressed as a percentage of patients in whom throat cultures taken

detection of pharyngeal gonorrhoea in either sex and should have priority of resources.

In all patients it is important to know which sites are infected in order that all infected sites can be sampled to assess the efficacy of treatment.

MICROSCOPY

This is important as it enables a presumptive diagnosis to be made in the clinic so that appropriate treatment can be given immediately. Immediate treatment facilitates the prevention of spread of infection and progression of the disease to its more serious sequelae, particularly in those patients likely to default.

The Gram-stained smear

A smear of secretion or discharge is prepared and Gram-stained by standard bacteriological technique (Collee et al 1988), but 0.1% neutral red is the preferred counterstain. The stained and dried slide is examined under a 2 mm oil-immersion objective lens. A typical positive Gram-stained smear of urethral discharge from a male patient with gonorrhoea usually shows a large number of characteristic kidney-shaped Gram-negative diplococci (GNDC) lying within the polymorphonuclear leucocytes with few extracellular organisms. If pleomorphic extracellular Gram-negative diplococci and bacilli with rare extracellular GNDC with morphology typical of *N. gonorrhoeae* are seen, the result of the smear examination is equivocal and not diagnostic. If no GNDC are seen the smear result is reported as negative.

Results in males

In patients whose Gram-stained smears of urethral discharge are unequivocally positive or negative this technique provides an immediate differential diagnosis between gonococcal and non-gonococcal urethritis in 85% of patients (Jacobs & Kraus 1975). When the Gram-stained smear shows typical intracellular GNDC the culture is positive in over 95% of cases. Similarly, when the smear is unequivocally negative, the culture is also negative in over 95% of cases. In general, the sensitivity of Gram-staining urethral smears from symptomatic men ranges from 83 to 96% and the specificity from 95 to 99% (Goodhart et al 1982). The majority of false positive smears are due to organisms, other than the pathogenic neisseriae, which fail to grow on selective medium. Very occasionally, however, usually in less than 0.1% of typical positive smears, the GNDC are shown to be meningococci on culture.

A diagnosis should not be made on the basis of equivocal results. As a general rule, Gram-staining is less reliable in the diagnosis of long-standing or asymptomatic infections or when the microscopist is inexperienced. Goodhart et al (1982) found that the probability of gonorrhoea in men whose smears were reported as containing intracellular GNDC dropped from 94.8% to 53.9% when an inexperienced technician interpreted smears from patients with urethritis. The probability of gonorrhoea in patients without symptoms whose smears were reported positive by an experienced observer was only 34.9%. This poor predictive value results from the low prevalence (2%) of gonorrhoea in the population of men without symptoms. Because of the complexity of the gut flora, rectal smears are only of value if pus or mucopus can be collected by proctoscopy. Gram-staining has no place in the diagnosis of pharyngeal infection.

Results in females

The sensitivity of Gram-staining of cervical smears ranges from 23 to 65% and the specificity from 88 to 100% (Goodhart et al 1982). According to Barlow & Phillips (1978) and Thin & Shaw (1979), Gram-staining of urethral smears made no significant difference to the diagnosis of gonorrhoea in women. Rectal smears are not examined microscopically as a routine in the female patient.

In infections without symptoms, commonly seen in women, the number of gonococci are less than in the male. The bacterial flora of the female genito-urinary tract, also, is both qualitatively and quantitatively greater than in the male. Many of these organisms are small Gram-negative cocci and cocco-bacilli, sometimes appearing in pairs, and occasionally intracellularly, making interpretation of the smear difficult. When extracellular GNDC were considered as positive the sensitivity of Gram-staining increased from 31% to 51%, while the specificity decreased from 99 to 86% (Goodhart et al 1982).

As the performance of Gram-staining is assessed against isolation of gonococci the quality of the culture system will influence the observed sensitivity of microscopy. A poor culture system which fails to detect infections with low numbers of gonococci (i.e. those infections not likely to be detected by microscopy) will result in microscopy giving a falsely high sensitivity.

In a small percentage of both male and female patients typical positive smear results will be obtained but gonococci will not be isolated on culture. This could arise when patients have taken an antibiotic before coming to the clinic, or be due to the particular strain of gonococcus having a pronounced sensitivity to vancomycin, one of the antibiotics used in certain selective media: vancomycin sensitivity may vary from 2% (Mirret et al 1981) to as high as 30% (Windall et al 1980).

tiation is even more important as the vast majority of the GNDC isolated will be meningococci. Simple, rapid, and accurate differentiation of gonococci from non-gonococcal neisseriae can be readily obtained by the Phadebact Monoclonal GC Test. All non-gonococcal neisseriae (monoclonal antibody test negative isolates) from an ano-genital site should be further identified to confirm that they are not gonococci which lack the usual protein I epitopes. If resources allow, it is good practice to identify all non-gonococcal neisseriae. Because of the problems associated with conventional sugar utilization methods this is best done using a rapid method.

A reliable method to detect gonococcal infection in women at their first visit to the clinic would make a most significant improvement to our current diagnostic approaches.

REFERENCES

Adler M W, Belsey E M, O'Conner B H, Catterall R D, Miller D L 1978 Facilities and diagnostic criteria in sexually transmitted disease clinics in England and Wales. British Journal of Venereal Diseases 54: 2–9

Amies C R 1967 A modified formula for the preparation of Stuart's transport medium. Canadian Journal of Public Health 58: 296–300

Anand C M, Kadis E M 1980 Evaluation of the Phadebact *Gonococcus* test for the confirmation of *Neisseria gonorrhoeae*. Journal of Clinical Microbiology 12: 15–17

Arko R J, Finley-Price K G, Wong K-H, Johnson S R, Reising G 1982 Identification of problem *Neisseria gonorrhoeae* cultures by standard and experimental tests. Journal of Clinical Microbiology 15: 435–438

Barlow D, Phillips I 1978 Gonorrhoea in women. Diagnostic, clinical and laboratory aspects. Lancet i: 761–764

Barlow D, Nayyar K, Phillips I, Barrow J 1976 Diagnosis of gonorrhoea in women. British Journal of Venereal Diseases 52: 326–328

Barr J, Danielsson D 1971 Septic gonococcal dermatitis. British Medical Journal 1: 482–485

Bhattacharyya M N, Jephcott A E 1974 Diagnosis of gonorrhoea in women: Role of the rectal sample. British Journal of Venereal Diseases 50: 109–112

Bhattacharyya M N, Jephcott A E, Morton R S 1973 Diagnosis of gonorrhoea in women: comparison of sampling sites. British Medical Journal 2: 748–750

Bonin P, Tanino T T, Handsfeld H H 1984 Isolation of *Neisseria gonorrhoeae* on selective and non-selective media in a sexually transmitted disease clinic. Journal of Clinical Microbiology 19: 218–220

Boyce J M, Mitchell E B 1985 Difficulties in differentiating *Neisseria cinerea* from *Neisseria gonorrhoeae* in rapid systems used for identifying pathogenic *Neisseria* species. Journal of Clinical Microbiology 22: 731–734

Boyce J M, Mitchell E B, Knapp J S, Buttke T M 1985 Production of ^{14}C-labelled gas in BACTEC *Neisseria* Differentiation Kits by *Neisseria cinerea*. Journal of Clinical Microbiology 22: 416–418

Catterall R D 1970 Diagnosis of vaginal discharge. British Journal of Venereal Diseases 46: 122–124

Chipperfield E J, Catterall R D 1976 Reappraisal of Gram-staining and cultural techniques for the diagnosis of gonorrhoea in women. British Journal of Venereal Diseases 52: 36–39

Collee J G, Duguid J P, Fraser A G, Marmion B D (eds) 1988 Mackie and McCartney's Medical Microbiology vol II, 13th edn. Churchill Livingstone, Edinburgh

Curtis G D W, Slack M P E 1981 Wheat-germ agglutination of *Neisseria gonorrhoeae*: A laboratory investigation. British Journal of Venereal Diseases 57: 253–255

Danielsson D, Forsum U 1975 Diagnosis of Neisseria infections by defined immunofluorescence. Methodologic aspects and applications. Annals of the New York Academy of Sciences 254: 334–349

Demetriou E, Sackett R, Welch D F, Kaplan D W 1984 Evaluation of an enzyme immunoassay for detection of *Neisseria* gonorrhoeae in an adolescent population. Journal of the American Medical Association 252: 247–250

Donegan E A 1985 Serological tests to diagnose gonococcal infections. In: Brooks G F, Donegan E A (eds) Gonococcal infection. Edward Arnold, London, p 168–177

Dossett J H, Appelbaum P C, Knapp J S, Totten P A 1985 Proctitis associated with *Neisseria cinerea* misidentified as *Neisseria gonorrhoeae* in a child. Journal of Clinical Microbiology 21: 575–577

Ebright J R, Smith K E, Drexler L, Ivsin R, Krogstad S, Farmer S G 1982 Evaluation of modified Stuart's medium in culturettes for transport of *Neisseria gonorrhoeae*. Sexually Transmitted Diseases 9: 44–47

Faur Y C, Weisburd M H, Wilson M E, May P S 1973 A new medium for the isolation of pathogenic *Neisseria* (NYC medium). I. Formulation and comparisons with standard media. Health Laboratory Science 10: 44–54

Goodhart M E, Ogden J, Zaidi A A, Kraus S J 1982 Factors affecting the performance of smear and culture tests for the detection of *Neisseria gonorrhoeae*. Sexually Transmitted Diseases 9: 63–69

Hookham A B 1981 Thayer-Martin medium and modified New York City medium for the cultural diagnosis of gonorrhoea. British Journal of Venereal Diseases 57: 213

Human R P, Jones G A 1986 Survival of bacteria in swab transport packs. Medical Laboratory Sciences 43: 14–18

Jacobs N F Jr, Kraus S J 1975 Gonococcal and non-gonococcal urethritis in men. Clinical and laboratory differentiation. Annals of Internal Medicine 82: 7–12

Janik A, Juni E, Hayn G A 1976 Genetic transformation as a tool for detection of *Neisseria gonorrhoeae*. Journal of Clinical Microbiology 4: 71–81

Jephcott A E, Rashid S 1978 Improved management in the diagnosis of gonorrhoea in women. British Journal of Venereal Diseases 54: 155–159

Knapp J S, Totten P A, Mulks M H, Minshew B M 1984 Characterization of *Neisseria cinerea*, a nonpathogenic species isolated on Martin-Lewis medium selective for pathogenic *Neisseria* spp. Journal of Clinical Microbiology 19: 63–67

Lawton W D, Battaglioli G J 1983 Gono Gen coagglutination test for confirmation of *Neisseria gonorrhoeae*. Journal of Clinical Microbiology 18: 1264–1265

Lawton W D, Koch L W 1982 Comparison of commercially available New York City and Martin-Lewis medium for recovery of *Neisseria gonorrhoeae* from clinical specimens. Journal of Clinical Microbiology 18: 1264–1265

McMillan A, Young H 1978 Gonorrhea in the homosexual man: frequency of infection by culture site. Sexually Transmitted Diseases 5: 146–150

McMillan A, McNeillage G, Young H, Bain S S R 1980 Detection of antigonococcal IgA in cervical secretions by indirect immunofluorescence: an evaluation as a diagnostic test. British Journal of Venereal Diseases 56: 223–226

Martin J E, Jackson R L 1975 Biological environmental chamber for the culture of *Neisseria gonorrhoeae*. Journal of the American Venereal Disease Association 2: 28–30

Martin J E, Lester A 1971 Transgrow: A medium for transport and growth of *Neisseria gonorrhoeae* and *Neisseria meningitidis*. Health Services and Mental Health Administration Health Report 86: 30–33

Martin J E, Lewis J S 1977 Anisomycin: improved antimycotic activity in modified Thayer-Martin medium. Public Health Laboratory 35: 53–60

Martin J E, Armstrong J H, Smith P B 1974 New system for cultivation of *Neisseria gonorrhoeae*. Applied Microbiology 27: 802–808

Mirret S, Keller L B, Knapp J S 1981 *Neisseria gonorrhoeae* strains inhibited by vancomycin in selective media and correlation with auxotype. Journal of Clinical Microbiology 14: 94–99

Noble R C, Cooper R M 1979 Meningococcal colonisation misdiagnosed as gonococcal pharyngeal infection. British Journal of Venereal Diseases 55: 336–339

Norins L C 1974 The case for gonococcal serology. Journal of Infectious Diseases 230: 677–679

Odugbemi T, Arko R J 1983 Differentiation of *Kingella denitrificans* from *Neisseria gonorrhoeae* by growth on a semisolid medium and sensitivity to amylase. Journal of Clinical Microbiology 17: 389–391

Oxtoby M J, Arnold A J, Zaidi A A, Kleris G S, Kraus S J 1982 Potential shortcuts in the laboratory diagnosis of gonorrhoea: a single stain for smears and nonremoval of cervical secretions before obtaining test specimens. Sexually Transmitted Diseases 9: 59–62

Philip A, Garton G C 1985 Comparative evaluation of five commercial systems for the rapid identification of pathogenic *Neisseria* species. Journal of Clinical Microbiology 22: 101–104

Philip S K, Ison C A, Easmon C S F 1984 Coagglutination identification of *Neisseria gonorrhoeae*. Correspondence. British Journal of Venereal Diseases 60: 66

Pollock H M 1976 Evaluation of methods for the rapid identification of *Neisseria gonorrhoeae* in a routine clinical laboratory. Journal of Clinical Microbiology 4: 19–21

Prior R B, Spagna V A 1981 Application of a Limulus test device in rapid evaluation of gonococcal and non-gonococcal urethritis in men. Journal of Clinical Microbiology 14: 256–260

Ratner H B, Tinsley H, Keller R E, Stratton C W 1985 Comparison of the effect of refrigerated versus room temperature media on the isolation of *Neisseria gonorrhoeae* from genital specimens. Journal of Clinical Microbiology 21: 127–128

Rice R J, Biddle J W, Jean Louis Y A, De Witt W E, Blount J H, Morse S A 1986 Chromosomally mediated resistance in *Neisseria gonorrhoeae* in the United States: Results of surveillance and reporting 1983–1984. Journal of Infectious Diseases 153: 340–345

Robinson M J, Oberhofer T R 1983 Identification of pathogenic *Neisseria* species with the RapID NH system. Journal of Clinical Microbiology 17: 400–404

Saez-Nieto J A, Fenoll A, Vazquez J, Casal J 1982 Prevalence of maltose-negative *Neisseria meningitidis* variants during an epidemic period in Spain. Journal of Clinical Microbiology 15: 78–81

Saginur R, Clecner B, Portnoy J, Mendelson J 1982 Superol (catalase) test for identification of *Neisseria gonorrhoeae*. Journal of Clinical Microbiology 15: 475–476

Seth A 1970 Use of trimethoprim to prevent overgrowth by *Proteus* in the cultivation of *N. gonorrhoeae*. British Journal of Venereal Diseases 46: 201–202

Smeltzer M P, Curran J W, Brown S T, Pass J 1980 Accuracy of presumptive criteria for culture dignosis of *Neisseria gonorrhoeae* in low-prevalence populations of women. Journal of Clinical Microbiology 11: 485–487

Sng E H, Rajan V S, Yeo K L, Goh A J 1982 The recovery of *Neisseria gonorrhoeae* from clinical specimens: effects of different temperatures, transport times and media. Sexually Transmitted Diseases 9: 74–78

Sng E H, Lim A L, Yeo K L 1984 Susceptibility to antimicrobials of *Neisseria gonorrhoeae* isolated in Singapore: implications on the need for more effective treatment regimens and control strategies. British Journal of Venereal Diseases 60: 374–379

Spagna V A, Prior R B, Perkins R L 1980 Rapid presumptive diagnosis of gonococcal cervicitis by the Limulus lysate assay. American Journal of Obstetrics and Gynecology 137: 595–599

Spence M R, Guzick D S, Katta L R 1983 The isolation of *Neisseria gonorrhoeae*: A comparison of three culture transport systems. Sexually Transmitted Diseases 10: 138–140

Stamm W E, Cole B, Fennell C, Bonin P, Armstrong A S, Herrmann J E, Holmes K K 1984 Antigen detection for the diagnosis of gonorrhoea. Journal of Clinical Microbiology 19: 399–403

Svarva P L, Maeland J A 1979 Comparison of two selective media in the cultural diagnosis of gonorrhoea. Acta Pathologica et Microbiologica Scandinavica 87B: 391–392

Talbot M D, Spencer R C, Kinghorn G R 1983 Vancomycin sensitive penicillinase producing *Neisseria gonorrhoeae*. Correspondence. British Journal of Venereal Diseases 59: 277

Tapsall J W, Cheng J 1981 Rapid identification of pathogenic species of *Neisseria* by carbohydrate degradation tests: importance of glucose in media for preparation of inocula. British Journal of Venereal Diseases 57: 249–252

Thayer J D, Martin J E 1966 Improved medium selective for cultivation of *N. gonorrhoeae* and *N. meningitidis*. Public Health Reports, Washington 81: 559–562

Thin R N, Shaw E J 1979 Diagnosis of gonorrhoea in women. British Journal of Venereal Diseases 55: 10–13

Thin R N, Williams I A, Nicol C S 1971 Direct and delayed methods of immunofluorescent diagnosis of gonorrhoea in women. British Journal of Venereal Diseases 47: 27–30

Totten P A, Holmes K K, Handsfield H M, Knapp J S, Perine P L, Falkow S 1983 DNA hybridization technique for the detection of *Neisseria gonorrhoeae* in men with urethritis. Journal of Infectious Diseases 148: 462–471

Tronca E, Handsfield H H, Wiesner P J, Holmes K K 1974 Demonstration of *Neisseria gonorrhoeae* with fluorescent antibody in patients with disseminated gonococcal infection. Journal of Infectious Diseases 129: 583–586

Welborn P P, Uyeda C T, Ellison-Birang N 1984 Evaluation of Gonocheck II as a rapid identification system for pathogenic *Neisseria* species. Journal of Clinical Microbiology 20: 680–683

Wilkinson A E 1977 The sensitivity of gonococci to

penicillin. Journal of Antimicrobial Chemotherapy 3: 197–198

Windall J J, Hall M M, Washington J A, Douglass T J, Weed L A 1980 Inhibitory effects of vancomycin on *Neisseria gonorrhoeae* in Thayer-Martin medium. Journal of Infectious Diseases 142: 775

Wood I A, Young H 1986 Identification of pathogenic *Neisseria* by enzyme profiles determined with chromogenic substrates. Medical Laboratory Sciences 43: 24–27

World Health Organization Scientific Group 1978 *Neisseria gonorrhoeae* and gonococcal infections. Technical Report Series 616. World Health Organization, Geneva

Yajko D M, Chu A, Hadley W K 1984 Rapid laboratory identification of *Neisseria gonorrhoeae* with lectins and chromogenic substrates. Journal of Clinical Microbiology 19: 380–382

Young H 1981 Advances in routine laboratory procedures for the diagnosis of gonorrhoea. In Harris J R W (ed) Recent advances in sexually transmitted diseases 2. Churchill Livingstone, Edinburgh, p 59–71

Young H 1978 Identification and penicillinase testing of *Neisseria gonorrhoeae* from primary isolation cultures on New York City medium. Journal of Clinical Microbiology 7: 247–250

Young H, Reid K G 1987 Immunological diagnosis of gonococcal infection. In: Young H, McMillan A (eds) Immunological diagnosis of sexually transmitted diseases. Marcel Dekker, New York, p 77–116

Young H, Reid K G 1984 Immunological identification of *Neisseria gonorrhoeae* with monoclonal and polyclonal antibody coagglutination reagents. Journal of Clinical Pathology 37: 1276–1281

Young H, Bain S S R 1983 Neisserial colonisation of the pharynx. British Journal of Venereal Diseases 59: 228–231

Young H, McMillan A 1982 Rapidity and reliability of gonococcal identification by coagglutination after culture on modified New York City medium. British Journal of Venereal Diseases 58: 109–112

Young H, Paterson I C, McDonald D R 1976 Rapid carbohydrate utilisation test for the identification of *Neisseria gonorrhoeae*. British Journal of Venereal Diseases 52: 172–175

Young H, Harris A B, Urquhart D, Robertson D H H 1979 Screening by culture for the detection of gonorrhoea in women. Scottish Medical Journal 24: 302–306

Young H, Harris A B, Tapsall J W 1984 Differentiation of gonococcal and non-gonococcal neisseriae by the superoxol test. British Journal of Venereal Diseases 60: 87–89

16

Gonorrhoea: clinical features and treatment

The clinical features of gonorrhoea reflect the inflammatory changes induced by infection of mucosal surfaces by *Neisseria gonorrhoeae*; in some cases the inflammation may be so mild that the patient may be unaware of being infected. A chronic inflammatory process of mucous membranes may have serious sequelae, however, particularly in women, in whom infertility or an increased risk of ectopic pregnancy may result. An infrequent but serious complication is systemic dissemination of the organism.

CLINICAL FEATURES

CLINICAL FEATURES IN THE ADULT MALE (UNCOMPLICATED GONOCOCCAL INFECTION)

Urethral infection

The patient complains of urethral discharge and an often mild dysuria in about 90% of cases. If infection has spread proximally to the posterior urethra there may be symptoms of frequency of micturition, urgency and painful erections. Clinical examination may reveal a reddened urethral meatus with a purulent or mucopurulent discharge. Inguinal lymph nodes may be enlarged on both sides. Examination of the urine by the two glass test will show pus in the first glass if the anterior urethra is mainly affected, or in both glasses if the posterior urethra and/or bladder is involved. If the inflammatory process in the urethra is less severe 'threads' may be found in the urine. These threads are casts of mucus-secreting urethral glands, located in the submucosa and called Littré's glands. Invariably inflamed in urethral gonorrhoea, the ducts of Littré's glands shed casts, composed of pus cells and desquamated tubular cells, into the urine.

It is now clear that a considerable number (possibly as many as 15% in some localities) of males with urethral gonorrhoea have few symptoms if any (Neilsen et al 1975).

Post-gonococcal urethritis may occur in at least 20% of males adequately treated with penicillin (Ch. 17).

Oropharyngeal infection

Infection of the pharynx results from transfer of organisms from the genitalia during fellatio or, less commonly, cunnilingus. Although there is a significant correlation between symptoms of pharyngitis and the practice of fellatio, the isolation of *N. gonorrhoeae* from the pharynx does not correlate with symptoms of pharyngitis (Wiesner et al 1973). Symptoms may be present in only about 20% of cases (Stolz & Schuller 1974), when there may be sore throat, perhaps with referred pain in the ear. Clinical examination may reveal no abnormalities, or a mild pharyngitis or tonsillitis.

Ano-rectal infection

Infection in this site in the male is invariably the result of a homosexual act. The clinical and histological features of ano-rectal gonorrhoea are discussed in detail in Chapter 38. The majority of patients (more than two-thirds) with ano-rectal gonorrhoea have no symptoms of infection. In others there may be a history of pruritus and mucoid or mucopurulent anal discharge, anal pain, bleeding and tenesmus.

Proctoscopic examination may show a normal appearance, or there may be either patchy or generalized erythema of the rectal mucosa with mucopus in the lumen of the anal canal and rectum. The histology is that of a non-specific proctitis (McMillan et al 1983). The inflammatory reaction does not extend into the sigmoid colon. In some cases the mucous membrane is friable, bleeding to the touch, and in others may present a granular appearance. The anal canal, constructed of stratified cuboid or squamous epithelium, is not affected by the gonococcus.

The differential diagnosis of ano-rectal gonorrhoea includes ulcerative colitis, Crohn's disease, ischaemic colitis, radiation or drug-induced colitis, amoebic proctitis, giardiasis and lymphogranuloma venereum.

Local complications of untreated ano-rectal infection include perianal and ischio-rectal abscesses and anal fistulae.

Local complications of gonorrhoea in the male

Inflammation and abscess formation in the parafrenal glands (Tyson's glands)

This is not common (less than 1%) but, when it occurs, it usually produces painful tender swellings on one or both sides of the frenum. Pus may be expressed from the duct.

Gonococcal balanitis

As the gonococcus tends not to attack the squamous epithelium of the glans penis this complication is uncommon.

Inflammation and abscess formation in the para-urethral glands on either side of the urethral meatus

This is rare now in areas where medical attention is easily available. A painful swelling develops on one or both sides of the urethral meatus. Pus may be expressed from the duct of the gland.

Periurethral cellulitis and abscess formation

This is rare except when medical help is delayed. The inflammatory reaction to the gonococcus in the subepithelial tissues of the urethra is particularly marked in the region of Littré's glands and ducts, which may become obstructed resulting in the formation of small cysts and abscesses. Coalescence of these small abscesses results in the formation of periurethral abscess (Harkness 1948). These abscesses may rupture into the urethra or to the exterior, or may heal with scarring.

There is pain and swelling at the site of the abscess and there may be some restriction in urine flow if it bulges into the urethra. If the corpus spongiosum is affected, painful erections will be experienced, and there may be ventral angulation of the penis. On examination there is a tender fluctuant swelling, most commonly at the site of the fossa navicularis or bulb.

If untreated the abscess may point; the overlying skin becomes inflamed and oedematous and the abscess may rupture, producing a fistula.

Urethral strictures

Although rare in developed countries, urethral strictures and fistulae as late complications are common in tropical countries (Osoba & Alausa 1976). Fibrous strictures develop from healing of areas of periurethral cellulitis or abscesses. Further periurethral abscesses may develop proximal to the area of the stricture and their rupture to the exterior results in the formation of urinary fistulae. Fistulae, either single or multiple, are most commonly found in the perineum or scrotum.

Strictures usually develop many years after infection, but may be found within five years of the initial infection (Osoba & Alausa 1976). Symptoms of urinary obstruction include straining at micturition, poor force of the urine stream, prolonged micturition with dribbling. Increased frequency of micturition occurs from incomplete emptying of the bladder or from cystitis. Urinary retention eventually develops and death can result from ascending urinary infection and renal failure.

Inflammation and abscess formation of the bulbo-urethral glands (Cowper's glands)

This complication is uncommon in countries with good medical services. The patient complains of fever, throbbing pain in the perineum, painful defaecation and frequency of micturition. Reflex spasm of the sphincter urethrae may produce acute retention of urine. An abscess, which is usually unilateral, may point in the perineum. The inflamed glands and abscess are palpable on rectal examination and are exquisitely tender.

Prostatitis and seminal vesiculitis

Acute gonococcal prostatitis and seminal vesiculitis are rare. There are usually constitutional disturbances, fever, perineal discomfort, urgency of micturition, haematuria and painful erections. Occasionally acute retention of urine results from reflex spasm of the external sphincter of the bladder. A tender swollen gland is detected on rectal examination. With abscess formation, symptoms become more severe with painful defaecation and suprapubic pain. Pyrexia becomes more pronounced. Rectal examination shows a large, tense swelling bulging into the rectum. The abscess may rupture into the urethra or rectum.

Chronic prostatitis, inflammation of the bulbo-urethral glands (Cowperitis) and chronic inflammation of the seminal vesicles may be found in long-standing infections and can produce vague symptoms of local inflammation such as urethral discharge in the morning and perineal discomfort. Palpation of the glands may reveal irregular thickening, and the prostatic fluid expressed often contains large numbers of pus cells which may exhibit 'clumping' (Ch. 18).

Epididymitis

This is usually unilateral, when the patient complains of a painful swollen testis. On examination there may be erythema of the scrotum on the affected side; the epididymis is enlarged and tender; and there is often a secondary hydrocele. Inflammation of the testis itself is rare (Ch. 18).

Infection of the median raphe of the penis

This is rare, but when it occurs a bead of pus may be

expressed from a duct opening on to the skin on the ventral surface of the penis.

CLINICAL FEATURES IN THE ADULT FEMALE (UNCOMPLICATED GONOCOCCAL INFECTION)

In most cases females with gonorrhoea (70% or more) have few, if any, symptoms. They may occasionally complain of vaginal discharge, but this may be attributable to concomitant vaginitis caused by *Trichomonas vaginalis*. Uncommonly, inflammation of the trigone of the bladder produces urinary frequency. The sites infected in the uncomplicated cases are:

Cervix	85–90%
Urethra	65–75%
Rectum	25–50%
Oropharynx	5–15%

The affected cervix may appear normal on inspection, or there may be signs of inflammation with mucopus exuding from the external os. There may be no clinical evidence of urethritis but occasionally pus may be expressed from the orifice. Rectal gonorrhoea in the female, as in the male, usually produces few symptoms. Oropharyngeal gonorrhoea in the female results from fellatio, and the features are similar to those in the male.

Local complications of gonorrhoea in the female

Inflammation and abscess formation of the para-urethral glands, including those lying externally on either side of the external meatus (Skene's glands)
Abscess formation is not common, but involvement of these glands by the gonococcus is probably mostly present in urethral infection in the female.

Inflammation and abscess formation of the greater vestibular glands (Bartholinitis and Bartholin's abscess)
The glands may be involved on one or both sides. There may be few symptoms of Bartholinitis but, in the routine examination, on compressing the gland, pus may be expressed from the orifice of the duct. When an abscess forms, the patient may complain of pain in the vulva, and examination reveals a tender cystic swelling of the posterior half of the labium majus, the skin of which may be reddened. In less acute and partially treated cases a chronic inflammation may result, causing palpable thickening of the glands.

Pelvic inflammatory disease and salpingitis
These complications are considered in Chapter 23. The incidence of salpingitis in untreated cases is generally given as 10%.

DISSEMINATED GONOCOCCAL INFECTION, INVOLVING BOTH SEXES

This uncommon complication, occurring in less than 1% of cases, is usually seen in women and in homosexual males in whom the infection has been asymptomatic and untreated (Graber et al 1960). Dissemination may occur from any infected site and more often during or just after menstruation and in pregnancy.

Gonococcal strains associated with disseminated infection usually belong to serogroup WI and auxotype AHU$^-$, are extremely sensitive to benzylpenicillin and resistant to the complement-dependent bactericidal action of normal human serum (see Ch. 14). To what extent factors in the host or factors in the organism. or a combination of both, are responsible for causing disseminated gonococcal infections, is as yet unknown. Disseminated gonococcal infection due to beta-lactamase producing gonococci has been recorded in a case report (Thompson et al 1981).

The clinical manifestations of disseminated gonococcal infection usually take the form of fever, rash and arthralgia or arthritis. The spectrum of clinical features of this complication is fairly broad but two forms possibly represent successive stages of the disease.

In the initial bacteraemic stage or form, symptoms are usually of short duration, the patient complaining of fever, rigors, joint pains and perhaps a skin rash. There are characteristic skin lesions and polyarticular arthritis involving usually the knees, wrists, small joints of the hands, ankles and elbows, without sufficient joint effusion present to allow aspiration. If obtained, the fluid from joints is sterile on culture, but blood cultures are often positive for *N. gonorrhoeae* (Holmes et al 1971) if taken within two days of onset of the illness. There may be a tenosynovitis.

In the second form, involvement of one joint is usual, a considerable effusion is present and *N. gonorrhoeae* may be recoverable from the synovial fluid, which contains many polymorphonuclear neutrophil leucocytes. This form, sometimes called the 'septic-joint stage', occurs usually after symptoms have been present for at least four days. A large joint, especially of the upper limb, tends to be affected, e.g. shoulder, elbow. The sternoclavicular or temporomandibular joint may also be affected. Systemic features are usually milder than in the bacteraemic form, skin lesions are seldom found and blood cultures are usually negative for *N. gonorrhoeae*.

Intermediate stages of the disease may be seen and

in the 'septic-joint stage' if untreated, the articular surfaces of the joint may be destroyed and fibrous or bony ankylosis may follow.

The skin lesions in disseminated gonococcal infection

These are usually associated with constitutional disturbance, including fever and polyarthritis. There are essentially two types of skin lesion (Ackerman et al 1965): (i) haemorrhagic lesions, (ii) vesiculopapular lesions on an erythematous base.

Both types of lesion begin as erythematous macules, but in the haemorrhagic type the lesions become purpuric, especially on the palms and soles. In the second type lesions become papular and progress through vesicles to pustules.

Generally resolution occurs in 4–5 days, but cropping may occur during febrile episodes. The lesions, often painful, have an asymmetrical distribution over the body and are particularly noticeable on the extremities and around affected joints. Histological examination of a skin lesion (Seifert et al 1974) shows a small vessel vasculitis in the dermis and subcutis and marked fibrinoid change. There is a perivascular infiltration of polymorphonuclear and mononuclear cells. Degenerating polymorphonuclear leucocytes and evidence of haemorrhage are commonly seen. Using conventional staining techniques, *N. gonorrhoeae* is rarely found in these skin lesions, although antigenic material may be detected by direct immunofluorescent staining. It is possible that the skin lesions result from alternative pathway complement activation by endotoxin (Scherer & Braun-Falco 1976).

The lesions of a disseminated gonococcal infection are clinically and histologically similar to those seen in meningococcal septicaemia.

Meningitis, endocarditis and pericarditis

Meningitis is an uncommon manifestation of disseminated gonococcal infection and is usually found associated with arthritis and dermatitis (Holmes et al 1971).

Gonococcal endocarditis is also a rare but often lethal complication (John et al 1977). The degree of severity of the condition lies between the endocarditis due to *Staphylococcus aureus* and that due to oral streptococci, conventionally but inaccurately referred to as '*Streptococcus viridans*' (Report of a Working Party of the British Society for Antimicrobial Chemotherapy 1985). Most commonly the aortic valve is involved. Maculopapular skin lesions are common and appear in crops. Emboli to cerebral, renal and peripheral arteries may occur (Williams 1938).

Myocarditis and pericarditis may occur more commonly than hitherto recognized. Transient electrocardiographic abnormalities appear to be common in disseminated infection (Holmes et al 1971, Stolz & Schuller 1974). As discussed later in this chapter, in the section on treatment, early referral in endocarditis for expert management by a cardiologist and cardiac surgeon is essential since deterioration may be rapid even when there is apparent response to antibiotic therapy.

Perihepatitis and hepatitis

Acute perihepatitis usually occurs in association with pelvic inflammatory disease in women, and a detailed account of the condition is found in Chapter 23. This complication is very rarely found in men (Kimball & Knee 1970). The patient complains of pain in the right hypochondrium and sometimes in the right shoulder from irritation of the right side of the diaphragm.

Hepatitis may occur following the bacteraemia of disseminated infection (Holmes et al 1971). The hepatic histology is not diagnostic, there being scattered foci of mononuclear and polymorphonuclear leucocyte infiltrates in the parenchyma, with enlarged portal zones infiltrated with lymphocytes.

GONOCOCCAL CONJUNCTIVITIS

This is rare except in the newborn and presents as a purulent conjunctivitis affecting one or both eyes. If untreated, keratitis or panophthalmitis with blindness may result.

GONORRHOEA IN INFANTS AND CHILDREN UNDER THE AGE OF PUBERTY

Gonococcal ophthalmia neonatorum (gonococcal conjunctivitis of the newborn)

This is a conjunctivitis with a purulent discharge in an infant which appears within 21 days of birth and is a notifiable disease in the United Kingdom. Ophthalmia neonatorum was formerly caused chiefly by *N. gonorrhoeae*, but is now more commonly caused by other organisms, including *Chlamydia trachomatis*. Gonococcal ophthalmia usually manifests itself within 48 hours of birth but it may be delayed for as long as a week and, if untreated, has dangerous consequences. The eyelids swell and pus collects in the conjunctival sac. Keratitis with corneal scarring may result if the condition is not treated.

Acute vulvo-vaginitis

This is uncommon in the United Kingdom nowadays. The parents usually notice discharge on the child's underwear and on examination a purulent vaginal discharge, with reddening and oedema of the vulva, may be found.

Oropharyngeal and rectal infection

Workers in the United States of America have described the occurrence of gonorrhoea in these sites in a number of children from lower socio-economic groups (Nelson et al 1976). Infection did not necessarily suggest sexual assault.

TREATMENT

Since its introduction into medical practice in 1944, penicillin has been widely and successfully used in the treatment of gonorrhoea and, more recently, semi-synthetic penicillins and other antimicrobial agents have been added to the therapeutic armamentarium. Although the proportion of strains with reduced sensitivity to penicillin has been rising slowly since the 1960s, the problem of resistance to penicillin has become more ominous with the recent discovery of beta-lactamase producing strains.

PRINCIPLES OF TREATMENT

The aim of treatment is to eradicate the organism from the body as quickly as possible. Ideally the treatment used should be based on the pattern of sensitivity to antibiotic and chemotherapeutic agents observed amongst the strains of the organism in the population served. Regimens of treatment should be constantly reviewed, account being taken of the results of continuous monitoring of isolates for the emergence of drug resistance.

A course of treatment with almost any antimicrobial drug to which the organism is sensitive will cure the majority of patients with gonorrhoea. Patient compliance, however, is often unsatisfactory and tablets may be inadvisably shared with a consort. For example, within one or two days of commencing oral treatment with ampicillin in doses, say, of 250 mg four-hourly, symptoms of gonococcal urethritis may resolve and lead the patient to assume wrongly that he has been cured. Strains of organisms with increased resistance to antimicrobials may emerge when courses of treatment prescribed are not completed.

For these reasons a single large dose of antibiotic, given under supervision either orally or parenterally, is preferred as treatment of uncomplicated infection. In most cases blood and tissue concentrations of drug reach a high level and are maintained for sufficient time to eradicate the organism. Oral administration of antibiotics is preferred to intramuscular injections, which

are not only painful but more liable to cause hypersensitivity reactions. Single-dose therapy with penicillins has not proved satisfactory, however, in the treatment of oropharyngeal or complicated gonococcal infections; in male ano-rectal gonorrhoea single-dose treatment with spectinomycin, ciprofloxacin and the newer cephalosporins is generally satisfactory (Table 38.7).

BENZYLPENICILLIN AND ITS PARENTERAL USE

In UK practice benzylpenicillin (synonym: penicillin G), freshly prepared in aqueous solution for parenteral use, is frequently given by intramuscular injection at regular intervals (2–4 times daily as a rule) — and is also given by intravenous injection; intrathecal injection is best avoided (British National Formulary, No.ll, 1986, p. 188–189). In United States practice, in contrast, the use of benzylpenicillin, freshly prepared in aqueous solution, is restricted to use by the intravenous route (Mandell & Sande 1985a). These differences in practice between the UK and the US are reflected in the various schedules of treatment, as for example those given in the British National Formulary and those given by the Centers for Disease Control, in their STD Treatment Guidelines (CDC 1985). Intravenous use of benzylpenicillin in doses above 1.2 g (2 million units) should be administered slowly at not more than 300 mg per minute to avoid irritation of the central nervous system (Reynolds 1985). Other considerations in its intravenous use are discussed in Chapter 10.

TREATMENT SCHEDULES

Uncomplicated infections in men and women

a. With N. gonorrhoeae (not beta-lactamase producing strains viz. non-PPNG)

Various regimens for single-dose treatment currently used in the treatment of uncomplicated gonorrhoea are given in Table 16.1. The sensitivity of the infecting organisms may vary geographically and hence cure rates may not approach those cited. For example, in Glasgow a single oral dose of 300 mg of minocycline hydrochloride cured 95% of infected patients (Masterton & Schofield 1976) whereas cure rates of only 75% were obtained in the United States (Duncan et al 1971) and only 50% in Australia (Baytch 1974).

Some antibiotics, such as spectinomycin or the cephalosporins, are also specifically useful in the treatment of infections caused by PPNG; to minimize the risk of extending microbial resistance to these antibiotics the authors consider that their use should be restricted to

Table 16.1 Single-dose treatments available for uncomplicated genital gonorrhoea in localities where the prevalence of beta-lactamase producing *N. gonorrhoeae* is low.

Antimicrobial agents		Dosage	Number of patients			Reference
			Treated	*Cured*	*(%)*	
Penicillin						
Ampicillin	*(R)	2 g orally	121	118	98	Waugh et al (1979)
Talampicillin	**(R)	1.5 g orally	101	98	98	Al-Egaily et al (1978)
Amoxycillin	*(R)	3 g orally	54	51	94	Thin et al (1977)
Procaine penicillin		3.78 g i.m.	109	106	97	Taylor & Seth (1975)
Cephalosporin						
Cefoxitin		2 g i.m.	140	136	97	Veeravahu et al (1983)
Cefuroxime		1.5 g i.m.	67	66	99	Price & Fluker (1978)
Cefuroxime axetil ester	*	1.5 g orally	67	66	99	Wanas & Williams (1986)
Ceftriaxone		250 mg i.m.	28	28	100	Handsfield & Murphy (1983)
Cefaclor	*	3 g orally	64	62	97	Panikabutra et al (1983)
Ceftizoxime		500 mg i.m.	100	99	99	Spencer et al (1984)
Miscellaneous						
Rosoxacin		300 mg orally	40	36	90	Lim et al (1984a)
Spectinomycin hydrochloride	(H)	2 g i.m.	30	25	83	Porter & Rutherford (1977)
Ciprofloxacin	(H)	250 mg orally	18	18	100	Shahmanesh et al (1986)

* with 1 g probenecid by mouth
** with 2 g probenecid by mouth
(R) = recommended regimens for those not hypersensitive to penicillin
(H) = treatment suitable for those who are hypersensitive to penicillin
i.m. = intramuscularly

treatment of PPNG infections. In Edinburgh, where only 2% or less of isolates are PPNG, ampicillin in a single oral dose of 2 g given with 1 g of probenecid remains the treatment of choice. Treatment with other antimicrobials is reserved for those in whom the first treatment fails; for those infected in a locality with a high prevalence of PPNG; or for those giving a history of penicillin hypersensitivity. Where the prevalence of PPNG exceeds 5% it is probably justified to use a beta-lactamase stable antimicrobial agent as first-line treatment (McCutchan et al 1982).

b. With beta-lactamase producing N. gonorrhoeae (PPNG) Antimicrobial agents, evaluated for the treatment of PPNG infections, are shown in Table 16.2. Patients with uncomplicated genital infection should be treated with one of these: (i) if their infection is known to be caused by PPNG; or (ii) if they are the sexual partners of such patients, or (iii) if individuals have acquired their infection in areas of the world where the prevalence of PPNG is known or suspected to be high.

Spectinomycin was the first drug to be used widely in the treatment of gonorrhoea caused by PPNG and is still recommended as treatment of choice by the Centers for Disease Control of the US Department of Health and Human Services (CDC 1985). The fact that some isolates of PPNG are resistant to spectinomycin (Ashford et al 1981, Easmon et al 1982) necessitates the use of the second or third generation cephalosporins,

which are effective but expensive. Furthermore 8% of patients with hypersensitivity to penicillin are also allergic to cephalosporin.

Clavulanic acid, a product of *Streptomyces clavuligerus*, is a potent inhibitor of many beta-lactamases although by itself it has little anti-bacterial activity. When given with an antibiotic such as amoxycillin it blocks the beta-lactamase enzymes rendering the organisms sensitive to amoxycillin's rapid bactericidal effect. Prescribed as Augmentin (Beecham) — each tablet containing potassium clavulanate equivalent to 125 mg clavulanic acid with amoxycillin trihydrate equivalent to 250 mg amoxycillin — it is effective in the treatment of PPNG infection (Table 16.1).

Sulbactam, a penicillanic acid sulphone, similar in structure to and like clavulanic acid, is also an irreversible inhibitor of several bacterial penicillinases and cephalosporinases. Having little intrinsic anti-bacterial activity, sulbactam when given with benzylpenicillin extends the effectiveness of the benzylpenicillin to treatment of PPNG (Crider et al 1984). As Sultamicillin, sulbactam in covalent union with ampicillin is effective in the oral treatment of PPNG infections (Farthing et al 1985).

Rosoxacin (Eradacin, Sterling Research Laboratories, Guildford, Surrey), a pyridylquinolone derivative chemically related to nalidixic acid (Idanpaan-Heikkila & Tuuomisto 1985) causes central nervous system side effects such as headache, dizziness, drowsiness and

Table 16.2 Drugs available for the treatment of uncomplicated genital gonorrhoea caused by beta-lactamase producing *Neisseria gonorrhoeae* (PPNG).

Drug		Dosage	Number of patients			Reference
			Treated	*Cured*	*(%)*	
Spectinomycin		2 g i.m.	23	22	96	Arya et al (1978)
		2 g i.m.	50	50	100	Calubiran et al (1982)
		2 g i.m.	52	52	100	Tupasi et al (1983)
		2 g i.m.	51	47	92	Crider et al (1984)
Cephalosporins						
Cefoxitin	★	1 g i.m.	51	50	98	Sanchez et al (1983)
	★	2 g i.m.	39	38	98	Zajdowicz et al (1983)
Cefuroxime	★	1.5 g i.m.	59	58	98	Tupasi et al (1983)
Cefuroxime axetil ester	★	1.5 g orally	10	10	100	Schift et al (1986)
Cefotaxime		0.5 g i.m.	33	33	100	Boakes et al (1981)
		1.0 g i.m.	102	102	100	de Koning et al (1983)
Ceftriaxone		250 mg i.m.	42	42	100	Panikabutra et al (1985)
Ceftizoxime		1 g i.m.	26	26	100	Harrison et al (1984a)
Cefaclor	★	3 g orally	27	25	93	Panikabutra et al (1983)
Cefamandole	★	1 g i.m.	42	30	71	Panikabutra et al (1983)
Rosoxacin		300 mg orally	60	58	97	Lim et al (1984a)
		300 mg orally	45	40	89	Panikabutra et al (1984b)
		300 mg orally	24	21	88	Harrison et al (1984b)
Amoxycillin/clavulanic acid		Amoxycillin 3 g, clavulanic acid 250 mg; two doses at 4-hourly intervals	29	28	97	Lim et al (1984b)
			23	20	87	Lim et al (1986)
Sulbactam	★	Ampicillin 750 mg, Sulbactam 750 mg	14	10	71	Farthing et al (1985)
	★	(Ampicillin 1.125 g, Sulbactam 1.125 g)	6	6	100	Farthing et al (1985)
Thiamphenicol	★★	2.5 g orally	58	57	98	Tupasi et al (1983)
		2.5 g orally	44	19	33	Kim (1984)
		0.5 g i.m. followed by 2.0 g orally	33	32	97	Panikabutra et al (1984a)

★with probenecid in a single oral dose of 1 g
★★not available in United Kingdom or USA
i.m. = intramuscular injection

euphoria in about half of patients treated with a single oral dose of 300 mg; mostly these adverse reactions occur within 1–3 hours and subside within 3 hours (Calubiran et al 1982, Cohen et al 1984). Clearly patients should not drive or operate machinery after taking rosoxacin. Treatment at bedtime may be useful as a way of dealing with these adverse effects. Occasionally there may be gastrointestinal upsets.

Rosoxacin has been shown to induce lesions in weight-bearing joints of young animals receiving high, single or repeated doses. The relevance of this to man is unknown but the manufacturers recommend that frequent repeat doses should not be given to those under 18 years of age (ABPI Data Sheet Compendium 1988–89).

Thiamphenicol is identical in chemical structure to chloramphenicol except that the nitro group of chloramphenicol is replaced by a sulphomethyl group. The therapeutic attention that has been devoted to the drug rests largely on the claim that it does not cause irreversible bone marrow aplasia — dose-dependent reversible depression of haemopoiesis and immunogenesis occurs rarely, but to a greater extent than with chloramphenicol (Garrod et al 1981). Its main advantage over other drugs in PPNG infections is that it is less costly. Ferrari, in his review (Ferrari 1984), came to the conclusion that extensive clinical experience has indicated that a single dose of 2.5 g thiamphenicol causes no detectable blood anomalies and is safe for the treatment of gonococcal infections. Its apparent lack of delayed toxicity, unrelated to dose, the seriously limiting factor in the use of chloramphenicol, appears not to apply to thiamphenicol. Midvedt (1982) comments that, although a case of fatal aplastic anaemia associated with thiamphenicol has been reported in the literature, the incidence of aplastic anaemia in patients taking the drug is close to the background rate for idiopathic aplastic anaemia. It is used effectively and widely in some countries of Europe and in South America. In single dosage the drug appears to have no effect against *C. trachomatis* (Loo et al 1983). Thiamphenicol is not commercially available in the UK or in the United States.

c. With chromosomally-mediated resistant N. gonorrhoeae (CMRNG)
Patients who fail with standard treatments or who are infected with penicillin resistant strains that do not produce beta-lactamase (CMRNG) may be treated with spectinomycin 2.0 g intramuscularly or ceftriaxone 250 mg intramuscularly (CDC 1985).

With the high in vitro resistance of gonococcal strains isolated in Bangkok to a number of antimicrobials (penicillin, tetracycline, erythromycin, trimethoprim/sulphamethoxazole, kanamycin, spectinomycin, thiamphenicol) it has been considered that the adaptation of the gonococcus to antimicrobial selective pressures may mean that single drug treatments of the condition are no longer appropriate and 'combination therapies' need to be evaluated to delay further antimicrobial resistance. The regimen spectinomycin 2.0 g and cefuroxime 1.5 g intramuscularly plus probenecid was suggested for Bangkok and wherever such trends may be found in other countries (Brown et al 1982).

Oropharyngeal and rectal gonorrhoea
The treatment of rectal gonorrhoea in men is discussed also in Chapter 38. Single-dose treatment is generally considered to be less effective in the treatment of oropharyngeal infection in both sexes and in rectal infection in the male than in uncomplicated genital gonorrhoea (Scott & Stone 1966, Ödegaard & Gundersen 1973). Infection in these sites usually can be eliminated by a course of antibiotics given by mouth; either ampicillin or talampicillin (250 mg) may be given

4 times daily for 5 to 7 days (John & Jefferiss 1973). About 95% of gonococcal infections in homosexual men are serogroup WII, which is associated with the Mtr phenotype; such strains appear to have been selected as a result of selective pressure such as antibiotic usage, and their characteristics could account for the high failure rate when single dosage regimens are used in homosexual men (see Ch. 14).

Pharyngeal infection with PPNG has been treated successfully with cefuroxime in a dosage of 1.5 g daily by intramuscular injection for 3 days (Lindberg et al 1982). Ceftriaxone 250 mg intramuscularly once is also recommended for PPNG infections of this anatomical site (CDC 1985).

Co-trimoxazole has been accorded by the Centers for Disease Control a special role for the treatment of pharyngeal infections due to PPNG (CDC 1985). It is recommended to be given in a single dose of 9 tablets (each tablet containing 80 mg trimethoprim and 400 mg sulphamethoxazole, total daily dose trimethoprim 720 mg, sulphamethoxazole 3600 mg) daily for 5 days. In the 1985 CDC Guidelines it is, however, given second place to ceftriaxone. It should be remembered that co-trimoxazole is specially liable to induce cutaneous reactions in patients with the Acquired Immune Deficiency Syndrome, whether or not they have Kaposi's sarcoma (Idanpaan-Heikkila & Tuomisto 1985) and that its toxic effects are at least equal to those of sulphonamides (Mandell & Sande 1985b).

Post-gonococcal urethritis (PGU) in the male
The management of this complication is dealt with in Chapter 17. In an attempt to reduce the incidence of post-gonococcal urethritis, a 5 to 7-day course of oxytetracycline may be given, starting on the day after giving treatment for gonorrhoea, to avoid the mutually antagonistic effects of penicillin and tetracycline.

Complicated gonorrhoea

1. Epididymitis
If inflammation is severe, the patient should be admitted to hospital and kept in bed. A scrotal support should be worn to relieve pain. It may be necessary during or after treatment to aspirate a secondary hydrocele. Antimicrobial therapy consists of either benzylpenicillin 600 mg (1 million units) 6-hourly intramuscularly; co-trimoxazole B.P. 2 tablets twice-daily; or doxycycline 100 mg 8-hourly until the condition has resolved; ordinarily treatment will not be continued for longer than 5–10 days. The treatment of epididymitis caused by PPNG has not been adequately assessed. The authors recommend cefuroxime in a dosage of 1.5 g daily by intramuscular injection for 5 to 7 days.

2. Bartholinitis and abscess

The patient may need admission to hospital if the inflammation is severe and she should be treated with benzylpenicillin in the dosage given for epididymitis. In less severe cases there is usually a response to a course of oral antibiotics. If an abscess persists, this is best treated by aspiration during antimicrobial therapy or by marsupialization if this fails.

3. Pelvic inflammatory disease including salpingitis

See Chapter 23.

4. Disseminated gonococcal infection (DGI) with or without arthritis and/or skin lesions

The patient should be admitted to hospital, the affected joint(s) rested in a position of function, and treatment with benzylpenicillin 600 mg (1 million units) 6-hourly intramuscularly instituted. Usually within 48 hours the condition of the patient improves and oral treatment may be substituted and continued for 10–14 days. In such cases the gonococci have been found to be very sensitive to penicillin. In the case of those allergic to penicillin, co-trimoxazole may be suitable in a dose of 2 tablets twice-daily by mouth. When vomiting is troublesome co-trimoxazole may be given, diluted as an infusion, intravenously. Two 5 ml vials of co-trimoxazole (e.g. Bactrim for infusion, Roche; Septrin for infusion, Wellcome), each containing 80 mg trimethoprim B.P. and 400 mg sulphamethoxazole B.P. are diluted with 250 ml infusion solution (e.g. sodium chloride injection B.P. 0.9%) and given intravenously over a period of approximately one and a half hours (ABPI Data Sheet Compendium 1988–89, Datapharm, London).

For the treatment of disseminated gonococcal infection due to beta-lactamase producing *N. gonorrhoeae* (PPNG) a number of alternative treatments are available and given for 7 days:

a. Cefuroxime 750 mg given by intramuscular 8-hourly injection for 7 days; or
b. Cefotaxime 500 mg given by intravenous injection 6-hourly for at least 7 days (CDC 1985); or
c. Ceftriaxone 1.0 g given by intravenous injection once-daily for 7 days (CDC 1985).

Following these schedules of treatment it is often essential to deal with a possibly co-existent chlamydial infection by giving afterwards the following: doxycycline 200 mg initially by mouth after food, followed by 100 mg once-daily for 7 days. Tetracycline, oxytetracycline and erythromycin may be given alternatively for 7-day courses.

Endocarditis and meningitis

In the pre-antibiotic era 4–10% of all cases of endocarditis were due to *N. gonorrhoeae* (John et al 1977) and in one series of 38 cases encountered over a 12-year period, 10 (26%) infections were due to this organism (Williams 1938). Since deterioration may occur rapidly in endocarditis — despite apparently appropriate antibiotic treatment — and delay in valve replacement therapy may prove fatal, it is strongly recommended that such patients should be referred early for expert management by a cardiologist and a cardiac surgeon (Report of a Working Party of the British Society for Antimicrobial Chemotherapy 1985). Patients with fever and a heart murmur should have blood cultures — three specimens taken at intervals of several hours — without delay before any antibiotic treatment is given, even if this necessitates referral to hospital. In endocarditis, since in two-thirds of cases the infection is streptococcal, the combination recommended is benzylpenicillin and the aminoglycoside gentamicin, of which the latter will require regular monitoring of blood levels. If the gonococcus isolated has a minimal bactericidal concentration (MBC) of 1 mg or less/l the gentamicin may be stopped in 2 weeks as recommended for penicillin-sensitive streptococcal infections. The benzylpenicillin should be given by intravenous bolus injection of 7.2 g (12 million units) daily in 6 divided doses (4-hourly). A total of one month's treatment is advised, and probenecid may be administered concurrently. Whether the gonococcus has or has not a reduced sensitivity to penicillin (MBC more than 1 mg/l) eradication of the infection in endocarditis is frequently impossible and valve replacement will be necessary.

In meningitis, treatment with intravenous penicillin should continue for 2 weeks.

In the case of PPNG infections, CMRNG infections, or in patients allergic to penicillin, treatment for these serious conditions will require to be devised on an individual basis with consultations between microbiologist, cardiologist and cardiac surgeon. As in all gonococcal infections contact-tracing is essential.

TREATMENT OF PREGNANT WOMEN WITH GONORRHOEA

Care is needed in giving any drug in pregnancy. Penicillin is considered generally safe, and benzylpenicillin given intramuscularly in a dose of 1 million units 6-hourly for 12 doses is effective. Erythromycin is also considered to be safe although cure rates may be low, say 70% (Brown 1978) and absorption uncertain; a dose of 500 mg erythromycin base 6-hourly orally for 7 days is an alternative in patients hypersensitive to penicillin.

Ceftriaxone 250 mg intramuscularly as a single dose will be necessary for PPNG infections. Pregnant women who are allergic to penicillin, cephalosporins or probenecid should be treated with spectinomycin 2.0 g intramuscularly as a single dose and be given erythromycin (base) 500 mg by mouth 4 times daily for 7 days (CDC 1985).

CONJUNCTIVITIS OF THE NEWBORN (OPHTHALMIA NEONATORUM)

Combined local and parenteral therapy is necessary:

Local: frequent, repeated instillations of sterile normal saline into affected eye. Topical antibiotic treatment may produce sensitization reactions and should on this account be avoided.

Parenteral: benzylpenicillin should be given in a dosage of 30 mg (50 000 units) per kg body weight per day in 2 or 3 divided doses by intramuscular injection until cure is obtained, generally within a week (McCracken & Eichenwald 1974).

For the treatment of neonatal conjunctivitis associated with PPNG, cefuroxime in a dosage of 100 mg/kg/day by intramuscular injection in 3 divided doses for 7 days has proved useful (Dunlop et al 1980). In developing countries where hospital facilities are limited, kanamycin given as a single intramuscular injection of 75 mg or 150 mg, with gentamicin eye ointment (1% w/v) applied every 30 minutes for the first 10 hours and then 4 times per day (Fransen et al 1984) for 3 days is effective in treating infection with PPNG and non-PPNG. Possible ototoxicity of kanamycin, however, must be taken into account.

Both parents must be examined and treated appropriately.

TESTS OF CURE

After treatment every patient should be carefully examined to ensure that the infection has been cured.

Follow-up tests in the male

In any given area it is essential first to assess the cure rate of the treatment schedule adopted as a routine. In general these assessments are made by the rapid disappearance of signs and/or symptoms and their continued absence over 14 days. Persistence of urethral signs and/or symptoms necessitates urethral cultures, taken preferably after the urine has been retained for three hours, or the immediate culture of exudate from the first urine voided. Such trials are possible only in some centres.

When confidence in a schedule has been obtained the following routines are satisfactory: any urethral discharge should be examined and the urine inspected for the presence of pus and/or 'threads' on the seventh day. These tests should be repeated three weeks later and serological tests for syphilis should be carried out then and again two months later.

To determine the efficacy of treatment of rectal and pharyngeal gonorrhoea, cultures should be taken from the anatomical sites affected until three consecutive cultures, taken at weekly intervals, are negative.

Follow-up tests in the female

Two consecutive series of cultures from the urethra, cervix and rectum should be taken at weekly intervals before assuring cure. If positive on first attendance, the culture from the fauces should be taken twice, one and two weeks after treatment.

It is often difficult to distinguish between treatment failure and reinfection. By convention, the finding of positive tests within two weeks of treatment is regarded as a failure of treatment if the patient does not admit to further sexual intercourse. Where facilities exist this convention could be very usefully supplemented by the use of serovar determination to differentiate between reinfection and treatment failure (see Ch. 14).

TREATMENT WHEN DIAGNOSIS OF GONORRHOEA IS SUSPECTED ON EPIDEMIOLOGICAL GROUNDS

Accurate diagnosis and treatment is the approach of choice when adequate facilities exist. Treatment before diagnosis is not desirable as a routine even in contacts, except when there are special problems. For example a contact of a known case of gonorrhoea may be treated if unlikely to re-attend. In such a case a form of treatment known to produce high cure rates in that locality (say of 95%) may be justified. In the case of contacts of patients with an infection due to PPNG, then treatment with spectinomycin or cephalosporin is justified. Follow-up is important also.

REFERENCES

CLINICAL FEATURES

Ackerman A B, Miller R C, Shapiro L 1965 Gonococcemia and its cutaneous manifestations. Archives of Dermatology 91: 227–232

Graber W J, Sanford J P, Ziff M 1960 Sex incidence of gonococcal arthritis. Arthritis and Rheumatism 3: 309–313
Harkness A H 1948 The pathology of gonorrhoea. British Journal of Venereal Diseases 24: 137–147

Holmes K K, Counts G W, Beaty H N 1971 Disseminated gonococcal infection. Clinical review. Annals of Internal Medicine 74: 979–993

John J F, Nichols J T, Eisenhower E A, Farrar W E 1977 Gonococcal endocarditis. Sexually Transmitted Diseases 4: 84–88

Kimball M W, Knee S 1970 Gonococcal perihepatitis in a male. The Fitz-Hugh-Curtis syndrome. New England Journal of Medicine 282: 1082–1084

McMillan A, McNeillage G, Gilmour H M, Lee F D 1983 Histology of rectal gonorrhoea in men, with a note on anorectal infection with *Neisseria meningitidis*. Journal of Clinical Pathology 36: 511–514

Neilsen R, Søndergaard J, Ullman S 1975 Asymptomatic male and female gonorrhoea. Acta Dermato-venereologica 55: 499–501

Nelson J D, Mohs E, Dajani A S, Plotkin S A 1976 Gonorrhea in preschool- and school-aged children. Report of the Prepubertal Gonorrhea Cooperative Study Group. Journal of the American Medical Association 236: 1359–1364

Osoba A O, Alausa O 1976 Gonococcal urethral stricture and watering-can perineum. British Journal of Venereal Diseases 52: 387–393

Report of a Working Party of the British Society for Antimicrobial Chemotherapy (Simmons N A, Cawson R A, Eykyn S J, Geddes A M, Littler W A, Oakley C M, Shanson D C) 1985 Antibiotic treatment of streptococcal and staphylococcal endocarditis. Lancet ii: 815–817

Scherer R, Braun-Falco O 1976 Alternative pathway complement activation: a possible mechanism inducing skin lesions in benign gonococcal sepsis. British Journal of Dermatology 95: 303–309

Seifert M H, Warin A P, Miller A 1974 Articular and cutaneous manifestations of gonorrhoea. Annals of the Rheumatic Diseases 33: 140–146

Stolz E, Schuller J 1974 Gonococcal oro- and nasopharyngeal infection. British Journal of Venereal Diseases 50: 104–108

Thompson J, Dunbar J M, van Gent A, van Furth R 1981 Disseminated gonococcal infection due to a beta-lactamase producing strain of *Neisseria gonorrhoeae*. A case report. British Journal of Venereal Diseases 57: 325–326

Wiesner P J, Tronca E, Bonin P, Pedersen A H B, Holmes K K 1973 Clinical spectrum of pharyngeal gonococcal infection. New England Journal of Medicine 288: 181–185

Williams R H 1938 Gonococcic endocarditis. A study of twelve cases with ten postmortem examinations. Archives of Internal Medicine (Chicago) 61: 26–38

TREATMENT

Al-Egaily S, Dunlop E M C, Rodin P, Seth A D 1978 Talampicillin and probenecid compared with ampicillin and probenecid for the treatment of gonococcal urethritis in men. British Journal of Venereal Diseases 54: 243–246

Arya O P, Rees E, Percival A, Alergant C D, Annels E H, Turner G C 1978 Epidemiology in treatment of gonorrhoea caused by penicillinase-producing strains in Liverpool. British Journal of Venereal Diseases 54: 28–35

Ashford W A, Potts D W, Adams H J W et al 1981 Spectinomycin-resistant penicillinase-producing *Neisseria gonorrhoeae*. Lancet ii: 1035–1037

Baytch H 1974 Minocycline in single dose therapy in the treatment of gonococcal urethritis in male patients. Medical Journal of Australia 1: 831–832

Boakes A J, Burrows J, Eykyn S J, Phillips I 1981 Cefotaxime for spectinomycin resistant *Neisseria gonorrhoeae*. Correspondence, Lancet ii: 96

Brown S 1978 *Neisseria gonorrhoeae* and gonococcal infections. Technical Report Series 616, World Health Organization, Geneva, p 99

Brown S, Warnnissorn T, Biddle J, Panikabutra K, Traisupa A 1982 Antimicrobial resistance of *Neisseria gonorrhoeae* in Bangkok: is single drug treatment passé? Lancet ii: 1366–1368

Calubiran O V, Crisologo-Vizconde L B, Tupasi T E, Torres C A, Limson B M 1982 Treatment of uncomplicated gonorrhoea in women: Comparison of rosoxacin and spectinomycin. British Journal of Venereal Diseases 58: 231–235

Centers for Disease Control (CDC) 1985 STD treatment guidelines. Morbidity and Mortality Weekly Report (supplement) 34; No.4S

Cohen A I, Rein M F, Noble R C 1984 A comparison of rosoxacin with ampicillin and probenecid in the treatment of uncomplicated gonorrhoea. Sexually Transmitted Diseases 11: 24–27

Crider S R, Kilpatrick M E, Harrison W O, Kerbs S B J, Berg S W 1984 A comparison of penicillin G plus a beta-lactamase inhibitor (Sulbactam) with spectinomycin for treatment of urethritis caused by penicillinase-producing *Neisseria gonorrhoeae*. Sexually Transmitted Diseases 11: 314–317

de Koning G A J, Tio D, van den Hoek J A R, van Klingeren B 1983 Single lg dose of cefotaxime in the treatment of infections due to penicillinase-producing strains of *Neisseria gonorrhoeae*. British Journal of Venereal Diseases 59: 100–102

Duncan W C, Glicksman J M, Knox J M, Holder W R 1971 Treatment of gonorrhoea with a single oral dose of minocycline. British Journal of Venereal Diseases 47: 364–366

Dunlop E M C, Rodin P, Seth A D, Kolator B 1980 Ophthalmia neonatorum due to beta-lactamase producing gonococci. Short reports, British Medical Journal 281: 483

Easmon C S F, Ison C A, Bellinger C M, Harris J W 1982 Emergence of resistance after spectinomycin treatment for gonorrhoea due to beta-lactamase-producing strain of *Neisseria gonorrhoeae*. British Medical Journal 284: 1604–1605

Farthing C, Thin R N, Smith S, Phillips I 1985 Two regimens of sultamicillin in treating uncomplicated gonorrhoea. Genitourinary Medicine 61: 44–47

Ferrari V 1984 Introductory address — salient features of thiamphenicol: review of clinical pharmacokinetics and toxicity. Sexually Transmitted Diseases 11: 336–339

Fransen L, Nsanze H, D'Costa L, Brunham R C, Ronald A R, Piot P 1984 Single dose kanamycin therapy of gonococcal ophthalmia neonatorum. Lancet ii: 1234–1236

Garrod L P, Lambert H P, O'Grady F 1981 Antibiotic and chemotherapy, 5th edn. Churchill Livingstone, Edinburgh, p 165–168

Handsfield H H, Murphy V L 1983 Comparative study of ceftriaxone and spectinomycin for treatment of uncomplicated gonorrhoea in men. Lancet ii: 67–70

Harrison W O, Sanchez P L, Lancaster D J, Kerbs S B J, Berg S W 1984a Ceftizoxime (FK-749) in effective therapy for urethritis caused by penicillinase-producing *Neisseria gonorrhoeae*. Sexually Transmitted Diseases 11: 30–31

Harrison W O, Wignall F S, Kerbs S B J, Berg S W 1984b Oral rosoxacin for the treatment of penicillin-resistant gonorrhoea. Lancet i: 566

Idanpaan-Heikkila J E, Tuuomisto J 1985 Sulphonamides and trimethoprim. Other urinary antiseptics — nalidixic acid and congeners. In: Dukes M N G, Beeley L (eds)

Side effects of drugs, Annual 9, Ch 30, Miscellaneous antibacterial and antiviral drugs, p 261–265

John J, Jefferiss F J G 1973 Treatment of ano-rectal gonorrhoea with ampicillin. British Journal of Venereal Diseases 49: 362–363

John J F, Nichols J T, Eisenhower E A, Farrar W E 1977 Gonococcal endocarditis. Sexually Transmitted Diseases 4: 84–88

Kim J-H 1984 Comparison of thiamphenicol and spectinomycin in the treatment of uncomplicated gonorrhea in men. Sexually Transmitted Diseases 11: 386–390

Lim K B, Rajan V S, Giam Y C, Lui E O, Sng E A, Yeo K L 1984a Treatment of uncomplicated gonorrhoea with rosoxacin (acrosoxacin). British Journal of Venereal Diseases 60: 157–160

Lim K B, Rajan V S, Giam Y C, Lui E O, Sng E A, Yeo K L 1984b Two dose Augmentin treatment of acute gonorrhoea in men. British Journal of Venereal Diseases 60: 161–163

Lim K B, Thirumoorthy T, Lee C T, Sng E H, Tan T 1986 Three regimens of procaine penicillin G, Augmentin and probenecid compared for treating acute gonorrhoea in men. Genitourinary Medicine 62: 82–85

Lindberg M, Ringeritz O, Sandström E 1982 Treatment of pharyngeal gonorrhoea due to beta-lactamase-producing gonococci. British Journal of Venereal Diseases 58: 101–104

Loo P S, Felmingham D, Ridgway G L, Oriel J D 1983 Treatment of gonococcal infections in men with single dose thiamphenicol. Correspondence, British Journal of Venereal Diseases 59: 407

McCracken G H, Eichenwald H F 1974 Antimicrobial therapy: Therapeutic recommendations and a review of newer drugs. Journal of Pediatrics 85: 297–312

McCutchan J A, Adler M W, Berrie J R H 1982 Penicillinase-producing Neisseria gonorrhoeae in Great Britain 1977–1981: alarming increase in incidence and recent development of endemic transmission. British Medical Journal 285: 337–340

Mandell G L, Sande M A 1985a The penicillins. In: Gilman A G, Goodman L S, Rall T W, Murad F (eds) The Pharmacological basis of therapeutics, 7th edn. Macmillan New York, p 1115–1137

Mandell G L, Sande M A 1985b Trimethoprim-sulfamethoxazole. In: Gilman A G, Goodman L S, Rall T W, Murad F (eds) The pharmacological basis of therapeutics, 7th edn. Macmillan, New York, p 1104–1108

Masterton G, Schofield C B S 1976 Minocycline hydrochloride (Minocin) as a single-dose oral treatment of uncomplicated gonorrhoea in men. British Journal of Venereal Diseases 52: 43–45

Midvedt T 1982 Other antibiotic drugs. In: Dukes M N G, Ellis J (eds) Side effects of drugs, Annual 6. Excerpta Medica, Amsterdam, 247–252

Ödegaard K, Gundersen T 1973 Gonococcal pharyngeal infection. British Journal of Venereal Diseases 49: 350–352

Panikabutra K, Ariyarit C, Chitwarakorn A, Saensanoh C 1983 Cefaclor and cefamandole as alternatives to spectinomycin in the treatment of men with uncomplicated gonorrhoea. British Journal of Venereal Diseases 59: 298–301

Panikabutra K, Ariyarit C, Chitwarakorn A, Soonthararak A, Saensanoh C 1984a Single-dose treatment of uncomplicated gonorrhea in men with intramuscular and oral thiamphenicol. Sexually Transmitted Diseases 11: 404–406

Panikabutra K, Ariyarit C, Chitwarakorn A, Saensanoh C 1984b Rosoxacin in the treatment of uncomplicated gonorrhoea in men. British Journal of Venereal Diseases 60: 231–234

Panikabutra K, Ariyarit C, Chitwarakorn A, Saensanoh C, Wongba C 1985 Randomised comparative study of ceftriaxone and spectinomycin in gonorrhoea. Genitourinary Medicine 61: 106–108

Porter I A, Rutherford H W 1977 Treatment of uncomplicated gonorrhoea with spectinomycin hydrochloride (Trobicin). British Journal of Venereal Diseases 53: 115–117

Price J D, Fluker J L 1978 The efficacy of cefuroxime for the treatment of acute gonorrhoea in men. British Journal of Venereal Diseases 54: 165–167

Report of a Working Party of the British Society for Antimicrobial Chemotherapy (Simmons N A, Cawson R A, Eykyn S J, Geddes A M, Littler W A, Oakley C M, Shanson D C) 1985 Antibiotic treatment of streptococcal and staphylococcal endocarditis. Lancet ii: 815–817

Reynolds F E F (ed) 1985 Martindale, the extra pharmacopoeia. The Pharmaceutical Press, London, p 1101–1110

Sanchez P L, Wignall S, Zajdowicz T R, Kerbs S, Berg S W, Harrison W O 1983 One gram of cefoxitin cures uncomplicated gonococcal urethritis caused by penicillinase-producing Neisseria gonorrhoeae (PPNG). Sexually Transmitted Diseases 10: 135–137

Schift R, van Ulsen J, Ansink-Schipper M L, van Joost Th, Michel M F, Woudstra R K, Stolz E 1986 Comparison of oral treatment of uncomplicated urogenital and rectal gonorrhoea with cefuroxime axetil ester or clavulanic acid potentiated amoxycillin (Augmentin). Genitourinary Medicine 62: 313–317

Scott J, Stone A H 1966 Some observations on the diagnosis of rectal gonorrhoea in both sexes using a selective culture medium. British Journal of Venereal Diseases 42: 103–106

Shahmanesh M, Shukla S R, Phillips I, Westwood A, Thin R N 1986 Ciprofloxacin for treating urethral gonorrhoea in men. Genitourinary Medicine 62: 86–87

Spencer R C, Smith T, Talbot M D 1984 Ceftizoxime in the treatment of uncomplicated gonorrhoea. British Journal of Venereal Diseases 60: 90–91

Taylor P K, Seth A D 1975 Ampicillin plus probenecid compared with procaine penicillin plus probenecid in the treatment of gonorrhoea. British Journal of Venereal Diseases 51: 183–187

Thin R N, Symonds M A E, Shaw E J, Wong J, Hopper P K, Slocombe B 1977 A double blind trial of amoxycillin in the treatment of gonorrhoea. British Journal of Venereal Diseases 53: 118–120

Tupasi T E, Crisologo L B, Torres C A, Calubrian O V, De Jesus I 1983 Cefuroxine, thiamphenicol, spectinomycin and penicillin G in uncomplicated infections due to penicillinase-producing strains of Neisseria gonorrhoeae. British Journal of Venereal Diseases 59: 172–175

Veeravahu M, Sumathipala A H T, Clay J C 1983 Cefoxitin v procaine penicillin in the treatment of uncomplicated gonorrhoea. Correspondence. British Journal of Venereal Diseases 59: 406

Wanas T M, Williams P E O 1986 Oral cefuroxime axetil compared with oral ampicillin in treating acute uncomplicated gonorrhoea. Genitourinary Medicine 62: 221–223

Waugh M A, Cooke E M, Nehaul B B G, Brayson J 1979 Comparison of minocycline and ampicillin in gonococcal

urethritis. British Journal of Venereal Diseases
55: 411–414

Williams R H 1938 Gonococcic endocarditis. A study of
twelve cases with ten postmortem examinations. Archives
of Internal Medicine (Chicago) 61: 26–38

Zajdowicz T R, Sanches P L, Berg S W, Kerbs S B J,
Newquist R L, Harrison W O 1983 Comparison of
ceftriaxone with cefoxitin in the treatment of penicillin-
resistant gonococcal urethritis. British Journal of Venereal
Diseases 59: 176–178

17

Non-gonococcal urethritis, chlamydial infections and other related conditions

Non-gonococcal urethritis (NGU) — synonym, non-specific urethritis (NSU) — is a convenient term to describe the very common condition seen in men and presenting clinically as a purulent or mucopurulent urethral discharge, associated often with the symptom of dysuria, and occurring a few days to a few weeks after intercourse. The urethral discharge in a patient with NGU contains pus cells but *Neisseria gonorrhoeae* cannot be detected by microscopy of Gram-stained films or culture. The term non-specific genital infection (NSGI) has been introduced to include with non-specific urethritis in the male the clinically less clearly defined infection in the female, who may have neither symptom nor easily detected sign.

Non-gonococcal urethritis in males is the most frequently reported sexually transmitted disease in men; in 1983 there were 108 503 cases recorded in the United Kingdom, for example, compared with 75 711 in 1973. As relapses are very common, particularly in those believed to be non-chlamydial in origin, and as primary as well as recurrent infections are recorded as 'new cases' in quarterly returns from clinics the upward trend may be exaggerated since it has occurred at a time when a fall in the number of cases of gonorrhoea has been recorded. NGU varies widely in severity from the clinical point of view, and asymptomatic infections are common. Other genital or ocular infections, likely to share the same aetiology include, in the male, epididymitis and possibly, although not proven to be so, chronic abacterial prostatitis and, in the female, cervicitis and pelvic inflammatory disease. In some forms of non-gonococcal ophthalmia neonatorum (conjunctivitis of the newborn) chlamydia is the infecting organism and is transmitted from the genital tract of the mother during parturition. A chlamydial conjunctivitis is seen also in all age groups and in male homosexuals a proctitis may occur.

AETIOLOGY

There is experimental evidence that at least two organisms, *Chlamydia trachomatis* (Ch. 2) and to a lesser extent *Ureaplasma urealyticum* (Ch. 2) have a role in the aetiology of NGU, although the extent of their involvement or indeed what other agents, e.g. *Mycoplasma hominis* and *M. genitalium*, may have a role is not yet clear.

FAMILY: CHLAMYDIACEAE

Genus: Chlamydia

Organisms belonging to the genus *Chlamydia* are the cause of ocular, genital and systemic diseases in man. Once regarded as viruses because of their obligate intracellular growth, many of their fundamental properties, however, are those of bacteria. Two species are recognized, viz. *Chlamydia trachomatis* and *Chlamydia psittaci*: both are obligate intracellular parasites which cannot by themselves alone synthesize the high energy compounds adenosine triphosphate (ATP) and guanosine triphosphate (GTP) and multiply by binary fission. Now regarded as Gram-negative bacteria, *Chlamydia* contain DNA and RNA; possess enzymes; contain cell wall material; have a developmental cycle; and share common antigens. DNA homology between *C. psittaci* and *C. trachomatis*, however, is only 10%, showing that these two organisms are derived from different ancestors (Kingsbury & Weiss 1968, Becker 1978); placed in the same genus, however, on the basis of their similarities they may be considered as examples of convergent evolution. *C. trachomatis*, unlike *C. psittaci*, is sensitive to sulphadiazine and D-cycloserine and forms compact glycogen-containing inclusions that can be stained with iodine. DNA homology within *Chlamydia trachomatis* strains lies between 96–100% (Kingsbury & Weiss 1968, Becker 1978) and supports their classification as a single species. As obligate intracellular parasites chlamydia can only be isolated and grown in suitable host cells. Early workers used the yolk sac of the embryonated chicken egg, but tissue culture is more suitable. Insofar as sexually transmitted diseases are concerned, *C. trachomatis* is the more important of the two species. Of the three biovars of this species known, one is found as a latent infection in mice and two which concern man have no animal reservoir, viz. *C. trachomatis biovar trachoma* and *C. trachomatis biovar lymphogranuloma*.

Developmental cycle of Chlamydia

All chlamydiae, unique among prokaryotic cells, undergo a developmental cycle in the cytoplasm of eukaryotic cells. Two main structures in the growth cycle are recognized: the elementary bodies (EB) which are the infectious stage of the developmental cycle; and the reticulate bodies (RB) which are concerned solely with the multiplication of chlamydial populations within the eukaryotic cell.

The EB are spherical rigid-walled structures 200–300 nm in diameter, packed tightly with DNA, thus rendering the core electron dense when examined with the electron microscope. The dense DNA core is surrounded by a cytoplasmic membrane, external to which is an outer envelope, which in *C. psittaci* has been shown to have small surface projections topographically related to 'button' structures on the concave inner surface of the outer envelope. These structures may be concerned with the adhesion of chlamydiae to the host cell (Ward 1983).

Infection of the host cell is initiated by close adhesion of EB to the host cell surface and entry of the attached EB is by endocytosis, where the invading organisms lie within a vacuole formed by the host membrane. The susceptibility of the cell to infection has been found to be altered by prostaglandins and other substances; an observation which may be of clinical importance, given the biochemical changes observed during the menstrual cycle for example (Ward 1983).

Within 6–9 hours of ingestion the EB enlarge to form RB with a diameter of about 1 μm. Electron microscopy shows the structure of the mature RB to be essentially that of a Gram-negative bacterium. RB multiply by binary fission which is kept in balance with host cell metabolic activity since the organism requires ATP from the host cell. The outer envelope, a highly flexible structure, interacts with the host cell and large amounts of the envelope bud off the RB surface to form vesicles and inclusions containing chlamydial antigens which may become incorporated into the host cell membranes to be excreted by the host cell during the chlamydial developmental cycle (Richmond & Stirling 1981). A characteristic of infection with both *C. trachomatis* and *C. psittaci* is the tendency of both species to produce persistent infection. It has been found in vitro that chlamydia competes with the host cell for nutrients but the host cell is not killed and infected cells can divide although they have a longer generation time than uninfected cells, and give rise to infected progeny (Horoshak & Moulder 1978). Limiting of essential nutrients may greatly extend the duration of the growth cycle. In this way factors compromising the host's capacity for macromolecular synthesis may spare essential precursors in the host's soluble pools for the biosynthetic needs of the infection; alternatively factors stimulating proliferation of host cells may raise the level of the intracellular pools above subsistence levels and thereby activate latent infection (Hatch 1975). Such mechanisms may give rise to persistently infected cells, and chlamydial antigens incorporated into host cell membrane may offer continuing stimulation for the immune system as well as a target for immune attack (Ward 1983).

By 20 hours after infection some of the RB undergo reorganization within the expanding inclusion to form infectious EB; these reorganizing RB have been termed 'intermediate bodies'. Ultimately the mature inclusion may occupy some three-quarters of the host cell volume and contain up to 10^4 chlamydial particles; release of these particles results from cell lyses. In persistently infected cells small numbers of EB may be released by budding through the host cell membrane.

Biovars and serovars of Chlamydia trachomatis

Chlamydia contain genetic information for several hundred different proteins and as a result are antigenically complex. Sensitive immunoblotting and radioimmune precipitating techniques have enabled the identification of some chlamydial antigens reactive both with patients sera and monoclonal antibodies. A commonly used complement fixation test (CF) for example is genus-specific, and chemical characterization of the genus-reactive antigen indicates that it is a lipopolysaccharide similar to that of Gram-negative bacteria (Ward 1983).

On the basis of a micro-immunofluorescent test (micro IF) *C. trachomatis* is classified into 15 serotypes, and the type-specific antigens have been identified as trypsin-labile proteins at the surface of the EB. Clinically distinct infections are associated with different serovars of *C. trachomatis*.

In hyperendemic trachoma *C. trachomatic biovar trachoma* contains serovars A, B, Ba and C; in ocular infection of sexually transmitted origin (paratrachoma) or genital tract infection *C. trachomatis biovar trachoma* contains serovars D, E, F, G, H, I and K; and in lymphogranuloma venereum, isolates contain the LGV serovars L-l, L-2 and L-3. Cross-reactions to a lesser titre in the micro-IF tests are found, with other serotypes forming part of the antigenic complex being studied (e.g. C, J, H, I and A are serologically related to the C complex). Molecular explanation of these and other reactions will require detailed characterization of proteins at the EB surface. Since chlamydial antigens show little serological cross-reaction with other bacterial genera the prospects of developing a useful diagnostic test for chlamydia antibody are thought to be good (Ward 1983).

Disease due to Chlamydia trachomatis biovar trachoma
(tropical trachoma, serovars A, B, Ba and C)
In hyperendemic tropical trachoma, due to *biovar trachoma* (serovars A, B, Ba and C), the organisms are spread by eye-to-eye transmission particularly in unhygienic conditions, affecting about 500×10^6 people and causing blindness in some 2×10^6. Chlamydia require rapid transmission in moist conditions and hyperendemic trachoma occurs in conditions of 'ocular promiscuity' — that is to say in conditions that favour the frequent, unrestricted and indiscriminate mixing of ocular contacts or of ocular discharges (Jones 1975, Note 17.1)

Disease due to C. trachomatis biovar trachoma (ocular or genital infections) serovars D, E, F, G, H, I, K
The ocular or genital infections of western countries, on the other hand, tend to occur when there is frequent mixing of genital contacts or discharges with occasional transfer to the eye (Jones 1975). These chlamydial infections, due to serovars D–K, are predominantly genital and the incidence of both adult chlamydial conjunctivitis and conjunctivitis of the newborn, with or without involvement of other sites e.g. nasopharynx, are dependent upon the incidence of genital infections in the adult population and, in the case of infants, in their mothers (Viswalingam et al 1983).

Although mainly genital and, either alone or with *N. gonorrhoeae*, causes of pelvic inflammatory disease, these organisms may also cause perihepatitis in the form of the Curtis-Fitz-Hugh syndrome (Ch. 23). In this syndrome the combination of right upper quadrant abdominal pain and perihepatitis occurs in association with genital tract infection (Bolton & Darougar 1983).

There is evidence also which suggests that chlamydiae may be a cause of peripheral and axial forms of human arthritis, either in association with lymphogranuloma venereum or as a reactive arthritis (Keat et al 1983), as in Reiter's disease (Ch. 19).

Disease due to C. trachomatis biovar LGV
(lymphogranuloma venereum) serovars L-1, L-2 and L-3
Biovar LGV is sexually transmitted (serovars L-1, L-2 and L-3) and in contrast to *biovar trachoma*, which is pathogenic to the squamocolumnar cells of mucous membrane, it causes primarily a disease of the lymphatic tissue, involving characteristically the lymph nodes of the genito-anal region (Ch. 23).

Psittacosis, a disease due to Chlamydia psittaci
Chlamydia psittaci causes a disease (psittacosis) in parrots and certain other birds. Psittacosis in man may arise when infected dust or droplets are inhaled; illness ranges from an 'influenza-like' syndrome with general malaise, fever, anorexia, rigors, sore throat and head-ache and photophobia, to a severe illness with delirium and a pneumonia with numerous well-demarcated areas of consolidation.

All chlamydial infections have a tendency to be persistent as chronic or clinically inapparent forms.

FAMILY: MYCOPLASMATACEAE

Genus I: *Mycoplasma*
Genus II: *Ureaplasma*

The two genera within this family, *Mycoplasma* and *Ureaplasma*, are characterized by being totally devoid of cell walls and being bounded by a plasma membrane only (Razin & Freundt 1984). Although Gram-negative they stain poorly with aniline dyes and are best observed in Giemsa-stained smears. Both genera can grow in cell-free medium, requiring cholesterol or a related sterol for growth. The basic medium required is a peptone-enriched beef heart infusion broth containing also horse serum and yeast extract as well as penicillin to inhibit bacterial growth. In broth colonies grow best under atmospheric conditions, but solid media are best incubated in a carbon-dioxide enriched atmosphere. The metabolic activity of mycoplasmas can be used to detect their growth in broth. Mycoplasmas metabolize *arginine* to form ammonia, and ureaplasmas produce urease that breaks down *urea* to form ammonia.

Mycoplasma
A number of species of *Mycoplasma* are found in association with human infection or disease, and in the case of urogenital infection interest has concentrated on *Mycoplasma hominis* and *Mycoplasma genitalium*. In the case of non-gonococcal urethritis, attention is, however, centred on *Ureaplasma urealyticum* where evidence suggesting that this species is a cause is strong although the organism is of low invasiveness, causing a recognizable infection in a small proportion of colonized men (Taylor-Robinson & McCormack 1980).

Ureaplasma
Members of the genus *Ureaplasma* are distinguished by their ability to hydrolyse urea and this is the minimum requirement for assigning a new isolate to the genus. The name *Ureaplasma urealyticum* has been given to the single human species so far identified in this new genus. Serologically distinct serovars are recognized and include in Group A, serovars 2, 4, 5, 7, 8, 9, K2 and U24 and in Group B, serovars 1, 3 and 6. The subdivision is consistent with the results of DNA hybridization. The species occurs predominantly in the mouth, respiratory tract and urogenital tract (Ch. 2).

Both *M. hominis* and *U. urealyticum* are present on the genital mucosa of over half of sexually experienced adults (Taylor-Robinson & McCormack 1980) and it is against this background that their role, and particularly that of *U. urealyticum*, in non-gonococcal urethritis will be considered in later paragraphs. Colonization of the newborn is detected more often in those delivered vaginally than in those delivered by caesarean section (Klein et al 1969). Colonization does not persist and there is a progressive decrease with age in the proportion of infants colonized. Both mycoplasmas and ureaplasmas are seldom found in the genito-urinary tact in prepubertal boys (e.g. 2%) but more often in prepubertal girls (e.g. 11%) (Lee et al 1974).

Colonization, however, increases as a result of sexual contact. Thus, in a study of 156 young American women who had never had genital contact, about 6% yielded ureaplasmas, compared with about 27% who had experienced genital apposition without vaginal penetration. In the case of those who had experienced sexual intercourse, in those who had one partner the colonization rate was about 38%; two partners about 55%; and three or more partners 75% (McCormack et al 1975). In the case of normal men, Boston college students, those who had not experienced sexual intercourse were found to be virtually free from mycoplasmas. Amongst those who had experienced sexual intercourse colonization with ureaplasma was significantly more prevalent and rose in relation to the number of sexual partners, ranging from about 19% in those who had had sexual intercourse with one woman to about 56% of those who had experienced intercourse with more than 14 (McCormack et al 1973). Subsequent work suggests that the prevalence of both *M. hominis* and *U. urealyticum* diminish after the menopause (Taylor-Robinson & McCormack 1980).

CLINICAL AND MICROBIOLOGICAL STUDIES ON THE AETIOLOGY OF NGU

Results of studies in NGU in men have given overall isolation rates for *C. trachomatis* varying from 23 to 57% (Oriel et al 1976), while an isolation rate aproaching 70% was found in patients with a 'frank' urethral discharge (Alani et al 1977). The isolation rate in patients with gonococcal urethritis is approximately 10 to 30% (Oriel et al 1976) while in control groups it is usually less than 5%. Significantly more pairs of sexual partners give the same chlamydial culture result than give different results, and the chlamydial isolation rate is higher among men admitting a casual sexual contact than in men claiming only regular partners (Alani et al 1977). These findings provide evidence for sexual trans-

mission of *C. trachomatis* and for its aetiological role in NGU.

Indirect evidence for the association of *C. trachomatis* with NGU is provided by serological studies. The micro-immunofluorescence test used to demonstrate the existence of serotypes (3 of LGV, 4 of tropical trachoma, and 7 associated with sexually transmitted oculogenital and genital infections) can be used also to detect serum antibody (Holmes et al 1975). With this technique the positivity rates in patients with NGU, gonococcal urethritis, and no urethritis were 55%, 79% and 38% respectively; the corresponding isolation rates for *C. trachomatis* were 42%, 19% and 7% respectively. The serotype of the chlamydial isolate correlated with the specificity of the serum antibody.

An increase in serum antibody gave good correlation with the isolation of *C. trachomatis*. When paired sera were examined, conversion from negative to positive was found in 54% and a four-fold rise in titre in 30% of patients from whom *C. trachomatis* was isolated, whereas only 4% of patients with negative culture demonstrated sero-conversion or a four-fold rise in titre (Holmes et al 1975). In *C. trachomatis* infection of the urethra the antigenic stimulus is weak and results in a modest antibody response, with some 10–20% of men developing no detectable specific antibodies at all, although many studies have reported antibodies more frequently at higher titres in men with urethritis than in those with no apparent disease. In men experiencing their first attack, a number develop an IgM response (Wang et al 1977); in subsequent attacks IgG may develop early in the infection but IgM may not be demonstrated. The complement fixation test has proved of little value (Treharne et al 1983).

Among patients whose cultures failed to yield *C. trachomatis*, antibody prevalence correlated with the number of past sex partners and with previous NGU: this could, in part, account for the high prevalence of antibody in patients with gonococcal urethritis. There is also an association between the presence of *C. trachomatis* in the urethra and the development of post-gonococcal urethritis.

Although these cultural and serological studies suggest that *C. trachomatis* is a significant cause of NGU, its exact pathological role is difficult to establish unequivocally: it could be argued that chlamydiae normally lead a commensal existence in the genital tract but may, on occasions, act as opportunistic pathogens. Alternatively, their numbers may simply increase when another infection develops, making their detection easier.

The same arguments can be applied to the role of *Ureaplasma urealyticum* in NGU. Studies on the isolation of *U. urealyticum* have given isolation rates ranging from approximately 20 to 80% in patients with NGU, and approximately 10 to 50% in control groups (McCormack et al 1973). Antibody against *U. urealyticum* has not been shown to develop with any regularity in NGU (McCormack et al 1973).

The failure to provide unequivocal conclusions about the role of *C. trachomatis* and *U. urealyticum* in the aetiology of NGU is due, in part, to the impossibility of finding control groups whose sexual behaviour can be matched with that of the group of patients with urethritis being tested. Also, variations in the efficiency of sampling and isolation techniques and the tendency of organisms to become latent are likely to be important considerations. For these reasons attempts have been made in recent times to come to a firmer conclusion about the role of these organisms by studying the effect of antibiotics in alleviating the clinical manifestations of the disease, and to determine whether there is a relationship between improvement and the disappearance of organisms from the urogenital tract.

In one clinical trial there was statistically significant evidence that sulphonamides, with some activity against *C. trachomatis* but not *U. urealyticum*, were effective in treating chlamydia-positive cases, whereas spectinomycin, active against *U. urealyticum* but relatively inactive against *C. trachomatis*, was successful in ureaplasma-positive cases but not in chlamydia-positive cases. These results (Bowie et al 1976) support the theory that *C. trachomatis* was an important cause of NGU and also suggest that *U. urealyticum* was implicated. In later quantitative culture studies also, response to therapy suggested that *U. urealyticum* may be the cause of cases of chlamydia-negative NGU (Bowie et al 1977).

M. hominis does not seem to have an important pathogenic role in NGU, and ureaplasmas are unlikely causes in some men since organisms persist sometimes despite complete clinical recovery. Notwithstanding this situation, Coufalik et al (1979) were able to show by the use of *differential antibiotics* that ureaplasmas might be the cause in at least 10% of their patients. Basing their study on the fact that minocycline inhibits the multiplication of both *C. trachomatis* and *U. urealyticum* whereas rifampicin inhibits only chlamydiae, it was observed *inter alia* that patients in whom ureaplasmas disappeared recovered more frequently than those in whom the organisms persisted. Although the observation might be used as evidence for a causative role of ureaplasmas it is not, as the authors explain, possible to know whether the patients improved because the organisms disappeared or whether the organisms were not recoverable because the disease subsided spontaneously, isolation being less easily achieved in the absence of discharge.

Taylor-Robinson & McCormack's analytical discourse (1980) on the aetiology of NGU refers to the occurrence

of naturally occurring tetracycline-resistant ureaplasmas and of a case of non-specific urethritis associated with such (Ford & Smith 1974) and to the probability that more observations of this kind might be possible and useful (Evans & Taylor-Robinson 1978).

Experimental inoculation of humans with organisms is not to be undertaken lightly; even in NGU the problem of repeated relapses, Reiter's disease and other syndromes with less clear-cut effects associated with urethritis or conjunctivitis make experimental inoculation a matter for serious consideration from an ethical point of view. Notwithstanding such issues, two medical men, Dr Taylor-Robinson and Dr Csonka inoculated themselves with two strains of *U. urealyticum*. In this experiment special precautions were taken to be sure that the inoculum contained *U. urealyticum* only, and that these were not in numbers of organisms in excess of what might be introduced during sexual intercourse.

In one subject, the ureaplasma multiplied in the urethra and dysuria developed soon. Pus cells were detected in the urine and an immunological reaction of short duration was detected serologically. Tetracycline given six days after inoculation brought about rapid clearance of organisms from the urine and a more gradual disappearance of symptoms and signs. In the second subject another ureaplasma 'strain' was inoculated and similar effects followed although there was evidence that prostatic involvement occurred. Although treatment with tetracycline a month after inoculation eliminated the organisms, urinary threads of epithelial cells and polymorphonuclear leucocytes persisted for at least six months (Taylor-Robinson et al 1977).

As a result of their experiment it can be concluded that *U. urealyticum* is able to cause urethritis and may initiate chronic disease, but whether it is responsible for a major or insignificant part of the naturally occurring NGU remains unanswered. Nevertheless, among causes of NGU other than *C. trachomatis*, *Ureaplasma urealyticum* is the most favoured (Taylor-Robinson & McCormack 1980). Other mycoplasmas, *Mycoplasma fermentans*, a rare inhabitant of the lower genital tract, and *M. hominis*, a common inhabitant of this site, are not generally regarded as significant in the aetiology of NGU, although the latter may have an aetiological role in inflammatory pelvic disease in women. *M. genitalium* similarly, on laboratory evidence in primates, has this potential (Møller et al 1984 (Ch. 2)).

Urethritis caused by organisms other than those discussed is very uncommon (less than 1%) in relation to the mass of patients with NGU. Herpes simplex virus, *Candida albicans* and *Trichomonas vaginalis* have been considered as causes. Cystitis due to *Mycobacterium tuberculosis* is now a very rare cause of urethritis in this country, but in urinary tract infections due to other bacteria a urethrocystitis is not uncommon. Both trauma and foreign bodies are occasional factors and hypersensitivity may be involved.

In summary, cultural, serological and therapeutic studies demonstrate that *C. trachomatis* and *U. urealyticum* are associated with a major proportion of cases of NGU although unequivocal evidence for their pathological role in this condition is not yet available. By serotyping isolates of *U. urealyticum* by Black's growth-inhibition method Shephard & Lunceford (1978) found that, of eight so classified, type 4 was associated most frequently with NGU among the US personnel stationed at Camp Lejeune, N.Carolina. In this study, however, as Taylor-Robinson & McCormack (1980) pointed out, the control organism had been collected some 1–3 years earlier and stored in the frozen state at −85°C and temporal changes in serotypes could not therefore be excluded.

These studies must be evaluated against a background of improving methodology and it may be that in future, quantitative studies will help to provide unequivocal results. The aetiology of a proportion of cases of NGU is still far from clear as no organisms can be isolated.

POST-GONOCOCCAL URETHRITIS (PGU)

After treatment for gonorrhoea with the penicillins or aminoglycosides up to about 50% of men can be expected to develop post-gonococcal urethritis (PGU) (Vaughan-Jackson et al 1977), their urethral discharge recurs and an excess of polymorphonuclear leucocytes is seen on microscopy but *N. gonorrhoeae* cannot be found on microscopy or on culture.

The sexually transmissible serotypes of *C. trachomatis* have been implicated in the aetiology of PGU. *C. trachomatis* has also been isolated from urethral material in approximately 50% of men who developed urethritis following treatment for gonorrhoea; the organism could not be demonstrated in the control group of patients who did not develop PGU (Vaughan-Jackson et al 1977). Others (Oriel et al 1975) have noted that men with gonococcal urethritis who also have a chlamydial infection are more liable to develop PGU. It may be that *N. gonorrhoeae* and *C. trachomatis* are sexually transmitted at the same time. It is not clear whether *U. urealyticum* or other mycoplasmas have a role in the aetiology of PGU (Holmes et al 1975, Vaughan-Jackson et al 1977) but in one study among men who were not colonized by *U. urealyticum*, post-gonococcal urethritis was significantly associated with a *C. trachomatis* infection; among those with *C. trachomatis* infection PGU developed in about two-thirds of those who had *U. urealyticum* infection and in less than one-third of those who did not (Bowie et al 1978).

It has been suggested that defective cell wall forms

of gonococci (L-forms) may be a cause of PGU, but the presence of such L-forms in clinical specimens has still to be proved (Waitkins & Geary 1977). L-forms of gonococci can be produced in vitro by treatment of cultures with penicillin and it has been suggested that sub-lethal levels of penicillin could cause this change in vivo (Holmes et al 1967a). L-forms are able to multiply in osmotically favourable surroundings and, because of their defective cell wall, are resistant to antibiotics which affect cell wall synthesis.

PATHOLOGY OF CHLAMYDIAL INFECTION

In conjunctivitis due to chlamydiae the formation of a follicle commonly occurs, but this is a tissue reaction to irritation and is not specific. Cellular inclusions were first described in trachoma by Halberstaedter & von Prowazek in 1907 and later, in 1910, in urethral discharge (Halberstaedter & Prowazek 1910). In histological sections of cervical mucosa similar inclusions appear as cytoplasmic vacuoles when examined by light microscopy and are most easily seen in columnar endocervical cells. The vacuoles may occupy nearly the entire volume of the cell and, on electron microscopy, are seen to contain numerous small spherical bodies about 1 μm in diameter; these represent infectious elementary bodies, non-infectious reticulate bodies and transitional stages (Swanson et al 1975). The pathology of the urethra and conjunctiva is not easy to study as biopsy is not justified; urethral follicles however have been seen with the operating microscope in some men with *Chlamydia*-positive NGU (Dunlop et al 1967). Changes are not necessarily attributable wholly to chlamydiae as other organisms commonly colonize the cervix. Neutrophil polymorphonuclear leucocytes are dominant in the early stages of eye infections and are similarly found in urethritis and cervicitis.

CLINICAL FEATURES OF NON-GONOCOCCAL URETHRITIS

In the male NGU usually presents clinically as a mucopurulent urethral discharge associated with dysuria. The dysuria tends to be variable in severity with the discomfort or pain localized to the shaft of the penis or to the region of the meatus. The onset may occur within a few days to a month or more after the infecting intercourse. The urethral discharge may be small in quantity and mucoid, or it may be copious and frankly purulent. Sometimes the discharge may dry at the urethral meatus to form a greyish crust and the discharge may appear to be more copious in the morning than at other times. Occasionally dysuria is very severe and the urethral discharge blood-stained. When there is a urethrocystitis, frank haematuria may occur with blood dispersed throughout the urinary stream. In patients, particularly in those whose symptoms or signs are mild, it is important to examine the urethra for discharge before the patient has passed urine in the morning.

In acute haemorrhagic cystitis the patient may complain of malaise and of passing blood after urinating, when dysuria may occur at the end of micturition (terminal dysuria). There may be frequency, urgency and strangury.

The term non-specific genital infection (NSGI) in the male includes the commonest clinical presentation of non-gonococcal urethritis (NGU) as well as less common effects such as cystitis, epididymitis and prostatitis. Non-gonococcal proctitis is seen in male homosexuals, where *C. trachomatis* may be isolated in about 10%.

Associated disease, complications of a generalized nature, or distant from the original genital site are uncommon (less than 1%) and include acute follicular conjunctivitis, in which *Chamydia* may be isolated, Reiter's disease, anterior uveitis and possibly ankylosing spondylitis. It has been suggested also that subfertility may be related to ureaplasma infection, the organisms attaching themselves to the spermatozoon and inhibiting fertilization (Gnarpe & Friberg 1972).

NON-SPECIFIC GENITAL INFECTION (NSGI) IN WOMEN

Non-specific genital infection (NSGI) is a term that extends to the theoretically-expected involvement of the female, although it is a less precise clinical entity than NGU in the male. The diagnosis may be unsatisfactorily based on the existence of a non-gonocccal urethritis in the partner, symptoms of vaginal discharge or dysuria and the evidence of inflammation of the cervix, vagina, urethra or greater vestibular gland (Bartholinitis). In chlamydial infection the cervix may occasionally have a follicular or 'cobblestone' appearance. Pelvic inflammatory disease, involving the Fallopian tubes, can be found in some patients considered to have NSGI and infertility may result from tubal involvement. In STD-associated salpingitis, especially in young women, the aetiological agents in decreasing order of frequency, at least in Scandinavian countries, were thought to be *C. trachomatis*, *N. gonorrhoeae* and *M. hominis* (Westrom & Mardh 1983). Perihepatitis may occur, when a genital infection with either *N. gonorrhoeae* or *C. trachomatis* or both may be unsuspected.

Aetiology
It is likely that *C. trachomatis* is responsible for a proportion of cases of NSGI in women. *C. trachomatis*

can be isolated from the cervix in 20–40% of women who have gonorrhoea or who have been contacts of men with NGU (Oriel et al 1974, Burns et al 1975). In the case of female contacts of men with *Chlamydia*-positive NGU, *C. trachomatis* has been recovered from the cervix in about 57.5%, compared with only 23% of contacts of men with *Chlamydia*-negative NGU (Oriel & Ridgway 1982). Clinical findings, although not reliable criteria for diagnosis, do suggest that oedema, congestion and mucopurulent discharge are associated with chlamydial infection of the cervix in a proportion of cases, and that these signs regress after treatment (Rees et al 1977). Although some degree of an inflammatory reaction is induced by *C. trachomatis* it is unwise, however, to imply that chlamydial infections can be diagnosed from these appearances (Hare & Thin 1983). *C. trachomatis* is to be regarded as a pathogen of the female genital tract, conventional rather than conditional or opportunistic, in that it provokes, in some cases, a well-marked tissue response to infection of the cervix: it can be found also in the Fallopian tubes in salpingitis (Mardh et al 1977). Chlamydial infection of the female genital tract is widespread and may induce subclinical infections. In the presence of a co-existing infection with *N. gonorrhoeae* the organism may be more readily detected by culture (Oriel & Ridgway 1982).

There is some evidence to suggest that *U. urealyticum* and *Mycoplasma hominis* may be implicated in a few cases of pelvic inflammatory disease, although the precise extent of their involvement is not clear (McCormack et al 1973).

DIAGNOSIS OF NGU IN MEN AND NSGI IN WOMEN

C. trachomatis is implicated in the aetiology of many cases of NGU in the male and related infections in the female and it can be detected by microbiological tests as outlined below, but this service is often much less available than is desirable. In the case of men, presentation with a non-gonococcal urethritis with urethral discharge will lead to the prescription of the appropriate effective antibiotic (e.g. a tetracycline), whereas diagnosis in women on the grounds of clinical signs is quite unreliable and appropriate therapy will often not be given. Clearly an organismal diagnosis in the case of women at risk of a chlamydial infection is an essential service. The use of reagents based on monoclonal antibody techniques should make possibilities of definitive diagnosis accessible in localities where tissue culture methods are not easily provided. Single serum samples have no diagnostic value in chlamydial infection of the urethra, but in epididymitis, acute pelvic inflammatory disease, perihepatitis, high-titre or rising titre results will give support to a diagnosis of a chlamydial infection.

In the case of *M. hominis* and *U. urealyticum*, half of genital specimens will contain these ubiquitous organisms. With the interpretation of positive findings being difficult to assess in the individual patient, routine isolation is difficult to justify (Taylor-Robinson & McCormack 1980) although quantitative cultures may give some help to the clinician.

NGU in men

In the case of urethritis in the male it is the clinician's prime duty to exclude the presence of the gonococcus, initially by careful microscopy of the Gram-stained smear but backed up by inoculation of a culture plate at the same time. If the laboratory is distant then a swab may be sent in Amies' transport medium.

If the initial examination of a good sample of pus from the urethra shows numerous pus cells but no Gram-negative diplococci then a presumptive diagnosis of non-gonococcal urethritis may be made.

This diagnosis of NGU of the anterior urethra is strengthened by finding of haziness with or without urethral threads in the first glass in the urine test and a clear urine in the second and third. In the case of a urethrocystitis, all specimens of urine in this crude clinical test show a haze due to pus cells. A haze in urine due to precipitated phosphates may be differentiated from the haze due to pus cells by adding 10% acetic acid to dissolve the phosphates.

Routine tests need not be taken to exclude *T. vaginalis* and *C. albicans* or other yeasts in the male, as cultures are frequently negative and the role of these organisms as a cause of NGU is probably not important. In the case of cystitis in the male, however, a midstream specimen should be taken for bacteriological investigation and plans must be made for an excretion urogram, as bacterial cystitis in the male is almost invariably associated with a functional or anatomical abnormality in the urinary tract (Ch. 24).

NSGI in women

A diagnosis of NSGI in women implies that *Neisseria gonorrhoeae* has been excluded as a cause. Although attempts may be made to eradicate *C. trachomatis* it must be emphasized that other organisms such as *Bacteroides fragilis* may be pathogenic on occasions, such as after surgical procedures, and treatment of anaerobic bacterial infections with metronidazole may be necessary. Streptococci, staphylococci, Gram-negative bacilli, anaerobes or facultative anaerobes, can be pathogens in the genital tract and antibiotic or chemotherapeutic treatment may be required, depending on the sensitivity of these organisms.

In the case of pelvic inflammatory disease, although it is common practice to define the aetiology by isolating potential pathogens from the endocervix, the aetiology is probably better defined by examining tubal flora when possible. The cervix and vagina of normal women may contain all the species of anaerobic bacteria capable of causing pelvic infection. Endocervical cultures are of limited value in suggesting the species of organisms responsible for tubal infections, although these may be due to mixed infections or anaerobes (Thompson & Hager 1977). Classically in salpingitis *N. gonorrhoeae* was considered to be the only pathogen for which recovery from the cervix is correlated with recovery from the Fallopian tubes, but *Chlamydia trachomatis* has been isolated more often from both sites in this condition (Mardh et al 1977). Pelvic inflammatory disease is dealt with more fully in Chapter 23.

Evidence is strong in pelvic inflammatory disease for an aetiological role for *C. trachomatis* and *M. hominis*; in the case of *U. urealyticum* evidence for an association is weak. Similarly for post-abortal fever, postpartum fever, evidence for *M. hominis* having an aetiological role is strong. In the case of chorioamnionitis and low birth weight the evidence for the ureaplasma having an association is strong although the causal relationship is not proved (Taylor-Robinson & McCormack 1980).

ISOLATION OF *CHLAMYDIA TRACHOMATIS*

In the male, after moistening the swab with transport medium, an endo-urethral swab (Medical Wire and Equipment Co. Ltd.) is passed gently into the anterior urethra to a depth of 5 cm and withdrawn, and the tip of the swab is then agitated in a container of 2SP (Note 17.2) or 10% sorbitol (Evans & Woodland 1983). Excess fluid is removed by rotating the swab while gently pressing against the inside of the container. After moistening, the swab can be passed gently along the anterior urethra for 5–10 cm. On final removal the swab may be cut off with disposable scissors.

In the female, specimens may be obtained for testing after exposing the cervix with a bivalve speculum. The cervix should be cleaned with sterile gauze and a sample obtained by rotating a swab in the cervical canal at the squamocolumnar junction, concentrating on any inflamed area or where 'follicles' are seen. Similarly, material may be obtained from the rectum or from the oropharynx.

In the case of the conjunctiva, in the neonate particularly, the lower lid of each eye should be everted and a specimen taken by drawing a cotton wool-tipped swab along its mucosal surface. Specimens should be taken from the upper lids also if possible

Antibiotic treatment given to patients before specimens are taken adversely affect chances of isolation. Tetracyclines and erythromycin will reduce the likelihood of isolating the organism, and in patients treated with cephalosporins or penicillin the chances of negative results in primary isolation are increased (Evans & Woodland 1983). Specimens should be sent to the laboratory within 2 hours when possible: otherwise they should be taken in a cryoprotectant transport medium (e.g. 2SP or sorbitol 10%) and stored at −70°C before inoculating monolayers. If this is not possible specimens should be transported in liquid nitrogen.

METHODS FOR THE LABORATORY DIAGNOSIS OF CHLAMYDIAL INFECTION (Evans & Woodland 1983)

1. Detection of inclusion bodies by direct microscopy

In addition to Giemsa and immunofluorescence staining, iodine may also be used to detect the glycogen-containing inclusion bodies of *C. trachomatis* in smears made from urethral, cervical and vaginal scrapings or swabs. Unfortunately, direct microscopy by any of these techniques is too insensitive to be of practical value.

2. Detection of *Chlamydia* antigen by immunocytochemical methods

Although polyclonal antibodies against *C. trachomatis* have been developed and used successfully in the detection of chlamydial antigens in clinical specimens (Mumtaz et al 1985), the use of monoclonal antibodies in test systems has advantages because they react only with single antigenic determinants. Monoclonal antibodies against *C. trachomatis* were first produced by Stephens and colleagues (1982). Antibodies that reacted with genus-specific antigens reacted preferentially with reticulate body antigens whereas those that reacted to species, subspecies or type-specific antigens reacted with both reticulate body and elementary body antigens. Monoclonal antibodies have been used in fluorescent antibody and ELISA (enzyme-linked immunosorbent assay) methods for the detection of chlamydial antigens in conjunctival, urethral and endocervical material (Taylor et al 1984, Thomas et al 1984, Pugh et al 1985) and, in general, the results have shown good correlation with those of conventional culture. The major advantages of immunocytochemical methods over culture are that they are simpler, quicker and a little more sensitive. Problems of transport are also circumvented. A disadvantage is that non-viable organisms are likely to be detected.

3. Culture

Isolation of *C. trachomatis* on McCoy (Note 17.3) cells,

irradiated to stop their replication, is a sensitive method, whereas the isolation in the yolk sac of an egg is insensitive and prone to contamination (Darougar et al 1974). As irradiation is inconvenient for some laboratories alternative methods of comparable sensitivity have been described, e.g. treatment of cells with the nucleoside analogue 5-iodo-2-deoxyuridine (IDU) or with the fungal metabolite cytochalasin B (Stirling & Richmond 1977).

Treatment of the cells with these agents favours intracellular parasitism by preventing host cell replication and thus making more of the nutrients and precursors in the medium available to the chlamydiae. A simplified culture technique (Ripa & Mardh 1977) uses cycloheximide, an inhibitor of protein synthesis in eukaryotic but not in prokaryotic cells, to favour the growth of chlamydiae. This technique is suitable for routine isolation of *C. trachomatis* on a large scale as it does not involve pretreatment of the cells; cycloheximide is added after the chlamydiae have been taken up by the cells.

The clinical specimen is inoculated into flat-bottomed tubes containing the cell monolayers on cover-slips, and the tubes are then centrifuged for 1 hour at 3000 g at a temperature of 35°C to enhance the intracellular uptake of chlamydiae. The inoculated monolayers are then incubated for 48–72 hours, the cover-slips fixed with methanol and stained with iodine or Giemsa's stain. Inclusions may be demonstrated in positive cases.

It should be noted that culture of *C. psittaci* should not knowingly be attempted if the laboratory is not equipped for the culture of micro-organisms defined as being of category B1 (Department of Health and Social Security 1978, Evans & Woodland 1983).

4. Serology

Information on antibody responses during chlamydial infections is based largely on micro-immunofluorescence (micro-IF) tests, in which reactions between antibodies and acetone-fixed organisms are detected by fluorescent antiglobulin conjugate. In this micro-IF test (Grayston & Wang 1975) sera are screened against several antigens, either singly or in groups, representative of the many chlamydial serotypes. Only a few laboratories offer this test at present. A simpler test using a single antigen (*C. trachomatis* serotype E) is capable of detecting antibodies to a group antigen as well as type-specific antibodies to *C. trachomatis* serotypes (Richmond & Caul 1977). Using this test, single serum specimens from patients can be readily screened. Although the test may yield useful epidemiological information on the extent to which a particular population has been exposed to genital chlamydiae infections, it is of little value in the assessment of individual patients, since antibody could be due to a past infection.

A four-fold rise in titre or conversion from sero-negative to seropositive correlates well with the isolation of *C. trachomatis*, but this does not provide rapid diagnosis.

Detection of quantitative differences in antibody by an objective test such as radioimmunoassay or enzyme-linked immunosorbent assay may prove of value in future, as may the investigation of secretory IgA. A single method to detect chlamydial antigen in genital secretions would also provide a useful diagnostic test.

ISOLATION OF *MYCOPLASMA* SPP AND *UREAPLASMA UREALYTICUM*

For optimal isolation of mycoplasmas specimens must not be allowed to become dry and should therefore be inoculated directly into medium, kept at 40°C and transported to the laboratory as soon as possible. Urine samples should also be kept cool and, for best isolation, centrifuged to deposit epithelial and other cells.

In the male, mycoplasmas may be found to colonize the urethra and the subpreputial sac (Taylor-Robinson & McCormack 1980). In the case of women, 'vaginal specimens' are more likely to contain these organisms than the urethra, endocervix, posterior fornix or urethra. The technique of obtaining 'vaginal' specimens involves simply spreading the labia with the gloved hand to expose the introitus and inserting a swab (2.5–5.0 cm) into the vagina with the other hand and rubbing the swab against the vaginal wall (McCormack et al 1972). First voided urine samples (40 ml) are an indirect less sensitive method of sampling genital mucosa in both sexes.

In the laboratory the *liquid-to-agar technique* is based on the fact that *U. urealyticum* metabolizes urea to ammonia (Shepard & Lunceford 1970) and *M. hominis* arginine to ammonia. Aliquots of medium showing raised pH are then added to an agar medium containing urea and a sensitive indicator of ammonia, namely manganese II sulphate. After incubation the colonies of *U. urealyticum* are dark brown. Colony morphology is not reliable. Serological tests for detecting antibody produced are based on the *metabolism inhibition test*, specific for metabolites — arginine for *M. hominis* and urea for *U. urealyticum*.

The NYC medium, devised in the New York City Department of Health, primarily for the isolation of pathogenic neisseriae, also readily supports the growth of *U. urealyticum* and mycoplasmas. The medium permits direct isolation and identification of these organisms as well as *N. gonorrhoeae* without interference from contaminating saprophytes (Faur et al 1974).

Liquid cultures are normally incubated aerobically at 37°C, while solid media are incubated in an atmosphere containing 95% nitrogen and 5% carbon dioxide. Results are usually available within 1–5 days.

CHEMOTHERAPY OF CHLAMYDIA AND UREAPLASMA INFECTIONS

The results of a laboratory evaluation of anti-bacterial agents against chlamydia suggest that oxytetracycline is most effective (MIC, 0.06 μg/ml) and erythromycin has a useful second place (MIC, 0.03 μg/ml) (Ridgway et al 1976). Gentamicin, spectinomycin, trimethoprim/ sulphamethoxazole are not likely to be effective, and the effects of penicillin G and ampicillin are relatively poor.

The results of a laboratory evaluation of anti-bacterial agents against ureaplasma showed that minocycline was the most active antibiotic, with a median MIC (0.03 μg/ml). well below reported blood serum concentrations attained after therapeutic doses (Spaepen et al 1976). Doxycycline and demeclocycline, although not as active in vitro as minocycline against the majority of strains tested, still gave low median MIC values (0.125 μg/ml). Tetracycline was less active than its analogues (MIC, 0.25 μg/ml). Erythromycin required the highest concentration, MIC 2.0 μg/ml.

In the case of ureaplasma, approximately 10% of ureaplasma isolated may be resistant to oxytetracycline and minocycline (Evans & Taylor-Robinson 1978). Resistance to erythromycin does not seem to be linked to tetracycline resistance (Evans & Taylor Robinson 1978) although strains resistant to both antibiotics have been isolated (Spaepen et al 1976).

Treatment of NGU in the male
The value of tetracycline in the treatment of NGU was investigated in patients who were members of a 5500-man crew of a large aircraft carrier in the US Navy (Holmes et al 1967b). After 6 days of liberty in the Philippines the men returned for 30 consecutive days at sea where discipline was strong and opportunities for further sexual intercourse very remote. In this experiment, now regarded as a classic, it was established that tetracycline was better than placebo and that a 7-day course was better than a 4-day course, that is to say with a follow-up limited to 20 days or less.[*]

In the long term, however, the effects are less clear, and in a trial in Birmingham there was only about a 10% difference between placebo and a short course of tetracycline when an assessment was made over a 10-week period (Fowler 1970). In the case of NGU treated with placebo, the patient will tend to suffer symptoms longer, so treatment with a tetracycline is justified on this ground alone. Although optimum drug, dosage and duration of therapy have still not been decided (Oriel

*All US. Naval ships are "dry"

& Ridgway 1983) it is recommended that oxytetracycline is prescribed in a dose of 250 mg 4 times daily for a minimum of 7 days. The patient may then be assessed after 1 week and 2 weeks, when a further week's course may be prescribed if symptoms or signs of urethritis persist or if numerous urethral threads containing pus cells are seen in the first glass in the urine test. As the value of a 21-day course has not been proved to be greater than a 7-day course it is not accepted routine practice to prescribe a long course.

Compliance in taking prescribed treatment is difficult to secure in men with NGU who otherwise feel well. Patients must be told not to take milk, milk products or antacids which prevent absorption and to take their oxytetracycline tablet(s) half an hour before meals. In addition to the tetracycline treatment the patient is advised to abstain from alcohol for 2 weeks and to abstain from intercourse for the same period. The former is advised on the basis that the inflammation is believed to be aggravated by taking alcoholic beverages and to subside more readily with rest. Relapse after coitus and/or excessive alcohol consumption is often reported by patients with NGU.

A long-acting tetracycline, minocycline, is effective and blood levels of 2 μg per ml can be maintained with a 12-hourly dose. A course of 200 mg followed by 100 mg 12-hourly for 6 days in one trial (Prentice et al 1976) produced a short-term cure in 89% (41 patients) and failed to do so in 11% (5) who had discharge after a 6-day period.

With minocycline the complaint of vertigo is a recognized complication. In up to 89% of cases treated with the drug there have been symptoms of nausea, vomiting, anorexia, abdominal cramp, weakness, ataxia, vertigo, dizziness, which start during the first 48 hours of treatment and disappear shortly after cessation of therapy. This experience is not unusual and there is a very low incidence of reactions when the syrup is used; problems seem to be related to the formulation used (Hoigné et al 1984). An isolated case of a hypersensitivity-like acute interstitial nephritis has been reported in a 43-year-old woman, occurring 10 days after treatment with minocycline (250 mg 4 times daily for 5 days) for an upper respiratory infection (Walker et al 1979). The patient recovered spontaneously, after withdrawing minocycline, which had been prescribed again before admission to hospital. There is preferential concentration of minocycline in the thyroid gland and reports of melanin-like substance in the thyroid gland (black thyroid) are difficult to evaluate in clinical terms (Midtvedt 1984).

Doxycycline (Vibramycin, Pfizer Ltd.) is sometimes effective in a dose of 200 mg once on day 1 and 100 mg daily for 6 days afterwards, and compliance is easier to secure. The capsules should be taken immediately after meals to avoid abdominal pain which may occur when the stomach is empty, and the possibility of photosensitivity has to be taken into account.

At present it is suggested that, when eradication of ureaplasma is deemed to be advisable, a tetracycline should be used although resistance to this antibiotic has been found in 10% of isolates. Isolation facilities for diagnosis, antibiotic sensitivity testing and tests of cure are not widely available.

Treatment of NSGI in the female

In the case of a regular partnership, or where *C. trachomatis* has been isolated, treatment of both male and female partners is recommended. In females with signs or symptoms suggestive of NSGI then such treatment may also be justified even if isolations are not obtained. Treatments and dosages are similar to those for the male, except that erythromycin stearate is preferred as a routine treatment and should be used in women who are pregnant or lactating. The duration of erythromycin stearate treatment (500 mg twice-daily) should be at least a week, when subsequent test of cures are available for assessing the results of therapy, or continued for 2 weeks if such assessments are not possible.

NON-GONOCOCCAL CONJUNCTIVITIS OF THE NEWBORN (non-gonococcal ophthalmia neonatorum)

Mild inflammation of the conjunctiva is common a few days after birth and resolves generally without treatment. This may be due to trauma or a transitory infection acquired during birth. In the case of gonococcal conjunctivitis, acquired from the infected maternal cervix, blindness will result if no treatment is given, and diagnosis in the child will require also examination, diagnosis and treatment of the mother and her sexual contacts, whether consort or husband. The social consequences of this intervention are to be endured in all cases because the dangers of omission of treatment are very serious.

In non-gonococcal conjunctivitis not caused by bacteria the condition is commonly due to one of the sexually transmissible serotypes of *C. trachomatis*. The steps taken to ensure treatment of the mother and father or partner are highly desirable.

INFECTIONS IN THE NEWBORN DUE TO *CHLAMYDIA TRACHOMATIS*

Conjunctivitis is the most obvious clinical form of neonatal chlamydial infection since contamination can occur from the mother's infected cervical excretions during birth or by shedding of chlamydia in inflammatory discharges from an infected eye in the newborn. Infection is not confined to the conjunctiva, and the respiratory tract, the middle ear, the gut and the vagina can be contaminated (Schachter et al 1979).

The increase in incidence of NGU in men, and the increasing isolation rate of certain serotypes of *C. trachomatis* in some 40% or more in this condition, is likely to be associated with a large number of women acting as carriers. As chlamydial infection can be asymptomatic in men with minimal signs of urethritis, and is ordinarily so in women, conjunctival infection of the newborn is to be expected. Chlamydial conjunctivitis in the newborn is likely to be associated also with spread of chlamydia to the nasopharynx; involvement of the lung and middle ear, causing respectively pneumonia or otitis media, occurs in a very small proportion.

Conjunctivitis
In the United Kingdom, where prophylactic treatment of the eyes is not given at birth, clinical conjunctivitis in maternity units was found in 2.6% (71 of 2700 infants in Cambridge in 1968, and in 139 of 5282 infants in Liverpool in 1980) (Hobson et al 1983).

There are difficulties in assessing the true incidence of conjunctivitis because babies are rarely in hospital for the full incubation period of the order of 3 to 13 days, or longer when the inoculum is small. In the case of gonococcal conjunctivitis diagnosis is usually made 24–48 hours after birth.

Clinical features
The infection usually presents as a mucopurulent conjunctivitis which may vary from mild to severe within the incubation period already stated. The discharge may be only scanty and not obviously purulent but it is sometimes more copious and frankly purulent, or on occasions blood-stained (Rees et al 1977). On examination the palpebral conjunctiva shows mild to severe infiltration and papillary hyperplasia. In its more severe form there is also oedema of the eyelids and palpebral conjunctiva, particularly of the lower lid. Signs may be minimal and inflammatory reaction apparently transitory but in some cases conjunctival scarring develops (Watson & Gairdner 1968).

In the absence of specific treatment, the course is usually benign, but may be protracted. The sight is not compromised, although micropannus and conjunctival scarring may be found on long-term follow-up (Hobson et al 1983).

Diagnosis
The discharge should be wiped gently away from the surface of the eyelids with a swab and the lower lids everted. A cotton-wool swab should be passed gently but firmly along the lower and upper palpebral conjunctiva and then agitated gently in 2SP transport medium. The sample should reach the laboratory within 2 hours or be stored at a temperature of −70°C until cultured.

Similar samples are taken from the posterior pharyngeal wall, particularly in older children and on follow-up.

The earlier the provisional diagnosis, the earlier the full investigation and treatment, not only of the baby but also of the mother who is at risk of pelvic inflammatory disease (Hobson & Rees 1977) and of the father.

In the investigation of neonatal conjunctivitis the following are essential steps:

1. Microscopy of Gram-stained smear from the palpebral conjunctiva for Gram-negative diplococci (*N. gonorrhoeae*).
2. Direct inoculation of selective medium with material from the palpebral conjunctiva to detect or exclude *N. gonorrhoeae*.
3. Swab from palpebral conjunctiva placed in 2SP or other chlamydial transport medium for the isolation of *Chlamydia*.
4. Swab taken in Amies' transport medium for isolation of other bacterial pathogens.
5. Pelvic examination of the mother to exclude *N. gonorrhoeae*, *C. trachomatis* and other pathogens.
6. Examination of sexual partner of the mother.

Infection of the nasopharynx by *Chlamydia trachomatis* in the newborn
It is difficult to be certain whether the isolation of *Chlamydia* from the nasopharynx of infants represents an 'established infection' or pathological condition of the pharynx rather than contamination by tears. The infection is usually light in terms of numbers of infectious units and is often clinically inapparent and without sequelae but it can persist for up to 200 days in the absence of chemotherapy (Harrison et al 1978).

Pneumonia
It is difficult to establish an aetiological relationship between chlamydial infection of the conjunctiva or of the nasopharynx and neonatal pneumonia.

Treatment
Once *N. gonorrhoeae* has been excluded, it is justifiable to treat a mild neonatal conjunctivitis with a 0.5% (w/v) solution of neomycin prescribed as single dose sterile eye drops ('Minims' Neomycin Sulphate, Smith and Nephew Pharmaceutical Ltd., 20 units in each single dose), instilled into the eye every 4 hours. Neomycin is effective against most isolates of staphylococci and some strains of *Proteus vulgaris* and *Pseudomonas aeruginosa*. It has no action against fungi, viruses or intra-

cellular chlamydia. If the conjunctivitis is marked and does not respond to neomycin then isolation of chlamydia should be attempted and if this organism is *discovered, or suspected*, 1% tetracycline eye ointment is applied (Achromycin eye ointment) along the lower lid 4-hourly on 4 occasions daily for 21 days (Charters & Rees 1976). Since topical treatment may well be insufficient, consideration should be given to the strong case for the use of systemic treatment.

Infants with chlamydial infections frequently have concurrent pharyngeal infection which is likely to persist after topical chemotherapy alone with eye oint-ments, and may be a focus for reinfection of the eye (Rees et al 1981). In addition, the eye infection may be associated with concurrent or subsequent pneumonia and otitis media and even myocarditis (Grayston et al 1981).

There is therefore a very strong case for systemic treatment of all infants with chlamydial conjunctivitis, and erythromycin ethylsuccinate given in divided doses to a total of 40–50 mg per kg body weight per day for 2–3 weeks is reliable. There appears to be no advantage in giving systemic and topical treatment simultaneously (Hobson et al 1983).

NOTES TO CHAPTER 17

Note 17.1

The word promiscuous derives from *pro* — for, or in favour of; *miscere* — to mix: hence promiscuous conditions are conditions that favour mixing.

Note 17.2

'2SP', transport medium for *Chlamydia*; see Note 6.1.

Note 17.3

The McCoy cell line, originally used because it was thought to be a line of human synovial cells, is now known to be closely related in karyotype and antigenic constitution to the mouse fibroblastic tumour cell line L929, used for the laboratory growth of *C. psittaci* (Hobson 1977).

REFERENCES

Alani M D, Darougar S, Burns D C MacD, Thin R N, Dunn H 1977 Isolation of *Chlamydia trachomatis* from the male urethra. British Journal of Venereal Diseases 53: 88–92

Becker Y 1978 The chlamydia: molecular biology of procaryotic obligate parasites of eucaryotes. Microbiological Reviews 42: 274–306

Bolton J P, Darougar S 1983 Perihepatitis. British Medical Bulletin 39(2): 159–162

Bowie W R, Floyd J F, Miller Y, Alexander E R, Holmes J, Holmes K K 1976 Differential response of chlamydial and ureaplasma associated urethritis to sulphafurazole. Lancet ii: 1276–1278

Bowie W R, Wang S-P, Alexander E R et al 1977 Etiology of nongonococcal urethritis. Evidence for *Chlamydia trachomatis* and ureaplasma. Journal of Clinical Investigation 59: 735–742

Bowie W R, Alexander E R, Holmes K K 1978 Etiologies of post-gonococcal urethritis in homosexual and heterosexual men; roles for *Chlamydia trachomatis* and *Ureaplasma urealyticum*. Sexually Transmitted Diseases 5: 151–154

Burns D C MacD, Darougar S, Thin R N, Lothian L, Nicol C S 1975 Isolation of *Chlamydia* from women attending a clinic for sexually transmitted disease. British Journal of Venereal Diseases 51: 314–318

Charters D W, Rees E 1976 Chlamydial ophthalmia neonatorum. New Zealand Medical Journal 83: 82–84

Coufalik E D, Taylor-Robinson D, Csonka G W 1979 Treatment of nongonococcal urethritis with rifampicin as a means of defining the role of *Ureaplasma urealyticum*. British Journal of Venereal Diseases 55: 36–43

Darougar S, Cubitt S, Jones B R 1974 Effect of high-speed centrifugation on the sensitivity of irradiated McCoy cell culture for the isolation of *Chlamydia*. British Journal of Venereal Diseases 50: 308–312

Department of Health and Social Security 1978 Code of practice for the prevention of infection in clinical laboratories and postmortem rooms. HMSO, London

Dunlop E M C, Freedman A, Garland J A et al 1967 Infection by Bedsoniae and the possibility of spurious isolation: 2. Genital infection, disease of the eye, Reiter's disease. American Journal of Ophthalmology 63: 1073–1081

Evans R T, Taylor-Robinson D 1978 The incidence of tetracycline-resistant strains of *Ureaplasma urealyticum*. Journal of Antimicrobial Chemotherapy 4: 57–63

Evans R T, Woodland R M 1983 Detection of Chlamydiae by isolation and direct examination. British Medical Bulletin 39(2): 181–186

Faur Y C, Weisburd M H, Wilson M E, May P S 1974 NYC Medium for simultaneous isolation of *Neisseria gonorrhoeae*, large-colony mycoplasmas and T mycoplasmas. Applied Microbiology 27: 1041–1045

Ford D K, Smith J R 1974 Non-specific urethritis associated with a tetracycline-resistant T-mycoplasma. British Journal of Venereal Diseases 50: 373–374

Fowler W 1970 Studies in non-gonococcal urethritis. The long-term value of tetracycline. British Journal of Venereal Diseases 46: 464–468

Gnarpe H, Friberg J 1972 Mycoplasma and human reproductive failure. The occurrence of different mycoplasmas in couples with reproductive failure. American Journal of Obstetrics and Gynecology 114: 727–731

Grayston J T, Wang S P 1975 New knowledge of chlamydiae and the diseases they may cause. Journal of Infectious Diseases 132: 87–105

Grayston J T, Mordhurst C H, Wang S-P 1981 Childhood myocarditis associated with *Chlamydia trachomatis* infection. Journal of the American Medical Association 246: 2823–2827

Halberstaedter L, von Prowazek S 1910 Ueber die bedeutung der chlamydozoen bei trachom und blenorrhoe. Berliner Klinische Wochenschrift 47: 661–663

Hare M J, Thin R N 1983 Chlamydial infection of the lower genital tract of women. British Medical Bulletin 39(2): 138–144

Harrison H R, English M G, Lee C K, Alexander E R 1978 *Chlamydia trachomatis* infant pneumonitis. Comparison with matched controls and other pneumonias. New England Journal of Medicine 298: 702–708

Hatch T P 1975 Competition between *Chlamydia psittaci* and L-cells for host isoleucine pools: a limiting factor in chlamydial multiplication. Infection and Immunity 12: 211–220

Hobson D 1977 Tissue culture procedures for the isolation of *Chlamydia trachomatis* from patients with non-gonococcal genital infections. In: Hobson D, Holmes K K (eds) Non-gonococcal urethritis and related infections. American Society for Microbiology, Washington D C, p 286–294

Hobson D, Rees E 1977 Maternal genital chlamydial

infection as a cause of neonatal conjunctivitis. Postgraduate Medical Journal 53: 595–597

Hobson D, Rees E, Viswalingam N D 1983 Chlamydial infections in neonates and older children. British Medical Bulletin 39(2): 128–132

Hoigné R, Keller H, Sontag R 1984 Penicillins, chloramphenicol, cephalosporins and tetracyclines. In: Dukes M N G (ed) Meyler's Side effects of drugs, Elsevier, Amsterdam, ch 26, p 446–491

Holmes K K, Johnson D W, Floyd T M, Kvale P A 1967a Studies of venereal diseases. II. Observations on the incidence, aetiology and treatment of the postgonococcal urethritis syndrome. Journal of the American Medical Association 202: 467–473

Holmes K K, Johnson D W, Floyd P M 1967b iii. Double-blind comparison of tetracycline hydrochloride and placebo in treatment of non-gonococcal urethritis. Journal of the American Medical Association 202: 467–473

Holmes K K, Handsfield H H, Wang S-P, Wentworth B B, Turck M, Anderson J B, Alexander E R 1975 Aetiology of non-gonococcal urethritis. New England Journal of Medicine, 292: 1199–1205

Horoshak K D, Moulder J W 1978 Division of single host cells after infection with chlamydiae. Infection and Immunity 19: 281–286

Jones Barrie R 1975 The prevention of blindness from trachoma. The Bowman Lecture. Transactions of the Ophthalmological Societies of the United Kingdom vol 95, 16–33

Keat A, Thomas B J, Taylor-Robinson D 1983 Chlamydial infection in the aetiology of arthritis. British Medical Bulletin 39(2): 168–174

Kingsbury D T, Weiss E 1968 Lack of deoxyribonucleic acid homology between species of the genus Chlamydia. Journal of Bacteriology 96: 1421–1423

Klein J O, Buckland D, Finland M 1969 Colonization of newborn infants by mycoplasmas. New England Journal of Medicine 280: 1025–1030

Lee Y-H, McCormack W M, Marcy S M, Klein J O 1974 The genital mycoplasmas. Their role in disorders of reproduction and in pediatric infections. Pediatric Clinics of North America 21(2): 457–466

McCormack W M, Rankin J S, Lee Y-H 1972 Localization of genital mycoplasmas in women. American Journal of Obstetrics and Gynecology 112: 920–923

McCormack W M, Braun P, Lee Y H, Klein J O, Kass E H 1973 The genital mycoplasmas. New England Journal of Medicine 288: 78–89

McCormack W M, Almeida P C, Bailey P E, Grady E M, Lee Y-H 1975 Sexual activity and vaginal colonization with genital mycoplasmas. Journal of the American Medical Association 221: 1375–1377

Mardh P-A, Ripa T, Svensson L, Westrom L 1977 Chlamydia trachomatis infection in patients with acute salpingitis. New England Journal of Medicine 296: 1377–1379

Midtvedt T 1984 Penicillins, cephalosporins and tetracyclines. In: Dukes M N G (ed) Side effects of drugs. Annual 8, Elsevier, Amsterdam, p 248–253

Møller B R, Taylor-Robinson D, Furr P M 1984 Serological evidence implicating Mycoplasma genitalium in pelvic inflammatory disease. Lancet i: 1102–1103

Mumtaz G, Mellars B J, Ridgway G L, Oriel J D 1985 Enzyme immunoassay for the detection of Chlamydia trachomatis antigen in urethral and endocervical swabs. Journal of Clinical Pathology 38: 740–742

Oriel J D, Ridgway G L 1982 Epidemiology of chlamydial infection of the human genital tract: evidence for the existence of latent infections. European Journal of Clinical Microbiology 1: 69–75

Oriel J D, Ridgway G L 1983 Genital infection in men. In: Darougar S (ed) Chlamydial disease. British Medical Bulletin, Churchill Livingstone, 39(2): 133–137

Oriel J D, Powis P A, Reeve P, Miller A, Nicol C S 1974 Chlamydial infections of the cervix. British Journal of Venereal Diseases 50: 11–16

Oriel J D, Reeve P, Thomas B J, Nicol C S 1975 Infection with Chlamydia Group A in men with urethritis due to Neisseria gonorrhoeae. Journal of Infectious Diseases 131: 376–382

Oriel J D, Reeve P, Wright J T, Owen J 1976 Chlamydial infection of the male urethra. British Journal of Venereal Diseases 52: 46–51

Prentice M J, Taylor-Robinson D, Csonka G W 1976 Non-specific urethritis: A placebo controlled trial of minocycline in conjunction with laboratory investigations. British Journal of Venereal Diseases 52: 269–275

Pugh S F, Slack R C B, Caul E D, Paul I D, Appleton P N, Gatley S 1985 Enzyme amplified immunoassay: a novel technique applied to direct detection of Chlamydia trachomatis in clinical specimens. Journal of Clinical Pathology 38: 1139–1141

Razin S, Freundt E A 1984 Mycoplasmataceae etc. In: Krieg N R, Holt J C (eds) Bergey's Manual of systemic bacteriology vol l. Williams and Wilkins, Baltimore/London, p 742–770

Rees E, Tait A, Hobson D, Byng R E, Johnson F W A 1977 Neonatal conjunctivitis caused by Neisseria gonorrhoeae and Chlamydia trachomatis. British Journal of Venereal Diseases 53: 173–177

Rees E, Tait I A, Hobson D, Kavaylannis P, Lee N 1981 Persistence of chlamydial infection after treatment for neonatal conjunctivitis. Archives of Diseases of Children 56: 193–198

Richmond S J, Caul E O 1977 Single-antigen indirect immunofluorescence test for screening venereal disease clinic populations for chlamydia antibodies. In: Hobson D, Holmes K K (eds) Non-gonococcal urethritis and related infections. American Society for Microbiology, Washington D C, p 259–265

Richmond S J, Stirling P 1981 Localization of chlamydial group antigen in McCoy cell monolayers infected with Chlamydia trachomatis or Chlamydia psittaci. Infection and Immunity 34: 561–570

Ridgway G L, Owen J M, Oriel J D 1976 A method for testing the antibiotic susceptibility of Chlamydia trachomatis in a cell culture system. Journal of Antimicrobial Chemotherapy 2: 71–76

Ripa T, Mardh P-A 1977 New simplified culture technique for Chlamydia trachomatis. In: Hobson D, Holmes K K (eds) Non-gonococcal urethritis and related infections. American Society for Microbiology, Washington D C, p 323–327

Schachter J, Grossman M, Holt J, Sweet R, Spector S 1979 Infection with Chlamydia trachomatis: involvement of multiple anatomic sites in neonates. Journal of Infectious Diseases 139: 232–234

Shepard M C, Lunceford C D 1970 Urease colour test medium U9 for the detection and identification of 'T' mycoplasmas in clinical material. Applied Microbiology 20: 539–543

Shepard M C, Lunceford C D 1978 Serological typing of Ureaplasma urealyticum isolates from urethritis patients by an agar growth inhibition method. Journal of Clinical

Microbiology 8: 566–574

Spaepen M S, Kundsin R B, Horne H W 1976 Tetracycline-resistant T-mycoplasmas (*Ureaplasma urealyticum*) from patients with a history of reproductive failure. Antimicrobial Agents and Chemotherapy 9: 1012–1018

Stephens R S, Tam M R, Kuo C C, Nowinski R C 1982 Monoclonal antibodies to *Chlamydia trachomatis* antibody specificities and antigen characterization. Journal Immunology 128: 1083–1089

Stirling P, Richmond S 1977 The developmental cycle of *Chlamydia trachomatis* in McCoy cells treated with cytochalasine B. British Journal of General Microbiology 100: 31–42

Swanson J, Eschenbach D A, Alexander E R, Holmes K K 1975 Light and electron microscopic study of *Chlamydia trachomatis* infection of the uterine cervix. Journal of Infectious Diseases 131: 678–687

Taylor-Robinson D, McCormack W M 1980 Medical progress: The genital mycoplasmas. New England Journal of Medicine 302: 1003–1010, 1063–1067

Taylor-Robinson D, Csonka G W, Prentice M J 1977 Human intra-urethral inoculation of ureaplasmas. Quarterly Journal of Medicine, New Series 46: 309–326

Taylor H R, Agarwala N, Johnson S L 1984 Detection of experimental *Chlamydia trachomatis* eye infection in conjunctival smears and in tissue culture by use of fluorescein-conjugated monoclonal antibody. Journal of Clinical Microbiology 20: 391–395

Thomas B J, Evans R T, Hawkins D A, Taylor-Robinson D 1984 Sensitivity of detecting *Chlamydia trachomatis* elementary bodies in smears by use of a fluorescein labelled monoclonal antibody: comparison with conventional chlamydial isolation. Journal of Clinical Pathology 37: 812–816

Thompson S E, Hager W D 1977 Acute pelvic inflammatory disease. Sexually Transmitted Diseases 4: 105–113

Treharne J D, Forsey T, Thomas B J 1983 Chlamydial serology. In: Darougar S (ed) Chlamydial disease. British Medical Bulletin 39(2): 194–200

Vaughan-Jackson J D, Dunlop E M C, Darougar S, Treharne J D, Taylor-Robinson D 1977 Urethritis due to *Chlamydia trachomatis*. British Journal of Venereal Diseases 53: 180–183

Viswalingam N D, Wishart M S, Woodland R M 1983 Adult chlamydial ophthalmia (paratrachoma). British Medical Bulletin 39 (No. 2): 123–127

Waitkins S A, Geary I 1977 Detection and identification of gonococcal L-forms using a direct immunofluorescence test. British Journal of Venereal Diseases 53: 161–169

Walker R G, Thomson N M, Dowling J P, Chisholm S O 1979 Minocycline-induced acute interstitial nephritis. British Medical Journal 1: 524

Wang S-P, Grayston J T, Kuo C-C, Alexander E R, Holmes K K 1977 Serodiagnosis of *Chlamydia trachomatis* infection with the micro-immunofluorescence test. In: Hobson D, Holmes K K (eds) Nongonococcal urethritis and related infections. American Society for Microbiology, p 237–258

Ward M F 1983 Chlamydial classification, development and structure. British Medical Bulletin 39: 109–115

Watson P G, Gairdner D 1968 TRIC agent as a cause of neonatal eye sepsis. British Medical Journal 3: 527–528

Westrom L, Mardh P-A 1983 Chlamydial salpingitis. British Medical Bulletin 39(2): 145–150

18

Prostatitis, orchitis and epididymitis

PROSTATITIS

In those with clinical features, particularly episodes of pain in the distribution believed to be characteristic of inflammation of the prostate, it may not be possible to confirm a diagnosis of prostatitis because histological findings and the results of examination of the prostatic fluid, including attempts to isolate organisms, are often inconclusive. Acute and chronic bacterial prostatitis due to organisms isolated by conventional bacteriological means, and referred to as 'eubacteria' in this discussion, are, however, more clearly defined as entities than in the case of 'chronic prostatitis', where no organisms can be isolated either by conventional bacteriological methods, or even by the special methods required for other organisms considered possibly to have an aetiological role. As the diagnosis of prostatitis tends therefore to be made on symptoms, it is necessary to consider first the symptom 'prostatic pain', recognizing also that there will be overlap in symptomatology with non-gonococcal urethrocystitis on the one extreme and with dysnergic bladder neck obstruction on the other.

PROSTATIC PAIN

'Prostatic' pain occurs as a symptom in inflammatory conditions of the gland and has its origins in the gland itself and in structures with which it is intimately related (urethra, the trigone and its urethral extension, the pre-prostatic sphincter and the musculature of the pelvic floor) (Blacklock 1978).

The pain may be felt in the suprapubic region, the groins and the spermatic cord and testis of one or both sides, and may radiate to the inner thighs. It may radiate to the perineum and to the penis, where it may be felt in the urethra and in the penile meatus, usually at the beginning and on completion of micturition. There may also be urgency, frequency, dysuria and painful ejaculation. Symptoms in prostatitis may include any one or all of these (Blacklock 1978, Meares 1978).

In view of the common segmental autonomic inner-

vation of the kidneys, urethra, bladder and prostate, the distribution of pain may be the same in pathology of any part of the upper and lower urinary tract; for these reasons excretion urography and cystourethroscopy will be necessary to exclude such pathology when the prostate itself, so far as can be ascertained, is not the cause of the pain (Blacklock 1978). Similar symptomatology is also seen in those with or without prostatitis but with dysnergic bladder neck obstruction detected by investigation or urinary flow during micturition (Warwick & Whiteside 1976). Prostatitis itself may cause intravesical obstruction, often localized to the bladder neck (Murnaghan & Millard 1984).

PROSTATITIS WITH DEMONSTRABLE EUBACTERIAL INFECTION

Acute prostatitis
This is characterized by pyrexia, rigors, frequency and urgency of micturition and dysuria. There is pain in the distribution described, although perineal pain itself is uncommon in the acute phase, since the accompanying malaise encourages bed rest and relaxation of pelvic floor musculature (Blacklock 1978). Gentle palpation of the gland per rectum may show that it is tender, swollen, irregular and indurated. If untreated a prostatic abscess may develop and cause perineal pain of great intensity. Bacteriological examination of the urine by conventional techniques generally demonstrates the causative organisms, which may be *Escherichia coli*, *Klebsiella* spp, *Pseudomonas aeruginosa* or *Proteus* spp.

Chronic prostatitis
This is one of the most common causes of relapsing urinary tract infection due to eubacteria in any age group but, more commonly, in middle age. It may be associated with a variety of organisms, most commonly Gram-negative bacilli but occasionally Gram-positive organisms. Chronic bacterial (eubacterial) prostatitis is characterized by a relapsing urinary tract infection due to the same pathogen (Meares 1978) and although some

patients present with an asymptomatic bacteriuria, symptoms of 'prostatic' pain and dysuria also occur.

PROSTATITIS WITHOUT DEMONSTRABLE EUBACTERIAL INFECTION

Chronic or 'non-acute' prostatitis with 'prostatic' pain

Clearly this is the most common form of prostatitis seen today in western developed countries. In its clinical presentation it is chronic, with recurrent episodes of pain, and it may be referred to in terms such as abacterial prostatitis, non-acute prostatitis, prostatosis, or chronic prostatitis. Symptoms are those already described under the heading of 'prostatic' pain but malaise and pyrexia are absent, and the perineal pain, particularly, is not as severe as in acute bacterial prostatitis. In contrast to chronic eubacterial prostatitis recurrent episodes of cystitis and epididymitis do not tend to occur.

As *Chlamydia trachomatis* is probably the cause of acute 'idiopathic' epididymitis, occurring particularly in men under 35 years of age, and as the organism may be isolated from material aspirated from the epididymis in such cases (Berger et al 1978) a similar aetiology might be suggested for chronic or 'non-acute' prostatitis. In an investigation of 53 cases of non-acute prostatitis in Sweden, Mardh et al (1978), however, isolated *C. trachomatis* from the urethra in only one case and failed to find this organism in any of the 28 specimens of prostatic fluid examined. From this result, and from those of micro-immunofluorescent tests, they considered that in their study *C. trachomatis* appeared to play only a minor role, if any, in 'non-acute' prostatitis: isolation difficulties might, however, be analogous to the situation of ocular hyperendemic trachoma, where it is possible to isolate *C. trachomatis* from 70% of acute cases but from only 5% of the chronic (Darougar et al 1977).

Prostatitis, chronic in form with a tendency to relapse and remission, is a difficult entity to define on criteria other than the presence of 'prostatic' pain as findings based on examination of the expressed prostatic secretion are not reliable; the overlap of its symptomatology with bladder neck dysnergia and sometimes with serious pathology of the urinary tract necessitate referral for urological advice and examination. When symptoms do not abate completely with antimicrobial treatment, given either speculatively or for what may be a coincidental infection with either *Chlamydia*, *Ureaplasma* or *Trichomonas*, referral for urological examination is necessary.

The discovery of excess leucocytes in the expressed prostatic secretion has been taken as the sole criterion in making a diagnosis of prostatitis in patients without prostatic pain. Using this finding 'prostatitis' has been diagnosed after treatment of urethritis, both gonococcal (Thin 1974) and non-gonococcal (King 1964), as well as in a number of conditions of uncertain aetiology, namely: most (83%) cases of ankylosing spondylitis (Mason et al 1958); most (95%) cases of Reiter's disease (Mason et al 1958), compared with 33% rheumatoid arthritis; and in many cases (64%) of anterior uveitis (Catterall 1961).

For reasons given below, there is doubt over the significance of both the diagnosis and of the findings of 'excess' pus cells in the expressed prostatic secretion.

DIAGNOSIS OF PROSTATITIS

Younger patients with symptoms of 'prostatitis' will tend, rather than the older, to be seen in departments of genito-urinary medicine, together with those whose sexual habits may bring anxiety about venereal disease. The symptom of 'prostatic' pain will generally be the reason for initiating fuller investigation, although the finding of significant bacteriuria usually with pyuria, in men will also necessitate such examinations.

The diagnosis of prostatitis due to eubacteria may be made by quantitative bacteriological techniques (Meares 1978, Meares & Stamey 1968). The following procedures are necessary.

Investigations in prostatitis

Urethral smears, including early morning urethral smears and cultures, should have been taken to exclude gonococcal infection; tests should also be taken, when possible, to exclude *Chlamydia trachomatis*, *Ureaplasma urealyticum*, *Trichomonas vaginalis* and herpes simplex virus.

Intercourse should be proscribed for at least 24 hours (Blacklock 1969), say as a routine, for 48 hours before testing; the patient should have a full bladder and a desire to micturate (e.g. after retaining urine overnight or for about 8 hours).

1. Skin preparation is usually unnecessary in the circumcised male. The uncircumcised man is instructed to retract his foreskin and maintain retraction throughout collection of the specimens. The glans is cleansed with detergent; all soap is washed away with a swab soaked in sterile saline.

2. The first 5–10 ml of urine passed is collected in a sterile tube (specimen 1).

3. A midstream specimen of urine (MSU) is obtained after the patient has urinated about 200 ml (specimen 2).

4. The patient stops voiding, and by gentle prostatic massage a few drops of prostatic fluid are collected in

a wide mouthed container (specimen 3: prostatic fluid).

5. The patient then voids, and 5–10 ml urine is collected (specimen 4, urine after prostatic massage).

Cultures for eubacteria should be quantitative.

The diagnosis of bacterial prostatitis (or, *sensu stricto*, eubacterial) is made when the bacterial counts in specimen 3 (prostatic fluid) or specimen 4 (urine after prostatic massage) are more than ten-fold those in specimen 1 and specimen 2.

Technique in obtaining specimens of prostatic secretion

As a general rule it is best for the patient to be placed in the left lateral position, with the buttocks at the edge of the bed and the knees well drawn up, although some doctors prefer to have the patient in the dorsal or knee-elbow position. The patient should be asked to breathe freely through the mouth, as this will relax the abdominal muscles and avoid the Valsalva manoeuvre (Leading Article 1970) i.e. causing increased intra-thoracic pressure by forcible exhalation effort against a closed glottis. The well-lubricated forefinger should be introduced slowly. Each lateral lobe of the prostate receives two or three gentle strokes with the palmar surface of the finger, commencing at the periphery of the gland and ending at the midline. This is followed by two downward strokes in the midline over the prostatic urethra. Finally the finger is withdrawn slowly through the anal canal. Slow insertion and withdrawal of the finger lessens discomfort considerably. If no secretion appears at the external urethral meatus, even after gentle milking of the penile urethra, a further attempt may be made at a later date.

A number of adverse reactions to prostatic palpation have been described. Bilbro (1970) recorded 8 episodes of syncope or faintness, occurring within 30 seconds to 2 minutes, in 2500 prostatic examinations on US Army personnel in Korea during a 13-month period. The patients turned pale and had a bradycardia of 36–48 beats per minute. As the patients showed a sudden loss of consciousness, if they were not placed supine, it must be assumed they were not lying down when rectal examination was carried out. In one case, a 30-year-old man complained of severe anal spasm after examination of the prostate and collapsed striking his head on the edge of a desk sustaining a scalp wound. While falling he had a mild tonic-clonic seizure and was subsequently apnoeic and pulseless. A sharp blow to the anterior chest produced a carotid pulse and a bradycardia of 46 beats per minute. The patient regained consciousness after 3 minutes and recovered uneventfully (Poleshuck 1970). Again it seems that this patient was not lying down during the examination.

An assessment of prostatic inflammation based on the number of leucocytes per high-power microscope field (x40 objective) and on the cell count in expressed prostatic secretions was reported by Simmons & Thin (1983). They estimated that the upper limit of normal for the number of leucocytes was 5 per oil immersion field or $0.5 \times 10^9/1$. These values are lower than those reported by others, but dilution of secretion with residual urine in the method may explain this discrepancy. A change in the pH (measured by Biotest pH papers, Camlab Ltd., Cambridge, England) is related to the inflammatory response and not to the organisms isolated (Blacklock & Beavis 1974, White 1975) and thus may be of value as a clinical test. To base a diagnosis on microscopy findings alone, however, is not reliable (Meares 1978); counts of more than 10 leucocytes per high-power field have been found in 6% of healthy volunteers in the Royal Navy (Blacklock 1969). Cellular content varies from day to day and on occasions not enough may be found in a sample. As infection appears to be focal, prostatic needle biopsy is also thought to be an unsatisfactory method of examination (Blacklock 1969, Meares 1978). Magnetic resonance imaging (MRI) provides precise delineation of the prostate — applied in the sagittal plane it demonstrates very clearly the relation of the gland to the base of the bladder, and in the coronal plane the gland's lateral margins. Confident differentiation, however, between prostatitis and neoplasm is not possible, and the application of MRI appears to be in the staging of prostatic carcinoma (see Note 18.1; Kean & Smith 1986).

In those cases of prostatitis not due to eubacteria, when there has been a poor response to courses of treatment with oxytetracycline or doxycycline, even when a course has been continued for a three week period, examination of the urine should be extended to include the examination of three specimens of early morning urine for *Mycobacterium tuberculosis* by microscopy and culture; a white blood cell count, plasma urea, creatinine and electrolytes are usefully obtained at this stage.

Consultation with a urologist is necessary in all men with a eubacterial urinary infection, whether or not there is also a prostatitis and whether or not the urinary tract infection has responded to a course of antibiotics. In prostatitis with 'prostatic' pain and without a demonstrable eubacterial cause a urological opinion is necessary, particularly when organisms thought to be associated with non-gonococcal urethritis, namely *C. trachomatis* or *U. urealyticum* have been eradicated without a permanent change in symptoms.

On cystoscopy the urologist may find little more than erythema of the bladder trigone to back the diagnosis of prostatitis. In urinary infections, whether due or not to eubacteria, causes of persistent prostatic pain include neoplasm, urethral stricture, glandular prostatic hyperplasia, radiolucent or opaque bladder calculi, and other causes of structural or functional obstruction to urinary flow. An excretion urogram may precede urethrocystoscopy. Because of the overlapping symptomatology with that of outflow obstruction the urologist may consider screening cases by a voiding flow record. Although transrectal ultrasonography has proved useful in the diagnosis of benign prostatic hyperplasia, and may be helpful in the confirmation of a diagnosis of acute prostatitis, there is great difficulty in distinguishing the features of prostatic cancer and chronic prostatitis (Peeling & Griffiths 1984). Rectal examination of the benign prostate (i.e. in the absence of carcinoma) does not raise the serum acid phosphatase concentrations (Daar et al 1981).

The pain of 'prostatitis' differs from that of proctalgia fugax, which may be defined as pain, seemingly arising in the rectum, recurring at irregular intervals and being unrelated to organic pain (Douthwaite 1962). Among the diagnostic features of this condition are:

1. unaccountable occurrence at very irregular intervals in the day or night in a patient in perfect health;
2. spontaneous disappearance of the pain;
3. localization of pain in rectal region above the anus, always in the same place in the same patient, but varying somewhat in different sufferers;
4. severity is variable but pain may be intense; and
5. the pain is described as gnawing, aching, cramp-like or stabbing.

TREATMENT IN PROSTATITIS

Treatment of eubacterial urinary tract infection has been considered in Chapter 24, but apart from doxycycline, erythromycin, oleandomycin, lincomycin and clindamycin, other antibiotics appear to diffuse poorly into prostatic fluid. For this reason co-trimoxazole has been suggested in a dose of 2 tablets twice-daily for 2–4 weeks in eubacterial prostatic infections. Trimethoprim alone 480 mg every 12 hours for 4 weeks is preferable, however, as side effects, particularly in older people, are less common. Long-term suppressive therapy with nitrofurantoin, 50–100 mg, once-or twice-daily, may control the infection (Meares 1978).

In those with 'non-acute' or chronic prostatitis with prostatic pain, not due to eubacteria, there is a case to be made to eradicate trichomonas, chlamydia or ureaplasma, if these organisms are to be found.

An attempt should be made also to clear such an infection in the sexual partner(s) when the relationships are long-term rather than casual. In those with constant changes in partners this approach may not be justifiable. When the infection is believed to have been a sequel to non-gonococcal urethritis or to have arisen *de novo* after sexual exposure, a course of doxycycline (200 mg initially followed by 100 mg daily for 14–21 days) which penetrates the prostate, may help when oxytetracycline or tetracycline have failed. If *T. vaginalis* is found in the patient or his partner metronidazole should be used in both. Similarly in vaginitis in the partner, whether due to *Candida* or of uncertain aetiology, attempts may be made to treat the vaginitis.

When no organismal cause has been demonstrated and/or if the possibility of sexual transmission is only speculative, sexual intercourse should not be proscribed. There is no place for regular prostatic massage in the treatment of 'non-acute' or chronic prostatitis. Symptoms will tend to wax and wane regardless of therapy.

In the individual patient, if ingestion of alcoholic or other beverages, or of spicy foods appear to have aggravated symptoms, restriction should be suggested. The same principle obtains regarding frequency of sexual intercourse (Meares 1978). Rest and reassurance may help when investigation has shown a disturbance of micturition and a deficient voluntary sphincter relaxation (Blacklock 1978). If there is evidence of bladder neck obstruction relief may be obtained by endoscopic bladder neck incisional procedures (Warwick & Whiteside 1976), although such surgical intevention will be restricted to those over 35 years of age to avoid possible interference with fertility in younger men, in whom symptoms may abate in time.

In cases when a diagnosis of prostatitis has been made on the sole basis of finding pus cells in numbers believed to be excessive, treatment is not indicated, unless a coincidental infection such as *N. gonorrhoeae* is also found, or unless a positive attempt is being made to eradicate, say, a chlamydial infection for the benefit of a female sexual partner. In the case of diseases such as anterior uveitis or ankylosing spondylitis, in which excessive numbers of pus cells in the prostate are a coincidental finding, there is no indication for treatment.

INFLAMMATION OF THE TESTIS AND EPIDIDYMIS

Acute epididymitis occurs as a complication of a urinary tract infection, usually due to coliform organisms in the case of older men (over 35 years of age); in the case of younger men, in whom such a coliform infection is rare, epididymitis is usually due to sexually transmitted organisms, *C. trachomatis* or *N. gonorrhoeae*. In countries where medical attention and antibiotic or chemotherapy are readily available, gonococcal epididymitis is rare. Acute epididymitis due to coliform organisms tends to extend into the testis only in advanced disease, when there may be abscess formation.

In epididymitis complicating a general infection, as in leprosy and mumps and in the now rare late-stage syphilis, there is almost invariably substantial testicular involvement also (Morgan 1976). It is therefore important to try to distinguish between acute epididymitis and orchitis by careful examination and to detect sexually transmitted infections.

Patients who have a frank urethral discharge may tend to reach departments of genito-urinary medicine, whereas those who do not have such a discharge or who may have only a slight discharge may be referred to surgical units. The approach to the diagnosis may therefore differ and there is a need for each discipline to collaborate in diagnosis and management of epididymitis as special microbiological facilities required for isolation of the organisms responsible are not always widely available.

Whenever there is uncertainty, however, as to the nature of any thickening, irregularity, nodule or enlargement of the testis or epididymis, referral to a surgeon is necessary as surgical exposure is required for the exclusion or detection of malignant neoplasm. In recent times, with the advent of high frequency real-time ultrasound and the high-resolution imaging of the scrotum and its contents that it provides, the diagnosis of scrotal pathology has become highly accurate. In the diagnosis of malignant disease scrotal ultrasonography is much superior to clinical examination (see p. 250: High frequency real-time scrotal ultrasonography.)

ACUTE EPIDIDYMITIS, A COMPLICATION ARISING FROM INFECTION OF THE URINARY TRACT

In countries where antibiotics are freely available acute epididymitis is an uncommon complication of gonorrhoea (Morgan 1976). In a London STD clinic, Rodin (1969) reported that in 1968 there was 1 case of epididymitis seen in 1214 cases of gonorrhoea, and 1 case among 1691 cases of NGU. In young men, however, acute epididymitis is clearly associated with sexually transmitted organisms, as, for example, in the investigation of a group of 18 men under 32 years of age with epididymitis, culture from the urethra yielded *N. gonorrhoeae* in 6 and *C. trachomatis* in six: both organisms were isolated in an additional patient. Isolations of herpes virus, cytomegalovirus and *U. urealyticum* were also made from urethral specimens in this group (Harnisch et al 1977).

In a study of acute epididymitis (in hospital clinics of the University of Washington) in 13 men under the age of 35 years and 10 over that age, it was found that in the case of the younger men *C. trachomatis* was the likely cause, as this organism was found in the aspirated material from the affected epididymis in 5 of the 6 tested. In 4 of the 5 patients with chlamydia isolated from the urethra the organism was also obtained from the epididymis. In 5 of the 10 older men examined, only coliform organisms were found in material aspirated from the epididymis (Berger et al 1978). In this investigation, also, in 9 of 15 men with epididymitis not due to coliform organisms, *U. urealyticum* was found in the first voided urine but aspirated material from the epididymis provided no evidence that *U. urealyticum* reached the epididymis.

In older men in their thirties or later, when there may have been no risk of a sexually transmitted infection, epididymitis is usually associated with bacteriuria due to *Escherichia coli*, *Klebsiella spp*, *Pseudomonas aeruginosa* or *Proteus spp*. In such cases urological investigation is indicated and this should include an excretion urogram and urethrocystoscopy. When epididymitis is associated with a chronic cystitis there is always some predisposing cause of the infection such as obstruction, stone or neurological disorder and it is important to exclude pyelonephritis, renal tuberculosis or analgesic nephropathy. Chronic eubacterial prostatitis may also be a cause.

ORCHITIS OR EPIDIDYMO-ORCHITIS IN GENERALIZED INFECTIONS

Orchitis and epididymo-orchitis secondary to generalized infections may be seldom seen in STD clinics but knowledge of their pathology (Morgan 1976) as well as that of other inflammatory lesions of the epididymis and testis, is necessary for differential diagnosis.

In syphilis the testicular lesion may be a diffuse chronic interstitial inflammation proceeding to atrophy or a gumma. Clinically, this now rare late-stage effect presents as a painless smooth enlargement of the testis, which is characteristically not tender. Eventually the testis becomes hard due to fibrosis.

In leprosy, particularly lepromatous leprosy, involvement of the testis and to a lesser extent the epididymis is very common. *Mycobacterium leprae* proliferates freely in the testes and testicular atrophy is associated with sterility, impotence and gynaecomastia.

Tuberculous epididymitis may begin quickly and be indistinguishable from the infections described but it is usually insidious. The epididymis enlarges and becomes hard and craggy but is only slightly tender. The vas deferens may be elongated and beaded. Later the epididymis becomes fixed to the skin.

A tuberculous orchitis, generally accompanied by an

epididymitis, is always secondary to lesions elsewhere especially in the lungs, bones, joints or lymph nodes. It is often preceded by tuberculosis of the prostate and seminal vesicles.

In mumps, epididymo-orchitis complicates 20% of cases in adults, with 1 in 6 showing bilateral involvement. Scrotal swelling is usually noted within a week of parotid enlargement, but sometimes only when the clinical signs of mumps have disappeared. Focal inflammatory changes in the testis become diffuse and there is suppuration in severe cases. The epididymis is involved in 85% of cases and on rare occasions epididymitis occurs by itself. Bilateral orchitis followed by atrophy results in sterility or serious impairment of fertility. If there is no atrophy, even in bilateral cases, fertility does not appear to be impaired. The onset of orchitis is associated with fever and headache. The testis is extremely painful and tender.

Appearing at any stage of the disease brucellosis, an orchitis is clinically more evident than an epididymitis. Morgan (1976) cites reports on an incidence of 5–18% and records that it may be five times commoner in *Brucella melitensis* infections than in those due to *Br. abortus*. In *coxsackie virus B* infections orchitis is common, sometimes involving one-third of those infected.

A sperm granuloma is due to extravasation of spermatozoa into surrounding tissue, causing a characteristic cellular reaction followed by fibrosis. Sometimes such a granuloma may be seen in the spermatic cord, especially since vasectomy has become commoner.

A granulomatous orchitis is a chronic inflammatory lesion of uncertain aetiology leading to a hard swelling of the testis in those of 50–60 years of age (Morgan 1976).

In an inflamed hydrocele, proliferation of mesothelial cells in the inflammatory exudate is frequently seen, and is an observation of importance to the pathologist, who wishes to differentiate this change from a true mesothelioma.

Hard non-tender masses of nodular periorchitis may be palpable through the scrotal wall. These may be 0.2–2.0 cm in diameter, projecting from either or both layers of the tunica. Sometimes they form loose bodies and histologically they consist of concentrically laminated hyalin collagen (Morgan 1976).

In infestations with *Wuchereria bancrofti*, *W. pacifica*, *Brugia malayi* and related filariae, the clinical manifestations are slow to develop and change in each successive age group. As the infection develops, the adult worms in the lymph nodes may be associated with an adenopathy and sometimes fever and an allergic inflammatory reaction in the catchment areas of the nodes. A lymphangitis spreads centrifugally, for example from the affected lymph glands in the abdomen, down the

spermatic cord and testis, producing a funiculitis and orchitis. An effusion may develop within the tunica vaginalis and eventually elephantiasis of the scrotum. Filariasis due to *W. bancrofti* will be seen in those from Africa and throughout the tropics. In filariasis due to *W. pacifica* (from the islands of the Southern Pacific, particularly Samoa) clinical manifestations are more severe. In filariasis due to *B. malayi* (from coastal regions of India, from Malaya, Indo-China, Indonesia and New Guinea) genital involvement is rare (Kershaw 1978).

MALIGNANT TUMOURS OF THE TESTICLE

Surgical exploration is very important when there is doubt about the diagnosis of any swelling of the testis; some 4–16% or more of seminomas or teratomas may present as inflammatory lesions (Blandy et al 1970), and 74% of testicular tumours occur in the age group 20–49 years (Pugh 1976). The new diagnostic technique, scrotal ultrasonography, has been shown to be highly accurate in comparison to clinical examination (see paragraph below).

The usual symptoms of testicular cancer include a lump in the testicle, painless swelling or altered consistency of the testis. In many cases the tumour is discovered incidentally during medical examination and the mildness of early symptoms together with fear of cancer may lead patients to delay seeking advice (Mettlin 1983). Typically testicular cancer is stony hard with 'a suggestion of weightiness' on palpation. It is of prime importance when the diagnosis is suspected to refer patients promptly for surgical advice (Weinerth 1986). In addition to assessment by inspection at operation the surgeon will have available the results of serum assays of various tumour markers of malignant germ-cell tumours, viz. alphafetoprotein, beta subunit of human chorionic gonadotrophin and placental alkaline phosphatase (Kohn & Raghavan 1981).

Ultrasonography and nuclear magnetic resonance are currently being evaluated as non-invasive methods of screening (Hargreaves 1987). The former has been shown to be highly accurate and of great value (Leading Article 1987, Fowler et al 1987).

The incidence and mortality rates for testicular cancer tend to be bimodal with prominent peaks in the age group 25–34 years and a lesser peak beginning after age 75. The incidence of testicular cancer is four times greater in whites than in blacks in the USA (Mettlin 1983). Generally higher in incidence in Europe than elsewhere, the number of newly diagnosed cases of cancer of the testicle per 100 000 population per annum is given for various countries as follows: Switzerland,

9.1–9.9; Denmark, 6.7; Hamburg, 5.4; Norway, 4.4; Scotland, 3.7. Worldwide there has been a rise in incidence in young men by about half over the last two decades, and in the age group 20–34 years testicular cancer is now the commonest malignancy although mortality has been reduced by improvement in treatment (Kemp & Boyle 1985).

The majority of testicular tumours are germ-cell tumours, broadly classified further into seminoma and malignant teratoma. At present cure rates for seminomas when patients are seen early approximate 80% and early-stage teratoma can be cured by orchidectomy. For metastatic disease effective cytotoxic chemotherapy is available (Peckham 1981).

Testicular maldescent is recognized as being associated with an increased risk of tumour formation and another recognized factor which predisposes to testicular cancer is a history of malignancy in the contralateral testis. Random biopsy with special histological techniques may show premalignant cells — carcinoma in situ — believed to be precursors of most germ-cell tumours. This technique applied more widely has revealed carcinoma in situ in about 5% of patients with unilateral testicular germ-cell cancer (Von Der Maase et al 1986); 2% of adult men with a history of maldescent of the testis; up to 1% of infertile men; and in up to 80% of men with the rare condition of gonadal dysgenesis (Hargreaves 1987).

High frequency real-time scrotal ultrasonography

The advent of high-frequency real-time ultrasound is now recognized as providing highly accurate investigation of scrotal pathology (Leading Article 1987, Fowler et al 1987) and is advocated in all patients referred with scrotal symptoms and signs. In the diagnosis of malignant disease its high accuracy, sensitivity and specificity are clearly superior to clinical methods (Note 18.2). Hypoechoic malignant lesions can be discovered within the testicular substance and small central and impalpable tumours can be revealed.

The analysis of use of scrotal ultrasonography in clinical practice provided by Fowler et al (1987) is illuminating. In orchitis the testis is diffusely hypoechoic. In acute epididymitis the epididymis is swollen and hypoechoic. The differentiation between solid and cystic lesions enables the easy diagnosis of epididymal cysts. Ultrasound is of great value in the examination of a testis rendered impalpable by a surrounding hydrocele. In varicoceles blood flow can be 'visualized'. Torsion of the testis, however, is not easy to diagnosis by real-time scrotal ultrasonograph, so that when torsion is suspected clinically, surgical exploration should not be delayed by diagnostic imaging (Leading Article 1987).

CLINICAL FEATURES OF ACUTE EPIDIDYMITIS

The onset of acute epididymitis due to pyogenic organisms, including *N. gonorrhoeae* or associated with non-gonococcal urethritis, is usually acute, and the pain on the affected side severe. An associated purulent or mucopurulent urethral discharge is usual in this condition in young men, and there may be malaise and fever. It tends to occur during the 2nd–3rd week of urethritis, affecting the tail first then the whole of the epididymis, which becomes painful, swollen and tender, while the overlying skin appears red and shiny. There may be an inflammatory hydrocele. After a few days the inflammation subsides but the epididymis may be left swollen and indurated.

After excluding the gonococcus as a cause, clinical findings may help to distinguish epididymitis due to coliform organisms from that due to chlamydia. Although a urethral discharge may be present in the majority of those with chlamydial infection, the patient may not be aware of it; the first urine specimen voided will contain more pus cells than the second, and threads may be present. In coliform urinary infection pyuria will be present in all urine specimens; there will often be visible turbidity in the first voided specimen as well as the second. Inguinal pain may be more pronounced in the chlamydia-positive cases than in the coliform. Scrotal oedema and erythema may be more pronounced in the coliform infection (Berger et al 1978).

DIAGNOSIS IN EPIDIDYMITIS

Gonococcal infections are recognized by the methods already outlined (Ch. 15). Non-gonococcal epididymitis may be associated with chlamydial infections although the diagnosis is usually reached by:

1. Detection or exclusion of the gonococcus as a cause.
2. Examination of urethral specimens for *C. trachomatis*. Epididymal aspirations are not advised as a routine procedure.
3. Detection or exclusion of *E. coli*, *Klebsiella* spp, *Pseudomonas* or *Proteus* spp by bacterial examination of a midstream specimen of urine.

Blandy et al (1970) advise that surgical exploration should be carried out in every apparent 'epididymitis' if there is no infection of the urinary tract, particularly when the swelling is not obviously confined to the epididymis. Acute inflammatory swelling of the testis is always a surgical emergency in a young man. The main differential diagnosis rests between epididymitis, torsion and tumour and, as clinical signs are not trustworthy, when urethritis, pyuria or bacteriuria are absent, surgical exposure is necessary. Ultrasound examination of the acute painful scrotum is useful in demonstrating the state of the underlying testes and epididymis (Michell et al 1985) and has been helpful when clinical assessment has been impossible. The differentiation of acute epididymitis from testicular torsion cannot be secured by ultrasonography, so that when torsion is suspected referral for surgical exploration should not be delayed by diagnostic imaging (Leading Article 1987, Fowler et al 1987).

Tuberculous epididymitis is rare, but the examination of three consecutive early morning specimens of urine by microscopy of the centrifuged deposit and by culture should detect *Mycobacterium tuberculosis*.

The diagnosis of infection with *W. bancrofti*, *W. pacifica* or *B. malayi* can be established with certainty only by identifying the microfilariae in the peripheral blood or by recovering an adult worm from an infected lymph node.

Once again it should be emphasized that *in any undiagnosed thickening, irregularity, nodule or enlargement of the testis or epididymis, surgical exposure of the testis is necessary for the exclusion or detection of malignant neoplasm* although the surgeon will have ultrasonography as a new and important aid to diagnosis. In the case of an *acute inflammatory swelling of the testis in a young man* the importance of *excluding torsion* is also emphasized and in this case surgical exploration should not be delayed by diagnostic imaging (see paragraph above).

TREATMENT OF ACUTE EPIDIDYMITIS

Treatment will depend upon the cause. In the case of acute epididymitis the patient should rest in bed. A bandage or jock strap with a cotton-wool pad supporting the testis will limit movement and prevent pain. In gonococcal infections a course of benzylpenicillin (600 mg or 1 million units) is given in 6-hourly dosage intramuscularly for the first 2–3 days and may be changed later to ampicillin 500 mg 6-hourly given orally. Alternatively co-trimoxazole 2 tablets may be given by mouth thrice-daily for 2–3 days initially and twice-daily afterwards. Treatment should continue for one to two weeks. As a chlamydial infection may co-exist with gonorrhoea, or will be suspected or proved in the case of those without a coliform urinary infection, a course of oxytetracycline or doxycycline may be given immediately after the specific treatment for gonorrhoea has been completed. If the aetiology is thought to be that of non-gonococcal urethritis or if *C. trachomatis* has been isolated from the urethra, oxytetracycline (250 mg 6-hourly) or doxycycline (100 mg twice-daily) may be given for one to two weeks. Improvement is rapid, but a cragginess or induration of the epididymis may persist for weeks or months. The tracing and treatment of contacts is essential in both gonococcal and chlamydial infections as well as in those in which the organismal diagnosis is uncertain.

In urinary tract infections where there is a significant bacteriuria, the investigations and management are discussed in Chapter 24.

NOTES TO CHAPTER 18

Note 18.1

Magnetic resonance imaging (MRI) is favoured in general by clinicians as an alternative term to nuclear magnetic resonance (NMR) imaging, the rationale being that the word 'nuclear' could have unfavourable connotations in the mind of the general public (Kean & Smith 1986).

Note 18.2

$$\text{Accuracy} = \frac{\text{True positive} + \text{True negative}}{\text{all}} \times 100\%$$

$$\text{Sensitivity} = \frac{\text{True positive}}{\text{True positive} + \text{False negative}} \times 100\%$$

$$\text{Specificity} = \frac{\text{True negative}}{\text{True negative} + \text{False positive}} \times 100\%$$

REFERENCES

Berger R E, Alexander E R, Monda G D, Ansell J, McCormick G, Holmes K K 1978 Chlamydia trachomatis as a cause of acute 'idiopathic' epididymitis. New England Journal of Medicine 298: 301–304

Bilbro R H 1970 Syncope after prostatic examination. New England Journal of Medicine 282: 167–168

Blacklock N J 1969 Some observations on prostatitis. In: Williams D C, Briggs M H, Standford M (eds) Advances in the study of the prostate. Heinemann, London, p 37–61

Blacklock N J 1978 Prostatic pain. British Journal of Hospital Medicine 20: 80–81

Blacklock N J, Beavis J P 1974 The response of the prostatic fluid in inflammation. British Journal of Urology 46: 537–542

Blandy J P, Hope-Stone H F, Dayan A D 1970 Tumours of the testicle. William Heinemann Medical Books, London

Catterall R D 1961 Significance of non-specific genital infection in uveitis and arthritis. Lancet ii: 739–742

Daar R S, Merrill C R, Moolla Clarke T N S 1981 Rectal examinations and acid phosphatase: evidence for persistence of a myth. British Medical Journal 1378–1379

Darougar S, Woodland R M, Forsey T, Cubitt S, Allami J, Jones B R 1977 Isolation of Chlamydia from ocular infections. In: Hobson D, Holmes K K (eds) Nongonococcal urethritis and related infections. American Society for Microbiology, Washington, p 295–298

Douthwaite A H 1962 Proctalgia fugax. British Medical Journal 2: 164–165

Fowler R C Chennells P M, Ewing R 1987 Scrotal ultrasonography: a clinical evaluation. British Journal of Radiology 60: 649–654

Hargreaves T B 1987 Carcinoma in situ of the testis. British Medical Journal 293: 1389

Harnisch J P, Bergen R E, Alexander E R, Monda G, Holmes K K 1977 Aetiology of acute epididymitis. Lancet i: 819–821

Kean D M, Smith M A 1986 Magnetic resonance imaging. Principles and Applications. Heinemann Medical Books, London, p 2–3, 130–131

Kemp I, Boyle P (eds) (1985) Atlas of cancer in Scotland 1975–1980. Epidemiological perspective. International Agency for Research on Cancer (IARC) Scientific Publications No 72, Lyon

Kershaw W E 1978 Filariasis due to infection with Wuchereria bancrofti, W. pacifica, Brugia malayi and related filaria. In: Jelliffe D B, Stansfield J P (eds) Diseases of children in the subtropics and tropics, 3rd edn. Edward Arnold, London, p 915–919

King A 1964 Non-gonococcal urethritis. Associated conditions and complications. In: Recent advances in venereology, ch 13. Churchill, London, p 375–378

Kohn J, Raghavan D 1981 Tumour markers in malignant germ-cell tumours. In: Peckham M J (ed) The management of testicular tumours. Arnold, London, p 50–69

Leading Article 1970 Prostatic syncope. British Medical Journal 3: 61

Leading Article 1987 Scrotal ultrasonography. Lancet ii: 1064

Mardh P-A, Ripa K T, Colleen S, Treharne J D, Darougar S 1978 Role of Chlamydia trachomatis in non-acute prostatitis. British Journal of Venereal Diseases 54: 330–334

Mason R M, Murray R S, Oates J K, Young A C 1958 Prostatitis and ankylosing spondylitis. British Medical Journal 1: 748–751

Meares E M 1978 Prostatitis: diagnosis and treatment. Drugs 15: 472–479

Meares E M, Stamey T A 1968 Bacteriologic localization patterns in bacterial prostatitis and urethritis. Investigative Urology 5: 492–518

Mettlin C 1983 Cancer of the prostate and testis. In: Bourke G J (ed) The epidemiology of cancer. Croom Helm, Kent, ch 14, p 245–259

Michell M J, Thompson R P, Bell A J Y, Pryor J C, Packham D A 1985 Ultrasound examination of the scrotum. British Journal of Urology 57: 346–350

Morgan A D 1976 Inflammation and infestation of the testis and paratesticular structures. In: Pugh R C E (ed) Pathology of the testis. Blackwell Scientific Publications, Oxford, p 79–138

Murnaghan G F, Millard R J 1984 Urodynamic evaluation of

bladder neck obstruction in chronic prostatitis. British Journal of Urology 56: 713–716

Peckham M J 1981 General introduction: biological diversity and predisposing factors. In: Peckham M J (ed) The management of testicular tumours. Arnold, London

Peeling W B, Griffiths G J 1984 Imaging of the prostate by ultrasound. Journal of Urology 132: 217–224

Poleshuck V A 1970 Prostatic prostration. Correspondence, New England Journal of Medicine 282: 632

Pugh R C B 1976 (ed) Pathology of the testis. Testicular tumours — introduction. Blackwell Scientific Publications, Oxford, p 139–159

Rodin P 1969 Incidence of epididymitis in a department of venereal diseases in the London Hospital. In: Blandy J P, Hope-Stone H F, Dayan A D (eds) Tumours of the testicle. Heinemann Medical Books, p 69

Simmons P D, Thin R N 1983 A method for recognising non-bacterial prostatitis: preliminary observations. British Journal of Venereal Diseases 59: 306–310

Thin R N T 1974 Prostatitis after urethritis in Singapore. British Journal of Venereal Diseases 50: 370–372

Von Der Maase H, Rørth M, Walbom-Jørgensen S et al 1986 Carcinoma in situ of contralateral testis in patients with testicular germ cell cancer: study of 27 cases in 500 patients. British Medical Journal 293: 1398–1401

Warwick R T, Whiteside C G 1976 A urodynamic view of clinical urology. In: Hendry W F (ed) Recent advances in urology. Churchill Livingstone, Edinburgh, p 60–61

Weinerth J L 1986 48. The male genital system. In: Sabiston D C (ed) Textbook of surgery. W B Saunders, Philadelphia, p 1676–1678

White M A 1975 Change in pH of expressed prostatic secretion during the course of prostatitis. Proceedings of the Royal Society of Medicine 68: 511–513

usually manifests itself 10 to 30 days after sexual inter-course or after an attack of dysentery. The mode of onset is variable, but commonly urethritis precedes the appearance of conjunctivitis, which is followed by arthritis. Any of the three features, however, may appear initially.

The duration of the first attack of Reiter's disease varies from between two weeks and several years. In general (more than 70%) first episodes resolve within 12 weeks.

At least half of patients develop recurrences, the interval between the initial episode and the recurrence varying between three months and up to 36 years. Although recurrence may be precipitated by urethritis or dysentery, other factors have been identified and include surgical operations on the urinary tract. The clinical manifestations may be classified as follows.

INFLAMMATION OF THE GENITO-URINARY TRACT IN THE MALE

1. Non-gonococcal urethritis (NGU)

Non-gonococcal urethritis is the most common form of urinary tract inflammation in this disease, and in about 70% of cases is also associated with the post-dysenteric form of the disease (Paronen 1948, Csonka 1960). In a series of 144 cases of Reiter's disease associated with urethritis, the urethritis associated with the initial episode was gonococcal in 17%; non-gonococcal in 43%; both gonococcal and non-gonococcal in 36% and undi-agnosed in 4%.

In patients who have a mixed gonococcal and non-gonococcal urethritis a urethral discharge usually persists following treatment of the gonorrhoea with penicillin. Occasionally a patient who has had gonor-rhoea and has been adequately treated develops Reiter's disease but shows no evidence of post-gonococcal ureth-ritis even on careful examination.

The clinical features of the associated non-gonococcal urethritis are identical to those of uncomplicated ureth-ritis; in both conditions the severity varies considerably. If untreated, the urethritis usually subsides after some two to four weeks, but occasionally may persist for several months.

During the recurrent episodes of Reiter's disease, there may be no clinical evidence of urinary tract inflammation. Csonka (1960), who studied 156 recur-rences of the disease, recorded urethritis in about 58% of these. When urethritis is associated with a recurr-ence, it is most often non-gonococcal in nature, and an integral feature of the recurrence, rather than the appar-ently initiating factor of the first attack. It is clear, however, that in some patients reinfection with gonor-rhoea or with NGU following sexual intercourse may

precipitate a recurrence of signs and symptoms of Reiter's disease. Urethritis resulting from reinfection may not always be followed by a recurrence of the arthritis.

2. Cystitis

Cystitis, often mild and causing little inconvenience, may be associated with Reiter's disease; Csonka (1965) reports an incidence rate of some 20%.

A much more severe, but fortunately rare, form of cystitis is that of acute haemorrhagic cystitis. This is characterized by the rapid onset of frequency of mictur-ition, nocturia, strangury, urgency, haematuria and suprapubic or perineal pain, which may radiate to the penis or testes. Occasionally the patient may be ill with pyrexia, malaise and a polymorphonuclear leucocytosis. In some patients there may be a preceding urethritis (Berg et al 1957). The urine contains many leucocytes and red cells, but is sterile by conventional bacterio-logical examination.

Cystoscopy ought to be avoided during the acute stage, but it has revealed oedema of the bladder mucosa (including the trigone), superficial membranous sloughs, diffuse petechial haemorrhages, and multiple discrete ulcers.

Intravenous urography in most cases of acute haemor-rhagic cystitis shows unilateral or bilateral dilatation of the ureters and renal pelves and calyces. This is prob-ably due to obstruction of the ureteric orifices by mucosal oedema, although in a few cases the inflam-matory process may extend proximally from the bladder. Following resolution of the cystitis, the hydro-nephrosis usually, but not always subsides, generally within two months.

Without treatment, haemorrhagic cystitis may persist for long periods, often with exacerbations and re-missions. Haemorrhagic cystitis may occasionally precede by weeks or months the appearance of other features of the syndrome or may be the sole feature of a recurrence.

3. Acute prostatitis

Acute prostatitis, which may be followed by the forma-tion of prostatic abscesses, has been described in Reiter's disease, but is excessively rare.

The incidence of 'chronic prostatitis' is difficult to determine as there is controversy as to how such a diagnosis is made. Chronic prostatitis has been defined as being present when there are 10 or more pus cells per high-power field in samples of the expressed pros-tatic fluid examined as a wet film. Using this criterion, chronic prostatitis has been diagnosed in 95% of cases of Reiter's disease (Mason et al 1958) (see also Ch. 17).

4. Epididymo-orchitis

Epididymo-orchitis, probably secondary to concomitant

non-gonococcal urethritis, occurs uncommonly (see also Ch. 17).

5. Renal parenchymal involvement

Renal parenchymal involvement in Reiter's disease is a rarity (Paronen 1948).

INFLAMMATION OF THE GENITO-URINARY TRACT IN THE FEMALE

In the female, evidence of inflammation of the urinary tract and/or reproductive system is less obvious and less easily defined. Urethritis rarely shows a definite discharge because the urethra of the female is shorter, relative to the male. Non-specific inflammation as a sign may show by cystitis, on occasions haemorrhagic and of intense severity, vaginitis or cervicitis (Oates & Csonka 1959).

OCULAR INFLAMMATION

The most common ocular manifestation of Reiter's disease is conjunctivitis (occurring in about 30% of cases), which may be unilateral or, more frequently, bilateral. The severity of the conjunctivitis varies widely, ranging from a mild irritation with few objective signs to a severe inflammation with subconjunctival haemorrhage. Resolution occurs spontaneously within one to four weeks, although occasionally conjunctivitis may persist for several months. Mild episcleritis may be associated with conjunctivitis.

During a recurrent episode of the disease, and occasionally late on in the course of an initial severe acute episode, anterior uveitis may develop in about 8% of patients. This complication is usually confined to one eye, when the patient complains of gradual onset of pain and blurring of vision in that eye. On inspection the affected eye is red, particularly at the margin of the cornea, because there is congestion of anterior ciliary blood vessels. As a result of oedema, the normal pattern of the iris is obscured, the pupil is small, reacting poorly to light, and is irregular due to adhesions forming between the iris and the anterior surface of the lens.

It has been demonstrated that anterior uveitis occurs more commonly when a patient has radiological evidence of sacro-iliitis than when he does not. In one study (Oates & Young 1959) of 15 patients with Reiter's disease who had anterior uveitis, 12 had sacro-iliitis.

In a patient with Reiter's disease, uveitis is frequently recurrent, and is often the sole manifestation of a recurrence, during which objective evidence of arthritis is found infrequently. Indeed, uveitis may be the presenting feature of the disease, and hence all young people with uveitis should have a full physical exam-

ination to determine the aetiology of the ocular inflammation.

ARTHRITIS AND OTHER CONNECTIVE TISSUE DISORDERS ASSOCIATED WITH REITER'S DISEASE

Arthritis

During the acute initial episode of Reiter's disease, some 95% of patients develop symptoms of joint involvement. Although a number of patients (about 15%) may complain of arthralgia without objective evidence of inflammation such as joint swelling, the majority develop acute arthritis. The histological appearance of the synovial membrane is not characteristic, being indistinguishable from that of rheumatoid arthritis.

There is rapid onset of pain in, and swelling of, the affected joint, with limitation of movement. The skin overlying the joint may be reddened. There is thickening of the joint capsule and evidence of effusion into the joint. Atrophy of the muscles adjacent to the joint develops rapidly.

Although occasionally only one joint, usually the knee, may be affected, Reiter's disease is most commonly associated with polyarthritis (more than 95% of cases), with asymmetrical involvement of the peripheral large joints. The incidence of joint involvement during the initial episode of Reiter's disease in 50 cases is illustrated in Table 19.2. The joints of the lower limbs are predominantly affected. Usually the arthritis does not involve the joints simultaneously, as there is generally an interval of some days between one joint and another becoming inflamed. After reaching maximum severity, 10 to 14 days after its onset, the arthritis

Table 19.2 Incidence of arthritis occurring during the initial episode of Reiter's disease (data from 50 cases, 48 in men and 2 in women).

Joint involved	Number (and percentage) of patients	
Knee	40	(80)
Ankle	32	(64)
Tarsometatarsal	10	(20)
Metatarsophalangeal	2	(4)
Interphalangeal	18	(36)
Hip	9	(18)
Temporomandibular	1	(2)
Acromioclavicular	1	(2)
Shoulder	5	(10)
Sternoclavicular	2	(4)
Elbow	5	(10)
Wrist	12	(24)
Carpometacarpal	9	(18)
Metacarpophalangeal Interphalangeal	14	(28)
Sacro-iliac	5	(10)

gradually resolves, but recovery may be punctuated by acute exacerbations, perhaps associated with recrudescence of other manifestations of the disease.

Following the acute arthritis of the initial episode, there may be no clinical evidence of joint damage. In some cases, with each recurrent episode of arthritis, permanent damage is done to the joint which may ultimately show the features of chronic arthritis. Uncommonly, in less than 5% of cases, following the initial episode of arthritis, resolution of the inflammatory process is incomplete, and chronic arthritis rapidly develops in the affected joints. The patient complains of pain, stiffness and swelling of the joint, the severity of symptoms being subject to exacerbations and remissions; deformity is the ultimate fate of joints affected in this way. Most frequently it is the joints of the lower limbs and the sacro-iliac joints which bear the brunt of chronic arthritis in this disease. Generally, as chronic arthritis develops, other manifestations of the disease become less obvious, with the possible exception of anterior uveitis.

In a disease in which there may be periods of activity separated by long periods of apparent quiescence, it is not possible to give an accurate prognosis after a single episode of Reiter's disease. In one study of 100 patients who had suffered from Reiter's disease some 20 years previously, 18% had chronic arthritis (Sairanen et al 1969).

As a rare complication, spontaneous rupture of a joint, usually the knee joint, may occur; joint rupture is thought to occur from a cystic formation in the popliteal fossa. There is sudden onset of pain in the calf, and examination reveals a swollen leg which feels warm; the signs resemble thrombophlebitis, which may itself also occur during the course of Reiter's disease (see below). Arthrography is of great value in differentiating between the two conditions (Garner & Mowat 1972).

Radiology of joints in Reiter's disease

In the early stage of an acute episode of Reiter's disease, no radiological abnormalities may be observed; alternatively there may be non-specific, reversible changes such as thickening of the peri-articular tissues (Murray et al 1958). If the inflammatory process is mild, no further changes may occur, but as the disease progresses, radiological abnormalities develop in at least one joint in more than 40% of cases. These changes are most noticeable in the joints and bones of the lower limbs, especially the feet and in the sacro-iliac joints.

Destructive lesions ('erosions') are found at the periphery of the articular surface of the affected joint, and appear as small well-demarcated areas of bone destruction. As the condition progresses, the area of destruction increases and the articular surface of the joint is eventually destroyed, with radiological narrowing of the joint space. Erosions are most commonly found in the metatarsal, tarsal and interphalangeal joints of the feet, and on the posterior aspect of the calcaneum.

In cases where radiological abnormalities are found, periostitis is frequent. Most commonly the periostitis affects the neck of the metatarsals and metacarpals, the distal parts of the tibia, fibula and the shafts of the proximal phalanges; it appears on X-ray as a thin linear opacity running parallel to the cortex of the bone. In the bones of the tarsus and carpus the sharp outline of the bone may be replaced by an irregular contour.

Periostitis affecting the calcaneum is a common radiological finding, occurring in more than 50% of cases (Murray et al 1958). The changes involve the postero-lateral and plantar aspects of the bone. In chronic cases, as periosteal new bone is formed on the plantar surface of the calcaneum at the insertion of the plantar fascia, a 'spur' develops with a characteristic 'fluffy' appearance due to the diffuse nature of the periostitis.

Plantar spurs of a different character may be found in normal individuals, in those suffering from osteoarthrosis, in rheumatoid arthritis and in ankylosing spondylitis. These spurs, representing ossification at the site of attachment of plantar ligaments, are clearly defined and not associated with changes beyond the base of the spur.

Interpretation of radiographs of the sacro-iliac joints is often difficult, as some asymmetry of the joints is common, and leads to differences in appearance of the joints. Sacro-iliitis is found in about 50% of cases, most frequently in recurrent cases, the incidence rising with duration of the disease. It is manifest radiologically as loss of the normal outline of the joint, irregularity of the joint margins due to erosions, and sclerosis beyond the area of the erosion. Although sometimes unilateral (less than 20%), these changes are usually seen in both joints. Complete obliteration of the joint, as is seen in ankylosing spondylitis, is uncommon, but when it occurs it is indistinguishable from that condition. Occasionally, radiological changes, in the form of narrowing of joint space, irregularity of the joint margin and ossification of joint ligaments may be noted in the symphysis pubis.

Spinal changes may be noted uncommonly in Reiter's disease. Syndesmophytosis (i.e. the appearance of strips of bone joining adjacent vertebrae) occurs in cases of longstanding Reiter's disease. Rarely radiological changes indistinguishable from those found in ankylosing spondylitis are found in Reiter's disease.

In the chronic arthritis of Reiter's disease, joint deformities such as lateral dislocation of the proximal phalanges on the metatarsals may be noted on X-ray.

Plantar fasciitis

Clinical evidence of plantar fasciitis is found in about

20% of patients suffering an acute episode of the disease. The patient complains of pain in the sole of the foot. In the most severely affected cases, the skin overlying the fascia is reddened and swollen. More commonly, there is only tenderness of the fascia, particularly close to the heel. Although usually involving both feet, one may be more severely affected than the other. Plantar fasciitis generally resolves within several weeks of its onset, but occasionally may be very persistent.

Tendonitis and bursitis

Although any tendon and its synovial sheath may become inflamed during the course of Reiter's disease, the tendo achilles most often produces clinical signs (about 10% of cases in the acute stage). Tendonitis is most often accompanied by adjacent bone or joint disease.

Rarely inflammation of bursae, especially the pre-

patellar bursa, may occur during the acute stages of the disease. On a radiograph tendonitis and tenovaginitis may appear as a broad soft tissue shadow.

SKIN LESIONS

Keratoderma blenorrhagica (Figs. 19.1, 19.2) is the typical skin lesion found in Reiter's disease, occurring in about 10% of cases. Although the soles of the feet are most commonly affected, keratoderma may also occur anywhere on the body (dorsa of the feet, palms, extensor surfaces of the legs and forearms, trunk, scalp, scrotum, shaft of penis, umbilicus) and occasionally presents as a generalized skin rash.

The initial lesion is a brown macule 2–4 mm in diameter which rapidly becomes papular. The centre of the papule becomes pustular, and the roof becomes thickened. Increase in size occurs from the accumu-

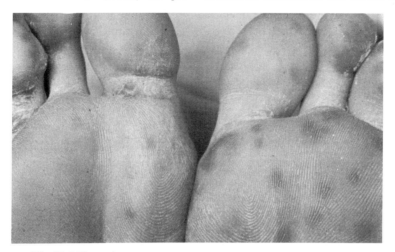

Fig. 19.1 Keratoderma blenorrhagica at an early stage in Reiter's disease.

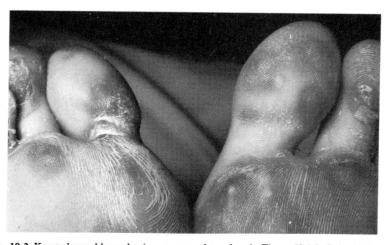

Fig. 19.2 Keratoderma blenorrhagica at a stage later than in Figure 19.1 in Reiter's disease.

lation of parakeratotic scales on the surface of the lesion, and lateral growth of the base; this is the typical limpet-like lesion of keratoderma. Most commonly lhe skin manifestations of Reiter's disease are less florid, and few typical keratoderma lesions are to be seen. In such cases, pustular lesions on the soles may be the only skin lesions to be found, and these subside generally within 3–4 weeks of their appearance. On the weight-bearing areas of the soles, lateral spread of the pustule produces a thick-walled bulla. Generally lesions on the trunk, arms, legs and shaft of penis are less typical, and consist of firm, dull-red papules (the hard parakeratotic nodule).

Keratoderma usually heals within 6 to 10 weeks from its onset, but may occasionally take much longer. 'Cropping' is characteristic during the course of an acute episode, various stages of development of the lesions of keratoderma being present at the same time.

Although the physical appearance of keratoderma may cause the patient distress, the lesions themselves do not usually produce discomfort, unless there is secondary bacterial infection.

The finger and toe nails may be involved in Reiter's disease. In mild cases, the nail plate becomes opaque, thickened, ridged and brittle. When the nails are more severely affected, in addition to the latter changes, sterile, subungual abscesses develop and, as these dry out, yellow debris accumulates under the distal half of the nail. As this process continues, the nail becomes elevated from its bed, turns brown and is often shed. The skin adjacent to the nail base, and the nail fold takes part in tne reaction. These changes may be mistaken for fungal infection of the nails.

The Köbner phenomenon has been described as occurring in Reiter's disease (non-specific trauma induces skin changes in the affected site of a type present at the same time elsewhere on the body). The Köbner phenomenon is found in many skin diseases e.g. psoriasis, lichen planus, warts (Rook et al 1986).

ORAL LESIONS

Lesions of the mucous membranes of the buccal cavity occur in about 10% of cases of Reiter's disease. The site most commonly affected is the palate, followed by the buccal mucosa, gingiva, and tongue. Such lesions are asymptomatic, have to be looked for carefully and generally heal within a few weeks of their appearance.

On the palate the lesions usually appear as whitish slightly elevated macules, not covered by inflammatory exudate, and surrounded by a narrow erythematous zone. Occasionally, multiple purpuric spots may appear.

Similar lesions may be noted on the buccal mucosa. On the tongue, round or oval reddened areas appear,

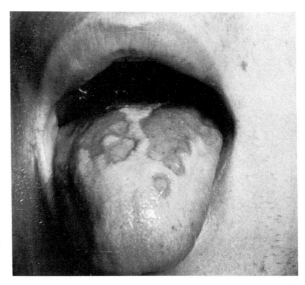

Fig. 19.3 Bald patches on the dorsum of the tongue in Reiter's disease.

sharply demarcated from the surrounding normal epithelium 'bald patches' (Fig. 19.3).

PENILE LESIONS

Reference has already been made to keratoderma of the shaft of the penis and the outer aspect of the prepuce. Lesions may also be found in about 25% of cases on the glans penis and on the mucous surface of the prepuce, which usually precede other mucocutaneous manifestations.

On the glans, the appearance of the lesion depends on whether or not the individual has been circumcised. If he is circumcised, the lesions are dry and appear as slightly elevated scaling macules sharply demarcated from the surrounding skin. When a prepuce is present, scale formation is inhibited, and the lesions appear as moist, glistening, red, sharply-defined macules which become confluent, producing a polycyclic margin known as circinate balanitis. Unless there is secondary bacterial infection, which is a common complication, pain is absent, and healing tends to occur within 4 weeks of the appearance of the lesions. Circinate lesions of the labia minora have also been described (Thamber et al 1977).

VISCERAL LESIONS OF REITER'S DISEASE

Clinical evidence of involvement of organs of the body, other than those previously mentioned, is uncommon.

It is quite possible that, in a disease with such a broad spectrum of symptoms and signs, many organs are involved in the inflammatory process, without producing obvious abnormalities.

Cardiovascular system

Pericarditis

This occurs uncommonly (less than 5%) during an acute episode of Reiter's disease. The patient may or may not have chest pain when there is pericarditis (Csonka & Oates 1957).

Myocarditis

The incidence of myocarditis is difficult to determine, but is less than 5%.

The most common finding is first degree heart block, i.e. a P-R interval of greater than 0.20 seconds. Rarely, other conduction defects such as second degree heart block, left bundle-branch block and complete heart block occur.

Although usually transient, these ECG abnormalities may persist unchanged for years, or one abnormality may supervene on another (Rossen et al 1975).

Aortitis

This is a rare complication, having been adequately described in the literature in fewer than 30 patients. It is usually associated with recurrent episodes of the disease, which has been present for at least eight years, with sacro-iliitis and with conduction defects (Block 1972). Aortic incompetence is the usual presenting feature.

Thrombophlebitis of the deep veins of the leg

This may be found during an acute episode of Reiter's disease in about 3% of cases (Csonka 1966). Patients complain of pain in the affected calf and there is tenderness, induration of the calf muscles, and oedema of the leg. Thrombophlebitis occurs within a few days of the onset of the arthritis and the knee joint on the affected side is always involved.

The most important condition to be distinguished from thrombophlebitis is spontaneous rupture of the knee joint. Arthrography, ultrasonic examination of the veins of the calf, and venography are useful aids to diagnosis.

RESPIRATORY SYSTEM

Pleurisy has been described as occurring in the acute stages of Reiter's disease, having been found in about 8% of cases described by Paronen (1948). Transient opacities may be observed on chest radiographs of patients, but their significance is uncertain (Gatler & Moskowitz 1962).

RETICULO-ENDOTHELIAL SYSTEM

Generalized enlargement of lymph nodes has been observed uncommonly in Reiter's disease (less than 1% of cases). Histological examination reveals non-specific reactive hyperplasia. Rarely there is moderate enlargement of the spleen.

NERVOUS SYSTEM

Various neurological abnormalities have been described in association with Reiter's disease, but these are seen in less than 2% of cases. Meningoencephalitis, multiple peripheral neuropathy, amyotrophic lateral sclerosis have been well-documented as occurring during an acute episode of the disease, occasionally reappearing during recurrences (Oates & Hancock 1959).

In longstanding cases of Reiter's disease, the occurrence of Parkinsonism and other neuro-psychiatric abnormalities is difficult to evaluate, as these disorders also affect the general population (Good 1974).

AMYLOIDOSIS

This is a very rare complication of severe Reiter's disease (Caughey & Wakem 1973).

LABORATORY TESTS IN REITER'S DISEASE

There is no diagnostic test for Reiter's disease, but the investigations given aid differential diagnosis.

Blood

Haemoglobin concentration, packed cell volume (PCV), mean corpuscular haemoglobin concentration (MCHC) and mean corpuscular volume (MCV)

In severe cases, the results of these tests indicate mild normocytic, normochromic anaemia, i.e. the haemoglobin concentration is less than 13.5 g/dl but the MCV is normal (76–96 fl; fl = femtolitre = μm^3) as is the MCHC (30–35 g/dl).

White cell count

In the acute episode of Reiter's disease, there is a polymorphonuclear leucocytosis (i.e. a white cell count of greater than $11.0 \times 10^9/l$) in 25 to 30% of cases.

Erythrocyte sedimentation rate (ESR)

This is elevated in more than 90% of cases of acute Reiter's disease, being in the early stages greater than 50 mm per hour (Westergren) in about 40% of cases. The ESR falls slowly during the first month of the acute episode, and, although becoming normal by about the sixth to tenth week after the onset, may remain elevated in about 15% of patients for much longer.

Plasma-protein changes

During the acute episode in about 30% of cases the plasma albumin is lower than normal, and the alpha globulin fraction elevated. There is only slight elevation in the gamma globulin fraction. In the acute stage, serum IgM may be raised, but falls to normal as the inflammatory process resolves.

Rheumatoid factor

The incidence of rheumatoid factor in the normal population is about 4%, and in Reiter's disease the incidence is similar. The rheumatoid arthritis latex particle agglutination test and the sheep red cell agglutination tests are usually negative (96%) in Reiter's disease. Although these tests for IgM rheumatoid factor are usually negative, IgG antiglobulin may be demonstrated in the serum of patients with Reiter's disease.

Anti-streptolysin O titre

The results of this test are within normal limits (less than 200 units per ml).

LE cells and antinuclear antibodies

These tests usually give negative results.

Uric acid

The differential diagnosis from gout may be difficult in 2% of cases of Reiter's disease when the serum uric acid is elevated.

Smooth-muscle antibody

This may be detected in about 50% of cases, and it should be noted that this test is not specific for active chronic hepatitis.

Synovial fluid

Joint aspiration is needed only if the diagnosis is in doubt, or if there is considerable discomfort from a large effusion. Fluid aspirated from an affected joint is yellow and turbid, clotting spontaneously. The white cell count varies considerably from 1000 to 5000 × 10^6 per litre. The normal white cell count in joint fluid is less than 200 × 10^6 per litre. Although the inflammatory exudate is initially composed mainly of polymorphonuclear leucocytes, as the duration of the arthritis increases, lymphocytes predominate.

The protein content of the fluid is high, about 40 to 50 g per litre (reference value for synovial fluid 10 to 20 g per litre). Synovial fluid glucose concentration is low (about 4.2 mmol litre) in about a third of patients. The total haemolytic complement activity in synovial fluid in Reiter's disease is normal or high (cf. rheumatoid arthritis where it is low). Recently, complement deposits have been demonstrated in the synovium.

Studies of cellular immunology

Reference has already been made earlier in this chapter and in Table 19.1 to the data on HLA-associated disease.

DIFFERENTIAL DIAGNOSIS OF THE ACUTE EPISODE OF REITER'S DISEASE

Although the diagnosis is clear when all three features of the triad are present, when there are only one or two signs, the following diseases must be considered in the differential dignosis.

Gonococcal arthritis

This is the disease with which Reiter's disease is most often confused. Both conditions have urethritis and arthritis in common. In any urethritis it is important to exclude the gonococcus, but it should be remembered that there may be dissemination of this organism from the pharynx or rectum, in the absence of urethral infection.

In gonococcal arthritis, isolation of *N. gonorrhoeae* from the synovial fluid is often unsuccessful.

The skin lesions of the bacteraemic stage of a disseminated gonococcal infection should not be confused with keratoderma.

Urethral gonorrhoea may be a precipitating factor in Reiter's disease and immediate differentiation may be difficult. Within two to three days of commencing antibiotic treatment, however, a gonococcal arthritis will have improved considerably, whereas improvement does not necessarily occur in Reiter's disease.

Rheumatoid arthritis

This disease is more commonly found in females, and usually presents in middle age. In contrast to Reiter's disease, the onset tends to be insidious and joints are affected in a symmetrical fashion. Any synovial joint may be involved, but particularly the metacarpophalangeal (80%); wrist (85%); elbow (70%); metatarsophalangeal (70%) and knee joints (80%). Although sacro-iliitis may be demonstrated radiologically, the appearances are rarely as striking as those found in Reiter's disease. Chronic prostatitis may be diagnosed in about 20% of males with rheumatoid disease. Anterior uveitis may occur in about 20% of patients. Rheumatoid factor is present in the serum in at least

80% of patients. Subcutaneous nodules, which occur in 30% of cases of rheumatoid arthritis, are never found in Reiter's disease.

Rheumatic fever

Although usually preceded by pharyngitis, a proportion (up to 30%) of patients with rheumatic fever do not give this history. The onset of arthritis, which is usually polyarticular, is acute, when large joints are chiefly affected. Classically the arthritis is migratory, affected joints returning to normal within a few days of the onset. Joints, however, may remain inflamed for weeks.

Erythema marginatum is found in about 10% of children affected, and in severe cases, subcutaneous nodules of various sizes may be found. Erythema nodosum may also be associated with rheumatic fever.

Ocular and urinary tract inflammation do not occur. Serum antistreptolysin O titres rise above normal limits in 80% of patients with rheumatic fever.

Acute septic arthritis (excepting gonococcal arthritis)

Acute septic arthritis may be caused by numerous organisms, e.g. *Staphylococcus aureus*, *Streptococcus pyogenes*, *Neisseria meningitidis*, *Salmonella* spp., *Streptococcus pneumoniae*.

Any joint may become inflamed, but most often the knee, wrist and elbow are affected. Aspiration of the effusion, with appropriate bacteriological examination of the aspirated fluid, is usually diagnostic.

Other reactive arthritides

Reactive arthritis may follow intestinal infection with *Yersinia enterocolitica*, *Shigella* spp, *Salmonella* spp and *Campylobacter* spp and is a feature of systemic viral infections, including rubella, EB virus and human parvovirus. The diagnosis is made by culture of the bacteria from the faeces or, in the case of yersinia and viral infection, by the detection of IgM antibodies in acute phase sera. Interestingly the majority of patients with yersinia arthritis have HLA-B27 in their tissue type.

Tuberculous arthritis

In the United Kingdom this is a rare disease, encountered most commonly in the elderly. The onset is insidious and most often the arthritis is monoarticular. Synovial biopsy, with bacteriological and histological examination is necessary for diagnosis.

Brucellosis

Bone and joints are frequently affected in this disease. Peripheral arthritis, sacro-iliitis and spondylitis occur. The arthritis may affect any joint, but commonly the shoulders, knees and elbows. Sacro-iliitis occurs in about 30% of patients, and may affect one or both sides.

In a patient with arthritis, particularly if there has been contact with farm animals, the following serological tests for brucellosis should be done to exclude this infection: a standard agglutination test; the anti-human globulin (Coombs) test for non-agglutinating antibodies; and the complement fixation test.

Trauma

Non-gonococcal urethritis is common in young men, and it is not uncommon to find urethritis in association with a traumatized joint.

Erythema multiforme and Stevens-Johnson syndrome

Erythema multiforme is a self-limiting skin disease associated in many cases with some underlying condition, such as herpes simplex infection or drug idiosyncrasy. When severe, the condition is termed Stevens-Johnson syndrome and is associated with mucous membrane ulceration (oral and genital) bullous lesions of the skin, conjunctivitis and arthritis.

Disseminated lupus erythematosus (DLE)

Usually females are affected by this condition. LE cells and antinuclear factor are found in the blood. DNA antibodies are present in the active stage of this disease. Antibody to double-stranded DNA is characteristic (Roitt 1988).

Other seronegative spondarthritides

Acute arthritis may be associated with ankylosing spondylitis, psoriatic arthritis, ulcerative colitis, Crohn's disease, Behçet's syndrome and Whipple's disease. The relationships of these conditions require separate consideration and may be important in the differential diagnosis, particularly of the chronic episode of arthritis.

DIFFERENTIAL DIAGNOSIS OF THE CHRONIC EPISODE OF REITER'S DISEASE

Idiopathic ankylosing spondylitis

Ankylosing spondylitis and Reiter's disease share many features. Both are associated with a peripheral arthritis, about 98% in the case of Reiter's disease and about 60% in ankylosing spondylitis. Sacro-iliitis is found in all patients with ankylosing spondylitis and in at least 50% of all cases of Reiter's disease in the chronic stages. Spinal involvement may occur in Reiter's disease, when the radiological appearance may be indistinguishable from ankylosing spondylitis. Rarely, those with all the manifestations of Reiter's disease develop the features of idiopathic ankylosing spondylitis later in life.

Evidence of inflammation of the urinary or reproductive system is found in all patients with Reiter's disease, and as 'chronic prostatitis' in at least 80% of cases of ankylosing spondylitis. Anterior uveitis, too, is a complication of about 20% of cases of both conditions and aortitis is a rare complication of both.

Idiopathic ankylosing spondylitis is not usually associated with keratoderma or other mucocutaneous lesions.

Psoriatic arthritis

This is the disease to which Reiter's disease bears a most striking resemblance. Psoriasis may uncommonly be associated with a seronegative, radiologically-erosive polyarthritis (about 5% of cases). Except in those patients with distal interphalangeal joint involvement, the anatomical distribution of joints affected by arthritis is not a helpful factor in reaching a diagnosis. Radiological evidence of sacro-iliitis is found also in at least 20% of patients with psoriatic arthritis.

There are close clinical and histological similarities between pustular psoriasis and keratoderma blenorrhagica. Peripheral arthritis and sacro-iliitis occur in the two conditions, so separation of psoriatic arthritis from Reiter's disease is not possible on every occasion. Not uncommonly, the features of one condition may predominate over the other. Sometimes, patients diagnosed as suffering from psoriatic arthritis may develop the later manifestations of Reiter's disease, and vice versa (Wright & Reed 1964, Maxwell et al 1966).

Ulcerative colitis, Crohn's disease, Whipple's disease and Behçet's disease

These conditions share with Reiter's disease peripheral arthritis, sacro-iliitis, anterior uveitis and diarrhoea. The skin and oral lesions tend to be somewhat different clinically and histologically from keratoderma and the oral lesions of Reiter's disease. Table 19.3 shows the comparative incidence of these abnormalities in this group.

Familial aggregation

Within Reiter's disease itself
Familial aggregation has been observed in both post-

dysenteric type Reiter's disease and the type associated with urethritis. It is difficult to be certain whether accumulation of cases within families is due to genetic factors or infectious agents or both.

Between Reiter's disease and other members of the group
It has been shown that psoriasis is 14 times more common in male relatives of Reiter's disease patients than in the general population. Clinical ankylosing spondylitis is eight times, and radiologically bilateral sacro-iliitis three times as frequent in male relatives of patients with Reiter's disease, as in the general population (Lawrence 1974).

TREATMENT

At present, treatment for Reiter's disease is not curative but is aimed at relieving symptoms. When the patient first attends, other STD should be excluded and the course of the disease fully explained to him. He should be told particularly that the acute episode may last for at least six weeks, but that sometimes it may last for twice as long.

URETHRITIS

The management of non-gonococcal urethritis has already been discussed (Ch. 17). The presence of the complication of Reiter's disease does not alter the general approach. Although of value in aiding resolution of urethritis, treatment with a tetracycline does not alter the course of the disease.

CONJUNCTIVITIS

This is a self-limiting condition, generally resolving within a few weeks of its onset. Although the use of topical steroid preparations may produce symptomatic relief, it is generally agreed that they should be withheld to prevent a possible viral keratitis.

Table 19.3 Incidence of common features in Reiter's disease and four members of the group of seronegative spondarthritides.

| Disease | Percentage incidence | | | | | |
	Peripheral arthritis	Sacro-iliitis	Anterior uveitis	Diarrhoea	Skin lesions	Oral lesions
Reiter's disease	97	50	8	*	10	10
Ulcerative colitis	10	20	5	80	2	15
Crohn's disease	5	20	5	50	2	10
Whipple's disease	65	20	0	90	**	**
Behçet's disease	45	**	70	40	80	98

* Incidence varies according to whether Reiter's disease follows urethritis or dysentery.
** Insufficient data.

IRITIS

In management of this complication advice should be obtained from an ophthalmologist. Mydriasis is maintained by the use of atropine sulphate eye drops, BNF, 1% w/v twice-daily, with phenylephrine eye drops, BNF, three times daily. Dilatation of the pupil produces relief of pain and reduces the risk of the development of iris adhesions.

Steroids should be applied topically, for example in the form of betamethasone sodium phosphate eye drops, three or four times daily.

ARTHRITIS

During the acute stage of the illness, when the joints are markedly inflamed, bed rest is advisable. It is of great importance to ensure that the correct posture is assumed during this period of rest (Boyle & Buchanan 1971). The patient should be nursed on a firm mattress, with adequate support given for his back. A bed cage to keep the weight of the bed clothes off the lower limbs is useful. Pillows must not be placed behind the knees as this favours the development of flexion deformities.

Local immobilization of an affected joint by means of a plaster of Paris splint, held in place by a bandage, may be a useful aid in relieving the patient's discomfort. Gentle active movement of the joint twice-daily reduces the risk of stiffness developing in the splinted joint. By supervising these exercises, a physiotherapist can help with the patient's management.

Various analgesics and anti-inflammatory drugs have been used in the management of the arthritis of Reiter's disease. A few drugs with which the authors have had experience are mentioned below.

Aspirin and salicylates

The dosage of aspirin must be determined by trial and error, the minimum dose effective in relieving the pain being used. To maintain adequate blood levels of the drug, four-hourly oral administration is necessary. The total daily dose varies between 3 g and 6 g.

Side effects of aspirin are common, and dyspepsia is the most common complaint (at least 30% of patients).

Aspirin administration may result in chronic gastrointestinal bleeding, and rarely acute massive haemorrhage. The use of salicylates should be avoided in all patients with a history of peptic ulceration. Hypersensitivity reactions to aspirin are very rare.

Indomethacin

This is a powerful analgesic and anti-inflammatory agent. The dosage is 25 mg three times daily by mouth. To relieve morning stiffness, a single tablet containing 75 mg indomethacin and given before retiring may be useful.

The side effects of this drug are dose-related and include headache, especially in the morning, dizziness, tinnitus, drug rashes, nausea and anorexia. Occasionally gastrointestinal haemorrhage from a peptic ulcer has occurred and sometimes even perforation.

It is recommended that, when a patient is seen with mild arthritis, aspirin should be used initially, and if there is a poor response to this drug, one of the other agents employed. In more severe cases, indomethacin may be required from the start, and continued until the inflammatory process begins to abate. Aspirin may then be substituted for these agents.

The use of corticosteroid preparations, such as prednisolone, is rarely necessary, most cases responding to the measures already outlined. When posterior uveitis or symptomatic pericarditis occur, specialist advice should be sought, as systemic steroids are indicated.

The aspiration of a tense effusion in the knee joint followed immediately by the instillation of 40 mg of methylprednisolone acetate (Depo-Medrone, Upjohn) has proved useful in alleviating joint symptoms, but prospective and controlled trials are difficult and have not yet been done.

CIRCINATE BALANITIS

This condition usually resolves spontaneously within a few weeks of its onset, but healing may be facilitated by the use of a topical steroid preparation, combined with an antimicrobial agent, e.g. betamethasone ointment with clinoquinol (Betnovate-C) applied twice-daily for 1–2 weeks.

When there is secondary bacterial infection, the use of local saline lavages, and dressings soaked in normal saline applied to the glans, are of value.

KERATODERMA BLENORRHAGICA

There is no specific treatment for this self-limiting manifestation. The skin should be kept dry.

THROMBOPHLEBITIS AND RUPTURE OF THE KNEE JOINT

The use of a supporting stocking and anti-inflammatory drugs (e.g. indomethacin) is sufficient to produce relief of symptoms. To reduce the possibility of phlebothrombosis developing in the deep veins of the calf, patients with this complication should not be immobilized longer than necessary. When synovial membrane rupture occurs, bed rest with immobilization of the joint for two to three days is all that is required.

NOTE TO CHAPTER 19

Note 19.1: Estimates of the strength of an association (Svejgaard et al 1983)

1. The 2 × 2 Table

	Number of individuals	
	Character present	*Character absent*
Patients	a	b
Controls	c	d

Frequency of character in patients: $h_p = \dfrac{a}{a + b}$

2. Relative risk (RR): $RR = \dfrac{a \times d}{b \times c}$

3. Etiologic fraction (EF): $EF = \dfrac{RR-1}{RR} \dfrac{a}{a + b} = \dfrac{RR-1}{RR} h_p$

(Positive associations: RR>1)

4. Preventive fraction (PF): $PF = \dfrac{(1-RR)h_p}{RR(1-h_p)+h_p}$

(Negative associations: RR<1)

REFERENCES

Aho K, Ahvonen P, Lassus A, Sievers K, Tiilkainen A 1974 HLA-A27 in reactive arthritis. A study of Yersinia arthritis and Reiter's disease. Arthritis and Rheumatism 17: 521–526

Bender K 1984 HLA system (2nd English edn) Section 5.2 HLA and Disease. Biotest Bulletin 2(2): 94–95

Berg R L, Weinberger H, Dienes L 1957 Acute haemorrhagic cystitis. American Journal of Medicine 22: 818–858

Block S R 1972 Reiter's syndrome and acute aortic insufficiency. Arthritis and Rheumatism 15: 218–220

Boyle J A, Buchanan W W 1971 Clinical rheumatology. Blackwell Scientific Publications, Oxford

Brewerton D A, Caffrey M, Hart F D, James D C O, Nicholls A, Sturrock R D 1973 Ankylosing spondylitis and HL-A 27. Lancet i: 904–907

Caughey D E, Wakem C J 1973 A fatal case of Reiter's disease complicated by amyloidosis. Arthritis and Rheumatism 16: 695–700

Csonka G W 1960 Recurrent attacks in Reiter's disease. Arthritis and Rheumatism 3: 164–169

Csonka G W 1965 Reiter's syndrome. Ergebnisse der Inneren Medizin und Kinderheilkunde 23: 139–189

Csonka G W 1966 Thrombophlebitis in Reiter's syndrome. British Journal of Venereal Diseases 42: 93–95

Csonka G W, Oates J K 1957 Pericarditis and electrocardiographic changes in Reiter's syndrome. British Medical Journal 1: 867–869

Dawkins R L, Christiansen F T, Kay P H, Garlepp M, McCluskey J, Hollingsworth P N, Zilko P J 1983 Disease associations with complotypes, supratypes and haplotypes. Immunological Reviews 70: 5–22

Eastmond C J, Woodrow J C 1977 Discordance for ankylosing spondylitis in monozygotic twins. Annals of Rheumatic Diseases 36: 360–364

Garner R W, Mowat A G 1972 Joint rupture in Reiter's disease. British Journal of Surgery 59: 657–659

Gatler R A, Moskowitz R W 1962 Pneumonitis associated with Reiter's disease. Diseases of the Chest 42: 433–436

Geczy A F, Alexander K, Bashir H V, Edmonds J P, Uppold L, Sullivan J 1983 HLA-B27, Klebsiella and ankylosing spondylitis: biological and chemical studies. Immunological Reviews 70: 23–50

Good A E 1974 Reiter's disease: a review with special attention to cardiovascular and neurologic sequelae. Seminars in Arthritis and Rheumatism 3: 253–286

Keat A C, Thomas B J, Taylor-Robinson D, Pegrum G D, Maini R H, Scott J T 1980 Evidence of *Chlamydia trachomatis* infection in sexually acquired reactive arthritis. Annals of the Rheumatic Diseases 39: 431–437

Kinsella T D 1985 Review of research on the role of *Klebsiella* antigens in the spondyloarthropathies. In: Ziff M, Cohen S B (eds) Advances in inflammation research, vol 9. The Spondyloarthropathies. Raven Press, New York, p 139–149

Kousa M, Saikku P, Richmond S, Lassus A 1978 Frequent association of chlamydial infection with Reiter's syndrome. Sexually Transmitted Diseases 5: 57–61

Lawrence J 1974 Family survey of Reiter's disease. British Journal of Venereal Diseases 50: 140–145

Mason R M, Murray R S, Oates J K, Young A C 1958 Prostatin and ankylosing spondylitis. British Medical Journal 1: 748–752

Maxwell J D, Greig W R, Boyle J A, Pasieczny T, Schofield C B S 1966 Reiter's disease and psoriasis. Scottish Medical Journal II: 14–18

Moll J M H, Haslock I, MacRae I F, Wright V 1974 Associations between ankylosing spondylitis, psoriatic arthritis, Reiter's disease, the intestinal arthropathies and Behcet's syndrome. Medicine 53: 343–364

Murray R S, Oates J K, Young A C 1958 Radiological changes in Reiter's syndrome and arthritis associated with urethritis. Journal of the Faculty of Radiologists 9: 37–43

Oates J K, Csonka G W 1959 Reiter's disease in the female. Annals of Rheumatic Diseases 18: 37–44

Oates J K, Hancock J A H 1959 Neurological symptoms and lesions occurring in the course of Reiter's disease. American Journal of Medical Sciences 238: 79–83

Oates J K, Young A C 1959 Sacro-iliitis in Reiter's disease. British Medical Journal 1: 1013–1015

Oliver R T D 1977 Histocompatability antigens and human disease. British Journal of Hospital Medicine 18: 449–459

Paronen I 1948 Reiter's disease. Acta Medica Scandinavica 131: Suppl 212

Ponka A, Martio J, Kosunen J U 1981 Reiter's syndrome in association with enteritis due to *Campylobacter foetus* ssp *jejuni*. Annals of Rheumatic Diseases 40: 414–415

Reiter H 1916 Ueber eine bisher unerkannte Spirochateninfektion (Spirochaetosis arthritica). Deutsche Medizinische Wochenschrift 42: 1535

Roitt I 1988 Essential immunology. Blackwell, Oxford. Table 15.2, p 269

Rook A, Wilkinson D S, Ebling F J G, Champion R H, Burton J L (eds) 1986 Kobner reaction. Textbook of Dermatology, 4th edn. Blackwell Scientific Publications, Oxford. vol. 1, p 58, 587, vol. 2, p 1477

Rosenbaum J T, Theofilopoulos A N, McDevitt H O, Cereira A B, Carson D, Calin A 1981 Presence of circulating immune complexes in Reiter's syndrome and ankylosing spondylitis. Clinical and Experimental Immunology 18: 291–297

Rossen R M, Goodman D J, Harrison D C 1975 A.V. conduction disturbances in Reiter's syndrome. American Journal of Medicine 58: 280–284

Sairanen E, Paronen I, Mahonen H 1969 Reiter's syndrome: a follow-up study. Acta Medica Scandinavica 185: 57–63

Schlosstein L, Terasaki P I, Bluestone R, Pearson C M 1973 High association of HLA antigen W27 with ankylosing spondylitis. New England Journal of Medicine 288: 704–706

Svejgaard A, Platz P, Ryder L P 1983 HLA and disease 1982 — a survey. Immunological Reviews 70: 193–218

Thamber N, Dunlop R, Thin R N, Huskisson E C 1977 Circinate vulvitis in Reiter's syndrome. British Journal of Venereal Diseases 53: 260–262

Weiss J J, Thompson G R, Good A 1980 Reiter's disease after *Salmonella typhimurium* enteritis. Journal of Rheumatology 7: 211–212

Wright V, Reed W B 1964 The link between Reiter's syndrome and psoriatic arthritis. Annals of Rheumatic Diseases 23: 12–21

20

Vaginal infection with prokaryotes

Vaginal infection with prokaryotes consists of a number of aetiologically separate clinical conditions of greatly differing clinical significance. The question of transmissibility by sexual intercourse as well as pathogenicity in the case of these organisms is a controversial subject although the principle applies that organismal flora of the genitals will bear some relationship to the degree of 'sexual mixing' practised by the individual or the partner. Vaginal infections due to prokaryotes may be classified as follows:

1. vaginal infection or colonization with *Streptococcus agalactiae*, more commonly referred to as the beta-haemolytic streptococcus, Lancefield Group B;

2. bacterial vaginosis (synonym non-specific vaginitis). an imperfect diagnosis based mainly on the bacterial flora, the pH and amine content of the vaginal fluid;

3. vaginal infection with *Actinomyces israelii* associated with the long-term use of chemically inert intra-uterine contraceptive devices; and

4. the toxic shock syndrome in menstruating women associated with the continuous use of tampons during menstruation and vaginal infection with toxin-producing strains of *Staphylococcus aureus*.

1. VAGINAL INFECTION WITH *STREPTOCOCCUS AGALACTIAE* (beta-haemolytic Lancefield Group B)

Streptococcus agalactiae (see Ch. 2) is the name applied to human members of group B streptococci (Parker 1978) although there are reasons to believe that they form a population group distinct from bovine Group B — classified by Lancefield on the basis of cell-wall carbohydrate antigens — streptococci (Ross 1978).

In the last 15 years *S. agalactiae* has been a serious cause of bacteraemia and other invasive infection in the newborn within the first few days of life. Dense vaginal colonization seems to make transmission more likely, and prematurity and a prolonged labour after rupture

of the membranes are important risk factors. Promiscuity in the female or that in her male partner is one determinant of the organismal flora of the genital tract; in the case of Group B streptococci, carriage rates of about 12–36% have been noted in the case of women attending STD clinics (Christensen et al 1974, Finch et al 1976). Carriage in adult women appears to be best detected by bacteriological examination of a urethral swab. Since the organism is to be found also on the penis, a presumptive case for its transmission sexually can be made out. Christensen et al (1984) found that prolonged urogenital carriage of group B streptococci in women (n = 88) who used tampons during menstruation was twice that in women who did not (respectively 49% & 24%), and thought that there was a causal relationship between the use of tampons and the persistence of Group B streptococci.

In relation to the problem of the newborn, however, positive cultures during pregnancy (6–28% recorded) may be less frequently found at delivery and a few patients may first acquire the organism at delivery. Invasive infections develop only in about 1% of colonized babies (Editorial (Lancet) 1984).

Two clinical syndromes, 'early-onset' and 'late-onset', are recognized in the newborn. The early-onset disease, although septicaemic in type, may also be meningitic, whereas the late-onset disease is almost always meningitic. Early-onset disease may occur within five days of birth, but usually within the first 24–36 hours. There is a close association between early-onset infection in the newborn and maternal complications, particularly premature labour and a prolonged period between rupture of the membranes and delivery. Infants of low birth weight tend to be affected. The late-onset disease presents usually after the tenth day of life as a purulent meningitis and can affect apparently healthy babies after normal labour with a mortality rate, although lower than early-onset disease, of 15–20% (Ross 1978).

Prevention of early-onset streptococcal infection seems possible. By using a monitor to count the respiratory rate of all newborn infants for the first 36 hours it has been noted that about 1% have a raised rate. Most of these will receive antibiotics, although only about 10% are later proved to have a streptococcal infection. With this procedure Valman & Wright (1984) have had no deaths from Group B streptococci, and the regimen is to be preferred to dosing all newborns indiscriminately with antibiotics.

2. BACTERIAL VAGINOSIS (synonym NON-SPECIFIC VAGINITIS)

Bacterial vaginosis, also referred to by the term 'non-specific vaginitis', is recognized clinically by the presence of an often scanty but characteristic homogeneous grey discharge, a vaginal fluid with a pH value of greater than 4.5, and commonly a complaint of a 'fishy odour', often noticed particularly during and after sexual intercourse. As an aid to recognition by the clinician the 'fishy odour' can be intensified by the addition of 10% potassium hydroxide solution to a small sample of vaginal fluid from untreated patients. The odour released by the potassium hydroxide solution suggested the presence of amines, a finding now confirmed by chemical analysis. *Bacterial vaginosis* is preferred as a term to cover this clinical entity because of its association with bacteria rather than fungi or protozoa; because no single bacterial agent can be regarded as solely responsible for the condition; and because a true inflammatory response of 'vaginitis' is absent in most cases.

Aetiology
Organisms associated with bacterial vaginosis.

Gardnerella vaginalis and the 'clue cell'
In 1954 Gardner & Dukes published a brief report that an organism, assigned the name *Haemophilus vaginalis* (Dunkelberg 1977), had been isolated from 81 of 91 cases of non-specific vaginitis. Subsequent reports from independent and geographically diverse sources referred to this small Gram-negative bacillus, which could grow on blood agar and could be isolated from the urogenital tract (Zinnemann & Turner 1963). Initially classified as a species of *Haemophilus* (Dunkelberg 1977), it was later shown, in conflict with the definition of the genus *Haemophilus*, that growth requirements did not include haemin (factor X), nicotinamide adenine dinucleotide (factor V), or other definable co-enzyme-like substances (Frampton & Lee 1964). Later Zinnemann & Turner (1963), basing arguments on morphology, recommended that the organism should be reclassified in the genus *Corynebacterium* and suggested the name *Coryne-*

bacterium vaginale. In 1980, Greenwood & Picket studied 78 clinical isolates and found that although the cell-wall morphology is not that of a 'typical' Gram-negative organism, e.g. *Escherichia coli*, it does resemble more closely that of a Gram-negative organism than a Gram-positive. Chemical analysis of the cell wall supports this view. DNA-hybridization showed that the organism had no genetic relationship with other genera, and this and other detailed studies led them to propose that the organisms hitherto designated as *Haemophilus vaginalis* or *Corynebacterium vaginale* should be assigned to a new genus, *Gardnerella*, and given the name *Gardnerella vaginalis*. Due to the unusual cell wall of the organism the new genus could not be assigned to a particular family.

Gardner & Dukes (1955) found that the microscopic appearance of epithelial cells in a wet preparation (vaginal fluid mixed with saline) gave a clue to the presence of the species now named *G. vaginalis*. The cytoplasm was described as especially granular in appearance with small bacilli, uniform in size, regularly spaced upon the surface of the cells. Not all cells were involved and some cells show only partial involvement. Frampton & Lee (1964) described particularly the Type I 'clue cell' with a dense layer of bacilli, uniform in size, covering the cell surface; when Type I 'clue cells' were found cultures were nearly always positive for *G. vaginalis*. In Type II clue cells, however, bacteria of variable size and shape were unevenly distributed over the cell surface. Although both Type I clue cells and high concentrations of *G. vaginalis* are almost invariably found in the vaginal fluid in bacterial vaginosis, *G. vaginalis* has long been known to present in the vaginal flora of normal women from geographically widely separated areas, e.g. in London (Frampton & Lee 1964); Halifax, Nova Scotia (Robinson & Mirchandani 1965); and, more recently, in the United States (Sautter & Brown 1980), and for this reason the significance of a positive culture for this organism in an individual patient is uncertain.

Recent studies on the morphology of the Gram-stained film from vaginal fluid showed that there is an inverse relationship between the quantity of large Gram-positive rods (*Lactobacillus* morphotype) and the small Gram-negative rods (*Gardnerella* morphotype). When the *Lactobacillus* morphotype is absent or present in low numbers, the *Gardnerella* morphotype may be numerous but is not used as a basis for diagnosis. When other forms of Gram-negative rods (possibly *Bacteroides* spp); Gram-positive cocci (possibly peptostreptococci); and Gram-negative or Gram-variable curved rods (possibly the motile *Mobiluncus* spp) are present, then the diagnosis is consistent with bacterial vaginosis (Spiegel et al 1983a, b).

Anaerobic bacteria

In bacterial vaginosis the anaerobic bacteria often present in highest concentrations are the so-called anaerobic vibrios (Blackwell et al 1983, Spiegel et al 1983a) now designated *Mobiluncus curtisii* and *M. mulieri*. These curved motile Gram-negative to Gram-variable rod-shaped bacteria are characteristically more resistant to alkaline solutions than most bacteria in vaginal discharge. Isolations can be best achieved from the vaginal discharge which has been diluted in a buffer of pH 12.0–12.6 (Pahlson & Forsum 1985; see also Section P4 p. 27). High concentrations of other anaerobic non-haemolytic peptostreptococci (e.g. *Streptococcus intermedius*; Ch. 2) and *Bacteroides* spp other than *B. fragilis*, e.g. *B. bivius*, have also been found to be present in high concentrations (Blackwell et al 1983). Other organisms include catalase-negative coryneforms like *G. vaginalis*, aerobes such as alpha- and beta-haemolytic streptococci (Group B), and occasionally coliforms. *Mycoplasma hominis* and *Ureaplasma urealyticum* are also often present. After a 7-day course of treatment with metronidazole (400 mg twice-daily by mouth) the vaginal flora changes radically, anaerobes diminish and lactobacilli become the predominant organism (Blackwell et al 1983), but the previous pattern of bacterial flora may return in a high proportion of patients.

Putrescine, cadaverine and gamma-amino-n-butyric acid in the vaginal fluid of bacterial vaginosis

The 'fishy' odour, associated with bacterial vaginosis and recognized or intensified by the addition of 10% potassium hydroxide to a sample of the vaginal fluid (Pheifer et al 1978), suggested the presence of amines. Their presence has been confirmed by qualitative analysis and, after dansylation — the addition of dansyl chloride to the vaginal washings — a number of amines have been identified by chromatography, of which putrescine and cadaverine are the most abundant (Chen et al 1978) and may be partly responsible for the 'fishy' odour. These diamines are to be found in trichomonal vaginitis as well as in bacterial vaginosis (Chen et al 1982). The presence of putrescine and cadaverine in the vaginal fluid have a *predictive value* (percentage of women with a positive result who have been diagnosed on clinical examination as having bacterial vaginosis or vaginitis due to *Trichomonas vaginalis*), found in one study to be 84% (Chen et al 1982). In the case of a negative result for the two diamines, the *predictive value* (percentage of women with a negative result who did not have bacterial vaginosis or vaginitis due to *T. vaginalis*) was estimated by the same research group as 92%. The presence of another substance frequently found (gamma-amino-n-butyric acid, GABA) gave a less secure predictive value (73%).

In vitro studies have shown that the amines, putrescine and cadaverine, can be produced by metronidazole-sensitive organisms isolated anaerobically from patients with bacterial vaginosis, presumably through the decarboxylation of ornithine and lysine, but diamines are not produced by *G. vaginalis* so isolated. Similarly, GABA, produced in vitro by the mixed anaerobic growth of organisms from bacterial vaginosis, is not so produced by *G. vaginalis*.

The pH value of vaginal fluid in bacterial vaginosis

In bacterial vaginosis the pH range of vaginal washings is from 4.7–6.5. Any amines in this range exist in the protonated form (salt) and are not volatile. After addition of 10% potassium hydroxide, the amines are converted to an unprotonated form (free base), become volatile and give a characteristic odour. It is possible that during and after intercourse the alkaline prostatic fluid may convert part of the amines to the unprotonated form and thus cause the characteristic odour (Chen et al 1978).

Conclusion

After a 7-day course of treatment with metronidazole there is clinical improvement, and the organisms (*G. vaginalis*, anaerobes such as *Mobiluncus*, 'Peptostreptococci' and *Bacteroides*), the fishy odour together with amines, such as putrescine and cadaverine, and gamma-amino-n-butyric acid, diminish or disappear, at least in the short term. The pH of the vaginal fluid is reduced to below 4.5 and *Lactobacillus* regains its predominance (Pheifer et al 1978, Spiegel et al 1980, Blackwell et al 1983). In bacterial vaginosis before treatment, vaginal flora contains large numbers of *G. vaginalis* ($> 10^6$ per ml) and anaerobes ($> 10^6$ per ml) in virtually all patients, whereas afterwards these organisms are markedly reduced or absent and the lactobacilli predominate (Blackwell et al 1983). The inverse relationship between the quantities of the *Lactobacillus* morphotype and the *Gardnerella* morphotype observed on microscopic examination of Gram-stained vaginal films by Spiegel et al (1983a, b), suggests an inter-relationship between the populations of these organisms. Diagnosis of bacterial vaginosis, in their view, depends more on a microscopically detectable change in the vaginal microflora from the *Lactobacillus* morphotype, with or without *Gardnerella* morphotype (normal), to a mixed flora with few or no *Lactobacillus* morphotypes.

In a sequential study of vaginal cultures from sexually active young women, Sautter & Brown (1980) challenged the view that the 'normal' vaginal flora should be regarded as solely *Lactobacilli*. Generally the flora was found to be polymicrobial (at least 37 species were recovered in the study) with an average of 10^8 colony-forming units per ml of vaginal fluid, and the number of species recovered in counts exceeding 10^4 varied between 1 and 10. The situation could be described as dynamic and subject to change. *Bacteroides* spp tended to be more prevalent during the first half of the menstrual cycle. The pH value varied from 4–6, with *Lactobacilli* and other acidophilic species such as *C. albicans* and *Ureaplasma urealyticum* being more numerous at the lower pH values. Other species (e.g. *Eubacterium contortum*, *E. lentum* and *B. melaninogenicus*) were isolated without any correlation to pH. *G. vaginalis* was present in a high proportion.

The question of 'normality' in relation to vaginal flora remains unanswered. Essentially bacterial vaginosis should be regarded as a statement of the state of the vaginal flora at a given time. Should the patient complain of discharge or spontaneously refer to an unpleasant odour then metronidazole treatment is justified for its value in the short term, although relapse rate may be high. Awareness of 'vaginal odour' may be heightened by advertisements of perfumes and deodorants, and a patient's attention may be drawn to the symptom. The concept of bacterial vaginosis relates only to the flora and chemical content of vaginal fluid, but as yet nothing is known about histopathology, immunology or possible precipitating cause. Organisms found in the vagina have a complex and dynamic inter-relationship and the degree of sexual mixing by the individual patient will play its role.

Diagnosis

Before considering the diagnosis of bacterial vaginosis it is necessary to screen patients to exclude *Neisseria gonorrhoeae*, *Chlamydia trachomatis*, *Candida albicans* and *Trichomonas vaginalis* and to examine the patient vaginally to exclude physical signs of pelvic inflammatory disease. Diagnosis of bacterial vaginosis does not rest upon the detection of any single specific organism. Essentially it is an imperfect diagnosis based on the state of the vaginal fluid, its complex bacterial flora and its amine products.

Symptom. A complaint of an unpleasant or 'fishy' odour often noticed particularly during or after sexual intercourse.

Range in pH of vaginal fluid. Vaginal fluid in bacterial vaginosis is alkaline with a pH in the range 4.7–6.5 (tests are invalid if made in the presence of blood or excess of cervical mucus); for practical purposes the pH tends to be > 5.0.

Release of volatile amines by potassium hydroxide. The characteristic smell can be recognized if a drop of potassium hydroxide solution is added to a drop of vaginal discharge. This is a subjective test and not recommended as a practice in the clinic or laboratory.

Biochemical diagnosis of bacterial vaginosis. An objective biochemical diagnosis of bacterial vaginosis is generally not available on account of its cost, viz. thin layer chromatography for the determination of the amines, putrescine or cadaverine, or gamma-amino-n-butyric acid.

Microscopy of the wet vaginal film. Epithelial cells in a wet preparation give a 'clue' to the presence of *G. vaginalis*. The cytoplasm of the clue cell is especially granular in appearance with small bacilli, uniform in size, regularly spaced on the surface of the cell.

The clue cell is best recognized by the addition of 0.1% methylene blue in saline to wet smear preparations. The bacteria are stained deep blue and can be distinguished from the normal flora (lactobacilli) (Petersen & Pelz 1984).

Microscopy of Gram-stained vaginal film. The morphological basis for microscopic diagnosis of bacterial vaginosis from a Gram-stained film has been discussed. As a technique it was derived from early experience and reports, but it has been more fully studied and developed by Spiegel et al (1983a, b). The features of use in microscopy are given in Table 20.1. Here the diagnosis of bacterial vaginosis rests more on diminished numbers of the *lactobacillus* morphotype and increase in the 'mixed' flora; *Gardnerella* is accorded minor importance showing only its inverse relationship in quantity to that of the *lactobacillus* morphotype.

Table 20.1 Microscopical assessment of Gram-stained film in the diagnosis of 'vaginosis'.

Vaginal content	Morphology of organisms in Gram-stained film			Diagnosis on appearance of film
(Gram-stained film)	*Lactobacillus* morphotypes	*Gardnerella* morphotypes (if present)	Mixed flora	
Microscopic assessment	+	+++	0 +++	normal 'vaginosis'
	++	++	0 +++	normal 'vaginosis'
	+++	+	0	normal

Treatment

Metronidazole

Clinical evidence shows that metronidazole is effective in the short-term treatment of bacterial vaginosis (Pheifer et al 1978, Balsdon et al 1980, Blackwell et al 1983) although relapse is common (14–39%). Its therapeutic effect is, however, difficult to evaluate and account for in specific terms, but its efficacy is more related to its effect on obligate anaerobes rather than on the facultative organism, G. vaginalis (Spiegel et al 1980).

Although G. vaginalis is not an anaerobe its growth in the laboratory is inhibited by metronidazole (Smith & Dunkelberg 1977, Ralph et al 1979) although the organism is less susceptible than are most anaerobes. The hydroxy-metabolite of metronidazole (1-[2-hydroxyethyl]-2-hydroxymethyl-5-nitroimidazole) is more active against G. vaginalis than is metronidazole itself (Ralph & Amatnieks 1980, Easmon et al 1982).

Obligate anaerobes, including Bacteroides melaninogenicus and B. corrodens, against which metronidazole has been shown to be effective experimentally and clinically (May & Baker 1980), were isolated in the majority of cases in the study by Pheifer et al (1978).

A treatment regimen based on 500 mg metronidazole twice-daily for 7 days is effective in bacterial vaginosis (Spiegel et al 1980, Blackwell et al 1983) although the relapse rate is high (14–40%). G. vaginalis, as has been discussed above, is sexually transmitted but it is not necessarily the primary pathogen (see above), and the activity of metronidazole appears to be more related to the effect of the drug on anaerobes.

Contact-tracing

Tracing and treatment of contacts with the view of eradicating G. vaginalis in the urethra of the male partners has been suggested as important (Dawson et al 1981). The high concentrations of the hydroxy metabolite of metronidazole in the urethra suggest that metronidazole should be effective in eradicating such carriage — possibly after only one or two doses of, say, 800 mg twice-daily.

In patients who complain of a vaginal discharge or of an unpleasant odour during or after intercourse and in whom the diagnosis of bacterial vaginosis is made on the basis of the high pH of vaginal fluid, the presence of amines or the finding of anaerobes, then metronidazole is appropriate treatment in a dose of 400 mg twice-daily for 1 week. The question of trial of treatment of the partner may be raised in a close-coupled partnership when relapse, after attention to hygiene in the case of the male, has caused problems. Care should be taken not to fix unduly the patient's attention on the subjective symptom of genital odour.

3. COLONIZATION OF THE UTERINE TRACT AND VAGINA WITH ACTINOMYCES ISRAELII

(associated particularly with the use of the chemically inert intrauterine contraceptive device)

In the vagina or endocervix, Actinomyces spp do not proliferate to form recognizable colonies in the absence of a foreign body, particularly an intrauterine contraceptive device (IUCD). The most commonly found species, Actinomyces israelii (Section P12 in Ch. 2) was isolated from patients in the Dundee, Scotland, area during the years 1978–1981 and was always associated with the long-term (more than 2 years) use of a chemically inert IUCD. Patients with copper-containing devices had a low prevalence — 2% (209 patients examined) — compared with 42% (197 patients examined) of those using a plastic (inert) device. It was considered that this was related to the known bacteriostatic action of copper or to the practice of replacing devices containing copper at regular, usually 2-yearly, intervals (Duguid et al 1982a, b, 1984). Bacteriostasis, however, in the case of copper-containing IUCD, is not likely to be absolute since the organism Eikenella corrodens may be found and act as a conditional or opportunistic pathogen in association with such an IUCD (see under Section P6 in Ch. 2).

Actinomyces spp and organisms of the related genus Arachnia produce masses of interwoven filaments sufficient to erode but not invade surface membranes and the mere finding of these organisms may have no clinical significance. The organism rarely spreads to involve the upper genital tract but when it does it causes a chronic suppurative condition known as actinomycosis, a cause of serious morbidity.

Detectable in wet mounts or Gram-stained smear, it may be identified by staining with fluorescein isothiocyanate (FITC)-labelled species-specific antiserum. Immunoassays are available and initial electrophoretic separation by SDS-PAGE (polyacrylamide gel electrophoresis) followed by electrophoretic transfer of separated antigens in the gel matrix to a nitrocellulose membrane is a method (see also explanation under 'Immunoblot assay for antibody to HIV antigens' in Ch. 31) which promises to distinguish colonization and superficial actinomycosis from invasive disease (see review by Holmberg 1987).

4. TOXIC SHOCK SYNDROME IN MENSTRUATING WOMEN

The toxic shock syndrome was first described in 1978 in children, and toxin-producing strains of Staphylococcus aureus, Phage Group 1 were recovered in most cases from various anatomical sites. Later, most cases of the toxic shock syndrome were found to occur in women of reproductive age and there was a striking association with the menstrual period. The clinical picture was described fully in 1980 by the United States Public Health Services Center for Disease Control (Shands et al 1980).

The risk of acquiring the disease appeared mainly to be associated with the use of a brand of highly absorbent tampons which contained a form of carboxymethylcellulose liable to enzymic degradation by vaginal organisms to yield glucose. The tampon may obstruct menstrual flow and, when digested, provide nutrient for the rapid growth of staphylococci. Exotoxins (Type C) or enterotoxin F, low molecular weight proteins produced by staphylococci, may be the agents responsible for the clinical manifestations of the syndrome (see 'Staphylococcal toxic shock syndrome' in Parker 1984).

Clinical features
The toxic shock syndrome typically, and in almost all patients, begins abruptly with fever, vomiting, diarrhoea and sometimes rigors (25%). The temperature is frequently (85%) above 40°C and patients may have abdominal pain. Hypotension develops within 72 hours and the fall in blood pressure may occur abruptly. A diffuse macular erythematous rash may go unnoticed or evolve into a more discrete macular rash. Headache and sore throat may be a presenting symptom or may develop in the course of the illness. A vaginal discharge, perhaps obscured by menstruation, may be observed (28%). Tampons on removal often emit a foul odour. Diffuse myalgia is almost always present, and many complain of skin or muscular tenderness when touched or moved. Recovery in the majority of patients occurs in 7–10 days although individuals may require 8–12 litres of fluid parenterally per 24 hours to maintain perfusion, and many become oedematous.

Desquamation occurs within 1–2 weeks, particularly on the palms of the hands and the soles of the feet and sometimes also on the face, trunk and tongue. Peeling of the skin may be extensive and the denuded finger tips may be sensitive as a result. Hair and nail loss may be seen in some patients.

The serum creatinine is typically (69%) elevated. Thrombocytopenia, hypocalcaemia, raised plasma bilirubin and elevated plasma enzymes are seen in 60%. Creatine kinase is elevated in about 40% (Shands et al 1980).

Treatment
Effective steps in therapy are not yet clearly defined. It is not known what roles, if any, antimicrobial therapy, vaginal irrigation, corticosteroid therapy or dialysis, play in reducing morbidity or mortality during the acute illness (Shands et al 1981).

Clearly, removal of the tampon or its debris, if present, and vaginal irrigation would eliminate foreign material capable of supporting growth of *Staphylococcus aureus* and promote drainage. Patients may require parenteral administration of enormous volumes of fluid (8–12 litres in the 24 hours) and vasopressor therapy to maintain perfusion. Much of this fluid is sequestered outside the intravascular space, and many patients become oedematous (Shands et al 1980). Early dialysis as a useful adjunct to the treatment of refractory hypotension has been advocated on the grounds that molecules of the size found in bacterial toxins are known to be readily dialysed (Fraley et al 1981).

Correction of hypocalcaemia by the parenteral administration of calcium chloride (12.0 g in 24 hours) was followed in one case by dramatic reversal of previously refractory hypotension (Nasser et al 1981). Naloxone, a drug which may act on one of several populations of opiate receptors to produce blockade of endorphin, has been found to reverse hypotension (in 8 patients with the toxic shock syndrome) when given parenterally (30 μg per kg body weight initially, followed by continuous infusion for one hour). (Hughes et al 1983).

Recovery occurs in the majority within 7–10 days. Desquamations occur within 1–2 weeks, most prominently on the palms and soles, but also on the face, trunk and tongue. The skin may peel in large sheets and there may be loss of nails and hair (Shands et al 1981).

Prevention
The toxic shock syndrome is associated with continuous use of tampons throughout the menstrual period. Women who have had the toxic shock syndrome may have recurrences and should not use tampons until *Staphylococcus aureus* has been eradicated from the vagina. Recurrences, if multiple, tend to have progressively less intense episodes. Toxin-producing staphylococci might be carried in the nares. Women who have not had the toxic shock syndrome have a low risk of its development (6.2 cases per 100 000 menstruating women). Since risk can be reduced further by using tampons for only part of the day or night or part of the menstrual cycle, individuals who have had the toxic shock syndrome should be advised accordingly (Davis et al 1980).

REFERENCES

Balsdon J, Taylor G E, Pead L, Maskell R 1980 *Corynebacterium vaginale* and vaginitis: a controlled trial of treatment. Lancet i: 501–504

Blackwell A L, Fox A R, Phillips I, Barlow D 1983 Anaerobic vaginosis (non-specific vaginitis): clinical, microbiological and therapeutic findings. Lancet ii: 1379–1382

Chen K C S, Forsyth P S, Buchanan T M, Holmes K K 1978 Amine content of vaginal fluid from untreated and treated patients with nonspecific vaginitis. Journal of Clinical Investigation 63: 828–835

Chen K C S, Amsel R, Eschenbach D A, Holmes K K 1982 Biochemical diagnosis of vaginitis: determination of diamines in vaginal fluid. Journal of Infectious Diseases 145(3): 337–345

Christensen K K, Christensen P, Flamhole L, Ripa T 1974 Frequencies of streptococci in Groups A, B, C, D and G in urethra and cervix swab specimens from patients with suspected gonococcal infection. Acta Pathologica et Microbiologica Scandinavica, Section B 82: 470–474

Christensen K K, Dykes A-K, Christensen P 1984 Relation between the use of tampons and urogenital carriage of group B streptococci. British Medical Journal 289: 731–732

Davis J P, Chesney P J, Wand P J, La Venturi M, and the Investigation and Laboratory team 1980 Toxic shock syndrome epidemiologic features, recurring risk factors and prevention. New England Journal of Medicine 303: 1429–1435

Dawson S G, Ison C A, Easmon C S F 1981 Vaginitis revisited. British Medical Journal 2: 1333–1334

Duguid H L D, Parratt D, Traynor R, Taylor D, Duncan I A, Elias-Jones J, Duguid R 1982a Studies on uterine tract infections and the IUCD with special reference to actinomycetes. IUCD Work Shop, London, 1982. British Journal of Obstetrics and Gynaecology, Suppl 4: 32–40

Duguid H L, Duncan I, Parratt D, Traynor R 1982b Actinomyces and intrauterine devices. Journal of the American Medical Association 248: 1379

Duguid H L D, Duncan I D, Parratt D, Taylor D 1984 Risks of intrauterine contraception devices. Correspondence, British Medical Journal 289: 767

Dunkelberg W E 1977 *Corynebacterium vaginale* review. Sexually Transmitted Diseases 4: 69–75

Easmon C S F, Ison C A, Kaye C M, Timewell R M, Dawson S G 1982 Pharmacokinetics of metronidazole and its principal metabolites and their activity against *Gardnerella vaginalis*. British Journal of Venereal Diseases 58: 246–249

Editorial 1984 Prevention of early onset Group B streptococcal infection in the newborn. Lancet i: 1056–1057

Finch R G, French G L, Phillips I 1976 Group B streptococci in the female genital tract. British Medical Journal 1: 1245–1247

Fraley D S, Bruns F J, Segel D P, Adler S 1981 Hypotension in the toxic shock syndrome. Annals of Internal Medicine 95: 124

Frampton J, Lee Y 1964 Is *Haemophilus vaginalis* a pathogen in the female genital tract? Journal of Obstetrics and Gynaecology of the British Commonwealth 71: 436–442

Gardner H L, Dukes C D 1954 New etiologic agent in nonspecific vaginitis. Science 120: 853

Gardner H L, Dukes C D 1955 *Haemophilus vaginalis* vaginitis. American Journal of Obstetrics and Gynecology 69: 962–976

Greenwood J R, Pickett M J 1980 Transfer of *Haemophilus vaginalis* Gardner and Dukes to a new genus, *Gardnerella: G. vaginalis* (Gardner and Dukes) comb nov. International Journal of Systematic Bacteriology 30: 170–178

Holmberg L 1987 Diagnostic methods for human actinomycosis. Review. Microbiological Sciences 4(3): 72–78

Hughes G S, Porter R S, Max R, Harkes C C 1983 Naloxone and septic shock. Annals of Internal Medicine 98: 559

May and Baker 1980 Anaerobicidal-agent, Flagyl (metronidazole) 2nd edn. ISBN 0 950 0352 7 0. May and Baker, Essex, p 1–15

Nasser R, Rowe P, Frierson J G, Murphy C 1981 Hypotension in the toxic shock syndrome. Annals of Internal Medicine 95: 124–125

Pahlson C, Forsum U 1985 Rapid detection of Mobiluncus species. Lancet i: 927

Parker M T 1978 The pattern of streptococcal disease in Man. In: Skinner F A, Quesnel L B (eds) Streptococci. Academic Press, London, p 71–106

Parker M T 1984 Staphylococcal diseases. In: Smith G R (ed) Topley and Wilson's Principles of bacteriology, virology and immunity, 7th edn, vol 3: Bacterial Diseases 259–260

Petersen E E, Pelz K 1984 Anaerobic vaginosis. Correspondence, Lancet i: 337–338

Pheifer T A, Forsyth P S, Durfee, M A, Pollock H M, Holmes K K 1978 Nonspecific vaginitis — role of *Haemophilus vaginalis* and treatment with metronidazole. New England Journal of Medicine 298: 1429–1434

Ralph E D, Austin T W, Pattison F L, Schieven B C 1979 Inhibition of *Haemophilus vaginalis* (*Corynebacterium vaginale*) by metronidazole, tetracycline and ampicillin. Sexually Transmitted Diseases 6: 199–202

Ralph E D, Amatnieks Y E 1980 Relative susceptibilities of *Gardnerella vaginalis* (*Haemophilus vaginalis*), *Neisseria gonorrhoeae* and *Bacteroides fragilis* to metronidazole and its two major metabolites. Sexually Transmitted Diseases 7: 157–160

Robinson S C, Mirchandani G 1965 Observations on vaginal trichomoniasis IV. Significance of vaginal flora under various conditions. American Journal of Obstetrics and Gynecology 91: 1005–1012

Ross P W 1978 Ecology of Group B streptococci. In: Skinner F A, Quesnel L B (eds) Streptococci. Academic Press, London, p 127–142

Sautter R L, Brown W J 1980 Sequential vaginal cultures from normal young women. Journal of Clinical Microbiology 22: 479–484

Shands K N, Schmid G P, Dan B B et al 1980 Toxic-shock syndrome in menstruating women. Association with tampon use and *Staphylococcus aureus* and clinical features in 52 cases. New England Journal of Medicine 303: 1436–1442

Shands K N, Dan B B, Schmid G P 1981 Task Force, Bacterial Diseases Division, Centers for Disease Control, Atlanta, Georgia 1981 Editorial, toxic shock syndrome: the emerging picture. Annals of Internal Medicine 94: 264–266

Smith R F, Dunkelberg W E 1977 Inhibition of

Corynebacterium vaginale by metronidazole. Sexually Transmitted Diseases 4: 20–21

Spiegel C A, Amsel R, Eschenbach D, Schoenknecht F, Holmes K K 1980 Anaerobic bacteria in nonspecific vaginitis. New England Journal of Medicine 303: 601–607

Spiegel C A, Eschenbach D A, Amsel R, Holmes K K 1983a Curved anaerobic bacteria in bacterial (nonspecific) vaginosis and their response to antimicrobial therapy. Journal of Infectious Diseases 148: 817–822

Spiegel C A, Amsel R, Holmes K K 1983b Diagnosis of bacterial vaginosis by direct gram stain of vaginal fluid. Journal of Clinical Microbiology 18(1): 170–177

Valman H B, Wright B M 1984 Prevention of early-onset Group B streptococcal infection in newborn. Lancet i: 1353

Zinnemann K, Turner G C 1963 The taxonomic position of 'Haemophilus vaginalis' (*Corynebacterium vaginale*). Journal of Pathology and Bacteriology 85: 213–219

21

Candidosis of the genitalia

Candidosis (synonyms — candidiasis (see Note 21.1), thrush) is a convenient generic term for infections caused by yeasts, acting as opportunistic pathogens in individuals whose host defences are impaired. Taxonomically the yeasts have been mostly assigned to a single genus *Candida*, but this 'genus' should be regarded as an artificial one comprised of non-sexually reproducing forms of members of a variety of other genera, some of which have now been identified (see Section E1b in Ch. 2). The most important member of the group, *Candida albicans*, is capable of causing the very common superficial infections of the mouth and vagina as well as widespread or more deep-seated disease, viz. systemic candidosis, an important hazard in modern medical procedures such as transplantation surgery, intravenous hyperalimentation and immunosuppressive surgery (Odds 1979) as well as in the emergent epidemic retrovirus infection (human immunodeficiency viruses HIV; synonyms — LAV/HTLV-III/ARV) leading to the Acquired Immune Deficiency Syndrome (AIDS) (see Ch. 31).

Although vulvo-vaginal candidosis, characterized by pruritus with or without vaginal discharge, tends often to be regarded as a minor condition in that it is transitory and its physical effects are not seriously damaging, it is a frequent cause of irritation and annoyance in women and — on account of its tendency to recur — an important cause of morbidity. Men tend to be less affected as the milieu of the glans and preputial sac is less favourable as a site for colonization by *Candida*.

AETIOLOGY

Morphology

Pathogenic yeast cells are typical of aerobic eukaryotes possessing intracellular organelles including mitochondria and ribosomes and a double membraned nucleus containing chromosomes. All pathogenic *Candida* and *Torulopsis* species multiply by the production of buds from a thin walled ovoid *blastospore* (yeast cell) 1.5–4.0 μm in diameter. The new growth or bud enlarges then stops as mitosis takes place and a septum is laid down between the parent and daughter cell unit.

A *hypha* is a long microscopic tube made up of multiple fungal cell units divided by *septa*. Hyphae arise as branches of existing hyphae or by the germination of spores. A *mycelium* is an entire fungal cellular aggregate including a hypha with all its branches. A *pseudohypha* arises by a budding process in which each generation of buds remains attached to its parent; the buds of the first and subsequent generations are narrow elongated cells that do not resemble the parent blastospore. The end-to-end aggregation of elongated blastospores or pseudohypha are distinguished from true *hyphae* in that there are constrictions at the septal junctions. *Chlamydospores* are an in vitro form of a yeast pathogen induced by low temperature incubation under poor nutritional conditions and have thick double-layered cell walls.

The formation of germ tubes is accepted as a reliable property for identifying *Candida albicans* and is used in medical laboratories because of its rapidity. The germ tube of *C. albicans* is a thin filamentous outgrowth from the cell without a constriction at its point of origin. Presumptive identifications based on the formation of germ tubes are 95–100% accurate when compared with stricter taxonomic methods, although their formation is influenced by temperature, amount of inoculum, composition of the medium and strain. Cells from a 24-hour-old culture (10^5–10^6 cells per ml) are suspended in bovine serum and examined microscopically for germ tubes after 1–3 hours incubation at 37°C (van der Walt & Yarrow 1984).

Taxonomy

Reference has been made in Chapter 2 to the fact that molecular studies have shown that the 'genus' *Candida* should be regarded as an artificial one in that its name does not imply descent from a common ancestor. The extreme diversity of its genetic material with base compositions (guaninine + cytosine) ranging from 30–64 mol % suggest that the genus should be considered to be comprised of non-sexually reproducing forms of members of a variety of other genera, some of which have now been identified. Perfect forms of *C. pseudotropicalis* (*Kluyveromyces fragilis*) and *C. kreusei* (*Issatchenkia orientalis*) have been established or confirmed by DNA hybridization techniques (Riggsby 1985). Looking more closely at the base compositions of various species of medical interest, the ranges of guanine plus cytosine (G + C) content in the nuclear DNA have been recorded in molecules %: *C. albicans*, 34.3–35.6; *C. tropicalis*, 35.9–36.1; *C. parapsilosis*, 40.5; *C. guillermondii*, 44.1–44.4; *C. glabrata*, 39.6–40.2 — the name of this species is synonymous with *Torulopsis glabrata*. In the case of the genus *Rhodotorula*, characterized by the property of synthesizing on malt agar culture red or yellow carotenoid pigments, the wide ranges in G + C content of 51.4–70.0 mol % are recorded for the various species. Many issues of generic differentiation are clearly still problematic (Kreger-van Rij 1984).

Distribution of species

Yeasts that are the principal agents of human candidosis are to be found in most warm-blooded animals and *Candida albicans* has been recovered from a wider range of animal hosts than any other species (Odds 1979). Using terminology not yet modified by findings already described, Do Carmo-Sousa (1969) considers that *C. albicans*, *C. stellatoidea*, and *Torulopsis glabrata* are obligatory animal saprophytes; that *C. guilliermondii*, *C. krusei*, *C. parapsilosis* and *C. tropicalis* are facultative saprophytes, being species that, although recoverable from sources other than animal, are able to build up populations mainly in the digestive tract of animals; and that others are simple transients sometimes ingested but unable to grow inside the animal host.

Using data from human sources in Europe and North America collected from the literature by Odds (1979) the anatomical distribution of yeast species is illustrated diagrammatically in Figure 21.1 and contrasted with data on isolations from the vagina in patients with vaginitis. It can be seen that *C. albicans* is the most commonly encountered of all species and that in the mouth it comprises over 70% of all isolates, with *Candida* (synonym — *Torulopsis*) spp, especially *T. glabrata*, being the next most commonly found. In the faeces *C. albicans* is again the most commonly encountered (48%) but proportionately less than in the mouth. The most striking difference between faecal and yeast isolates is the enormously higher proportion of *Rhodotorula* spp (13%) in the faeces than in the mouth (0.5%). In the vagina in those subjects without vaginitis the distribution of yeasts resembles the distribution in the faeces but *T. glabrata* forms a much greater proportion (18%) than it does in oral or faecal isolates. In the vagina in those with vaginitis *C. albicans* comprises a very high proportion of isolates (90%); in none of the studies reported by Odds was the proportion less than 70%. *T. glabrata* is less frequently found in those with vaginitis (6%) than in those without (17%); *Rhodotorula* spp appears never to be found in vaginitis (Odds 1979).

Colonization and adhesion

Adherence of micro-organisms to epithelial cells is a critical step in the colonization of mucosal surfaces and their subsequent capacity to cause disease. In particular Kimura & Pearsal (1978) demonstrated the capacity of *C. albicans* to adhere in vitro to human buccal epithelial cells and found that the adherence was significantly greater in human saliva than in phosphate-buffered saline. Enhanced adherence too was associated with germination of yeast cells (i.e. when germ tubes were formed) and under conditions conducive to germ tube formation. Similarly Sobel et al (1981) showed that although adherence of *C. albicans* in the yeast form to human buccal and vaginal epithelial cells occurred, conditions conducive to germ tube formation also increased the extent of adherence. The adherence of *C. albicans* to vaginal cells in vitro at pH 6 was considerably greater than at pH 3–4, a range corresponding to that of the normal vagina. Clinical observations have been correlated with the presence of filamentous forms with tissue invasion and the detection of germ-tube associated antigens have been exploited in the sero-diagnosis of invasive candidosis (Evans et al 1973).

In the early stages of attachment to and colonization of mucosal surfaces it is the yeast form which is invariably found, and for this reason yeasts are used in adhesion assays. Similarly, since candidosis of the mouth and vagina are the commonest clinical forms seen, in vitro adhesion to exfoliated buccal and vaginal epithelial cells is ordinarily measured. It has been found that adhesion of some strains of *C. albicans* is increased by growing the yeast in 'defined media' containing high concentrations of certain sugars (e.g. galactose, maltose, sucrose) and this enhancement appears to be related to the production of a fibrillar floccular layer on the yeast cell surface (McCourtie & Douglas 1984). Such evironmental changes may be important, particularly in the mouth.

The relative pathogenicity of the different *Candida* species is reflected in their individual ability to adhere to epithelial cells in vitro (King et al 1980) as well as to a variety of other cell surfaces; *C. albicans* also shows strain differences in adhesion and virulence. The avirulent seem to be unable to synthesize the fibrillar layer, whereas a strain of *C. albicans* responsible for a recent outbreak of systemic candidosis has been found to become exceptionally adhesive after growth in high-galactose medium (Douglas 1985). It is thought that

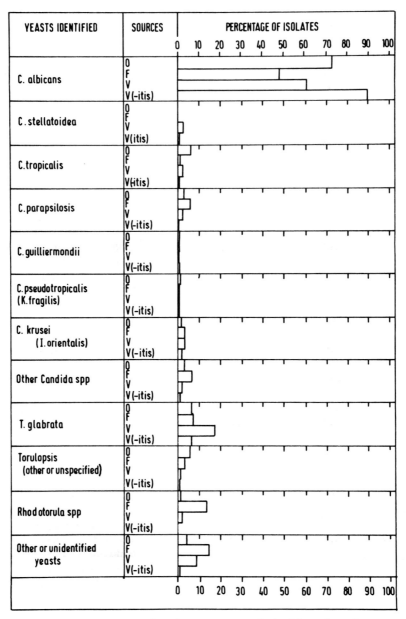

Fig. 21.1 Distribution of species among yeasts obtained from the oral cavity (0); the faeces or ano-rectum (F); the vagina — in those without vaginitis or in whom the presence or absence of vaginitis was not recorded (V); and the vagina in those with vaginitis (V(itis) from various studies recorded in detail by Odds 1979; the species given are those recorded by Odds (1979), rearranged in the approximate order of the classes described in Chapter 2. In those species now placed in new genera, and where the perfect form is known, the name is given in brackets.

Taxonomists now consider that the 'genus' *Torulopsis* should not be separated from the 'genus' *Candida*; *Torulopsis glabrata* is therefore synonymous with *Candida glabrata*. Furthermore, on the basis of DNA reassociation techniques, *Candida stellatoidea* is now regarded as synonymous with *C. albicans* (Meyer et al 1984).

adhesion is due to specific binding molecules (adhesins) on yeast surfaces, possibly analagous to bacterial fimbriae and multiple rather than single. *C. albicans* is the species best able to adhere to epithelial cells but others, such as *C. tropicalis* with respect to some denture material, are more adherent to inert materials (Douglas 1985).

Yeast-to-mycelium conversion

Changes in the in vitro growth environment lead to changes in the growth form of *C. albicans*. Blastospore production is much more easily obtained in laboratory media, and filament formation is unusual, but serum at 37°C is a good stimulant to filament formation, a property commonly applied in the germ tube test for *C. albicans*. Hyphal production in vivo is probably an indication of active growth but not necessarily of tissue invasion and therefore cannot be regarded as absolute diagnostic evidence for candidosis (Odds 1979); the case for the connection of yeast-to-mycelium conversion to pathogenicity continues to be debated (Sobel et al 1984). Stationary-phase cells can be induced to propagate either as a budding yeast or by germ-tube formation by allowing growth to resume in certain media at either 25°C (for yeast) or 37°C (for germ tubes). Among problems associated with temperture differences have been the detection of proteins analogous to 'heat shock' proteins in the cytoplasm of *C. albicans* cells when the temperature is shifted from 23°C to 37°C. As a result an alternative method of study of the process has been developed, where stationary-phase cells at 37°C develop at pH 4.5 as budding yeasts and at pH 6.7 as germ tubes (Riggsby 1985).

Factors predisposing to candidosis

Conditions which favour transition from saprophyte to pathogen and are relevant to vaginal candidosis particularly include pregnancy, diabetes mellitus, damage or maceration of the tissue, the use of immunosuppressive drugs, possibly also the oral contraceptive and oral antibiotics (Ridley 1975). Pregnancy is an undisputed factor in pathogenicity — possibly by virtue of changes in cell-mediated immunity, in glucose metabolism or by the provision of a glycogen-rich vaginal epithelium (Winner & Hurley 1966, Carroll et al 1973). In pregnancy there is a reduction of T-cell activity which may help to protect the fetus from rejection (Finn et al 1972) and there are changes in carbohydrate metabolism (Lind & Harris 1977) which may favour the growth of *Candida*. Vaginal carriage of yeasts is highest in the third trimester, and an abrupt reduction in the incidence of *Candida* in the vagina takes place in the post-partum period (Spellacy et al 1971, Odds 1979).

Oral contraceptives containing an oestrogen and a progestogen are the most effective preparations in general use and are called the 'combined' type. The oestrogen content ranges from 20–50 μg, and the progestogen content is dependent upon the chemical nature and biological activity of the six progestogens in use. The progestogen-only oral contraceptives, suitable for older patients who may be at risk from oestrogen, heavy smokers and in those in whom oestrogen causes severe side effects, have a higher failure rate (British National Formulary No.10, 1985). In respect to vaginal candidosis, assembled evidence indicates that the 'combined' type containing oestrogen enhances the susceptibility of the vagina to yeast overgrowth, leading sometimes to vaginitis (Odds 1979).

Antibiotics given orally appear to enhance the carriage of yeasts in the vagina but the evidence is more the matter of clinical consensus rather than by scientifically satisfactory controlled trials (Odds 1979). The theory that anti-bacterial antibiotics may eliminate certain microbial elements in the microflora of the vagina and that such alterations lead to yeast overgrowth because yeasts themselves are unaffected by antibacterial antibiotics, is difficult to substantiate. Contradictory evidence to the consensus view on the antibiotic-*Candida* relationship (Odds 1979) suggests that other factors may be involved in the aetiology.

Metronidazole treatment of trichomonal vaginitis may predispose patients to vaginal thrush (Moffett & McGill 1960). Corticosteroids depress cell-mediated immunity and as a result may predispose to candidosis. In respect to infection with the human immunodeficiency viruses (HIV) and the Acquired Immune Deficiency Syndrome, there is profound damage to the cell-mediated branch of the immune system and, although it is oropharyngeal candidosis spreading to cause oesophageal erosions that is often seen, disseminated candidosis occurs — although rarely (Ebbesen et al 1984).

PATHOLOGY

Histological study of infected vulvar and vaginal tissue is not part of routine clinical practice, and as a result reports are few. Gardner & Kaufman (1969) noted mild to moderate inflammatory changes without invasion of vaginal tissue by the yeast. It has been shown, however, that in the mouth at least, in acute and chronic candidiasis there is invasion of the epithelium by hyphae, which grow downwards in more or less straight lines without respect for epithelial boundaries. In this site electronmicroscopy examination confirmed that the growth of *Candida* is intracellular and that the fine structure of the epithelial cytoplasm shows minimal change (Cawson & Rajasingham 1972). Certain changes in squamous cells such as radial clumping and emptiness of stained material in the cytoplasm as well as increased nuclear activity and perinuclear haloes have been described in cervical vaginal Papanicolaou smears (Heller & Hoyt 1971).

CLINICAL FEATURES OF CANDIDOSIS

Symptoms and signs have diagnostic significance, and history-taking and examination are therefore important.

Candidosis of the female genitalia

Vulvar *pruritus* which may vary from slight to intolerable is the cardinal symptom of candidosis. When pruritus is intense vulvar erythema is pronounced. Sometimes patients complain of pruritus or burning after intercourse. On occasions, however, even when plaques or pseudomembrane involve the vagina widely there are no subjective symptoms or even evidence of vulvitis.

Burning is a common complaint, particularly upon micturition and especially when there is also local excoriation due to scratching. Sometimes complaints of dysuria and frequency can be erroneously attributed to cystitis.

Dyspareunia, especially in the nulliparous, may be severe enough to make intercourse intolerable. *Vulvar oedema* may cause ill-defined vulvar discomfort, and worry and apprehension may add to the patient's distress. A vaginal discharge is seldom the presenting complaint but the majority of patients have a discharge at some time and some patients may complain of dryness.

Erythema of the vulva is the commonest sign of candidosis and tends to be limited to the mucocutaneous surfaces between the labia minora. Although often limited to the vestibule, erythema may extend to the labia majora, the perineum, the perianal skin and occasionally to the mons veneris, the genito-crural folds, the inner thighs and even buttocks.

Oedema of the labia minora is commonly observed and is often more pronounced in candidosis during pregnancy. Fissuring may occasionally be noted at the fourchette and at the anus. Traumatic excoriations from scratching are often found in patients with severe itching.

The vagina is abnormally reddened in about 20% of cases. If adherent patches or plaques of 'thrush' or pseudomembrane are removed the vaginal skin underneath appears erythematous, and superficial ulceration with bleeding may be seen. The vaginal contents may be apparently normal but a characteristic curdy material

is found in 20% of the non-pregnant and in 70% of the pregnant. Although plaques may be small (1 mm) in size, larger (1 cm) and thick accumulations of exudate may be seen. A yeast odour is not thought to be characteristic in candidosis (Gardner & Kaufman 1969).

In contrast, primary cutaneous candidosis involves the outer parts of the labia majora and the genito-crural fold, and not infrequently the mons veneris, the perianal region and inner thighs. Vulvar lesions tend to be reddened and moist with defined scalloped edges. Cutaneous lesions tend to begin as small papules on a red base with outlying small satellite vesicles or pustules and progress to form shallow ulcerated areas resulting from ruptured vesicopustules.

T. vaginalis or *N. gonorrhoeae* may co-exist with the yeast infection, and on occasions all three organisms are found together.

Candidosis of the glans penis and prepuce

Characteristic symptoms of soreness and itching of the penis, accompanied sometimes by a discharge from under the prepuce, are seen in candidosis of the penis. On examination there may be a balanoposthitis with superficial erosions and sometimes eroded maculopapular lesions and preputial oedema. *C. albicans* may be isolated from the subpreputial sac, but on occasions there may be a balanoposthitis with erosions without detectable yeasts which appears to develop 6–24 hours after intercourse with a partner who has vaginal candidosis (Catterall 1966). Such a balanitis may be due to sensitivity to yeast-containing vaginal discharge. The balanoposthitis associated with diabetes has a similar appearance and *Candida* may not always be isolated.

Neonatal candidosis

Candidosis in the newborn may involve the umbilicus, mouth and napkin areas. The maternal vagina is only one source, as colonization may involve also the mouth and bowel. Attendants and environmental sources may also contribute to transmission.

DIAGNOSIS

Microscopy

Direct microscopy is essential as an 'on-the-spot' procedure in the diagnosis of candidosis of the vagina, and of the glans penis. In the case of the vagina, material is collected with a plastic loop or swab from the posterior fornix or from a characteristic plaque and smeared directly on a clean slide, as a dry preparation and as a wet preparation in a small quantity of saline, and covered with a glass cover-slip; alternatively, as a wet preparation, material is emulsified in 20% potassium hydroxide in water or dimethyl sulphoxide.

The smear is dried in air, fixed by heat and then Gram stained; all yeasts, like all fungi, are Gram-positive, and detected using the oil immersion (×100) objective. The wet saline mount is examined with the ×40 objective after racking down the condenser, or preferably with phase-contrast microscopy. In the case of the potassium hydroxide preparation, epithelial cells are cleared and the fungal elements revealed by direct or phase-contrast microscopy.

In medical practice yeast isolates are not regularly identified to species level sufficiently to satisfy taxonomists, although in deep-seated lesions particularly this is clearly desirable, and the characterization of isolates from superficial lesions would yield clinically and epidemiologically useful data. In recurrent candidosis the resulting morbidity is a serious problem for the individual and research is desirable. Yeasts are eukaryotes and identification is a complex subject, and only a brief discussion based on Odds (1979) is given here.

Candida spp grow well in culture media such as malt-extract or glucose-peptone agar at a lower pH than that required by bacteria (Gentles & La Touche 1969): the best known of the latter was first described by Sabouraud in 1894. The low pH (5.5) suppresses bacteria and the media can be made more inhibitory to bacteria by the incorporation of chloramphenicol (50 mg/1). The majority of clinical isolates from the genitalia will be *C. albicans*, for which two rapid specific tests are available.

1. *The germ-tube test.* *C. albicans* regularly produces hyphal shoots (germ tubes) after incubation in serum at 37°C for 3 hours. Occasional isolates of *C. stellatoidea* also produce germ tubes, but this is not surprising since its DNA is essentially identical to that of *C. albicans* and in present-day taxonomy the species is regarded as synonymous with the latter (see Ch. 2).

2. *Chlamydospore test.* Partially anaerobic conditions can be produced by the 'Dalmau' inoculation technique, by which the yeast isolate is partially scratched into the agar surface with the inoculation loop and glass cover-slips are pressed on to the inoculated surface. Incubation proceeds at 25°C. Chlamydospores are usually abundant under the edges of the cover-slips. The originally recommended media was corn-meal agar, but others are used and improved yields have been secured by incorporating the surfactant 'tween 80'.

For the determination of species it is necessary to characterize isolates further by determining certain physiological properties, viz. their abilities to assimilate and ferment individual carbon and nitrogen sources. Abbreviated tests are available which are sufficient as a means of making a presumptive rather than an absolute diagnosis (Odds 1979).

Emphasis has been given to the fact that yeasts are complex eukaryotes and that accurate identification of species may have important prognostic and therapeutic implications. New methods of characterization, such as the capacity of isolates to adhere to epithelial and other surfaces and DNA:DNA hybridization provide new methods for identification of *Candida* species and analysis of their genetic relationship (Riggsby 1985). The complex subject is provided for by the standard reference work edited by Kreger-van Rij (1984).

TREATMENT

In vaginal candidosis treatment is indicated on the basis of the symptoms of pruritus; the finding of vaginitis based on the clinical appearance, and the detection of *C. albicans* or other yeast species. This mycotic infection can be an annoyance that is difficult to tolerate but it is not invasive. Its tendency to recur, however, necessitates on occasions fuller investigation as a cause of local irritation as well as dysharmony in a personal sexual relationship.

Preparations widely used in the treatment of candidosis include the polyene antibiotics, nystatin and amphotericin B; the imidazoles, clotrimazole and miconozole; and, reserved for life-threatening systemic candidosis possibly the potentially hepatoxic imidazole, ketoconazole and 5-fluorocytosine.

The polyene antifungal antibiotics

The polyene antibiotics, nystatin and amphotericin B, are effective antifungal agents that bind to sterol components of cell membranes of susceptible fungi and act by increasing the permeability of the fungal membrane and causing a leakage of intracellular solutes. Cell death is secondary to the results of damage to the cell membrane.

Nystatin

Nystatin, discovered in 1950, was the first polyene to be used in the treatment of candidosis. With respect to vaginal candidosis it gradually replaced the topical use of 1% aqueous solution of gentian violet. Nystatin inhibits the in vitro growth of yeast pathogens at concentrations of 0.4–10 μg per ml, although higher minimum inhibitory concentrations have been quoted (Odds 1979). The sensitivity of yeasts to polyenes has not changed perceptibly over the years, although a slight increase in resistance would render them virtually useless as chemotherapeutic agents (Hamilton Miller 1973).

Isolates made resistant to polyenes are unlikely to survive in nature as they show profound differences in their morphology and are less pathogenic. The first amphotericin-resistant isolates, reported as having arisen due to therapy in a patient, showed that the usual ergosterol in the membrane had been replaced by other unidentified sterols, a change which apparently protected the fungi against polyenes. These isolates showed slow growth, impaired pseudomycelia formation and loss of pathogenicity, and therefore were unlikely to survive in nature (Drutz & Wood 1973, Woods et al 1974). The use of these polyenes in the short-term therapy of vaginal candidosis is not likely, therefore, to give rise to resistance in nature. Resistance induced experimentally appears to be reversed on withdrawal of the polyene, and there is no selective breeding of resistant strains (Hurley & Wright 1976).

The biological activity of nystatin is expressed in units, with the international standard for nystatin of 3 000 units per mg and with the pure compound having activity in excess of 5 500 units per mg (Hamilton Miller 1973). It is extremely toxic if given parenterally and therefore never used thus, but it is not absorbed from the gut and may be safely given by mouth.

Nystatin is prescribed as vaginal tablets, each containing 100 000 units, with instructions to insert one at night for 14 nights, continuing during menstruation. The patient should wash her hands and vulva before bedtime, lie down on the bed and gently insert the tablet into the upper third of the vagina. It should be explained that the nystatin is itself yellow in colour and that the appearance of a yellow discharge is not a cause for worry. Nystatin cream (100 units per gram) may be usefully applied to the skin on the vulva and, if required, to the adjacent skin. Should relapse occur, the administration of oral nystatin (500 000 units four times a day for a week) together with local treatment and the use of nystatin cream in the male partner is justified.

Amphotericin B

Amphotericin B, a polyene derived from *Streptomyces nuclosus*, inhibits in vitro growth of yeast pathogens at concentrations below 1 μg per ml (Odds 1979). Its interest as a polyene in the first decade after its introduction in 1966 lay in its use intravenously in systemic candidosis, although it is very toxic and liable to cause renal damage. For a review of its parenteral use, Odds (1979) should be consulted. Amphotericin B may be also used topically as a 3% cream (Fungilin, Squibb).

The fluorinated pyrimidine, 5-fluorocytosine

The fluorinated pyrimidine, 5-fluorocytosine, inhibits the in vitro growth of yeasts and many fungi. Once inside the yeast cell it is deaminated into 5-fluorouracil, which is then phosphorylated and incorporated into cellular RNA, thereby disrupting normal protein synthesis by the cell. Absorbed from the gut, and less toxic than amphotericin B, it may be given orally or systemically. Because of the high incidence of primary and secondary 5-fluorocytosine resistance among yeast pathogens, the drug should be solely reserved for use in systemic candidosis. Its use topically is strongly deprecated since this may lead to the introduction of resistant yeasts on such a scale that the drug could become worthless for its main role in the treatment of systemic candidosis (Holt 1974).

The anti-fungal imidazoles

The antifungal activity of the antifungal imidazoles differs from that of the polyenes (and 5-fluorocytosine) in that the imidazoles have a very broad spectrum of activity, affecting many filamentous fungi and dermatophytes as well as yeasts. Most *Candida* isolates are inhibited in vitro by concentrations in the range of 0.02 μg per ml, although results can vary as much as 200-fold in differing test media. The mechanisms of action are poorly understood but the permeability of susceptible organisms appears to become altered, causing visible damage to the structure and organization of cell organelles (Odds 1979).

Studies comparing the topical application of these imidazoles with nystatin are difficult to interpret, because the two drugs would have to be used for the same duration; therefore one or other drug could have to be given for a period that is not recommended (Milne 1978). As the imidazoles have an anti-bacterial action, clotrimazole or miconazole should not be used for vulvo-vaginal candidiasis when a gonococcal infection has to be excluded. Clotrimazole concentrations in the vagina are very substantial; a mean value of 447 μg/ml has been obtained 6–9 hours after the first 100 mg tablet of a 12-day course of once-daily vaginal tablets had been inserted. The gonococcus is, however, very resistant to clotrimazole, with a minimum inhibitory concentration of 64 to > 256 μg/ml and minimum 'cidal' concentration of > 256 μg/ml (Selwyn 1976).

Clotrimazole

Clotrimazole (Canesten, Bayer) is supplied as a 1% cream for topical use and as 100 mg vaginal pessaries. One 100 mg vaginal tablet inserted every night for 6 nights is an effective alternative to nystatin (Highton 1973) and more pleasant to use; a shorter course of one 200 mg vaginal tablet inserted for 3 consecutive nights may be sufficient in the uncomplicated case (Masterton et al 1977), and the insertion of a single 500 mg vaginal tablet at night may also suffice.

Miconazole (Gyno-Daktarin, Janssen)

Miconazole nitrate (Daktarin, Dermonistat) is supplied as a 2% cream for topical use, as a 2% intravaginal cream (Gyno-Daktarin, Monistat) and as vaginal pessaries, each containing 100 mg. The intravaginal cream is effective when it is introduced into the vagina by means of an applicator, which is filled to contain the required 5 g of cream (equivalent to 100 mg miconazole nitrate). The pessary or cream, introduced into the vagina once-nightly for 14 consecutive nights, is effective treatment, curing more than 80% of cases (Davis et al 1974, McNellis et al 1978). It is likely that shorter courses will prove to be effective in the uncomplicated case.

Econazole (Ecostatin, Squibb)
The therapeutic properties of another antifungal imidazole, econazole, are probably as good as clotrimazole or miconazole. It is supplied as pessaries containing econazole nitrate 150 mg and a cream — 1% econazole nitrate.

Treatment failure
Although treatment failure may occur, relapses are more frequent. It is possible that the mouth contributes to the continuing re-inoculation of the intestinal tract and is thus an indirect source of vaginal infection. Such cyclic reinfection from the bowel may require oral nystatin. The sexual partner may be examined and treated if there is evidence of candidiasis of the glans or preputial sac.

Vaginal absorption of imidazoles
The vaginal absorption of the imidazoles, in the three preparations used (viz. clotrimazole, miconazole and econazole) appears to be limited, and most is lost by vaginal leakage. About 2.5% of the dose of econazole and 1.5% of the dose of miconazole was recovered in the urine and faeces during a 96-hour period after the administration of a 5 g intravaginal dose (Vukovich et al 1977). These drugs should be avoided during the fetal organogenetic period in the first trimester of pregnancy, even though teratogenic effects have not been seen in laboratory animals treated with the drug. As nystatin does not appear to be absorbed from mucosal surfaces it should be used in preference, when treatment of candidiasis in the first trimester is essential. Local hypersensitivity to imidazole is rare and other side effects are very rare with topical use. Intravaginally clotrimazole may, however, cause serious burning and itching in about 1% (Weuta 1972).

Hepatotoxicity and ketoconazole (Nizoral, Janssen)
Ketoconazole, unlike the earlier antifungal imidazoles, is fairly well absorbed after oral administration; with a daily dose for adults of 200 mg a serum concentration of 2–4 μg per ml can be maintained. As its resorption is dependent upon the presence of some acid in the stomach, antacids and H_2-receptor antagonists inhibit its resorption. Its antifungal activity depends upon its effect on the cell membrane where it interferes with the biosynthesis of ergosterol. Ketoconazole is metabolized and eliminated by hepatic and renal routes (Tester-Dalderup 1984).

In May 1982 the United States Federal Drugs Administration took regulatory action following the notification of three cases of fatal massive hepatic necrosis (Astahova 1983), and in 1985 in the United Kingdom the Committee on Safety of Medicines drew attention to the danger of hepatotoxicity (Astahova 1985).

Symptoms usually occurred within the first few months of treatment, and the median time of onset of icteric reactions was 6 weeks (extremes 1 and 20 weeks); and of anicteric reactions 11 weeks (extremes 3 and 24 weeks) (Astahova 1983). Advice has been given to the effect that because of the idiosyncratic hepatotoxicity, and because most data have been derived from uncontrolled trials and case reports, ketoconazole should be used cautiously, avoiding it particularly in those with hepatic failure or an antecedent history of hepatic failure (Astahova 1983). Hepatotoxic effects still continue to be reported, and a reaction has been described pointing to the possibility of a late onset developing after withdrawal of ketoconazole (Astahova 1985). The risk of hepatotoxicity (Cohen 1982, Hay 1982, Jones 1982) makes the oral use of ketoconazole unjustified in cases of superficial genital candidosis, although it is valuable in some of the systemic mycoses such as certain forms of paracoccidiodomycosis and in histoplasmosis. The monitoring of the plasma bilirubin and liver-related enzyme tests are indicators of liver cell damage, but Rollman & Loof (1983) found that with serum 'liver function tests' (viz. enzyme tests for hepatocellular damage and bilirubin) it is not possible to predict from the first observed abnormal result whether a progressive reaction has been initiated.

Gynaecomastia and loss of libido and potency have occasionally been observed in men taking ketoconazole and may be related to a decrease in testosterone available to target organs (Schurmeyer & Nieschlag 1982). Careful attention is advised to the possible development of side effects secondary to diminished testicular, ovarian or adrenal steroid synthesis, especially in patients being given higher doses. Ketoconazole also has an inhibitory action on cortisol secretion both in vitro and in vivo, showing that patients with autonomous cortisol production caused by an adrenal tumour are prone to dangerous hypoadrenalism if treated with ketoconazole (Astahova 1983).

In addition to the risks of potentially serious liver effects in ketoconazole treatment, gastrointestinal complaints ranging from anorexia, nausea and gastralgia to constpation are the most frequently recurring side effects. Pruritus and exanthemata have been reported but do not cause major problems (Tester-Dalderup 1984). No unwanted effects affecting the haemopoietic and lymphatic systems have been reported.

In summing up the therapeutic position of ketoconazole, physicians should weigh potential benefits of treatment against the risk of liver damage, which may be irreversible by the time it is recognized, and carefully monitor their patients clinically and biochemically. With respect to therapy in candidal vulvo-vaginitis, ketoconazole is not advised. Although a regimen of 200 mg orally twice-daily for 5 days produces very high mycological cure rates and rapid relief of symptoms and signs, similar to those produced by the topical use of clotrimazole (Bingham 1984), relapse rates may be high (24.1%) and the potentially serious liver effects, which may appear unpredictably, make the use of ketoconazole unacceptable as treatment in superficial candidal vulvo-vaginitis.

Balanitis due to *Candida*

Balanitis due to *Candida* will generally settle with saline lavage (approximately 0.9% w/v being used) twice or three times daily; separation of the skin surfaces of the glans and inner surface of the prepuce is made by means of a strip of gauze (about 3.5 cm × 12 cm) soaked in saline which is renewed twice or three times daily. If such a measure fails, nystatin, clotrimazole, miconazole or econazole cream is effective.

Systemic candidosis

In life-threatening systemic candidosis, 5-fluorocytosine is an extremely effective drug, particularly when this condition is associated with organ transplant or cardiac prosthetic surgery, although not all 'wild' strains of yeast-like fungi are sensitive to it. It is likely that topical use of 5-fluorocytosine could induce an increase in the number of *Candida* strains with enhanced resistance to it and the drug could lose much of its therapeutic value (Holt 1974).

NOTE TO CHAPTER 21

Note 21.1

The suffixes '-asis', '-iasis' and '-osis' are of Graeco-Latin origin and mean a 'condition' or 'state of'. Since the medical terms for most other fungal infections end in -osis (exception pityriasis versicolor, synonym tinea versicolor) 'candidosis' has been preferred as it emphasizes a distinction between parasitic infections — names mostly ending in -iasis — and mycoses (Odds 1979). 'Candidosis' or 'candidiasis' are terms used for clinical convenience, and in scientific studies binomial nomenclature with reference to the imperfect (asexual) or perfect (sexual) states may be required. Since molecular studies have shown that the 'genus' *Candida* should be regarded as an artificial one, in that its name does not imply descent from a common ancestor, a rigidity in day-to-day language in respect to this subject is not necessary or helpful as the synonymous terms do not lead to confusion. Candidiasis is a term which remains in current usage in American (Emmons et al 1977, Holmes et al 1984) as well as British medical literature (Marks 1983).

REFERENCES

Astahova A V 1983 Drugs; ketoconazole and the liver. In: Dukes M N G (ed) 1983 Side effects of drugs annual 7, Ch 8. Excerpta Medica, Amsterdam, p 287–293

Astahova A V 1985 Antifungal agents. In: Dukes M N G (ed) 1985 Side effects of drugs annual 9, ch 28. Elsevier, Amsterdam, p 246–250

Bingham J S 1984 Single blind comparison of ketoconazole 200 mg oral tablets and clotrimazole 100 mg vaginal tablets and 1% cream in treating acute vaginal candidosis. British Journal of Venereal Diseases 60: 175–177

Carroll C J, Hurley R, Stanley V G 1973 Criteria for the diagnosis of *Candida* vulvovaginitis in pregnant women. Journal of Obstetrics and Gynaecology of the British Commonwealth 80: 258–263

Catterall T F 1966 Urethritis and balanitis due to *Candida*. In: Winner H I, Hurley R (eds) Symposium on *Candida* infections. Livingstone, Edinburgh, p 113–118

Cawson R A, Rajasingham K C 1972 Ultrastructural features of the invasive phase of *Candida albicans*. British Journal of Dermatology 87: 435–443

Cohen J 1982 Antifungal chemotherapy. Lancet ii: 532–537

Davis J E, Frudenfield J H, Goddard J L 1974 Comparative evaluation of Monistat and Mycostatin in the treatment of vulvovaginal candidiasis. Obstetrics and Gynecology 44: 403–406

Do Carmo-Sousa L 1969 Distribution of yeasts in nature. In: Rose A H, Harrison J S (eds) The yeasts, vol 1, Biology of yeasts. Academic Press, London, p 79–105

Douglas L J 1985 Adhesion of pathogenic *Candida* species to host surfaces. Microbiological Sciences 2(8): 243–247

Drutz D J, Wood R A 1973 Development of ergosterol-deficient amphotericin B resistant *Candida tropicalis* during therapy of *Candida* pyelonephritis. Clinical Research 21: 270

Ebbesen P, Biggar R J, Melbye M (ed) 1984 AIDS: a basic guide for clinicians. Munksgaard, Copenhagen, p 93

Emmons C W, Chapman H B, Utz J P, Kwon-Chung K J 1977 Medical mycology, 3rd edn. Lea and Febiger, Philadelphia

Evans E G V, Richardson M O, Odds F C, Holland K T 1973 Relevance of antigenicity of *Candida albicans* growth phases to diagnosis of systemic candidiasis. British Medical Journal 4: 86–87

Finn R, St Hill C A, Govan A J, Ralfs I G, Gurney F J, Denye V 1972 Immunological responses in pregnancy and survival of fetal homografts. British Medical Journal 3: 150–152

Gardner H L, Kaufman R H 1969 Benign diseases of the vulva and vagina. Mosby, St Louis, p 149–167

Gentles J C, La Touche C J 1969 Yeasts as human and animal pathogens. In: Rose A H, Harrison J S (eds) The yeasts, vol 1, Biology of yeasts. Academic Press, London ch 4, p 107–182

Hamilton Miller J M T 1973 Chemistry and biology of the polyene macrolide antibiotics. Bacteriological Reviews 37: 166–196

Hay R 1982 Ketoconazole. Leading article, British Medical Journal 285: 584–585

Heller C, Hoyt V 1971 Squamous cell changes associated with the presence of *Candida* sp. in cervical-vaginal Papanicalaou smear. Acta Cytologica 15: 379–384

Highton B K 1973 A trial of clotrimazole and nystatin in vaginal moniliasis. Journal of Obstetrics and Gynaecology of the British Commonwealth 80: 992–995

Holmes K K, Mardh P-A, Sparling P F, Wiesner P J 1984 Sexually transmitted diseases. McGraw-Hill, New York p 570

Holt R J 1974 Treatment of vulval candidiasis with 5-fluorocytosine. Correspondence, British Medical Journal 3: 523

Hurley R, Wright J T 1976 *Candida albicans* and polyene antibiotics. Correspondence, British Medical Journal 2: 522

Jones H E 1982 Ketoconazole. Editorial, Archives of Dermatology 118: 217–219

Kimura L H, Pearsall N N 1978 Adherence of *Candida albicans* to human buccal epithelial cells. Infection and Immunity 21: 64–68

King R D, Lee J C, Morris A L 1980 Adherence of *Candida albicans* and other *Candida* species to mucosal epithelial cells. Infection and Immunity 27: 667–674

Kreger-van Rij N J W (ed) 1984 The yeasts, a taxonomic study, 3rd edn. Elsevier, Amsterdam

Lind J, Harris V G 1977 Changes in the oral glucose tolerance test during the puerperium. British Journal of Obstetrics and Gynaecology 83: 460–463

McCourtie J, Douglas L J 1984 Relationship between cell surface composition of *Candida albicans* and adherence to acrylic after growth on different carbon sources. Infection and Immunity 45: 6–12

McNellis D, McLeod M, Lawson J, Pasquale S A 1978

Treatment of vulvovaginal candidiasis in pregnancy. A comparative study. Obstetrics and Gynecology 50: 674–678

Marks R 1983 Practical problems in dermatology. Martin Dunitz, London p 111

Masterton G, Napier J R, Henderson J N, Roberts J E 1977 Three day clotrimazole treatment in candidal vulvovaginitis. British Journal of Venereal Diseases 53: 126–128

Meyer S A, Ahearn D G, Yarrow D 1984 Genus 34 *Candida Berkhout*. In: Kreger-van Rij N J W (ed) The yeasts a taxonomic study, 3rd edn. Elsevier, Amsterdam p 841–843

Milne L J R 1978 The antifungal imidazoles: clotrimazole and miconazole. Scottish Medical Journal 23: 149–152

Moffett M, McGill M I 1960 Treatment of trichomoniasis with metronidazole. British Medical Journal 2: 910–911

Odds F C 1979 Candida and candidosis. Leicester University Press

Ridley C M 1975 The vulva. Saunders, London, p 120–130

Riggsby W S 1985 Some recent developments in the molecular biology of medically important *Candida*. Microbiological Sciences 2(9): 257–263

Rollman O, Loof L 1983 Hepatic toxicity of ketoconazole. British Journal of Dermatology 108: 376–378

Schurmeyer T H, Nieschlag E 1982 Ketoconazole-induced drop in serum and saliva testosterone. Lancet ii: 1098

Selwyn S 1976 Bacterial vaginitis and the rationale of clotrimazole therapy. Munchener Medizinische Wochenschrift 118: Suppl 1, p 49–52

Sobel J D, Myers P G, Kaye D, Levison M E 1981 Adherence of *Candida albicans* to human vaginal and buccal epithelial cells. Journal of Infectious Diseases 143: 76–82

Sobel J D, Muller G, Buckley H R 1984 Critical role of germ tube formation in the pathogenesis of candidal vaginitis. Infection and Immunity 44: 576–580

Spellacy W N, Zaias N, Buhi W C, Birk S A 1971 Vaginal yeast growth and contraceptive practice. Obstetrics and Gynaecology 38: 343–349

Tester-Dalderup C B M 1984 Antifungal agents. In: Dukes M N G (ed) Meyler's side effects of drugs. An encyclopedia of adverse reactions and interactions, 10th edn. p 516–524

van der Walt J P, Yarrow D 1984 Methods for the isolation, maintenance, classification and identification of yeasts. In: Kreger-van Rij N J W (ed) The yeasts a taxonomic study, 3rd edn. Elsevier, Amsterdam, p 45–104

Vukovich R A, Heald A, Darragh A 1977 Vaginal absorption of two imidazole antifungal agents, econazole and meconazole. Clinical Pharmacology and Therapeutics 21: 121

Weuta H 1972 Clotrimazol — Vaginaltablaten — Klinische Prufung im offenen-Versuch. Arzneim Forsch 22: 1291–1294

Winner H I, Hurley R 1966 Symposium on *Candida* infections. Livingstone, Edinburgh

Woods R A, Bard M, Jackson M, Drutz D J 1974 Resistance to polyene antibiotics and correlated sterol changes in two isolates of *Candida tropicalis* from a patient with an amphotericin B-resistant funguria. Journal of Infectious Diseases 129: 53–58

22

Trichomoniasis

Trichomoniasis is a common and sometimes distressing condition in women resulting from infection of the genito-urinary tract by the protozoon, *Trichomonas vaginalis*. The parasite may be found in the vagina, urethra, bladder, para-urethral ducts, and occasionally in the ducts of the greater vestibular glands. Although many women are symptomless, vaginal discharge, vaginitis, dyspareunia, dysuria and frequency are all common manifestations of infection with *T. vaginalis*.

Infection in men is often asymptomatic, but the protozoon may sometimes be found in those with signs of a urethritis or prostatitis. The ratio for cases of trichomoniasis in men and women respectively is difficult to determine, since in men the infection may be short-lived and the organism difficult to detect. With few exceptions, transmission is by sexual intercourse when the incubation period is in the range 4 days to 4 weeks. Neonates may occasionally develop a vulvovaginitis as a result of an infection acquired during passage through the birth canal.

AETIOLOGY

The causative organism, a flagellate protozoon of the urogenital tract, *Trichomonas vaginalis* was first described by Donné in 1836. Trichomonads vary in shape as a result of environmental conditions. In culture in vitro the organism is approximately 10 μm (range about 5–20 μm) in length and 7 μm in breadth (range about 3–13 μm) and tends to become ellipsoid or ovoid, whereas in the vagina the shape is very variable and the organism is often elongated. Pseudopodia-like extensions from its surface allow for feeding and attachment to solid objects. There are four anterior flagella which are about the same length as the body. Movement of the undulating membrane is vigorous and is controlled by the posterior flagellum which passes along its upper margin. The undulating membrane is about two-thirds that of the body length of the organism. The flagella originate from, and are intimately related to, a kinetosomal complex situated at the anterior end of the cell.

The costa, a slender chromatic basal rod, also originates from the kinetosomal complex, is uniform in diameter, tending to taper at its ends, and situated beneath the undulating membrane. A hyaline rod, the axostyle, is flattened into a capitulum closely applied to the nucleus and passes down the centre of the cell and appears to project posteriorly as a small spine. A single oval nucleus lies near the anterior end of the cell. A row of granules are to be seen on either side of both the costa (paracostal granules) and the axostyle (para-axostylar granules). Multiplication is by longitudinal binary fission. Cysts are not formed (Honigberg 1978).

T. vaginalis exhibits the characteristics of a microaerophile; in culture, anaerobic conditions prolong the period of population increase (Lowe 1978). The principal mode of nutrition is by pinocytosis or *sensu stricto* macropinocytosis (viz. 'cell-drinking' or ingestion of large molecules and tiny particles by cells) and phagocytosis ('cell-eating', a similar process to macropinocytosis except that particles are large enough to be seen in the light microscope) (Herbert et al 1985), which may proceed in any part of the body (Ovčinnikov et al 1975). First, an invagination appears in the cytoplasm and gradually its edges are drawn together. The wall of the vesicle thickens and acquires a villous pattern. Microorganisms and large particles are usually caught by pseudopodia: large and small particles including entire cells may be engulfed. Some, but not all entrapped organisms seem to be altered but it is impossible to say whether they have undergone changes after engulfment or have been phagocytosed in a poor condition. They are usually located in phagosomes but may lie freely in the cytoplasm with no evidence of a limiting membrane.

Ovčinnikov et al (1975) suggested that gonococci contained within trichomonads might be protected from the action of penicillin. Multiplication of gonococci within a phagosome could cause rupture and death of the trichomonad with release of the engulfed organisms. In their opinion, recurrences of gonorrhoea might be explained by ineffective treatment of a mixed infection but this situation has not been considered to be a problem in clinical practice. It has been shown also that organisms (e.g. *Neisseria gonorrhoeae*, *Mycoplasma hominis* and *Chlamydia trachomatis*), once ingested are degraded rapidly and are unlikely to form a source of persisting infection (Street et al 1984).

A sexually transmitted trichomonad, *Tritrichomonas fetus*, is seen in cattle and found in the preputial sac and on the glans penis of bulls; the organism, transmitted to cows during sexual intercourse, may cause vaginitis, endometritis and abortion.

Two other species of trichomonads, *Trichomonas tenax* and *Pentatrichomonas hominis* occur in man. Apart from *P. hominis* with its five anterior flagella, these organisms are morphologically similar to *T. vaginalis*. *T. tenax* is generally considered to be a harmless commensal of the mouth and is commonly associated with poor oral hygiene. It does not survive passage through the intestinal tract and cannot be established in the vagina. *P. hominis* is an inhabitant of the caecum and colon of man; a morphologically identical organism is found in other primates. Although it is considered to be a harmless commensal, it is often found in association with true pathogenic protozoa, e.g. *Entamoeba histolytica*. *P. hominis* does not survive in the mouth or vagina.

PATHOLOGY

In light and electron microscope studies of biopsies of the cervix in patients with trichomonal vaginitis, Nielsen & Nielsen (1975) found that trichomonads were gathered in small clusters on the stratified epithelium, but covered only a small area of the surface. Cells of *T. vaginalis* invaded superficial epithelial cells but did not penetrate to the deeper cell layer of epithelium. Epithelial damage tended to be located under clusters of trichomonads, but an intense vaginitis was present whether or not *T. vaginalis* cells were present on the epithelial surface. Their findings indicated that the interaction between cells of *T. vaginalis* and vaginal epithelium takes place primarily at a distance, probably by means of substances released into the vaginal fluid, and secondarily by a direct cell contact mechanism.

The biopsies showed chronic non-specific inflammation with subepithelial accumulation of plasma cells, lymphocytes and polymorphonuclear leucocytes. When inflammation was slight, neutrophils were found superficially in the epithelium, and when more severe the neutrophils were in the deeper layers also. There was sometimes ulceration of the surface, and all layers of the cervical epithelium showed some hyperchromasia and nuclear enlargement (Nielsen & Nielsen 1975).

On colposcopy, when inflammation due to *Trichomonas* is severe, magnification reveals patches of higher vascular density, which on naked-eye inspection are usually described as forming a 'strawberry cervix'. The inflammation produces significant changes in the pattern of the original squamous epithelium as seen through the colposcope. The stromal papillae are higher and reach almost to the surface of the epithelium. In these papillae the vessels are clearly visible and form simple capillary loops running vertically to the surface, but at the top of the loop two or more crests may be found. The shape of the loops may be described as fork-like or antler-like (Kolstad & Stafl 1977). As the capillaries are separated from the surface by only a few layers of epithelial cells contact bleeding is common (Slavin 1976).

Recently it has been reported that *T. vaginalis* causes striking retardation in motility of human spermatozoa when these were incubated in vitro (Tuttle et al 1977); the clinical significance of this observation has not been ascertained.

IMMUNITY

Trichomoniasis, like other mucosal infections, induces local production of secretory IgA in women (Ackers et al 1975), but this was seldom detected in men who harboured trichomonas or who were contacts of women who harboured the organism (Ackers et al 1978). This antibody response is not capable of eliminating infection. Untreated trichomoniasis in women tends to subside into a chronic low-grade infection with occasional reappearance of symptoms. Also, immune response to infection with *T. vaginalis* does not prevent reinfection, since repeated attacks of trichomoniasis are common.

Using a whole-cell antigen, antibody to *T. vaginalis* has been assayed using an enzyme-linked immunosorbent assay (ELISA). IgG antibody was detected in only 3% of children under 12 years of age. In contrast, IgG or IgM antibody or both were detected in about 80% of the women who had vaginal trichomoniasis and in about 14% of women considered to be uninfected on the basis of microscopy of wet or stained films. Although antibody was found in cervical and vaginal secretions, the correlation between current infection and the presence of antibody (IgG or IgA) was poorer than that found between circulating antibody and infection (Street et al 1982). Since the basis of diagnosis depended on the generally insensitive methods, viz. microscopy of films, the results of the ELISA test cannot be further evaluated.

EPIDEMIOLOGY AND TRANSMISSION OF INFECTION

In adults, infection with *T. vaginalis* is generally regarded as being sexually transmitted (Catterall &

Nicoll 1960, Morton & Harris 1975, Bramley 1976) Trichomoniasis is uncommon among children and virgins, but most common between the ages of 16 and 35 years, which is usually the period of greatest sexual activity. Trichomoniasis is commonly associated with other sexually transmissible diseases and up to 40% of women attending STD clinics with this infection may also have gonorrhoea (Tsao 1969).

A varying proportion, even up to 60%, of male sex partners of infected women may harbour the parasite and the majority are asymptomatic (Catterall 1977). In many instances, cure of women with recurrent trichomoniasis has only resulted after the parasite has been eradicated from the genital tract of their partner(s). There is often difficulty, however, at a single examination, in demonstrating the parasite in male patients who are contacts of women with *T. vaginalis* (Catterall & Nicoll 1960).

Trichomoniasis is mainly a sexually transmitted condition. Although direct female to female transmission, resulting from poor standards of sanitation and hygiene (e.g. contamination of baths, bidets, toilet seats, swimming baths and towels), has been proposed as a means of acquiring the infection, there is little evidence to support this view. Infection of a baby during delivery may result when the mother has vaginal trichomoniasis. Neonatal infestation followed by a long and variable period of latency could account for non-sexually acquired infection. However, neonatal infection in female babies, although a recognized clinical entity, is rare (Bramley 1976). It has also been suggested that intestinal trichomonads could become adapted to the vagina. There is, however, no evidence that these trichomonads can be successfully established in the human vagina.

There is an association between cervical carcinoma and infestation with *T. vaginalis* although a direct causal relationship is unproved (Ch. 25).

CLINICAL FEATURES IN WOMEN

Trichomoniasis is not readily recognized, nor are clinical manifestations reliable diagnostic parameters; only a minority of women with trichomoniasis show classic signs (Fouts & Kraus 1980). The prepatent period is difficult to determine although it has been estimated that clinical manifestations of the disease develop 4 to 28 days after sexual intercourse with an infected partner (Catterall 1972).

The clinical features of infection are very variable, the most common symptoms in those infected being vaginal discharge (56%) and dysuria 18% (Fouts & Kraus 1980). Vulval soreness and an unpleasant odour may also be present (Wisdom & Dunlop 1965). In many,

sometimes in 40% of cases, there may be no complaint of vaginal discharge (Fouts & Kraus 1980). The concept that all women infected with *T. vaginalis* have vaginal discharge should be discarded. Clinical features appear to differ according to the population and possibly age group studied.

The most common sign, occurring in about 70% of cases of trichomoniasis, is a vaginal discharge, varying in consistency from thin and scanty to thick and profuse; the classical sign of a frothy yellow discharge is found in proportions varying between 10 and 30%. Vulvitis and vaginitis are sometimes associated with a trichomonal vaginal discharge, and the cervix may be inflamed. When inflammation is severe, perhaps in only as few as 2% of those with trichomoniasis, as in the study by Fouts & Kraus (1980), patches of higher vascular density may give the appearance described as a 'strawberry cervix'. The tendency to contact bleeding from the surface is explained by the fact that only a few layers of epithelial cells separate capillaries from the surface. Urethritis is found in about a quarter of women. Bartholinitis is a rare complication, and is perhaps produced by bacterial infection rather than the protozoon. In above 5% of infected women there are no abnormal findings on clinical examination.

CLINICAL FEATURES IN MEN

Although *T. vaginalis* may be isolated from the urethra, urine or prostatic fluid of male contacts of women with trichomoniasis, more than 90% of these men will have no symptom of infection. Urethritis, prostatitis, cystitis and epididymitis have been given as manifestations of trichomoniasis (Harkness 1950, Fisher & Morton 1969) but the aetiology of these conditions may be more related to the aetiology of non-gonococcal urethritis and to pathogens, or potential pathogens, such as *Chlamydia trachomatis* and *Ureaplasma urealyticum*.

T. vaginalis may be isolated from the subpreputial sac and may be associated with balanoposthitis, which may rarely be ulcerative.

TRICHOMONIASIS AND CARCINOMA OF CERVIX

Infection with *T. vaginalis* is often associated with dysplasia and endocervical hyperplasia, changes which are reversible with treatment (Bertini & Hornstein 1970). Although the incidence of trichomoniasis was found to be four times higher in patients with carcinoma of the cervix than in control·patients in one study (Berggren

1969). There is no good evidence that the dysplasia observed in trichomoniasis is associated with malignancy. *T. vaginalis* may be associated with other sexually transmissible agents such as papillomavirus and herpesvirus.

DIAGNOSIS

The diagnosis of trichomoniasis relies upon both microscopy and culture for the demonstration of *T. vaginalis* in the secretions of patients. Repeated testing from a multiplicity of sites, especially in males, may be necessary to establish a diagnosis.

In women, vaginal exudate is collected from the posterior fornix with a sterile cotton-wool swab. If a urethral discharge is present in men, this can be collected with a bacteriological loop, otherwise an early morning scraping should be taken gently from the urethra before the patient passes the first morning urine. If these tests are negative then a centrifuged deposit of urine and prostatic secretion should be examined.

Polyester swabs, which are gentler on the urethral mucosa, have been recommended for taking specimens in men (Oates et al 1971) while small rectangles of polyester sponge (1 cm × 1 cm × 4 cm) can be used for collecting vaginal exudate in women (Robertson et al 1969); this sponge is more absorbent than cotton wool and a larger inoculum may be collected in this way.

The following diagnostic techniques may be applied.

Examination of a wet film

A fresh specimen of secretion may be examined rapidly as a wet preparation either directly, or after suspension in a few drops of isotonic saline or buffer. The actual technique of microscopy varies from clinic to clinic, but dark ground illumination, phase-contrast microscopy and ordinary light microscopy with reduced illumination are all used routinely. *T. vaginalis*, which is larger than a polymorphonuclear leucocyte but smaller than an epithelial cell, is readily recognized by its usually oval shape, its often rapidly moving flagella, the rippling movement of the undulating membrane, and the jerky movements of the organism. Ideally, the specimen should be examined immediately but if this is impracticable the swab should be placed preferably in Amies' transport medium; *T. vaginalis* does not survive well in Stuart's transport medium beyond 24 hours (Nielsen 1969). Although useful in diagnosis when the organism is numerous, half of the cases of trichomonal infection of the vagina may be missed if reliance is placed on examination of the wet film alone (Fouts & Kraus 1980).

Examination of stained films

Giemsa, Papanicolaou and Leishman's stains are commonly used for the diagnosis of trichomoniasis, while other methods such as Gram-staining with safranin as counterstain and staining with acridine orange have also been applied. Diagnosis by stained smear has the advantage that, once fixed, the specimen can be sent to a laboratory for processing, but it is insensitive and is not recommended.

When sufficiently numerous, and under good conditions of fixation and staining, *T. vaginalis* is recognizable in cervical smears taken for cytological examination, although variations in morphology due to artefacts of smear making and staining and the eosinophilic appearance of the parasite found in blood-stained smears, may make difficult a certain diagnosis. The protozoon nearly always loses its flagella during fixation and appears as a small sometimes pear-shaped cell, 10–30 μm in diameter, grey-blue in colour with multiple intracytoplasmic granules. Diagnosis depends on the recognition of the small dark grey ovoid nucleus, which can resemble degenerate nuclei of parabasal cells (Grubb 1977). Opinion varies as to the value of staining techniques in general and to Papanicolaou-stained cervical smears in particular. In one study, errors in diagnosis due to false-positive and false-negative findings when the Papanicolaou smear was used as the criterion for diagnosing and treating *T. vaginalis* infestation reached almost 50% (Pert 1972). When organisms are fewer in number, the discovery of the motile protozoon with its flagella and undulating membrane in a wet film, examined preferably by phase-contrast microscopy or by direct light microscopy, is the method of choice. Details of cellular changes associated with trichomonal infection are given by Hughes et al (1966).

False-negative results are also common in diagnosis by microscopy of the wet film, particularly if the numbers of trichomonads present are small. In one study, with a three-minute scrutiny of a wet film, positive diagnoses were only obtained in half the number detected by culture methods (Fouts & Kraus 1980).

Culture

Many media are available for the cultural diagnosis of trichomoniasis, but no one medium is consistently better than the others. These media are usually liquid and contain liver digest, serum and anti-bacterial and anti-fungal agents: commonly used media include cysteine-peptone-liver-maltose (CPLM) medium, Feinberg and Whittington's, Diamond's and commercially available Oxoid trichomonas medium. Cultures should be inoculated directly with specimens taken from the same sites as those for microscopy. Cultures are incubated at 37°C for 48 hours and examined microscopically for trichomonads: incubation should be continued and cultures examined daily for up to one week.

Opinion varies considerably as to the relative efficiency of culture and microscopy; techniques which work well in one area seem often to give poor results in other laboratories. Direct microscopic examination of a wet film of material obtained from the posterior fornix will detect infections where many trichomonads are present: lighter infestations should be detected within a few days by culture (Hess 1969).

Relying on modified Feinberg and Whittington's or Diamond's medium; incubating inoculated culture medium at 36.5°C; and microscopic examination of the sediment for *T. vaginalis* at 2–3, and again at 6–7, days after incubation, Fouts & Kraus (1980) identified the organism in 131 women whereas the infection was only detected in 66 (50.4%) by a three-minute microscopic scrutiny of wet film.

Accurate diagnosis of trichomoniasis followed by effective treatment is particularly important with respect to the interpretation of cervical cytology smears and biopsy specimens. Degenerative changes associated with trichomonal infection may mask the presence of dyskaryotic or malignant cells (Hughes et al 1966).

Immunocytochemical tests
Although the detection of trichomonads in vaginal exudate by direct immunofluorescence has proved superior to that by wet smear microscopy (Hayes & Kotcher 1960), difficulty in identification of the organisms amongst material which show non-specific fluorescence has limited its diagnostic usefulness. Enzyme-labelled immunocytochemical methods, however, have certain advantages over fluorescent antibody techniques, and O'Hara and colleagues (1980) reported the detection of *T. vaginalis* in cervical smears stained by an immuno-peroxidase method. Enzyme immunoassay systems for the detection of antigens may provide sensitive diagnostic methods in the future (Yolken 1982).

TREATMENT WITH 5-NITROIMIDAZOLES

The discovery in 1959 of the 5-nitroimidazole, metronidazole, as the first agent systemically active against trichomoniasis (Durel et al 1960) brought spectacular cure rates of 86–100% instead of the 10–20% of earlier treatments. Since 1969 the closely related 5-nitroimidazoles nimorazole, tinidazole, ornidazole, secnidazole and carnidazole have been introduced into clinical practice, although not all of them are available in every country. In the USA only metronidazole is approved by the Federal Drugs Administration for the treatment of trichomoniasis; in Britain nimorazole is also available. A review of the comparative data did not reveal clear advantage for one compound over another and cure rates lie within the range of 85–95% with symptoms generally being relieved within a few days (Meingassner & Heyworth 1981).

Metronidazole is the most extensively used drug of the group and although the other 5-nitroimidazoles differ somewhat in the pharmacological properties, the mode of antimicrobial activity is similar for all.

Mode of action
The majority of clinically important anaerobe genera such as *Bacteroides*, *Fusobacterium* and the spore-bearing *Clostridium* and metronidazole susceptible protozoa are inhibited by concentrations of approximately 3 μg per ml or less. Organisms such as anaerobic Gram-positive cocci and non-sporing bacilli are usually inhibited by 6 μg per ml or less (Ralph 1983).

The action of the 5-nitroimidazoles in anaerobic micro-organisms is thought to consist of four successive steps (Müller 1983, Müller & Gorrell 1983): 1. the entry of the drug into the cell; 2. its reductive activation to short-lived cytotoxic intermediates, a process inhibited by aerobiosis; 3. the toxic effect of these short-lived intermediates on intracellular components leading to cell death; 4. the release of biologically inactive end products. The main point of the hypothesis is the assumption that the nitro group of the drug has to be reduced in the target cell to form a toxic derivative; no cytotoxicity can be observed without such reduction.

The striking feature of the selectivity of metronidazole is that it affects anaerobic organisms, both prokaryotes and eukaryotes, where reduction of metronidazole, crucial to its action, appears to be achieved by redox mechanisms that are of great significance in the metabolism of anaerobes and play no, or only a minor, role in other organisms.

Cellular uptake of metronidazole appears to be passive and achieved by diffusion in both anaerobic and aerobic cells, but whereas in aerobic cells the drug remains unchanged, in anaerobic organisms it undergoes metabolic modification which decreases the intracellular concentration of unchanged drug and thus increases the concentration gradient across the cell membrane: this gradient promotes the continuous uptake of the drug and leads to an intracellular accumulation of its derivatives. The electrons necessary for the reduction of the nitro group of metronidazole origin and the direct donors of these electrons are thought to be ferredoxin-like electron transport proteins of low redox potential (doxins). Unstable intermediates in the process of reduction are thought to be cytotoxic, whereas end products such as acetamide and N-(2-hydroxyethyl) oxamic acid are not. The most significant competitor for available electrons is oxygen, as shown by diminished biological activity of metronidazole when susceptible organisms are present under aerobic conditions. Among other cytotoxic effects, metronidazole reduced in the presence of DNA binds to the nucleic acid and causes strand breakage with destabilization of the helix.

Resistance to metronidazole

Certain isolates of *T. vaginalis*, obtained from patients in whom several courses of metronidazole have failed, show normal susceptibility to metronidazole in in vitro assays performed under anaerobic conditions, but in certain aerobic in vitro assays their susceptibility is significantly lower than that of non-resistant isolates (Meingassner & Heyworth 1981, Müller 1983). There are marked differences in the effect of aerobiosis on metronidazole metabolism in various isolates of *T. vaginalis*. Aerobic conditions inhibit metronidazole uptake in resistant isolates to a greater extent than in susceptible ones, and changes in intracellular reduction may be responsible for relative resistance (Müller & Gorrell 1983).

Under completely anaerobic conditions, metronidazole may be effective against all *T. vaginalis* stocks, but under partially aerobic conditions its effects may vary widely (Müller 1979) and assays under aerobic conditions have been thought to give false results (Edwards & Shanson 1980). The crux of the matter seems to be that the activity of metronidazole in vitro under anaerobic conditions is little altered, but under aerobic conditions relative resistance is detected among ordinarily susceptible organisms and enhanced resistance among the resistant organisms. In the cytoplasm of *Trichomonas vaginalis* are to be found membrane-bound organelles, microbodies unique to this organism, called hydrogenosomes. All the enzymes responsible for the cleavage of pyruvate to acetate, CO_2 and H_2 appear to be located in these microbodies, which also enable the reduction of the 5-nitroimidazoles. The reduction products are unstable but their cytotoxic action appears to cause strand breakage in the DNA. This will only occur under anaerobic conditions and only with the reduced drug. There are data to suggest that in resistant trichomonads a low cytoplasmic nicotinamide adenine dinucleotide H oxidase may allow oxygen to permeate hydrogenosomes and interfere with their reductive action on the drug. The process is an example of selective toxicity, and intracellular concentration of drug metabolite is 50 to 100 times that of unchanged drug in body fluids. From the evolutionary point of view hydrogenosomes themselves may be organelles derived from clostridia.

The reduction of the nitro group of 5-nitroimidazoles and the production of cytotoxic intermediates is intimately connected with the functioning of the hydrogenosome, where the nitro group is reduced by electrons generated during hydrogenosomal pyruvate oxidation and donated to the drug by its doxins. Oxygen competes for these electrons, and as has been explained, under aerobic conditions the trichomonicidal activity of metronidazole is diminished (Meingassner & Heyworth 1981).

Mutagenicity and capacity to induce tumours in experimental animals

In some bacteria metronidazole can produce mutations, but a double-blind cross-over study showed that a daily dose of 0.8 g for 4 months did not induce an increase in the frequency of chromosomal aberrations in patients with Crohn's disease. Coulter (1979) indicated that the connection between mutation, a heritable change in DNA sequence, and gross changes in chromosome anatomy is not, however, understood.

As a nitro compound in widespread therapeutic use, metronidazole has been investigated in regard to its capacity to induce tumours in some laboratory animals. In connection with the effect on tumour incidence in mice, Roe (1977) writes that 'the effect involved the administration throughout the lives of the animals of total doses, on a mg per kg body weight basis, equivalent to between 350–1000 times that given to patients in the form of a 10-day course for the treatment of trichomoniasis'.

A more subtle discussion has developed about possible effects arising from disturbance in the gastrointestinal flora by the selective killing of organisms such as *Bacteroides*, which form a large proportion of lower intestine flora. As a result carcinogen-forming bacteria might be allowed to predominate and lead to a decrease in the capacity of intestinal flora to detoxicate potential carcinogens (Willson 1974).

In his review Roe (1977) writes that 'a small and indefinite cloud' hangs over the therapeutic use of metronidazole, as it does to many other drugs in relation to possible carcinogenicity and mutagenicity. Metronidazole, however, and another nitro compound, nitrofurantoin, have been in use for many years and in the United Kingdom for the years 1968, 1969 and 1970, more than 3 million prescriptions were written for the two drugs. So far no clinical evidence of carcinogenicity has been forthcoming (Hamilton-Miller & Brumfitt 1976). The cure of trichomoniasis and the control of secondary non-specific vaginal infection is highly desirable, and as a result may reduce the risk of cervical cancer itself (Roe 1977). The authors favour the use of metronidazole in the doses recommended for the treatment of trichomoniasis. More remote questions of carcinogenicity or effects on bowel flora cannot be completely answered yet: studies of populations with controls and data-linkage would be necessary for such an analysis.

At the Mayo clinic, 767 women, given at least one prescription of metronidazole for *T. vaginalis* infections between 1960 and 1969, have been followed up and no substantial increase in total cancer incidence, over that expected, has been found. In this study increased mobility, increase in divorces and remarriages with consequent name changes caused great difficulties in follow-up. The finding of 13 cases of in situ cancer of the cervix in this group and the discovery of 4 cases of cancer of the lung in heavy smokers (Medical News 1978), illustrate further difficulties in making comparisons.

Absorption, distribution and fate of metronidazole (Ralph 1983)

Peak serum concentrations of metronidazole are quite similar, whether after oral or intravenous administration, and average approximately 10 μg per ml after a single 500 mg dose. After an oral dose the peak serum concentration is reached about an hour after administration. Food does not significantly affect absorption, and bioavailability approaches 100%. Rectal administration of metronidazole by suppository results in peak concentrations approximately one half of those following equivalent oral doses and occurs at 4 hours after administration; the bioavailability of a rectal suppository is about 80%. The systemic absorption of intravaginal metronidazole is very slow with peak serum concentrations of approximately 2 μg per ml being attained 8–24 hours after administration of a 500 mg dose.

Metronidazole is excreted in the urine as unchanged drug and primarily oxidative metabolites, the major compounds being the hydroxy and acid metabolites. By specific and sensitive methods such as high pressure liquid chromatography (HPLC) in which unchanged metronidazole and the hydroxy and acid metabolites are measured separately, total excretion of these compounds after 48 hours is 30%, with the hydroxy metabolite being the primary excretion product.

Reductive metabolism of the nitro group of metronidazole occurs in humans, but to a very limited extent, probably by intestinal microflora and results in the formation of acetamide and N-(2-hydroxyethyl) oxamic acid. These compounds are detected in the urine and represent about 1–2% of the dose given.

The serum half-life of unchanged metronidazole (HPLC) averaged about 8 hours, and unchanged metronidazole is widely distributed throughout the body with tissue levels, in most cases, approximating serum levels.

Brown or reddish brown discoloration of the urine has been attributed to other formation of azoxy compounds secondary to the reduction of the nitro group of metronidazole, probably by intestinal microflora possessing nitroreductors.

In lactating women, after a single 2 g oral dose, peak concentrations in breast milk of 45–48 μg per ml are found at 2 hours, with elimination half-life in milk approximating that in serum. It has been estimated that an infant would consume about 25 mg of metronidazole in breast milk during the 48-hour period after the mother received a single 2 g dose. If breast feeding were to be deferred for 24 hours, consumption of metronidazole would fall to about 4 mg.

Treatment with metronidazole

Dosage

In the treatment of trichomonal vaginitis the single 2.0 g oral dose of metronidazole is as effective as a 250 mg dose administered three times daily for 7 days, and for ease of administration, better patient compliance and lower cost and since it achieved a cure rate comparable with the 7-day course, it has been recommended, although some patients may experience nausea and/or vomiting (Aubert & Sesta 1982). Although single-dose treatment is encouraged (American Medical Association 1983, British National Formulary 1985) it has not gained general acceptance. In the United Kingdom the conventional course ordinarily used is 200 mg thrice-daily for 7 days, although the 2.0 g single dose was put forward as a practical and acceptable alternative 15 years ago by Csonka (1971). In his cases some abdominal pain was reported by one patient and vomiting by another soon after taking the tablets. A randomized double-blind comparison of 2.0 g in a single oral dose and 400 mg twice-daily for 5 days led to a recommendation in favour of the single dose; nausea, vomiting and dizziness were reported by 1 of 96 patients treated with the single dose (Thin et al 1979).

Toxicity

At the dose generally used for trichomoniasis (200 mg thrice-daily for a week), metronidazole is well tolerated and during the 16 years of its widespread use, it has earned a reputation of being remarkably safe. Occasional side effects at these doses include nausea, an unpleasant taste in the mouth, furring of the tongue and gastrointestinal upsets; headache, dizziness, anorexia, depression and skin eruptions have been reported but rarely (Roe 1977). The single 2.0 g dose has been reported as producing nausea alone in 2% and with vomiting in 4%.

Metronidazole may produce a transient leucopenia in 4% of cases (Lefebre & Heseltine 1965) but this apears to be due to an accelerated disappearance of these elements from the blood, which temporarily exceeds bone marrow release, rather than to suppression of bone marrow (Taylor 1965); no serious blood dyscrasias have been reported.

Metronidazole in pregnancy

It is the first trimester of pregnancy that includes the stage of organogenesis in the embryo and during this stage certain drugs are teratogenic and cause congenital malformations. The most critical period for gross congenital defects is the somite stage of embryonic development, which in humans occurs between the 21st and 31st days of intrauterine life (35–45 days after the start of the last menstrual period). The central nervous system, heart, gut, skeletal system and muscle all begin to differentiate in the somite stage, and teratogenic drugs acting at this period may affect any of these systems. After the 8th to 10th week of intrauterine life the embryo is fully differentiated and drugs cannot, strictly speaking, be teratogenic although they can still cause disorders of growth and function. Thus, in the central nervous system particularly, damage after the first trimester can produce microcephaly and mental retardation. The total actual period for teratogenicity is usually believed to extend from about the third to the eighth or tenth week of intrauterine life, and during this time the mother may not know she is pregnant (Davies 1981).

There is no evidence that metronidazole is teratogenic in humans (Hawkins 1976) but it has been pointed out (Dunn et al 1979) that like disulfiram it inhibits aldehyde dehydrogenase and might theoretically increase the risk of the fetal alcohol syndrome in the offspring of women who drink during pregnancy.

Aldehyde, a breakdown product of alcohol, is cytotoxic and teratogenic at levels of over 35 μmol per 1 — levels, however, not ordinarily reached in most alcoholics. It is important therefore to avoid all drugs which inhibit aldehyde dehydrogenase and therefore it is best to avoid metronidazole during pregnancy. If essential for symptomatic trichomoniasis, treatment with metronidazole should be postponed until after the 16th week of pregnancy and the most strict injunction given to avoid all alcohol (Davies 1981).

As nitroimidazoles are excreted in breast milk, mothers who are breast feeding should not be given these drugs, although deferring breast feeding for 24 hours after giving the mother a 2.0 g dose would result in the baby only receiving about 4 mg (Ralph 1983). Metronidazole, however, appears safe for use in children (Rubridge et al 1970).

Drug interaction (alcohol and metronidazole)

In a study of 53 alcoholic patients on metronidazole, in which one case in a male was described as representative of the results obtained in the others, a decreased tolerance for alcohol, a diminished compulsion to drink intoxicants and an apparent aversion to ethanol were described (Taylor 1964). Mild to moderate disulfiram-like effects were also described (e.g. facial flushing, headache, nausea and sweating) with metronidazole, following alcohol ingestion. In vitro studies have shown that metronidazole can produce inhibition of aldehyde dehydrogenase and other alcohol-oxidizing enzymes, but a study in rats failed to substantiate the result of the in vitro studies (American Pharmaceutical Association 1976).

In recent well-controlled clinical studies the disulfiram-like reaction has not been reported, nor effects such as decreased craving for alcohol, described as occurring within one or two weeks of commencing metronidazole treatment (Semer et al 1966). Adverse effects of concurrent metronidazole and alcohol are apparently infrequent but patients should be advised about these possibilities in the event of alcohol being ingested during metronidazole therapy (American Pharmaceutical Association 1976).

Anti-treponeme activity of metronidazole

Metronidazole has only weak anti-treponemal activity, and it seems unlikely that the small doses of metronidazole used in the treatment of trichomoniasis would delay diagnosis in a patient incubating syphilis.

Nimorazole (Naxogin)

This nitroimidazole is similar to metronidazole. It is usually administered as 3 oral doses of 500 mg at 12-hour intervals.

TREATMENT FAILURE IN TRICHOMONAL VAGINITIS

Failure to cure trichomonal vaginitis with nitroimidazoles has distressing consequences because there is no certainly effective alternative treatment and palliatives are not satisfactory. With normal doses of metronidazole viz. 200 mg three times daily for 7 days, successful elimination of *T. vaginalis* is achieved in about 95% of women so infected; in some women repeated failure to achieve this has been thought to be due to a number of different factors: poor absorption of the drug; inability to produce trichomonicidal concentrations in vaginal tissue or contents; inactivation of the drug by micro-organisms in the vagina; non-compliance or failure to take the drug by the patient; reinfection; or enhanced resistance of the organism.

Individual idiosyncrasies in absorption of metronidazole from the gut lumen or in its passage into the vagina are, however, unlikely to be the cause of treatment failure (Robertson et al 1988). In this Edinburgh study of the concentrations of metronidazole in the plasma and vaginal content of 11 'treatment-failure' patients on usual dosage (200 mg 8-hourly by mouth given to the patient for two days in hospital under supervision) and high-dose metronidazole treatment (800 mg 8-hourly by mouth given subsequently under the same circumstances for 5 days) concurrent estimation by high pressure liquid chromatography of the concentrations of metronidazole in plasma and vaginal content showed that the two levels are closely related to each other and to the dose. These patients showed a normal level of plasma metronidazole (mean 8.3 mg per l, s.e. 0.7 mg per l) on the 200 mg dosage and on the high dosage a high plateau (mean 36.7 mg per l, s.e. 2.0 mg per l) was quickly reached. The simultaneous collection of vaginal content gave metronidazole concentrations in vaginal content averaging 80% of the corresponding plasma levels. The hydroxy metabolite, which has a lower anti-trichomonal activity than metronidazole (Lindmark & Muller 1976) was present in all plasma and vaginal content samples. When a single 2 g dose was administered to one 'treatment failure' patient no abnormality in metabolism was detected in the metabolism of the drug. The plasma concentration of metronidazole fell exponentially from 58 mg per litre at 75 minutes to 33 mg per l at 365 minutes giving an estimated half-life of 5.8 hours; concentrations of metronidazole in plasma at 184 and 305 minutes were 47 and 36 mg per l, similar to those in vaginal content, 47 and 31 mg per l respectively. The infection was not cleared in this patient.

Estimations of the in vitro sensitivity of *T. vaginalis* to metronidazole are not readily provided for clinical purposes, as methods are as yet of an experimental rather than a practical nature and show many variations in detail. The inocula are sometimes of organisms of unstated age or number; they are sometimes standardized in terms of the number inoculated; and the media are diverse in constitution, particularly with respect to the content of redox agents. Mostly no mention is made of the atmosphere superjacent to the cultures, whih has

an important influence on the metabolism and survival of the trichomonads (Meingassner et al 1978). Attempts have been made to control this feature (Meingassner & Stockinger 1981) and Lumsden et al (1988) have made some progress in finding a way of controlling the oxygenation of the test medium at some precise level, less than that of air, and in determining the level at which best compromise could be reached between good growth conditions for the organism and optimum oxygen tension for detecting resistance to the drug. Under these conditions, although there were occasional discordant results, it was possible to distinguish between *T. vaginalis* from 'treatment failure' patients who are likely to be cured by enhanced dosage and those who are not; *T. vaginalis* isolates which were very sensitive to mtronidazole could also be recognized.

TREATMENT OF SEXUAL PARTNERS OF WOMEN WITH TRICHOMONIASIS

Trichomonal infection is most readily found in the sexual partners of infected women, being demonstrable in 70% of the men who have had sexual contact within the past 48 hours; the percentage positive then appears to progressively decline, with 40% giving positive results if examined within 5 days and only 12% if examined after 21 days (Weston & Nicol 1963). Often asymptomatic or with mild clinical features of non-gonococcal urethritis it is, however, very often difficult to exclude the infection in the male, bearing in mind the variations in the efficiency of cultural methods and the difficulty in detecting trichomonas when either or both few in number or of low infectivity to culture. Using a 7-day standard course of metronidazole (250 mg thrice-daily) the relapse rate may be very low (5%) even if the sexual partners are not treated (Rein 1981). Single-dose treatment of 2.0 g metronidazole, in the latter's experience however, gave cure rates 6–12% lower than the 7-day standard regimen. The 7-day treatment may protect women from reinfection while the spontaneous reduction in numbers of *T. vaginalis* occurs in the infected male partner.

REFERENCES

Ackers J P, Lumsden W H R, Catterall R D, Coyle R 1975 Antitrichomonal antibody in the vaginal secretions of women infected with *T. vaginalis*. British Journal of Venereal Diseases 51: 319–323

Ackers J P, Catterall R D, Lumsden W H R, McMillan A 1978 Absence of detectable local antibody in genito urinary

tract secretions of male contacts of women infected with *Trichomonas vaginalis*. British Journal of Venereal Diseases 54: 168–171

American Medical Association 1983 Drug evaluations, 5th edn. Saunders, Philadelphia, p 1801–1802

American Pharmaceutical Association 1976 In: Evaluations of

drug interactions, 2nd edn. American Pharmaceutical Association, Washington D C, USA, p 158

Aubert J M, Sesta H J 1982 Treatment of vaginal trichomoniasis. The Journal of Reproductive Medicine 27: 742–745

Berggren O 1969 Association of carcinoma of the uterine cervix and *Trichomonas vaginalis* infestations. American Journal of Obstetrics and Gynecology 105: 166–168

Bertini B, Hornstein M 1970 The epidemiology of trichomoniasis and the role of this infection in the development of carcinoma of the cervix. Acta Cytologica 14: 325–332

Bramley M 1976 Study of female babies of women entering confinement with vaginal trichomoniasis. British Journal of Venereal Diseases 52: 58–62

British National Formulary 1985 British Medical Association and the Pharmaceutical Society of Great Britain, London

Catterall R D 1972 Trichomonal infections of the genital tract. Medical Clinics of North America 56: 1203–1209

Catterall R D 1977 The sexually transmitted diseases. In: Rook W (ed) Recent advances in dermatology. Churchill Livingstone, Edinburgh

Catterall R D, Nicoll C S 1960 Is trichomonal infestation a venereal disease? British Medical Journal 1: 1177–1179

Coulter J R 1979 Mutagenicity of metronidazole. Correspondence, Lancet i: 609

Csonka G W 1971 Trichomonal vaginitis treated with one dose of metronidazole. British Journal of Venereal Diseases 47: 456–458

Davies D M (ed) 1981 Disorders of the foetus and infant. Textbook of adverse drug reactions. Oxford University Press, Oxford, p 71–113

Donné A 1836 Research microscopiques. Comptes rendus hebdomadaire's des Seances de l'Academie des Sciences 3: 385–386

Dunn P M, Stewart-Brown S, Peel R 1979 Metronidazole and the fetal alcohol syndrome. Correspondence, Lancet ii: 144

Durel P, Roiron V, Soboulet A, Borel J Q 1960 Systemic treatment of human trichomoniasis with a derivative of nitro-imidazole. 8823 R.P. British Journal of Venereal Diseases 36: 21–26

Edwards D I, Shanson D 1980 Metronidazole inactivity by aerobes. Journal of Antimicrobial Chemotherapy 6: 402–403

Fisher I, Morton R S 1969 Epididymitis due to *Trichomonas vaginalis*. British Journal of Venereal Diseases 45: 252–253

Fouts A C, Kraus S J 1980 *Trichomonas vaginalis*: reevaluation of its clinical presentation and laboratory diagnosis. The Journal of Infectious Diseases 141(2): 137–143

Grubb C 1977 Colour atlas of gynaecological cytopathology. HM + M Publishers, Aylesbury, p 23, 28–29

Hamilton-Miller J M T, Brumfitt W 1976 The versatility of metronidazole. Leading article, Journal of Antimicrobial Chemotherapy 2: 5–8

Harkness A H 1950 In: Non-gonococcal urethritis. E and S Livingstone, Edinburgh, p 224–228

Hawkins D F 1976 Effects of drugs taken in pregnancy on the foetus. Journal of Maternal and Child Health, Aug, p 24

Hayes B S, Kotcher E 1960 Evaluation of techniques for the demonstration of *Trichomonas vaginalis*. Journal of Parasitology 46: suppl 45

Herbert W J, Wilkinson P C, Stott P C 1985 Dictionary of immunology, 3rd edn. Blackwell, Oxford, p 171, 173

Hess J 1969 Review of current methods for the detection of

Trichomonas in clinical material. Journal of Clinical Pathology 22: 269–272

Honigberg B M 1978 Trichomonads of importance in human medicine. In: Kreier J P (ed) Parasitic protozoa, vol 11. Intestinal flagellates, histomonads, trichomonads, amoeba, opalinids and ciliates. Academic Press, p 275–454

Hughes H E, Gordon A M, Barr G T D 1966 A clinical and laboratory study of trichomoniasis in the female genital tract. Journal of Obstetrics and Gynaecology, British Commonwealth 73: 821–827

Kolstad P, Stafl A 1977 Atlas of colposcopy. Universtetsforlaget, London, p 37

Lefebre Y, Heseltine H C 1965 The peripheral white blood cells and metronidazole. Journal of the American Medical Association 194: 127–130

Lindmark D G, Muller M 1976 Antitrichomonad action, mutagenicity and reduction of metronidazole and other nitroimidazoles. Antimicrobial Chemotherapy 10: 476–482

Lowe G H 1978 The trichomonads. Public Health Laboratory Service. Monograph Series 9, HMSO

Lumsden W H R, Harrison C, Robertson D H H 1988 Treatment failure in *Trichomonas vaginalis* in females. 2. In vitro estimation of the sensitivity of the organism to metronidazole. Journal of Antimicrobial Chemotherapy 21: 555–564

Medical News 1978 New metronidazole study: some reassuring findings for now. Journal of the American Medical Association 239: 1371

Meingassner J G, Stockinger K 1981 In vitro studies on the identification of metronidazole-resistant strains of *T.vaginalis*. Zeitschrift fur Haut Krankheiten 56: 7–15

Meingassner J G, Heyworth P G 1981 Intestinal and urogenital flagellates. Antibiotics and Chemotherapy (Karger, Basel) 30: 163–202

Meingassner J G, Mieth H, Lindmark D G, Müller M 1978 Assay conditions and demonstration of nitroimidazole resistance to *Trichomonas foetus*. Antimicrobial Agents and Chemotherapy 13: 1–3

Morton R S, Harris J R W 1975 Recent advances in sexually transmitted diseases. Churchill Livingstone, Edinburgh

Müller M 1979 Mode of action of metronidazole on anaerobic micro-organisms in *Metronidazole*. In: Phillips I, Collier J (eds) Academic Press, London, p 224–228

Müller M 1983 Mode of action of metronidazole on anaerobic bacteria and protozoa. Surgery: 165–171

Müller M, Gorrell T E 1983 Metabolism and metronidazole uptake in *Trichomonas vaginalis* isolates with different metronidazole susceptibilities. Antimicrobial Agents and Chemotherapy 24: 667–673

Nielsen M H, Nielsen R 1975 Electron microscopy of *Trichomonas vaginalis* Donné: interaction with vaginal epithelium in human trichomoniasis. Acta Pathologica et Microbiologica Scandinavica, Section B, 83: 305–320

Nielsen R 1969 *Trichomonas vaginalis* 1. Survival in solid Stuart's Medium. British Journal of Venereal Diseases 45: 328–331

Oates J K, Selwyn S, Breach M R 1971 Polyester sponge swabs to facilitate examination for genital infection in women. British Journal of Venereal Diseases 47: 284–292

O'Hara C M, Gardner W A, Bennett B D 1980 Immunoperoxidase staining of *Trichomonas vaginalis* in cytologic material. Acta Cytologica 24: 448–451

Ovcinnikov N M, Delektorskij V V, Turanova E N, Yashkova G N 1975 Further studies of *Trichomonas vaginalis* with transmission and scanning electron microscopy. British Journal of Venereal Diseases 51: 357–375

Pert G 1972 Errors in the diagnosis of *Trichomonas vaginalis* infection. Obstetrics and Gynecology 39: 7–9

Ralph E D 1983 Clinical pharmacokinetics of metronidazole. Clinical Pharmacokinetics 8: 43–62

Rein M F 1981 Current therapy of vulvovaginitis. Sexually Transmitted Disease 8: 316–320

Robertson D H H, Lumsden W H R, Fraser K F, Hosie D D, Moore D M 1969 Simultaneous isolation of *Trichomonas vaginalis* and collection of vaginal exudate. British Journal of Venereal Diseases 45: 42–43

Robertson D H H, Heyworth R, Harrison C, Lumsden W H R 1988 Treatment failure in *Trichomonas vaginalis* infections in females 2. Concentrations of metronidazole in plasma and vaginal content during normal and high dosage. Journal of Antimicrobial Chemotherapy 21: 373–378

Roe F J C 1977 Metronidazole: review of uses and toxicity. Journal of Antimicrobial Chemotherapy 3: 205–212

Rubridge C J, Scragg J N, Powell S J 1970 Treatment of children with acute amoebic dysentery: comparative trial of metronidazole against a combination of dehydroemetine, tetracycline and diloxanide furoate. Archives of Diseases in Childhood 45: 196–197

Semer J M, Friedland P, Vaisberg M, Greenberg A 1966 The use of metronidazole in the treatment of alcoholism. American Journal of Psychiatry 123: 722–724

Slavin G 1976 In: Jordan J P, Singer A (eds) The cervix. Saunders, London, p 260

Street D A, Taylor Robinson D, Ackers J P, Hanna N F, McMillan A 1982 Evaluation of an enzyme-linked immunosorbent assay for the detection of antibody to *Trichomonas vaginalis* in sera and vaginal secretions. British Journal of Venereal Diseases 58: 330–333

Street D A, Wells C, Taylor Robinson D, Ackers J P 1984 Interaction between *Trichomonas vaginalis* and other pathogenic micro-organisms of the human genital tract. British Journal of Venereal Diseases 60: 31–38

Taylor J A T 1964 Metronidazole — a new agent for combined somatic and psychotherapy of alcoholism: a case study and preliminary report. Bulletin o the Los Angeles Neurological Society 29: 158–162

Taylor J A T 1965 Metronidazole and transient leukopenia. Journal of the American Medical Association 194: 1331–1332

Thin R N, Symonds M A E, Booker R, Cook S, Langlet F 1979 Double blind comparison of a single dose and a five day course of metronidazole in the treatment of trichomoniasis. British Journal of Venereal Diseases 55: 354–356

Tsao W 1969 Trichomoniasis and gonorrhoea. British Medical Journal 1: 642–643

Tuttle J P, Holbrook T W, Fletcher C D 1977 Interference of human spermatozoal motility by *Trichomonas vaginalis*. Journal of Urology 118: 1024

Weston T E T, Nicol C S 1963 Natural History of trichomonal infection in males. British Journal of Venereal Diseases 39: 251–257

Willson R L 1974 Acute drug administration and cancer control. Lancet i: 810

Wisdom A R, Dunlop E M C 1965 Trichomoniasis study of the disease and its treatment. British Journal of Venereal Diseases 41: 90–96

Yolken R H 1982 Enzyme immunoassays for the detection of infectious antigens in body fluids: current limitations and future prospects. Reviews of Infectious Diseases 4(1): 35–68

23

Pelvic inflammatory disease and perihepatitis

Salpingitis or, more strictly, pelvic inflammatory disease (PID), resulting from ascending microbial infection of the cervix and uterus, is a well-recognized complication of infections due to *Neisseria gonorrhoeae* in which *Chlamydia trachomatis* may also play a part. In both gonococcal and non-gonococcal PID, various pathogenic or potentially pathogenic micro-organisms, including anaerobes in particular, may be involved aetiologically, and in non-gonococcal PID *C. trachomatis* may be the only pathogen to be found. An increasing incidence and renewed interest in the syndrome in which right upper quadrant abdominal pain due to perihepatitis occurs in association with PID require its consideration in this chapter.

PELVIC INFLAMMATORY DISEASE

Pelvic inflammatory disease, in its acute form, is mainly a disease of sexually active young women and usually results from an ascending microbial infection of the cervix and uterus. In developed countries, the annual incidence, which has been increasing over the past 25 years in women aged 15 to 39 years, varies between 10 to 13 per 1000, with a peak incidence of 20 per 1000 women in the 20 to 24-year age group (Westrom 1980).

In pathogenesis and in prognosis with regard to fertility, it differs from pelvic inflammatory disease arising as a sequel to previous surgical manipulation. Although inflammation of the uterine tubes (salpingitis) is clinically the most prominent feature, the supporting structures of the uterus share in the inflammation to a greater or lesser extent, so pelvic inflammatory disease (PID) is strictly the more accurate term and may be used synonymously.

AETIOLOGY

The complexity of the vaginal flora and the inaccessibility of the organs affected make it difficult to determine which organism(s) is/are aetiologically responsible for pelvic inflammatory disease. With the exception of *Neisseria gonorrhoeae*, it has not yet been possible to prove a causative relationship between organisms found in the cervical flora and those recovered from the Fallopian tubes; for this reason it is convenient to classify the condition either as gonococcal or non-gonococcal PID, a diagnosis based on the presence or absence of *N. gonorrhoeae* in the cervical culture. It is not always possible to determine the aetiology because it would be necessary to obtain cultures directly from the uterine tubes at laparoscopy or laparotomy, or from the pelvic peritoneal fluid by culdocentesis.

Gonococcal pelvic inflammatory disease

Salpingitis or, more strictly, PID is a complication in about 10% of women with untreated gonorrhoea (Eschenbach & Holmes 1975), the exact figure for incidence depending on the criteria used for diagnosis, the population group studied and accessibility to medical care. As already stated, *N. gonorrhoeae* is the only pathogen for which recovery from the endocervix is correlated with recovery from the Fallopian tubes (Thompson & Hager 1977). Even in this case the correlation is not good since the gonococcus is isolated from the uterine tubes in only about 10% of women with untreated gonorrhoea and salpingitis. This low recovery rate might be explained by a bactericidal action of the inflammatory exudate, or by a possibility that some other micro-organism is responsible. *Chlamydia trachomatis* may be isolated from the endocervix of about 40% of women with untreated gonorrhoea (Woolfitt & Watt 1977) but, although *Chlamydia* may play a part in the aetiology of PID (Rees et al 1977) the role of this organism in the aetiology of PID associated with gonorrhoea is not yet clear.

While recovery of *N. gonorrhoeae* from an endocervical culture of a patient with PID does not prove conclusively that the gonococcus caused the disease in the Fallopian tubes, there is little doubt that, at least in some cases, the gonococcus is the primary pathogen. In vitro studies have shown that *N. gonorrhoeae* can infect tubal mucosa, and invade and destroy epithelial cells (Ward et al 1974).

Non-gonococcal pelvic inflammatory disease
The aetiology of PID not associated with gonorrhoea remains enigmatic but is likely to have a multifactorial microbial aetiology (Eschenbach et al 1975). The study by Rees et al (1977) suggests a possible role for *Chlamydia*; a high incidence (16 of 24) of pelvic inflammatory disease, with an onset of pain between 13 and 38 days post-partum, was found in mothers of babies with chlamydial conjunctivitis. These workers also noted about 4% of cases of PID in 127 women with a chlamydial cervical infection. This organism has only been isolated from the peritoneal fluid of a variable proportion of women with PID (Sweet et al 1982). These differences may reflect a bactericidal action of the fluid, as in gonorrhoea, or lack of sensitivity of present sampling methods. Serological studies which have shown significant changes in serum IgM and IgG antibodies against *C. trachomatis* have been interpreted as indicating a causal role of that organism (Sweet et al 1982).

Mycoplasma hominis has been isolated from the uterine tubes of just under 10% of women with acute salpingitis (Mardh & Westrom 1970), and *Ureaplasma urealyticum* from 4%, but once again the role of these organisms is not clear.

Anaerobic organisms may play a part in the aetiology of PID seen in about 5% of sexually active young women (Mardh 1980). In the case of women with PID in the puerperal period and following surgery, including termination of pregnancy, anaerobes such as *Peptostreptococcus* and *Bacteroides spp* may be implicated, as can streptococci and, occasionally, enteric bacteria such as *Escherichia coli*. Often more than one organism is involved, particularly when anaerobes are isolated and trauma of surgery, residual blood clots, in situ sutures and vaginal packs are all predisposing factors.

Mycobacterium tuberculosis is now a rare cause of salpingitis, and is usually secondary to disease elsewhere, reaching the uterine tubes and uterus by means of the bloodstream (Jeffcoate 1975).

The role of viruses in the aetiology of PID is not clear, although Eschenbach et al (1975), demonstrated that herpes simplex virus and cytomegalovirus were not causative in his cases.

PATHOGENESIS

Organisms reach the uterine tubes by ascending from the endocervix. Rarely (less than 1%) tubal inflammation results from extension of inflammation from another pelvic organ, most commonly the appendix.

Several factors predispose to ascending infection. Surgical operations in the uterus, including hysterosalpingography, may lead to the development of PID in less than 5% of cases. Women using an intrauterine contraceptive device have a greater risk of developing salpingitis (Westrom et al 1976). Previous episodes of PID predispose to subsequent recurrences (Eschenbach & Holmes 1975). In the absence of surgical procedures, PID in pregnancy is uncommon.

In gonococcal and in non-gonococcal salpingitis, not associated with surgical operations, the inflammatory process affects chiefly the endosalpinx, the organisms having ascended by way of the endometrium, where a marked inflammation may be induced (Mardh et al 1981). There is destruction of tubal epithelium and a purulent exudate fills the lumen. Pus may escape from the fimbriated end of the tube and track down to the rectovaginal pouch, where a pelvic abscess may form. With continued inflammation, the ostia become occluded by oedema, and pus collects in the cavity of the tube forming a pyosalpinx. If untreated, fibrous adhesions form within the tube, with relatively few external adhesions. Occasionally a hydrosalpinx (an accumulation of serous fluid in the tube) is found; its pathogenesis is uncertain, but it may result from recurrent episodes of subacute salpingitis (Rees & Annels 1969).

Damage to the ciliated epithelium and the production of fibrous adhesions within the uterine tube, may delay the transit of a fertilized ovum to the uterus, and as a result, implantation may occur in the tube giving an ectopic pregnancy. Ectopic pregnancy is associated, in about half the cases, with changes suggestive of PID (Harralson et al 1973).

Infertility may result in about 20% of women who have been treated for PID (Westrom 1975) the prognosis being better when salpingitis is mild. Women who have had gonococcal salpingitis have a significantly higher chance of conceiving than those who have had non-gonococcal salpingitis.

Salpingitis associated with minor gynaecological operations is usually brought about by infection which ascends by means of the lymphatics in the outer layers of the uterus and tubes. Exosalpingitis results with the formation, in untreated cases, of extensive pelvic adhesions. The lumen of the tube is commonly little affected by the inflammatory process and therefore in such cases pyosalpinx and hydrosalpinx are uncommon; fertility is less often affected than after endosalpingitis.

CLINICAL FEATURES

Acute pelvic inflammatory disease
The symptoms of acute PID usually occur during or shortly after menstruation or in the puerperium.

The patient complains usually of lower abdominal pain, often exacerbated by movement of the psoas muscle, fever, rigors, malaise, anorexia and vomiting. With the increased use of laparoscopy, it has become apparent that whilst abdominal pain is the most reliable symptom, it may be minimal in at least 5% of cases (Jacobson & Westrom 1969). Pyrexia (temperature of 38°C or greater) may be found in only about two-thirds of women with acute PID, and more commonly in cases due to *N. gonorrhoeae* (McCormack et al 1977).

There is usually tenderness, and a variable degree of muscular guarding over the lower abdomen. Pain is elicited by moving the cervix during bimanual examination. Palpation of the uterus and tubes is usually impossible on account of tenderness and guarding.

In about half the cases of acute PID, the white cell count is elevated (Falk 1965). The erythrocyte sedimentation rate is raised in about 75% of cases (Jacobson & Westrom 1969), especially when the salpingitis is associated with gonorrhoea (McCormack et al 1977).

Paralytic ileus, presenting with abdominal distension and vomiting, may occur in 1% of cases. In such cases fluid levels are noted on the plain X-ray film of the abdomen, taken with the patient in an upright position.

Chronic pelvic inflammatory disease

Chronic PID may be asymptomatic and undiscovered until the patient is investigated for infertility. Symptoms, when they occur, consist of intermittent lower abdominal pain or discomfort; discomfort in the groins, backache, malaise and frequent heavy menstrual periods. The tubes may not be palpable, or they may be irregularly thickened; the uterus may be retroverted and fixed.

DIFFERENTIAL DIAGNOSIS

Ectopic pregnancy

There is usually sudden onset of pain in an iliac fossa or hypogastrium, often with syncope. Tracking of blood to the upper abdominal cavity may induce pain referred to the shoulder. Symptoms usually develop after a short period of amenorrhoea during which there may have been cramping discomfort in one iliac fossa. If intra-abdominal haemorrhage is severe, the patient presents a state of shock, with pallor, tachycardia and hypotension. There is tenderness over the lower abdomen, and on vaginal examination (which must not be performed in patients with signs of severe haemorrhage) there is irregular, tender enlargement of the tubes on the affected side. Pelvic haematoma may be detected in the rectovaginal pouch. Urine tests for pregnancy may be either positive or negative depending upon the secretory activity of the trophoblast (Note 6.5).

When available, radioimmunoassays for serum chorionic gonadotrophin (hCG) which becomes detectable within a few days of implantation, may be helpful in the diagnosis of ectopic pregnancy (Seppälä et al 1980). Linstedt et al (1981) indicate that ectopic pregnancy is unlikely if the serum hCG is close to that found in non-pregnant women. Occasional cases of ectopic pregnancy, however, will be missed. In their experience a decision limit of 2 μg per ml (13 units per 1, 2nd international standard) was set with a diagnostic sensitivity of 96%. Specialist gynaecological advice is indicated, however, in this surgical emergency.

Acute appendicitis

Abdominal pain commences usually in the umbilical area and after some hours localizes to the right iliac fossa. Menstrual irregularities are unusual, but nausea and anorexia is more pronounced than in acute pelvic inflammatory disease.

Ruptured ovarian or endometriotic cyst

There is usually sudden onset of lower abdominal pain, most commonly occurring about the time of menstruation. The patient is usually afebrile.

Acute pyelonephritis

There is generally a sudden rise in temperature, often with rigors, and pain in the loins and iliac fossae. Commonly there are urinary symptoms such as frequency of micturition, urgency, strangury, dysuria, nocturia and haematuria. The urine contains pus; there is a polymorphonuclear leucocytosis in most cases.

Intestinal obstruction

Pain is colicky in nature and is felt in the umbilical or hypogastric areas. It is associated with vomiting and absence of passage of flatus. Bowel sounds are hyperactive. There may be a history of previous abdominal surgery.

Septic abortion

A history of amenorrhoea is followed by symptoms and signs of abortion — either complete or incomplete. There is uterine bleeding, painful uterine contractions, pyrexia, tachycardia, offensive vaginal discharge, uterine tenderness and general systemic upset. The white cell count and erythrocyte sedimentation rate are raised. Vaginal examination may show a dilated cervix.

Diagnosis

A presumptive diagnosis of acute pelvic inflammatory disease may be made from the patient's history and the clinical and laboratory findings. Confirmation of acute PID requires the use of laparoscopy, except when a presumptive diagnosis of gonorrhoea has been made by smear examinations or confirmed by culture (see below). Jacobson & Westrom (1969), demonstrated that only 60% of clinically diagnosed cases of acute PID were confirmed by laparoscopy. In their series, acute appendicitis, pelvic endometriosis and intrapelvic haemorrhage were the conditions most commonly mimicking acute salpingitis.

Laparoscopy, however, requires the administration of a general anaesthetic, and is not without hazard. Rawlings & Balgobin (1975) reported a complication rate of 6%. Complications included perforation of the bowel wall, mesenteric haemorrhage, haematoma of the abdominal wall and pelvic abscess formation. Laparoscopy should only be undertaken by gynaecologists experienced in its use.

When a young woman attends a sexually transmitted diseases clinic complaining of lower abdominal pain whose onset has been within 10 days of the onset of menstruation, and when examination reveals tenderness in both fornices, the most likely diagnosis is acute pelvic inflammatory disease. Every effort must be made to identify gonococcal cases in the manner described elsewhere (Ch. 15). Where facilities exist, cultures from the cervix should also be taken for *Chlamydia trachomatis*. Treatment should be started on the result of examination of Gram-stained smears, and altered, if necessary, when culture reports become available.

Should there be any doubt about the diagnosis, particularly if symptoms fail to subside with treatment, advice from a gynaecologist should be sought as laparoscopy may be required.

TREATMENT

Cases of acute salpingitis with systemic disturbance should be admitted to hospital. The decision is not so straightforward in patients with less severe symptoms and signs. If there is any doubt as to the diagnosis, or about the patient's reliability in taking the antibiotic or chemotherapy prescribed, admission to hospital is indicated. In pregnancy, women are best cared for as inpatients.

Treatment of gonococcal pelvic inflammatory disease

In patients with acute salpingitis requiring admission to hospital, benzylpenicillin 600 mg (1 000 000 i.u.) by intramuscular injection every 6 hours results in improvement in the patient's condition, generally within 48 hours. After this time, provided resolution of the salpingitis is occurring, as judged by decreased tenderness in the iliac fossae and reduction in size and tenderness of the tubes, an oral antimicrobial agent may be substituted. Ampicillin given orally in a dose of 500 mg

6-hourly is satisfactory, and should be continued for at least 10 days. In patients with infections due to beta-lactamase producing gonococci, cefuroxime (2.0 g) intramuscularly in 8-hourly doses (or occasionally 6-hourly) is suggested as an approach to treatment, possibly preceded by spectinomycin 4.0 g as a single intramuscular dose.

In patients who fail to respond to penicillin treatment, reappraisal of the initial diagnosis must be made and a gynaecologist's advice sought, as laparoscopy and possibly removal of an IUCD may be necessary. The development of pelvic abscesses, a very rare occurrence in the United Kingdom, but common in the lower socio-economic groups in certain urban areas of the USA, may require drainage through the posterior fornix of the vagina.

Other antimicrobial agents may be used in the management of acute salpingitis. Co-trimoxazole given orally in a dosage of 2 tablets 8-hourly for at least 10 days is effective. Doxycycline in an oral dose of 200 mg 8-hourly for 48 hours followed by 100 mg 8-hourly for at least 14 days is satisfactory in some localities. Therapy with a tetracycline has the advantage of being effective against the potential or actual pathogens *C. trachomatis*, *M. hominis* and *U. urealyticum*; tetracyclines should not be used in pregnancy. In pregnant women who are hypersensitive to penicillin, erythromycin stearate orally, in a dosage of 500 mg 6-hourly may be used.

Although steroids may produce rapid resolution of the symptoms, there is no beneficial effect on future fertility or in preventing the development of chronic abdominal pain (Falk 1965).

Treatment of non-gonococcal pelvic inflammatory disease

Since non-gonococcal PID is now thought to be primarily a polymicrobial infection, broad spectrum antimicrobial cover is required. Tetracyclines should be the treatment of first choice in patients with non-gonococcal salpingitis. Doxycycline in the dosage given above has been found to be useful. In pregnancy, erythromycin stearate may be substituted.

In PID following surgical manipulation in particular, where trauma of the operation, residual blood clots, in situ sutures, and vaginal packs are all predisposing factors, the possibility of anaerobic infection will require treatment with antimicrobial agents, such as metronidazole. An oral dose of metronidazole 2 g immediately then 200 mg thrice-daily for 5–7 days has been found to be very effective (Study Group, Luton and Dunstable Hospital 1974). In this report, also, a similar course of metronidazole, given as a prophylactic, was dramatically effective in reducing vaginal carriage rate of non-sporing anaerobes such as *Bacteroides spp*. It is clear also that a bactericidal level of metronidazole in patients' blood sustained over the operative and immediate postoperative periods reduced the frequency of postoperative pelvic inflammatory disease. Metronidazole, in doses of 1 g, can be given as a suppository at 8-hour intervals in those who cannot take oral drugs (Study Group, Luton and Dunstable Hospital 1976). Currently it is advised that a 1 g metronidazole suppository is inserted into the rectum 8-hourly for 3 days in the treatment of anaerobic infections in the adult, and that oral medication with 400 mg 3 times daily should be substituted as soon as this becomes possible. Treatment should not ordinarily continue beyond a 7-day period. A fuller discussion on metronidazole is given in Chapter 22 and in Chapter 21.

The characteristics required in an antimicrobial agent to be effective in anaerobic infections include the ability to penetrate abscesses, resistance to inactivating enzymes in the infected site, activity against high inocula of organisms and activity under anaerobic conditions. Three drugs currently fulfil these criteria — clindamycin, cefoxitin and metronidazole.

Emerging resistance has been seen with clindamycin, and some strains are resistant to cefoxitin. Metronidazole, although inactive against aerobic components of mixed infections (Tally 1978), may render these organisms more susceptible to the phagocytic defence system by the elimination of anaerobes (Ingham et al 1977); see also discussion of metronidazole in Chapter 22.

PROGNOSIS

The earlier the patient is treated, and the milder the symptoms, the better is the prognosis with regard to fertility (Westrom 1975). Patients with treated gonococcal PID are less likely to be infertile than women with non-gonococcal PID. Abdominal pain, change in menstruation and deep dyspareunia may persist for many months in about a fifth of women treated for acute PID (Adler et al 1982).

PERIHEPATITIS

The increasing incidence of NGU in men, NSGI, including pelvic inflammatory disease, in women and the recognition of *C. trachomatis* as a causative organism in these conditions has focused attention on another manifestation of *C. trachomatis* disease, namely perihepatitis, with its main presentation of pain in the upper right quadrant of the abdomen and its association particularly with pelvic inflammatory disease in women. The relationship between upper abdominal peritonitis, perihepatitis and salpingitis was first described in 1919

in Uruguay by Carlos Stajano (Bolton & Darougar 1983). The recognition by Curtis (1930) of perihepatic adhesions resulting from perihepatitis, and their association with gonococcal salpingitis, was followed by a further description of the acute clinical features by Fitz-Hugh, of the University of Pennsylvania (1934).

Subsequently the condition of acute right upper quadrant abdominal pain in association with perihepatitis and gonococcal salpingitis became known as the Curtis-Fitz-Hugh syndrome. In more recent years renewed interest followed its increasing incidence and the recognition that *C. trachomatis* as well as *N. gonorrhoeae* may be causative organisms.

Curtis, a Chicago gynaecologist, noticed that he frequently found 'violin string' adhesions between the anterior surface of the liver and the adjacent anterior abdominal wall.

The use of the laparoscope has enabled confirmation of the findings of Curtis and Fitz-Hugh. In the acute stage of perihepatitis 'violin string' adhesions form which are fragile and friable and may be easily broken at laparoscopy either by insufflation of carbon dioxide or by instrumentation, leaving the appearance of white fibrous plaques and tiny haemorrhages (Bolton & Darougar 1983). In Curtis' description he emphasized that the adhesions were numerous, often of sufficient length to allow considerable movement between the liver and parietal peritoneum, and that they occupied an area of several inches in diameter. Characteristically the condition occurred in female patients with symptoms suggestive of gall bladder disease or pleurisy.

AETIOLOGY

The evidence assembled by Bolton & Darougar (1983) for the association between genital tract infection and perihepatitis is very strong. Stanley (1946) described the successful treatment of three female patients with perihepatitis in whom acute pain developed in the upper part of the abdomen, especially on the right side, in whom gonococci were cultured from the cervix or urethra or both. In the context of a surgical ward in Helsinki von Knorring & Nieminen (1979), describe six female patients with clinical symptoms indistinguishable from acute cholecystitis, and in all six the diagnosis was established by obtaining *N. gonorrhoeae* on culture from the cervix.

In recent years cases have been reported in which the clinical picture of the Curtis-Fitz-Hugh syndrome was present, the diagnosis of perihepatitis was supported by laparoscopy, but in whom the gonococcus could not be found. In these cases *C. trachomatis* is probably the cause. Of 11 cases in Zurich, women aged 17–38 years, reported by Müller-Schoop et al (1978) with acute peritonitis proved by laparoscopy, 7 also had perihepatitis, and only 2 had signs of salpingitis on gynaecological examination. Microimmunofluorescence tests showed extremely high titres (1/2048 or more) of IgG antibody in 6 patients, and in 4 there was strong evidence of recent chlamydial infection; the gonococcus was detected on cervical culture in 3.

In 1982, Wølner-Hanssen et al succeeded in isolating *C. trachomatis* by swabbing the surface of the liver capsule in a patient whose laparoscopic findings indicated acute salpingitis and perihepatitis, i.e. the Curtis-Fitz-Hugh syndrome, and who had presented because of a 10-day history of abdominal pain in the right upper quadrant. In this case *C. trachomatis* was also isolated from the cervix but not from the Fallopian tube; *N. gonorrhoeae* was not isolated from any site.

The route by which organisms affecting the genital tract may reach the liver surface has been the subject of much speculation. Transcoelomic, bloodstream and lymphatic spread have all been considered. *C. trachomatis* may ascend through the genital tract without causing salpingitis in some cases. A peritoneal reaction with exudate may facilitate spread of the organism.

The Curtis-Fitz-Hugh syndrome was first reported in a male in whom the gonococcus was cultured by Kimball & Knee (1970). In a case in Ibadan, Nigeria, the syndrome was accompanied by proven gonococcal urethritis, fever and arthritis of the left knee, both ankles and right wrist (Francis & Osoba 1972). In the case in a male bisexual described by Davidson & Hawkins (1982) *N. gonorrhoeae* was cultured from the throat, and the presence of a widespread pustular rash thought to be typical of a disseminated gonococcal infection suggested that spread had occurred by the bloodstream.

CLINICAL FEATURES

Characteristically the Curtis-Fitz-Hugh syndrome almost always occurs in young women. Pain, often severe and acute, is the main symptom and it is felt in the right upper quadrant of the abdomen. Similar severe pain may have been present in the preceding 1–2 weeks and occasionally there is a longer history of chronic pain. Patients with the acute and severe pain may be admitted as acute surgical emergencies and the condition confused with cholecystitis, biliary colic pleurisy, pneumonia or pulmonary embolism.

The pain is typical of peritoneal inflammation — being made worse by movement, deep breathing, and abdominal palpation — and patients prefer to lie still. The pain often radiates to the back and right shoulder. Nausea and vomiting sometimes accompany the pain, but vomiting is unusual. Tenderness of the right upper abdominal quadrant is always present and patients exhibit guarding and a positive Murphy's sign (Note 23.1). A hepatic friction rub may be heard over the right anterior costal margin. Signs of generalized peritonitis are usually absent but evidence of pelvic peritonitis should be sought. About half the patients have a low-grade pyrexia and the erythrocyte sedimentation rate may be raised.

Careful questioning will elicit a history of previous genital tract infection or pelvic inflammatory disease in at least two-thirds, and the majority will have symptoms and signs of pelvic infection (Bolton & Darougar 1983).

DIAGNOSIS

In patients with Curtis-Fitz-Hugh syndrome a sexual history should be obtained, and the examination necessary to exclude gonococcal, chlamydial infection and other sexually transmitted disease should be carried out. Haematological, biochemical and radiological investigations (white cell count, erythrocyte sedimentation rate, radiological and ultrasonic investigations of the biliary tract, radiological examination of the chest and liver-related enzymes and bilirubin) will enable the exclusion of alternative explanations of the patient's symptoms and signs.

Antichlamydial antibody levels in the blood may be useful retrospectively. Antibodies to *C. trachomatis* may also be sought in discharges from the cervix and urethra. A microimmunofluorescence test can be used to test serum for IgG and IgM antibodies and local discharges for IgG and IgA (Bolton & Darougar 1983).

TREATMENT

A gonococcal infection will require the appropriate antibiotic in doses recommended for pelvic inflammatory disease, and for proven or suspected chlamydial disease oxytetracycline or doxycycline may be used for a period of not less than 2–3 weeks.

Immediate relief of pain may be obtained when pain persists, in spite of antibiotic or chemotherapy, by the division surgically by cauterization and division of perihepatic adhesions under direct laparoscopic visualization (Reichart & Valle 1976).

NOTE TO CHAPTER 23

Note 23.1: Murphy's sign

The examining hand is placed just below the right costal margin midway between the xiphisternum and anterior axillary line. In patients with acute cholecystitis deep inspiration is associated with a sudden accentuation of pain.

REFERENCES

PELVIC INFLAMMATORY DISEASE

Adler M W, Belsay E H, O'Connor B H 1982 Morbidity associated with pelvic inflammatory disease. British Journal of Venereal Diseases 58: 151–157

Eschenbach D A, Holmes K K 1975 Acute pelvic inflammatory disease; current concepts of pathogenesis, etiology and management. Clinical Obstetrics and Gynecology 18: 35–56

Eschenbach D A, Buchanan T M, Pollock H M et al 1975 Polymicrobial etiology of acute pelvic inflammatory disease. New England Journal of Medicine 293: 166–171

Falk V 1965 Treatment of acute non-tuberculous salpingitis with antibiotics alone and in combination with glucocorticoids. Acta Obstetrica et Gynecologica Scandinavica 6 (suppl):1–118

Harralson J D, Van Nagell J R, Roddick J W 1973 Operative management of ruptured tubal pregnancy. American Journal of Obstetrics and Gynecology 115: 995–997

Ingham H R, Sisson P R, Tharagonnet D, Selkon J B, Codd A A 1977 Inhibition of phagocytosis in vitro by obligate anaerobes. Lancet ii: 1252–1254

Jacobson L, Westrom L 1969 Objectivized diagnosis of acute pelvic inflammatory disease. American Journal of Obstetrics and Gynecology 105: 1088–1098

Jeffcoate N 1975 In: Principles of gynaecology. Butterworths, London, p 292–301

Linstedt G, Janson P O, Thorburn J 1981 Sensitivity of serum gonadotrophin assay for ectopic pregnancy. Correspondence, Lancet i: 783–784

McCormack W M, Nowroozi K, Alpert S, Jackel S G, Lee Y-H, Lowe E W, Rankin J S 1977 Acute pelvic inflammatory disease: characteristics of patients with gonococcal infection and evaluation of their response to treatment with aqueous procaine penicillin G and spectinomycin hydrochloride. Sexually Transmitted Diseases 4: 125–131

Mårdh P-A 1980 An overview of infectious agents of salpingitis, their biology and recent advances in methods of detection. American Journal of Obstetrics and Gynecology 138 (suppl): 933–951

Mårdh P-A, Weström L 1970 Tubal and cervical cultures in acute salpingitis with special reference to mycoplasma and T-strain mycoplasmas. British Journal of Venereal Diseases 46: 179–186

Mårdh P-A, Moller B R, Ingerslev H J, Nussler E, Westrom L, Wolner-Haussen P 1981 Endometritis caused by Chlamydia trachomatis. British Journal of Venereal Diseases 57: 191–195

Rawlings E E, Balgobin B 1975 Complications of laparoscopy. British Medical Journal 1: 727–728

Rees E, Annels E H 1969 Gonococcal salpingitis. British Journal of Venereal Diseases 45: 205–215

Rees E, Tait I A, Hobson D, Johnson F W A 1977 Chlamydia in relation to cerv infection and pelvic inflammatory disease. In: Hobson D, Holmes K K (eds) Non-gonococcal urethritis and related infection. American Society for Microbiology, Washington D C, p 67, 76

Seppälä M, Tontti K, Ranta T, Stenman U-H, Chard T 1980 Use of a rapid hCG-beta-subunit radioimmunoassay in acute gynecological emergencies. Lancet i: 165–166

Study Group, Luton and Dunstable Hospital 1974 Metronidazole in the prevention and treatment of Bacteroides infections in gynaecological patients. Lancet ii: 1540–1543

Study Group, Luton and Dunstable Hospital 1976 Metronidazole in the prevention and treatment of Bacteroides infections after appendicectomy. British Medical Journal 1: 318–321

Sweet R, Schachter J, Robbie M 1982 Acute salpingitis: role of chlamydia in the United States. In: Mardh P A, Holmes K K, Oriel J D, Piot C, Schachter J (eds) Chlamydia infection. Elsevier Biomedical Press, Amsterdam, p 175–178

Tally F P 1978 Factors affecting antimicrobial agents in anaerobic abscess. Journal of Antimicrobial Chemotherapy 4: 299–301

Thompson S E, Hager D 1977 Acute pelvic inflammatory disease. Review. Sexually Transmitted Diseases 4: 105–113

Ward M E, Watt P J, Robertson J N 1974 The human fallopian tube; a laboratory model for gonococcal infection. Journal of Infectious Diseases 129: 650–659

Westrom L 1975 Effect of acute pelvic inflammatory disease in fertility. American Journal of Obstetrics and Gynecology 121: 707–713

Westrom L 1980 Incidence, prevalence and trends of acute pelvic inflammatory disease and its consequence in industrialized countries. American Journal of Obstetrics and Gynecology 138: 880–892

Westrom L, Bengtsson L P, Mardh P-A 1976 Estimations of the risk of acquiring pelvic inflammatory disease in women using intra-uterine contraceptive devices as compared to non-users. Lancet ii: 221–224

Woolfitt J M G, Watt L 1977 Chlamydial infection of the urogenital tract in promiscuous and non-promiscuous women. British Journal of Venereal Diseases 53: 93–95

PERIHEPATITIS

Bolton J P, Darougar S 1983 Perihepatitis. British Medical Bulletin 39(2): 159–162

Curtis A H 1930 A cause of adhesions in the right upper quadrant. Journal of the American Medical Association 94: 1221–1222

Davidson A C, Hawkins D A 1982 Pleuritic pain: Fitz Hugh Curtis syndrome in a man. British Medical Journal 284: 808

Fitz-Hugh T 1934 Acute gonococcic peritonitis of the right upper quadrant in women. Journal of the American Medical Association 102: 2094–2096

Francis T I, Osoba O 1972 Gonococcal hepatitis Fitz-Hugh-Curtis syndrome in a male patient. British Journal of Venereal Diseases 48: 187–188

Kimball M W, Knee S 1970 Gonococcal perihepatitis in the male. The Fitz-Hugh-Curtis syndrome. New England Journal of Medicine 282: 1082–1084

Müller-Schoop J W, Wang S P, Munzinger J, Schlapfer H U, Knoblauch M, Wammann R W 1978 Chlamydia trachomatis as possible cause of peritonitis and perihepatitis in young women. British Medical Journal 1: 1022–1024

Reichert J A, Valle R F 1976 Fitz-Hugh-Curtis syndrome. Journal of the American Medical Association 236: 266–268

Stanley M M 1946 Gonococcic peritonitis of the upper part of the abdomen in young women. Archives of Internal Medicine 78: 1–13

von Knorring J, Nieminen J 1979 Gonococcal perihepatitis in a surgical ward. Annals of Clinical Research 11: 66–70

Wølner-Hanssen P, Svensson L, Weström L, Mårdh P-A 1982 Isolation of Chlamydia trachomatis from the liver capsule in Fitz-Hugh-Curtis syndrome. Correspondence, New England Journal of Medicine 306: 113

24

Lower urinary tract infections

In this discussion the term urinary tract infection (UTI) is used to refer to an infection caused by micro-organisms, usually enterobacteria, isolated from the urine by conventional bacteriological methods. The causative organisms, not pathogenic when existing as bowel flora, will be referred to as 'eubacteria' to distinguish them from organisms, considered elsewhere in this book, such as chlamydia, mycoplasma or urea-plasma.

The diagnosis of UTI is based upon the discovery by quantitative culture methods of significant numbers of the causative eubacteria in the urine; diagnosis should not be based on the presence or absence of symptoms or signs, nor on the presence or absence of pus cells in the urine (Cattell 1980).

Since single-dose therapy is curative in 90% of female patients if the organism is susceptible to the antimicrobial agent used, and since treatment failure in these cases selects out a subset of patients with deep-seated renal infection (Sheehan et al 1984). this chapter will focus on the management of the former group. Urinary tract infections are very much less common in men than in women (Leigh 1983). In homosexual men the incidence in Seattle, USA, appears to be much higher than in heterosexual men (Barnes et al 1986) whereas in London, United Kingdom, this is not the case (Wilson et al 1986).

The term 'urethral syndrome' is used as a descriptive diagnosis in women with the urinary symptoms of dysuria and/or frequency, but in whom significant bacteriuria is not found.

AETIOLOGY

Significant bacteriuria

Clean-catch midstream voiding specimens will inevitably have the potential for contamination by organisms normally present in the anterior urethra or periurethral area, and for this reason quantitative culture is necessary to evaluate the significance of any bacterial growth (Cattell 1980). The demonstration of 10^5 or more of the same organism per ml of a freshly voided clean-catch midstream specimen of urine is regarded as evidence of significant bladder bacteriuria; the level 10^5 bacteria per ml is the dividing line between bacteriuria and contamination (Kass 1956, 1957).

Micro-organisms responsible

Micro-organisms responsible for UTI in adults cover a wide variety of species (Table 24.1), many having their origins in the large bowel. In this locality *Escherichia coli* comprised 71%; *Streptococcus faecalis* 4% and *Proteus mirabilis* 4%.

If a choice of therapy is to be made it is necessary to know the sensitivities to antimicrobial agents among the prevailing organisms isolated currently in the locality concerned. Among the organisms isolated from women

Table 24.1 Prokaryotes responsible for urinary tract infection in adults (see text).

Species identified in concentrations of 10^5 or more per ml	Numbers	(%)
Escherichia coli	302	(71.2)
Klebsiella pneumoniae	7	(1.6)
Klebsiella oxytoca	11	(2.5)
Serratia rubidea	2	(0.5)
Serratia marcescens	4	(0.9)
Enterococcus cloacae	6	(1.4)
Enterococcus aerogenes	2	(0.5)
Citrobacter freundii	6	(1.4)
Citrobacter diversus	2	(0.5)
Proteus mirabilis	18	(4.1)
Proteus vulgaris	3	(0.7)
Morganella morganii	1	(0.2)
Pseudomonas spp	10	(2.3)
Acinetobacter spp	2	(0.5)
Staphylococcus saprophyticus	10	(2.3)
Staphylococcus albus	5	(1.1)
Staphylococcus aureus	4	(0.9)
Streptococcus faecalis	19	(4.3)
Beta-haemolytic streptococcus Group B	1	(0.2)
No identification. Unacceptable profile	6	(1.4)
Low discrimination between tests Extended tests required	7	(1.6)
Total identified	438	

attending this Edinburgh clinic, it was found that out of 56 isolations, *Esch. coli* was identified on 40 occasions (71%) and of these isolates ampicillin resistance was detected in 65%; in 34/40 cases (85%) organisms were sensitive to trimethoprim; and of those resistant to trimethoprim 4 of 5 tested were sensitive to Augmentin (amoxycillin and clavulanic acid). For therapy in the case of *Streptococcus faecalis* (2 isolated) ampicillin was the preferred antibiotic. *Proteus* spp all were sensitive to ampicillin, trimethoprim and cephalexin. *Klebsiella pneumoniae* isolates (2) were resistant to ampicillin but sensitive to trimethoprim. Of the 4 *Staphylococcus albus* isolates, 2 were sensitive to ampicillin, 3 to trimethoprim and 4 to cephalexin. Of the 5 *Staphylococcus saprophyticus* isolates, 3 were sensitive to trimethoprim and those resistant were sensitive to Augmentin.

Regular scrutiny of the results of testing sensitivities enables the formulation of a rational antibiotic policy for a given locality at a given time. Surprisingly, however, it has been found that failures in treatment using single-dose therapy (with trimethoprim 400 mg or co-trimoxazole — trimethoprim 320 mg and sulphamethoxazole 1600 mg — or amoxycillin 3.0 g) were scarcely contributed to by antibiotic resistance in the urinary pathogens (Harbord & Gruneberg 1981).

Esch. coli strains, uropathogenic phenotypes

Observations made about 25 years ago suggested strongly that certain strains of *Esch. coli*, identifiable by their group-specific antigen, were better able than others to cause infection of the urinary tract (Rantz 1962, Turck & Petersdorf 1962). Organisms of the same species, in children with urinary tract infections, for example, were found to have on their surface 'P-fimbriae' in 33/35 (91%) of urinary strains examined. The ability of *Esch. coli* strains to adhere to periurethral cells correlated with their ability to cause a D-mannose-resistant specific haemagglutination with human erythrocytes (Kallenius et al 1981a). The receptor structure on epithelial cells for the fimbriae of 'pyelonephritogenic' *Esch. coli* strains has been identified as a glycolipid of the globoseries. A synthetic disaccharide has been found to inhibit the attachment of these organisms in vitro and may in time form the basis of a test for the recognition of 'pyelonephritogenic' strains of *Esch. coli* (Kallenius et al 1981b).

Host factors associated with UTI

ABO blood group, secretor state and susceptibility to recurrent urinary tract infection in women

Correlation between ABO blood group and susceptibility to certain infectious diseases is well-documented. In studies of a Chilean population patients of blood group B had 50% greater probability than those of non-B subjects, and 70% greater probability than O subjects, of contracting *Esch. coli* urinary tract infection (Cruz-Coke et al 1965).

The antigens of ABO blood groups are in two forms: a. alcohol-soluble in tissues of all subjects; and b. water-soluble in most body fluids and organs of secretors. The non-secretor state has been linked with the susceptibility to certain infectious agents. In an Edinburgh study of 319 women with recurrent urinary tract infection (control group 334 women of similar age ranges), it was found that women of blood groups B and AB who were non-secretors of blood-group substances showed a Relative Risk of recurrent urinary tract infection of 3.12 (95% confidence limits 1.49 and 6.52) in comparison with other types (Kinane et al 1982). This appears to be an example of synergy with both absence of anti-B isohaemagglutinin and secretor substances with increased risk of recurrent UTI in women. In the controls the prevalence of non-secretors of 26.6% reflected the increased incidence of non-secretors found in Scottish and in Irish ethnic groups compared with other regions in the United Kingdom. The belief is that isohaemagglutinins interact with blood-group like antigens on the bacterial cell wall, thus inhibiting attachment to uro-epithelial or periurethral cells. Thus persons capable of producing anti-B isohaemagglutinins may have a greater degree of protection against urinary tract infection. In general, the extent of bacterial cross-reaction with ABO blood group suggests that a selective advantage linked to ABO blood group might operate in combating infections. Determination of blood groups and secretor state may provide additional information in identifying individuals who are at risk.

P1 blood group phenotype and susceptibility to recurrent pyelonephritis

P1 blood group phenotype was found to be present in 97 of children with pyelonephritis, compared with 75% (84) age-matched children without UTI. The study suggested that in the absence of reflux, the Pl blood group contributes to susceptibility to recurrent pyelonephritis due to bacteria that bind to the glycolipid receptors of the globoseries. In the presence of reflux, uro-epithelial attachment does not seem to confer an advantage to the bacteria that infect the kidney (Lomberg et al 1983).

Sexual intercourse and urinary tract infection

10 to 20% of young sexually active women experience urinary tract infection, and the belief in the association between sexual intercourse and urinary tract infection in this group is commonly expressed (Loudon & Greenhalgh 1962, Sandford 1975, Kraft & Stamey 1977). 'Honeymoon cystitis' and pyelitis of pregnancy are

dramatic events that are often preceded by a history of urinary infection and antecedent sexual activity, but proof of association is lacking as physicians tend to see only patients with symptoms and generally have little information about sexually active women without symptomatic infection (Kunin 1978). In the investigations of Kunin & McCormack (1968), it was found that celibacy was associated with a lower frequency of infection. Bacteriuria was about half as frequent in the unmarried women of the 15–24 year age group (2.7%) compared with the married (5.9%) but the difference was only significant at the 0.1 level. It was more frequent among single women in this age group than among nuns of the same age (0.4%).

In a study in women by Bran et al (1972), the urethra was milked outwards 4–5 times during general anaesthesia and the urine obtained by suprapubic aspiration of the bladder. It was found that small numbers of bacteria may enter the bladder in association with urethral trauma, but in only 4 of the 10 patients examined did the suprapubic aspirates contain bacteria that are commonly associated with urinary tract infection. With respect to sexual intercourse specifically, it was shown to result in an increase in colony counts of bacteria of more than one log in clean-voided specimens in 30% of the 76 episodes studied (Buckley et al 1978). These intercourse-induced increases in bacterial counts were asymptomatic and transient, and the rate or duration of bacteriuria was not affected by the type of birth control used. Early voiding after intercourse did not prevent the development of the log increases in urine colony counts, but most of the population studied did not have a history of recurrent cystitis and the failure to prove the protectiveness of early voiding may not apply to a more susceptible population. In relation to the problem of women troubled by recurrent infections, a single dose of an anti-bacterial agent after intercourse can prevent such recurrences (Vosti 1975). In this study prophylaxis involved the intermittent use of antimicrobials over periods of 19–47 months; the antimicrobials used effectively after intercourse were: nitrofurantoin 50 or 100 mg; nalidixic acid 500 or 100 mg; or cephalexin monohydrate 250 mg, and the prophylactic period was usually continued for prolonged periods (1½–4 years).

Bacteriuria in young girls and women is probably preceded by colonization of the vaginal introitus by the specific species of bacteria causing the urinary infection. This vaginal colonization is more frequent and more prolonged and characterized by a greater number of bacteria in women susceptible to recurrent urinary infections than in normal women. *Esch. coli* adhere more avidly to the vaginal cells of women susceptible to urinary infections than those of normal women and this affinity may promote vaginal colonization by enterobacteria (Fowler & Stamey 1977). Host factors determining bacterial adherence (e.g. ABO blood group and secretor status; P1 blood group; see above) are possibly more important than bacterial adhesive factors in determining susceptibility to urinary infection (Fowler & Stamey 1978). Although individuals in whom introital enterobacteria are always recovered, viz. persistent carriers, seem to have more frequent urinary tract infection, such infection occurs also in non-carriers and conversely some persistent carriers do not suffer infection even over a follow-up period of some years. As a result O'Grady (1980) concluded that the results of introital culture cannot be used *routinely* to define women at risk.

Bladder defences and response to single-dose therapy

In some patients with lower urinary tract infection the infection clears spontaneously or with forced diuresis or may be cleared by a small dose of an anti-bacterial agent. In such cases histological study of the bladder shows only superficial inflammation, if any. In contrast, upper urinary tract disease is characteristically an entrenched infection in the renal medulla, an area particularly susceptible to infection because of decreased flow, hypertonicity which inhibits exudation of leucocytes, preventing killing of bacteria by antibody and complement and allowing survival of L-form cell wall damaged bacterial variants (Sheehan et al 1984).

PATHOLOGY

In patients with recurrent urinary infection or symptoms of cystitis bladder histology shows acute inflammatory changes which are inconstant and sometimes sparse. Bacterial cystitis appears to be a superficial mucosal infection with involvement of the transitional epithelium, and in some cases the subepithelial lamina propria, but seldom deeper tissues. The infection usually results in a diffuse accumulation of lymphocytes throughout the bladder epithelium, occasionally with dense lymphocyte infiltration and even follicle formation. On cystoscope examination, acute bacterial cystitis likewise appears to be a diffuse superficial process limited to bladder mucosa (Marsh et al 1974).

Leucocyturia

The belief that the presence of 'pus cells' in urine is essential as a sign of urinary infection is not justified as it has been shown that the correlation between bacteriuria and leucocyturia is weak. Bacteriuria may regularly be present in the absence of pyuria and conversely there are many causes of pyuria apart from bacteriuria. For this reason it has been argued that *routine* microscopy is unnecessary for the *routine* screening of urine for urinary infection. In the case of *symptomatic* patients, however, *selective* microscopy is valuable since the demonstration of marked pyuria in such patients is indicative of an inflammatory reaction within the urinary tract (Cattell 1980).

PHARMACOKINETICS OF ANTI-BACTERIAL AGENTS USED IN UNCOMPLICATED BACTERIAL URINARY TRACT INFECTION

Most of these antimicrobials used for the treatment of acute bacterial urinary tract infections are concentrated and excreted in the urine, thus bringing about very high antimicrobial levels in urine lying adjacent to the bladder mucosa. Sterilization of the urine, as well as the ultimate cure of the urinary infection, is directly dependent on the bactericidal urine level of the anti-bacterial agent and independent of the very much lower concentration in the serum or plasma (Stamey et al 1965). Single-dose treatment of other superficial infections caused by rapidly multiplying organisms, as in uncomplicated gonococcal infections, is also very effective (see Ch. 16) although the mechanism is probably not dependent on bactericidal urine levels.

Although used often in combination with sulpha-methoxazole, trimethoprim after a dose of 100 mg will provide urine levels far in excess of the minimal inhibitory concentrations for most urinary pathogens. A dose of 100 mg will provide levels of 30–100 μg per ml for the first 4 hours; 30–200 μg per ml for the next 4 hours; and levels of 10–90 μg per ml over the 8–24 hour period (Neu 1983). A single dose of 400 mg is known to be effective, producing 95% cure rates in UTI and comparable to single doses of 4 tablets of co-trimoxazole (trimethoprim 320 mg with sulphamethoxazole 1600 mg) or a suspension of amoxycillin 3.0 g (Harbord & Gruneberg 1981).

CLINICAL FEATURES

The sensation of discomfort on passing urine is extremely common in women of all ages. In a survey of 2933 women (age 20–64 years) in the Rhondda Valley, South Wales, 639 (21.8%) said they had had dysuria (burning pain on passing urine) during the past year. In 287 (9.8%) the dysuria lasted for a total of more than 2 weeks during the year. Significantly more common in the married than in the single, it was the younger age group which had consulted their doctor because of these symptoms (Waters 1969). A peak incidence, as recorded by visits to general practitioners (primary care physicians), was reported to have occurred in the 20-year age group, with about 90 phys-

ician visits for dysuria per 1000 patients per year. In the case of the men, very few were seen among the younger age groups but consultations were 10 per 1000 at the age of 40 years, rising to 40 per 1000 at the age of 60 years (Fry et al 1962). The apparent peak incidence is due to the fact that younger women with dysuria, rather than older, seek medical attention more frequently. In the case of the men their attendances are likely to be associated with bladder neck obstruction.

In patients with the symptoms of frequency and dysuria there are those who are always bacteriuric; those who are sometimes bacteriuric; and those who are never bacteriuric. In the latter group they may be conveniently considered to have the 'urethral syndrome' (the dysuria syndrome or symptomatic abacteriuria). provided that in all 'at-risk' women infections due to *Trichomonas vaginalis*, herpes simplex virus, *Chlamydia trachomatis*, *Neisseria gonorrhoeae* and candidosis have been excluded, and in the case of men examination has excluded non-gonococcal urethritis, whether chlamydial or non-chlamydial, gonococcal infection or herpes simplex virus infection. Clinical distinction between the urethral syndrome and bacteriuria cannot be made on clinical grounds and is dependent on the detection of significant bacteriuria by quantitative culture of the urine.

In an acute UTI, symptoms suggesting *lower urinary tract* involvement are frequency, burning and suprapubic pain whereas symptoms suggesting *upper urinary tract* infection are loin pain, raised temperature, rigors, nausea and vomiting and *macroscopic haematuria*. Some, however, may have the acute urethral syndrome; others bladder bacteriuria; and others renal bacteriuria, but differentiation on clinical grounds is not in fact possible (Sandford 1975).

DIAGNOSIS

Culture of midstream specimen of urine
Clean-catch midstream voiding specimens of urine are inevitably liable to contamination by organisms normally present in the anterior urethra or periurethral area, and for this reason the specimen of urine must undergo *quantitative* bacterial culture to evaluate the significance of bacterial growth. As previously discussed, significant bladder bacteriuria is present when 10^5 or more of the same organisms per ml of urine is demonstrated. Contamination is usually with commensal organisms and results in the growth of a very varied flora and is readily recognizable. In UTI growth is usually of a single bacterial species.

To avoid the problem of multiplication of bacteria after voiding, the laboratory must receive midstream specimens of urine promptly. If the laboratory is accessible within 3 hours, a clean-catch midstream urine collector (C R Baird International Ltd., Pennywell Industrial Estate, Sunderland, England SR4 9EW) may be given to the patient to use and to return promptly for laboratory testing. In recent years, however, problems in collecting and preserving urine samples have been largely overcome by the using of 'dip-slides', 'dip-spoons' or 'filter-strips'. These methods involve the immediate inoculation of culture medium with a defined amount of urine obtained immediately after voiding. In the case of the 'dip-slide' or 'dip-spoon' methods a fixed area is coated with nutrient agar medium on one side and MacConkey's agar on the other. It is dipped in fresh urine and drained and then may be sealed in the dry sterile container provided and dispatched to the laboratory, where after incubation the density of growth in the medium is compared with standard charts to determine the bacterial density. Following culture, identification of the organism and antibiotic sensitivity tests are carried out.

In the case of the 'filter-strip' technique a filter paper is immersed in the urine where it absorbs a finite volume of urine. The strip is then removed and placed on a plate of culture medium, thus delivering a reproducible volume of urine. The strip is then removed and the plate sent to the laboratory (Cattell 1980).

The antibody-coated bacteria test
The demonstration of antibody on bacterial surface using an immunofluorescent assay predicts renal infection in women (Jones et al 1974) but about one-fourth of women with renal infection do not give a positive response to the test. In addition, difficulties with standardization and varying interpretation have led to inconsistent results. As a result the test has not been recommended currently as a routine diagnostic tool for localization of a urinary infection (Ronald 1983).

Selective microscopy
In the rapid diagnosis of the acutely ill patient, the demonstration of Gram-negative bacteria on microscopy, particularly when associated with pyuria and little evidence of contamination, is good evidence of urinary tract infection.

When selective microscopy is indicated, part of the specimen is centrifuged and the deposit resuspended in a small volume. A wet film of this deposit is examined for the presence of pus cells, erythrocytes, 'casts' of kidney tubules and bacteria. The Gram-stained smear may be examined routinely, or alternatively only when bacteria are present in the wet film. A Gram-stained smear of the deposit helps distinguish between infected specimens (pus cells with Gram-negative bacilli or Gram-positive cocci) and contaminated specimens (squamous epithelial cells with mixed organisms

including Gram-positive bacilli, often lactobacilli). In some true infections bacteria may grow in the urine without the production of pus cells.

Proteinuria is a poor criterion upon which to base the diagnosis of UTI and its absence does not exclude infection.

MANAGEMENT OF UNCOMPLICATED URINARY TRACT INFECTION IN THE ADOLESCENT OR ADULT FEMALE

Among medical authorities of clinical, laboratory and other medical disciplines, worldwide, there is unanimity in enthusiasm for treating uncomplicated urinary tract infections with single-dose anti-bacterial therapy. The advantages of simplicity, effectiveness and cheapness are additional to those of good toleration, preference and compliance on the part of the patient. In addition the risk of organisms developing resistance is small, and the manoeuvre determines which patients need more intensive urinary tract investigation, treatment, or follow-up. In the case of pregnancy, also, the hazard to the fetus is less than with longer courses (Bailey 1983).

Single-dose therapy is suitable for ambulatory women, who are reliable, with easy access to medical care, with an uncomplicated UTI who are neither pregnant nor diabetic and are free from known renal disease. Those with acute pyelonephritis, an in-dwelling catheter or a major urinary tract abnormality will also be excluded. It can be used as both treatment and diagnostic manoeuvre to distinguish between upper and lower urinary tract infection. A follow-up midstream specimen of urine (clean-catch) is mandatory 3–7 days later to ensure adequacy of treatment and assess the need for further therapy or evaluation (Tolkoff-Rubin & Rubin 1983). Best studied regimens have been amoxicillin 3 g or a combination of trimethoprim 320 mg and sulphamethoxazole 1600 mg, viz. 2 co-trimoxazole double-strength dispersible tablets (British National Formulary 1985) (Sheehan et al 1984), but as an alternative in the case of the latter, trimethoprim is increasingly being used alone for the treatment of urinary tract infections since side effects are less than with co-trimoxazole, especially in older patients.

Our recommendations on the management of urinary tract infections due to eubacteria in non-pregnant adolescents and adults are given in Figure 24.1. Trimethoprim is the drug of choice in our locality because 1985 data showed there to be a low incidence of resistant organisms. In addition trimethoprim shows a low incidence of patient hypersensitivity, whereas with co-trimoxazole the sulphonamide component is responsible for the reaction in the patient. For those whom trimethoprim is not suitable viz. in pregnancy; allergy

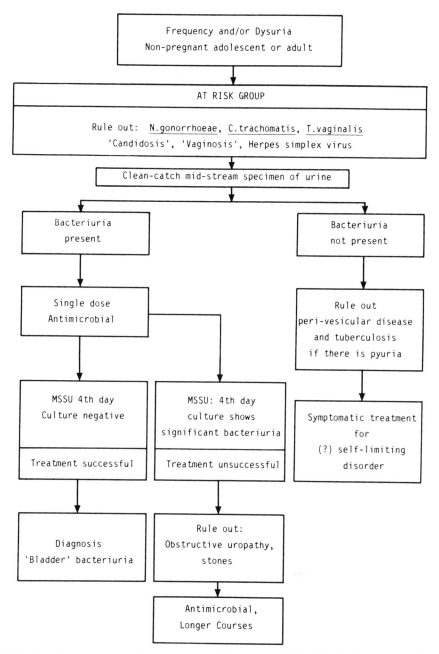

Fig. 24.1 A scheme for management of non-pregnant adolescent or adult female with frequency and/or dysuria.

on the part of the patient, or resistance in the micro-organism isolated, the second choice in treatment is amoxycillin (3.0 g) or ampicillin (3.0 g) given as a single dose.

PROGNOSIS

In UTI there is infrequent progression to chronic renal failure. Chronic pyelonephritis is often the primary cause of end-stage renal failure and is almost always associated with underlying structural defect. A UTI occasionally causes renal damage in some adults but appears to be infrequent in the absence of obstructive uropathy (Sandford 1975).

With single-dose treatment bladder bacteriuria will generally be cleared while renal bacteriuria will require more intensive treatment and investigation to exclude causes of obstructive uropathy.

THE URETHRAL SYNDROME

In a case control study of campus students (USA) Stamm et al (1980) found an association between the urinary symptoms of frequency and dysuria with pyuria and the presence of *Chlamydia trachomatis*, but in Llanedegrn, Cardiff, South Wales — in a randomized controlled trial of treatment of the urethral syndrome with intensive efforts to find a microbiological cause — O'Dowd et al (1984) were unable to isolate *C. trachomatis* from those presenting to their general practitioner with frequency and dysuria. In their cases each episode of the urethral syndrome was short — half were better by the fourth day and the rest by the 11th day. The condition was self-limiting, uninfluenced by treatment (e.g. doxycycline). Nearly half the patients 'got better' in the four-day interval while awaiting the result of the midstream specimen of urine, although in others the process took longer. Clearly the higher isolation rates for chlamydia in genito-urinary clinics are more in keeping with the nature of the population studied. The urethral syndrome when diagnosed on the basis of symptoms alone may have a psychosomatic basis.

In 'at-risk' groups it is nonetheless important to exclude *N. gonorrhoeae* and *C. trachomatis*. *Trichomonas vaginalis* and yeasts such as *Candida albicans* and herpes simplex virus may involve the periurethral tissues and should be excluded.

MANAGEMENT IN PREGNANT WOMEN WITH UTI

The plan of treatment based on the recommendations of Bailey (1983) is as follows:

1. Culture the urine of all pregnant women during the first trimester.

2. If bacteriuria is present, the patient is given a 5-day course of therapy. More recently single-dose treatment has been used as an alternative.

3. The urine is cultured 7 days later.

4. If the urine is sterile the woman is given no further treatment, but has her urine cultured at each clinic visit.

5. If the original infection is not eradicated the patient is given another 5-day course of therapy and is then immediately placed on prophylactic nitrofurantoin (50 mg each night) until the puerperium, when an intravenous urogram is undertaken.

6. If the initial infection is eradicated but a reinfection occurs, an antimicrobial either as a single dose or as a 5-day course is given, followed by prophylactic therapy as in 5 above. An intravenous urogram should be carried out after delivery.

Single-dose treatment of uncomplicated urinary tract infections holds a special attraction in pregnancy. If further trials confirm the effectiveness of a single dose, then this could become the treatment of choice for bacteriuria of pregnancy since, in addition, it would appear to identify those patients who require investigation of their urinary tract after delivery (Bailey 1983). Anti-bacterials suggested for single-dose treatments are as follows: amoxycillin 3.0 g; ampicillin 3.0 g; nitrofurantoin 100 mg.

MANAGEMENT OF THE UNCOMPLICATED URINARY TRACT INFECTION IN THE ADOLESCENT OR ADULT MALE

In the case of men a urinary tract infection will be suspected when there is dysuria and/or frequency, when both initial and second urine specimens are turbid, and when the turbidity is not due to phosphaturia. The presence or absence of purulent, mucopurulent or mucoid urethral discharge does not alter the diagnostic approach to such cases.

Microscopic examination of a Gram-stained film of the urethral discharge or of the centrifuged urine deposit will enable a presumptive diagnosis of UTI to be made, when Gram-negative bacteria are demonstrated in the presence of pus and when there is little evidence of contamination. Confirmation by quantitative culture, however, will be essential as well as the exclusion of *N. gonorrhoeae* and *C. trachomatis*. In the case of *all men with UTI or with haematuria, whether homosexual or heterosexual, intravenous urography is necessary* to detect functional or structural abnormality of the urinary tract, impaired bladder emptying or stone disease (Higgins 1978). Reference has been made to the findings in Seattle, USA, of a much higher prevalence of UTI among homosexual men than among heterosexual men (Barnes et al 1986), but this situation does not obtain in London. Currently the advice given is to refer for full urological investigation all men, whether heterosexual or homosexual, after their first attack of UTI. Clinic management in the case of males is currently as follows:

1. Suspect urinary tract infection in cases with the features already discussed. In addition, for homosexual males with NGU, send an MSSU for quantitative culture for eubacteria.

2. Take MSSU and if essential give tetracycline treatment — viz. if NGU is suspected — or preferably defer treatment until results of MSSU culture are available.

3. If MSSU shows bacteriuria the patient is seen in 3 days, when the MSSU is repeated. A single oral dose of trimethoprim 400 mg is given.

4. 4 days later (viz. 7 days after initial attendance) an MSSU is repeated to ascertain cure.

5. If infection persists, start on 6-week course of appropriate antibiotic.

6. In *all* cases of bacteriuria in males, excretion urography and cystoscopy are indicated.

FOLLOW-UP DEFINITIONS

In the management of urinary infection it is important to have clear criteria or definitions of cure, reinfection and relapse (Cattell 1976) as further investigations or different forms of treatment may be necessary.

Definition of cure

Cure is attained with the elimination of bacteriuria after treatment; persistently negative cultures of urine are necessary before a cure is pronounced. Disappearance of symptoms is not acceptable as a criterion.

Definition of relapse

A relapse is considered to have occurred when there is a recurrence of bacteriuria with the same organism immediately on stopping treatment, although urine cultures have been sterile during treatment.

Such a relapse may be due to wrong choice of antibacterial agent or its inadequate concentration in the urinary tract, emergence of resistant strains, anatomical abnormality, stone, renal calcification, scarred kidneys or bladder diverticula. A feature of *Proteus* infections is that the organisms may be converted to spheroplasts, particularly by penicillins, which change back to the original form after withdrawal of the drug.

Definition of reinfection

A reinfection is considered to have occurred when there is bacteriuria in patients where initial treatment has eliminated bacteriuria for weeks or months and urine cultures have been sterile.

INDICATIONS FOR EXCRETION UROGRAPHY

Intravenous urography (with a mortality rate of 1/20 000 examinations) is a means of detecting functional or structural abnormality of the urinary tract, impaired bladder emptying or stone disease. These abnormalities predispose to recurrent urinary infection, and intravenous urography is essential: 1. in children and adult males of any age with a urinary infection; 2. in adult females with recurrent bacteriuria who are not cured by single-dose antimicrobial treatment; 3. in both sexes with haematuria, which demands also both cytological examination of the urine and cystoscopy after control of the infection, unless in the case of the female, the haematuria is clearly associated with a coitus-related urinary infection (Higgins 1978).

In children and adult women a micturating cystogram is required to detect evidence of reflux in cases of uncontrolled bacteriuria.

REFERENCES

Bailey R R 1983 Single dose treatment for bacteriuria of pregnancy. In: Bailey R R (ed) Single dose therapy of urinary tract infection. Adis Health Science Press, Sydney, p 73–78

Barnes R C, Roddy R E, Daifuku R, Stamm W E 1986 Urinary-tract infection in sexually active homosexual men. Lancet i: 171–173

Bran J L, Levison M E, Kaye D 1972 Entrance of bacteria into the female urinary bladder. New England Journal of Medicine 286: 626–629

Buckley R M, McGuckin M, MacGregor R R 1978 Urine bacterial counts after sexual intercourse. New England Journal of Medicine 298: 321–324

Cattell W R 1976 Urinary tract infection. In: Hendry W F (ed) Recent advances in urology. Churchill Livingstone, London, p 232–244

Cattell W R 1980 Diagnosis and significance of urinary tract infection. In: Chisholm G D (ed) Urology, tutorials in postgraduate medicine. William Heinemann Medical Books, London, ch 2, p 19–36

Cruz-Coke R, Paredes L, Montenegro A 1965 Blood groups and urinary microorganisms. Journal of Medical Genetics 2: 185–188

Fowler J E, Stamey T A 1977 Studies of introital colonization in women with recurrent urinary infections. VII The role of bacterial adherence. Journal of Urology 117: 472–476

Fowler J E, Stamey T A 1978 Studies of introital colonization in women with recurrent urinary infections. X. Adhesive properties of *Escherichia coli* and *Proteus mirabilis*. Lack of correlation with urinary pathogenicity. Journal of Urology 120: 315–322

Fry J, Dillane J B, Joiner C L, Williams J D 1962 Acute urinary infections: their course and outcome in general practice with special reference to chronic pyelonephritis. Lancet i: 1318–1321

Harbord R B, Gruneberg R N 1981 Treatment of urinary tract infection with a single dose of amoxycillin, co-trimoxazole or trimethoprim. British Medical Journal 283: 1301–1302

Higgins P M 1978 Haematuria. British Journal of Hospital Medicine 19(4): 325

Jones S R, Smith J W, Sandford J P 1974 Localization of urinary tract infections by detection of antibody-coated bacteria in urinary sediment. New England Journal of Medicine 290: 591–593

Kallenius G, Svenson S B, Mollby R, Cedergren B, Hultberg H, Winberg J 1981a Structures of carbohydrate part of receptor on human uroepithelial cells for pyelonephritogenic *Escherichia coli*. Lancet ii: 604–606

Kallenius G, Molby R, Soenson S P, Helin I, Hultberg H, Cedergren B, Winberg J 1981b Occurrence of P-fimbriated *Escherichia coli* in urinary tract infections. Lancet ii: 1369–1372

Kass E H 1956 Asymptomatic infections of the urinary tract. Transactions of the Association of American Physicians 69: 56–64

Kass E H 1957 Bacteriuria and the diagnosis of infection of the urinary tract. Archives of Internal Medicine 100: 709–714

Kinane D F, Blackwell C C, Brettle R P, Weir D M, Winstanley F P, Elton R A 1982 ABO blood group, secretor state and susceptibility to recurrent urinary tract infection in women. British Medical Journal 285: 7–9

Kraft J K, Stamey T A 1977 The natural history of symptomatic recurrent bacteriuria in women. Medicine 56: 55–60

Kunin C M 1978 Sexual intercourse and urinary infections. Leading article, New England Journal of Medicine 298: 336–337

Kunin C M, McCormack R C 1968 An epidemiological study of bacteriuria and blood pressure among nuns and working women. New England Journal of Medicine 278: 635–642

Leigh D A 1983 A review of the published series of single dose therapy in urinary tract infection. In: Bailey R R (ed) Single dose therapy of urinary tract infection. Adis Health Science Press, Sydney, ch I, p 1–6

Lomberg H, Hanson L A, Jacobson B, Jodal U, Leffler H, Eden C S 1983 Correlations of P blood groups, vesicourethral reflux and bacterial attachment in patients with recurrent pyelonephritis. New England Journal of Medicine 308: 1189–1192

Loudon I S L, Greenhalgh G P 1962 Urinary tract infections in general practice. Lancet ii: 1246–1248

Marsh F B, Banerjee R, Panchamia P 1974 The relationship between urinary infection, cystoscopic appearnce and pathology of the bladder in man. Journal of Clinical Pathology 27: 297–307

Neu H C 1983 Single dose treatment of urinary tract infections: a pharmacologists view. In: Bailey R R (ed) Single dose therapy of urinary tract infection. Adis Health Science Press, Sydney, ch XIV, p 92–97

O'Dowd T C, Ribeiro C D, Munro J, West R R, Howells C H L, Harvard Davis R 1984 Urethral syndrome: a self-limiting illness. British Medical Journal 288: 1349–1352

O'Grady F W 1980 Factors affecting urinary tract infection. In: Bailey R R (ed) Single Dose Therapy of Urinary Tract Infection. Adis Health Science Press, Sydney, ch 1, p 3–18

Rantz L A 1962 Serological grouping of *Escherichia coli*: study in urinary traci infection. Archives of Internal Medicine 109: 37–42

Ronald A R 1983 Correlation of localisation of infection with response to single dose treatment. In: Bailey R R (ed) Single dose therapy of urinary tract infection. Adis Health Science Press, Sydney, ch V, p 25–32

Sandford J P 1975 Urinary tract symptoms and infection. Annual Review of Medicine 26: 485–498

Sheehan G, Harding G K M, Ronald A R 1984 Advances in the treatment of urinary tract infection. Proceedings of a symposium. Impact of the patient at risk on current and future antimicrobial therapy. The American Journal of Medicine 76(5A): 141–147

Stamey T A, Govan D E, Palmer J M 1965 The localization and treatment of urinary tract infections: the role of bactericidal urine levels as opposed to serum levels. Medicine 44: 1–35

Stamm W E, Wagner K F, Amsel R, et al 1980 Causes of the acute urethral syndrome in women. New England Journal of Medicine 303(8): 409–415

Tolkoff-Rubin N E, Rubin R H 1983 Single dose treatment of acute uncomplicated infections defined by the antibody-coated bacteria assay. In: Bailey R R (ed) Single dose therapy of urinary tract infection. Adis Health Science Press, Sydney, p 42–52

Turck M, Petersdorf R G 1962 The epidemiology of non-enteric *Escherichia coli*: prevalence of serologic groups. Journal of Clinical Investigation 41: 1760–1765

Vosti K L 1975 Recurrent urinary tract infections: prevention by prophylactic antibiotics after sexual intercourse. Journal of the American Medical Association 231: 939–940

Waters W E 1969 Prevalence of urinary tract infection in women. British Journal of Preventive and Social Medicine 23: 263–266

Wilson A P R, Tovey S J, Adler M W, Gruneberg R N 1986 Prevalence of urinary tract infection in homosexual and heterosexual men. Genito-Urinary Medicine 62: 189–190

25

Dysplasia and cancer of the cervix uteri

At the time of diagnosis of cervical cancer affected patients have a mean expected life of 13 years compared with the 24 years of life expected by the general population at the same age. The average patient will lose 45% of her remaining lifespan, the loss being respectively 39% for the localized and 69% for the non-localized. These calculations were made by Hakulinen and his colleagues (1981) from a study of the survival of cancer patients in Finland in 1953–1954 (Hakama 1982, 1983). Since those who attend departments of genito-urinary medicine are an 'at-risk' group, the staff of these units share with others an important role in prevention since precursors are detected at a stage long before the cancer becomes invasive.

EPIDEMIOLOGY

Multiple sexual partners and sexual intercourse in adolescence have been identified as key factors in the aetiology of squamous cell carcinoma of the cervix (Rotkin 1981). A case, however, can be made out for the belief that the sexual behaviour of the male partner may have an important or even crucial role in its aetiology (Skegg et al 1982). All observations on risk factors support the hypothesis that either one or more sexually transmissible agent is involved.

Cervical cancer has almost never been recorded in virgins. It is rare in nuns and common in prostitutes. Early marriage, multiple marriages, sexual intercourse beginning in adolescence and multiple sexual partners are variables more likely to be found in women with cervical cancer in comparison with controls. Frequency of coitus is not itself related to an increased risk (Rotkin 1981). The significantly higher concordance rate among monozygotes than among dizygotes with regard to cervical cancer could indicate a genetic influence which itself may also be a determinant of life style (Cedarloff & Floderus-Myrhed 1980).

Cancer of the cervix has a long period between puta-

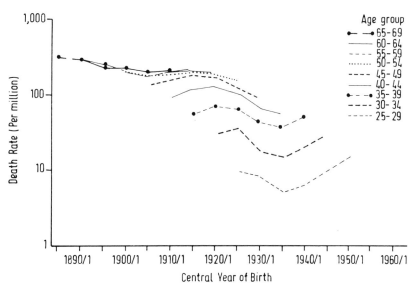

Fig. 25.1 Cancer of the cervix uteri. The graph shows changes in mortality rates in England and Wales during 1951–1980 within each five-year group for successive birth cohorts (Osmond et al 1983).

tive cause and effect (say death) so it is therefore useful to distinguish death rates which are identified with a particular generation from those that are related to a period. The trends in the mortality rates for England and Wales in successive generations are complex (Fig. 25.1). If the cohort values are interpreted in terms of year of birth there was a decline at the end of the last century which continued until the 1905 cohort (there had been an earlier peak around 1885). After this there was a rise until the 1920 cohort, followed by a further decline to the generation of women born around 1935. Subsequently there has been a pronounced upward movement with successive birth groups. Since cervical cancer is generally regarded as associated with the multiple sexual partners or with the transmission of one or more infectious agents from a male partner who has other sexual contacts, it is relevant to relate the cohort values to the times when generations of women reached maturity. Peaks relate to times when relevant generations of young women and/or their partners experienced freer sexual relationships, viz. during the first two World Wars. The rise in the most recent generations

is particularly steep (Fig. 25.2) but is based on smaller numbers and corresponds with a further recent profound change in sexual relationships (Osmond et al 1982, 1983). The cohort curve for cervical cancer is closely related to the incidence of gonorrhoea in related generations (Beral 1974). Again this probably reflects changes in sexual behaviour.

Focus exclusively on two factors specifically in female behaviour, namely those of sexual intercourse in adolescence and multiple sexual partners, has been criticized in a hypothesis which emphasizes the possible importance of the male factor in cancer of the cervix (Skegg et al 1982). This proposition is based on a number of epidemiological observations which are not explained by concentrating solely on factors in the female: 1. the very marked decline in mortality in many western countries, e.g. in England and Wales (Fig. 25.3) began long before any cytology screening programmes were introduced; 2. the very low risk in Jewish women (Fig. 25.4) — cancer of the cervix appears also to be very rare in Arab countries and Turkey (Parkin et al 1984) — and 3. the very high

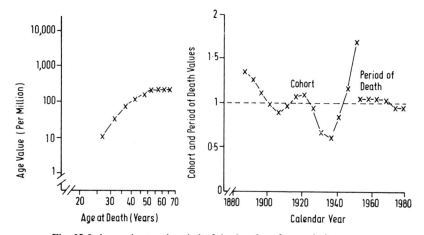

Fig. 25.2 Age, cohort and period of death values for cervical cancer (ages 25–69). On the left section of the figure the age value (similar to the age-specific death rate) is plotted against age at death on a log-log scale. A straight line would indicate a power relation of the rate with age. On the right section the cohort and period of death values are plotted against time with a horizontal dotted line indicating the average value. Cohort values are plotted against central year of birth and period of death values against central.year of death. If cohort values are interpreted in terms of year of birth there was a decline at the end of the last century which continued until the 1920 cohort, followed by a further decline to the generation of women born in the mid-1930s. Subsequently there was a pronounced upward movement with successive birth groups. The degree of variation in cohort values was substantially greater than that found in the period of death values, although the latter showed a gradual decrease. The peak shown relates to women who reached maturity (20–24 years) during the Second World War, and the nadir to the middle 1950s before the period of 'sexual liberation' (Osmond et al 1982, 1983).

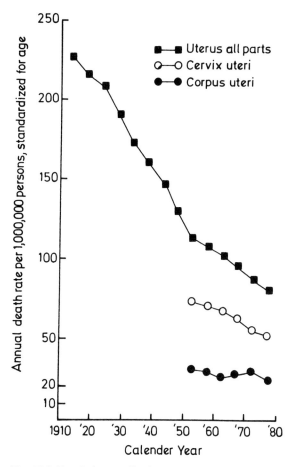

Fig. 25.3 Trends in mortality from cancer of the uterus (all parts, cervix and corpus) in England and Wales from 1911–1915 to 1976–1980, standardized for age using a world standard population (Skegg et al 1982).

incidence in Colombia (Fig. 25.4) and other South American countries (Fig. 25.5). Explanation of these three main points relies on the proposal that a factor introduced by the male into the female has been derived from a reservoir considered by Skegg et al (1982) to be female prostitutes. In western countries generally, over the period of time in question, men have tended to have less and less recourse to prostitutes. In the case of the Jewish men it is thought that although they may not have fewer extramarital partners than non-Jews they resort to prostitutes much less. That circumcision is a factor can be discounted as no difference was found between Lebanese Christians and Moslems despite their different circumcision status (Abou-Daoud 1966). In occupations that involve men in travel and absence from home the high mortality among their wives suggests too that the male factor is important (Beral 1974).

The very high incidence in Colombia, Cali (Fig. 25.4)

and elsewhere in South America is explained by the view, based on some evidence that men in these areas do tend, more than say, in Western Europe or in the United States, to patronize prostitutes (Alzate 1978, 1984). The authors of the hypothesis identify three types of sexual behaviour in society as a whole (see Fig. 1.6). In Type A, men and women are both strongly discouraged from extramarital relationships and such a pattern is seen among active members of religious groups such as the Mormons and the Amish (Cross et al 1968) where the incidence of cervical cancer is low. In Type B society there are double standards in sexual morality; the female is expected to have only one partner whereas the men are expected to have many. In some Latin American countries the Type B pattern exists today and was characteristic of many European and other societies both early in this century, but particularly in the last. Where there is social pressure which limits sexual expression in the female but encourages it in the male, prostitution tends to flourish. Type C society resembles present-day western society where value in the equality of male and female is emphasized and both sexes tend to have several partners during their lives.

The social class gradient in cervical cancer is pronounced and this may be related to difference in sexual behaviour of the female in lower socio-economic groups. Rotkin (1981) in his consideration of the epidemiology emphasizes the important influences on the young of poverty, overcrowding and abysmal deprivation, observable in many squalid urban dwellings in Latin America, such as the *barriada* of Lima in Peru, where prostitution at an early age is likely to be common.

The results of a case-control study in Toronto, Canada, demonstrated a two-fold risk of invasive squamous cell carcinoma of the cervix amongst current smokers relative to women who had never smoked. The significant effect of smoking was not diminished by simultaneously adjusting for age, education and indices of sexual behaviour. The association was further supported by observations that ex-smokers were at lower risk than current smokers (1.7 versus 2.3) and that the risk increased with the amount of cigarettes smoked (2.2 for less than half a pack per day to 2.9 for more than one pack per day) (Clarke et al 1982).

Professor Vessey and his colleagues from Oxford suggested that long-term use of the oral contraceptive pill might increase the risk of cancer of the cervix uteri (Vessey et al 1983). In their study of 6838 parous pill-using women and 3154 parous women using intrauterine contraceptive devices they found that the background risk for all types of cervical neoplasia (biopsy-proven dysplasia, carcinoma in situ and invasive cancer) was 0.9

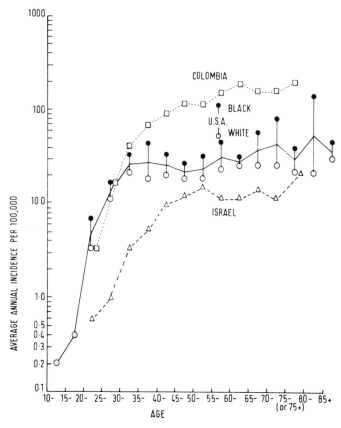

Fig. 25.4 Cancer of the cervix uteri. Age-specific incidence (average annual) in Colombia, Cali (1972–1976); United States of America, San Francisco Bay Area (1973–1977); and Israel (1972–1976). The figure illustrates the rates respectively for the black (●) and white (○) population in the San Francisco Bay Area. There were no cases in blacks in the age group 10–19. The rates for Israel are those for all Jews. (Waterhouse et al 1982.)

per 1000 woman years and that this was increased to 2.2 per 1000 woman years in those with more than eight years risk. These findings, as the authors admit, might be attributable to other important risk factors viz. age at first intercourse and number of sexual partners (Rotkin 1981) which were not documented in the study. Their finding that pill-users were slightly younger at marriage and at first-time pregnancy suggests the possibility that they began intercourse at an earlier age than women using the IUCD. All cancers in Vessey's study were detected at a curable stage, and regular screening is of course essential for pill-users at any age (Drife 1983). Adverse publicity about the pill can threaten the success of birth control programmes throughout the world and cause misgivings amongst those concerned in their planning, but clearly long-term effects on health need to be taken seriously and discussed rationally (Anonymous (Lancet) 1983).

AETIOLOGY

Carcinogenesis is a complex, process and understanding of the genetics of human cancer depends on very high technology biology. Studies on DNA tumour viruses of animals, for example, have shown that two separate genes are required to complete the tumorigenic transformation of normal cells in culture. One of the genes enables the cells to go on growing indefinitely; the other induces changes in the shape and behaviour of the cell that seem to be associated with the loss of any remaining constraints on growth. Two classes of gene, which have been identified in polyoma virus and adenovirus, have been categorized as immortalizing and transforming. Carcinogenesis appears to be generally a multistep process but the scientist may in time reduce the complex clinical problem to a system simple enough to be analysed in the laboratory (Robertson 1983).

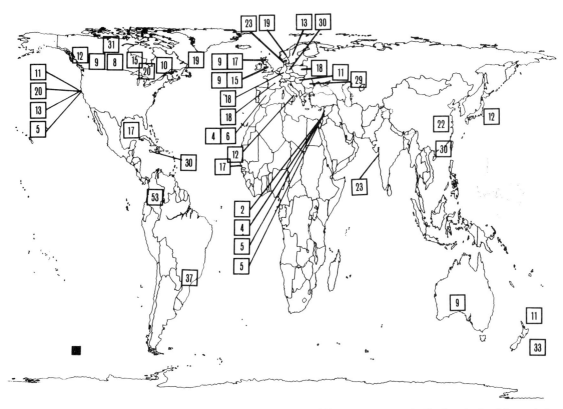

Fig. 25.5 Cancer of the cervix uteri. Average annual incidence per 100 000 — rates are standardized to the 'world' population (Waterhouse et al 1982).

It is relevant to consider the evidence for the association of two sexually transmitted viruses viz. herpes simplex virus Type 2 (HSV-2) and human papillomavirus (HPV) and their possible role in the causation of carcinoma of the cervix uteri. In connection with the role of herpesvirus, epidemiological data (Aurelian et al 1981) indicate that a woman with HSV-2 cervicitis has a 4–16 fold higher risk of developing this cancer than the HSV-2 negative. The prevalence of HSV-2 antibody is significantly higher in women with cervical cancer, carcinoma in situ, or dysplasia, than in controls. Infection with HSV-2 tends to precede by a mean period of five years the development of dysplasia.

More recently, in work that may prove to be valuable in the clinical management of cervical cancer, it has been found that cervical cancer patients are positive for antibody against at least two viral antigens, VP143 and AG-4, of which the latter is immunologically identical to an early viral protein. The antibody to AG-4 is IgM and appears to reflect growth of the cervical tumour from dysplasia to invasive cancer, to disappear following tumour removal — elimination of the antigen source — and to reappear with tumour recurrence. Other viral proteins (ICP-2 and ICP-14) are recognized by lympho-

cytes from 75% of patients with cervical dysplasia, carcinoma in situ or invasive cancer, compared with 13% of matched controls. Viral DNA sequences have been found in one cervical tumour and HSV-2 was isolated from a carcinoma in situ lesion. Specific RNA, an expression of HSV-2 DNA, has also been found in cancer cells. The virus or its DNA can transform cells in vitro and in a third of experimental monkeys, infected vaginally or cervically with HSV-2, severe dysplasia results after an interval of about 5 years (Aurelian et al 1981). Two separate immortalizing and tumorigenic functions have been identified in the genome of HSV-2 (Zuckerkandl 1984).

It has long been recognized that malignant conversion of warts, the benign tumours of skin and mucosa induced by papillomaviruses, may occur in animals and on rare occasions in man (zur Hausen 1977). Modern technology enabling the study of these viruses, the characterization by colposcopy of the lesions produced on the cervix and the recognition of the high prevalence of the human papillomavirus (HPV) in this anatomical site have all heightened interest in the possible role of HPV in the aetiology of cancer of the cervix. Papillomaviruses are produced in very low quantities and since no culture system has existed for their propagation the study and analysis of these viruses only became feasible with the discovery of molecular cloning (Pfister 1984) which enables their characterization into types on the basis of their DNA structure (see Ch. 27).

Cytological criteria for the identification of infection of the uterine cervix with HPV have been described, again only in recent times independently by Meisels & Fortin (1976) in Quebec and by Purola & Savia (1977) in Helsinki. Before these reports wart virus infection of the cervix was thought to be rare (Oriel 1971). Using the new diagnostic criteria Meisels et al (1977) found a prevalence of more than 70% for HPV infection of the cervix in patients who had been diagnosed previously as having mild dysplasia. Meisels and his colleagues (1982) identify on colposcopy four morphological types of wart lesion of the cervix, viz. the 'florid', the 'spiked', the 'flat' condyloma and 'condylomatous cervicitis'. In all lesions, irrespective of their gross morphology, the 'koilocyte' is the pathognomonic cell (see Ch. 27). These lesions of the cervix frequently co-exist in juxtaposition with or intermingled with dysplastic or neoplastic lesions. In their cases 68% of condylomatous lesions regressed spontaneously or after treatment, another 27% remained unchanged after a mean follow-up period of 14.5 months, and progression to more advanced lesions (moderate dysplasia, carcinoma in situ and invasive carcinoma) was observed in 10% of these condylomatous lesions with marked nuclear atypia and 5% of those without such atypia.

Nomenclature based on visual appearance, whether naked-eye or by colposcopy, in wart lesions which show such notable variety and complexity is liable to be confusing. 'Condyloma acuminatum' is the term used for a wart lesion in the genital area. The first word 'condyloma' is derived from the Greek word 'kondylos' meaning a knuckle and refers to its exophytic profile; the term 'flat condyloma' is, therefore, not appropriate and should be avoided. The Latin word 'acuminare' means to 'make pointed' and refers to the tapering profile of the new growth. Fletcher (1983) prefers the term 'flat koilocytosis' to describe the flat wart affecting the cervix uteri and to distinguish it from the exophytic wart lesions of other genital areas and occasionally of the cervix (see Ch. 27) which he refers to as 'condylomatous koilocytosis'. In brief he defines koilocytic cervical states as:

1. Condylomatous koilocytosis
2. Flat koilocytosis.

Koilocytosis is found in all warts, whether human or animal. The perinuclear halo of the koilocyte is a cytopathic effect of productive wart virus infection. Koilocytes are degenerating cells destined to die or to be shed from epithelium and cannot themselves generate a malignant cell line, although deeper cells may do so. Koilocytes are commonly associated with dysplasia and the connection may or may not be causal. Koilocytes may be adjacent to or coincident with a normal or dysplastic cell component (mild, moderate or severe dysplasia, carcinoma in situ or invasive carcinoma).

There is a close association between HPV and cervical cancer but it remains unclear as to whether the finding is casual rather than causal (Singer et al 1984). Of women with cancer of the cervix, 93% have in their sera an IgG antibody against a group-specific papillomavirus antigen; 60% of those with premalignant lesions have positive sera (Baird 1983). Zur Hausen's group in Germany and McCance and his colleagues in Britain have found evidence of certain human papillomavirus types in cervical precancer and cancer (Singer et al 1984) with techniques of DNA-DNA hybridization with radiolabelled HPV probes. HPV-6 has been found in 12 of 19 biopsy specimens of premalignant lesions in a group of London women (McCance et al 1983). HPV-11 was detected in every one of 5 similar lesions in Germany (Gissman et al 1983). HPV-16 genomes have been detected in about two-thirds of 18 cervical cancers (Durst et al 1983), and zur Hausen has found HPV-18, a newer type, in a fifth of cervical cancers (Singer et al 1984). The present hypothesis suggests that HPV-16 and HPV-18 represent high risk types for malignant progression and HPV-6 and HPV-11 low risk (Singer et al 1984). Co-factors such as herpes simplex virus may be necessary to enable HPV to induce malignancy in the cervix. Smoking cigarettes increases the relative risk of women developing carcinoma in situ (Trevathan et al 1983) (see Fig. 25.6).

On the basis of such nucleic acid studies, seven HPV types have been identified as specific to the urogenital tract, viz. the common types HPV-6, 11, 16 and 18 (Singer et al 1984) and the less common HPV-31, 33 and 35 (Beaudenon et al 1986, for discussion see Meanwell et al 1987). Available data suggest that in cervical carcinomas HPV-16 and 18 may be integrated into the cell genomes and integration of HPV-33 DNA sequences has been found in one case of vulvar carcinoma in situ (Bowen's Disease) (Beaudenon et al 1986). Although integration of HPV types 16 or 18 is a risk factor for the development of cervical cancer, conclusions about the biological significance of integration cannot be made. In the case of HPV-16 such integration was found to be common in those with cervical cancer and absent in those without, but in this study (Meanwell et al 1987) a number of points were made on the subject of HPV-16 DNA:

1. Positive and negative findings were obtained in adjacent areas of the same cervical cancer tumour;

2. HPV-16 occurred as episomal molecules in more than two thirds of these 31 carcinoma cases;

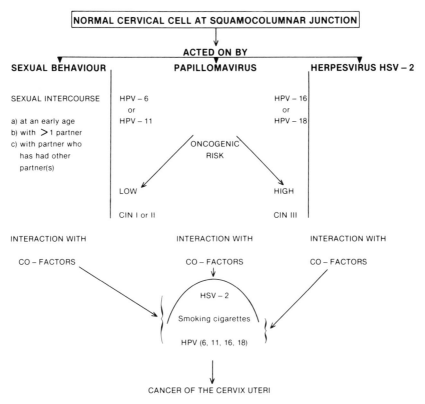

CANCER OF THE CERVIX UTERI
HYPOTHESES
ON
AETIOLOGY

Fig. 25.6 Cancer of the cervix uteri. Hypothesis on the possible role of papillomavirus types and other co-factors.

3. the HPV-16 integration, when found occurred at mostly single host-genome sites but once at multiple sites;

4. the association of HPV-16 and cervical neoplasia is age-related; the older the patient the more likely the virus is to be found.

In South Africa cervical papillomavirus infection has been found in two-thirds of the black women examined, and although this group have also a high risk of cervical cancer the high frequency of HPV in the normal cervix suggests that there may be events, other than HPV infection, required to initiate the cancerigenic process in the cervix (Leading Article (Lancet) 1987).

DIAGNOSTIC EXFOLIATIVE CYTOLOGY

Precancerous changes in the epithelium of the uterine cervix are well-known and can be detected by examining microscopically cells obtained by scraping the squamo-

columnar junction with a wooden spatula — the Ayre spatula is the best known, and others such as the Aylesbury and Lerner have advantages. This cytodiagnosis or 'cervical cytology' (see Note 25.2) has an established place among the methods for the early detection of cancer and is employed throughout the world as an efficient and highly successful large-scale screening technique (Hoffken & Soost 1981).

Dysplasia is the outward sign of heteroplastic changes in squamous or metaplastic epithelium and can be defined as disruption of the normal synchronism between nuclear and cytoplasmic maturation (Hoffken & Soost 1981). Follow-up studies have shown that mild, moderate and severe dysplasia and carcinoma in situ can be regarded as stages of one and the same disease. Richart & Barron (1969) thought that all dysplasia except evanescent ones (only those who had at least three abnormal smears were admitted to their study) would progress in the vast majority of cases to carcinoma in situ. In following the progression in their patients the transit times ranged from a median of 86 months for patients with mild dysplasia, to 48 months for those with moderate and to 12 months for those with severe. Estimates of regression and progression given in the literature, however, are widely discordant and Hoffken & Soost (1981) found that in their patients 61% of mild and moderate dysplasias regressed while 9% progressed to carcinoma in situ. About 60–70% of all carcinomas in situ are believed to develop into invasive carcinomas, the change occurring within a period of many years (5–20 years). From the point of view of the clinical management of the patient, severe dysplasia and carcinoma in situ may be regarded as precursors inevitably leading to squamous carcinoma. Dysplastic changes can develop directly into squamous cell carcinoma without going through the grades of increasing severity and there are also cases of carcinoma that arise *de novo*.

The terms dysplasia, carcinoma in situ, anaplasia, atypical metaplasia, have never been adequately and objectively defined and are the expression of a *subjective* microscopical assessment of these lesions by pathologists. The morphological graded diagnosis is not a reliable means of assessing the future behaviour of any given precancerous lesion; the lesions can either disappear, remain confined to the epithelium or in a relatively small proportion progress to invasive cancer (Koss & Greenebaum 1983).

Objective assessment of these lesions is possible, but the technology is not generally available to the clinician and depends for its application also upon the taking of tissue by biopsy. Fu et al (1981) have shown that the lesions can be divided into two groups according to their chromosome number and DNA quantitation; the one in which the lesions are more likely to have normal follow-up studies and rarely persist, in contrast to the other which mostly persist or progress to invasive carcinoma. Chromosomal karyotyping of cervical intraepithelial lesions has shown that the chromosome number (see Note 25.1) may be 46 (normal euploidy); 92 (polyploidy), or at abnormal levels (aneuploidy). Similarly, by nuclear DNA quantitation, the lesions may be euploid, polyploid or aneuploid.

In a retrospective study of 100 cases of cervical intraepithelial abnormalities (Fu et al 1981), in 34 cases with a normal follow-up 29 (85%) had a euploid or polyploid distribution. Of the 58 cases persisting, 55 (95%) had an aneuploid distribution and of the 8 cases which progressed to invasive carcinoma all had an aneuploid. Their findings suggested that euploid or polyploid lesions are more likely to have normal follow-up studies (91%) and rarely persist (9%). Of the aneuploid lesions 81% persisted as cervical intra-epithelial neoplasia, 12% progressed to invasive carcinoma, and 7% had a normal follow-up. The presence of abnormal mitoses was the most reliable histological criterion for aneuploidy. Mild to moderate dysplasia (CIN I and II) can be aneuploid, whereas some of the severe abnormalities (severe dysplasia, carcinoma in situ) may be diploid — tetraploid and hence a relatively favourable group.

Chromosomal karyotyping is not generally available as a technology for clinical use but cervical cytology screening (see Ch. 6) will enable the detection of the great majority of cases of cervical cancer long before the lesion becomes invasive. Virtually all cervical intraepithelial neoplasia (CIN) begins at the squamo columnar junction with one edge of the lesion bordering the columnar epithelium. The lesion begins on the anterior lip twice as often as the posterior lip and relatively infrequently at the lateral cervical angles. The changes seen in CIN are classified histologically into minimal dysplasia or carcinoma in situ (CIN III) (Richart 1973):

CIN Grade I: Minimal dysplasia characterized by disorderliness of maturation and cytological atypia which extends through the full thickness of the epithelium. There are many binucleated cells. Only the lowermost layers of cells are undifferentiated.

CIN Grade II: Moderate dysplasia. A precursor lesion of intermediate grade. The full thickness cytological atypia and lack of orderly maturation are obvious. 50–75% of the epithelium is composed of undifferentiated cells.

CIN Grade III: Severe dysplasia and carcinoma in situ. Carcinoma in situ is traditionally defined as a lesion composed of neoplastic cells extending through the full thickness of the epithelium and not penetrating the basement membrane. There are many mitotic figures at all levels and virtually no epithelial organization or maturation.

Similar classification is used by the cytologists, reporting on cells (Grubb 1977) scraped from the squamocolumnar junction, although more detailed reporting is used in the Munich schedule (Hoffken & Soost 1981). The British Society for Colposcopy and Cervical Cytology proposed that the classification CIN I, CIN II and CIN III should be universally adopted (Sharp et al 1983).

The collection of material from the cervix uteri suitable for study by the cytologist should precede any attempt at palpation and it is important that no medicament should be introduced into the vagina before taking the specimen. After introducing the speculum the external os is examined with the naked eye. The correct method of taking the smear, its immediate fixation (Note 25.2) and subsequent staining and reporting by an experienced cytologist are necessary to ensure accuracy of the report (Hoffken & Soost 1981). The success of cervical cytology as a means of diagnosing pre-invasive carcinoma is limited by the reluctance of many patients to have smear tests taken and by the false-negative rate. The use of the wooden Ayre spatula centred on the cervix and rotated through 360° is the conventional method of taking smears and is widely used in the United Kingdom. The use of paired sampling (two smears taken at the same attendance) improves the detection rate by 18.5% (Bourne & Beilby 1976, Beilby et al 1982) and could therefore contribute to the efficiency of screening.

In the hope that the use of immunocytochemical tumour-associated markers might improve the specificity and sensitivity of cervical smear testing Husain et al (1984) studied specimens collected from colposcopy, gynaecology and antenatal clinics. Positive staining with all monoclonal antibodies tested was present on a few apparently normal squamous cells, as well as both metaplastic and neoplastic cells of the cervix. It was concluded that the tests would not be useful in the detection and diagnosis of premalignant and malignant cervical cells but that the identification of metaplastic cells might be of some value. Research continues at present on the possible use of an automated screening staining method as a means of measuring quantitatively the expression of these markers.

Evidence for the effectiveness of screening is available from a number of countries (Draper & Cook 1983). Data from Nordic countries indicate that changes in the incidence correspond with the level of screening, the effect being most pronounced in Iceland which has the most intensive screening, followed by Finland and Sweden. A smaller effect was observed in Denmark, where only 40% of women are covered by an organized screening programme. In Norway where the organized programme covered only 5% of the population the disease showed an increasing trend during the period studied (Hakama 1982).

In Scotland in an analysis of mortality data for the years 1968–76, comparing Grampian and Tayside regions, where screening was most intensive, with the rest of Scotland, Macgregor & Teper (1978) concluded that the trends in mortality in these regions were attributable to the screening programme, although the results were based on small numbers.

In England and Wales cervical screening has brought little change to the overall mortality rates from cancer of the cervix uteri since 1968. Doubts have been expressed about the effectiveness of the present programme. The more intensive screening appears to have been carried out on younger women and among those of higher social class, groups with low mortality rates for the disease (Fig. 25.7). Although it is clearly important to reach those who have never been screened, the concept that cervical screening should be concentrated on women of 35 years of age or more has been criticized because it is the younger women who have in recent times the highest rates of 'positive' smears (Souter et al 1984) and of premalignant disease of the cervix (Cook & Draper 1984). Excluding colposcopy clinic specimens Souter et al (1984) noted among 22 245 women screened an overall detection rate of 12.1 per 1000 for positive smears and a rate of the order of 15–17 per 1000 in those 23–35 years old. Other reports of an upward trend in the incidence of, and mortality from, cancer of the cervix among young women come from Canada, Australia and New Zealand (Cook & Draper 1984)

POLICIES FOR DIAGNOSTIC EXFOLIATIVE CYTOLOGY

Recommendations for cervical cancer screening in Canada (Canadian Task Force 1982) include the following:

1. Health authorities should encourage and support the development of cytology screening programmes designed to detect the precursors of clinical invasive carcinoma of the cervix.

2. Women who have had sexual intercourse should generally be advised to have screening annually between the ages of 18 and 35 and thereafter every five years until the age of 60.

3. Women over the age of 60, who have had repeated satisfactory smears without significant atypia may be dropped from a screening programme for squamous cell carcinoma of the cervix.

4. High priority should be given to encouraging women at risk who have never had a cervical cytology examination to have one and to enter a screening programme.

5. The recommended screening frequencies apply to women whose smears show no epithelial atypia. Once such changes are detected schedules for repeat examinations should be dictated by the requirements for surveillance, diagnosis, treatment and follow-up.

6. Appropriate means should be employed to inform women of their degree of risk of carcinoma of the cervix. However, no attempt should be made to categorize women at high risk on a group basis.

7. Women over 35 years of age whose contact with the health care system is through venereal disease clinics or penal institutions and who, in their own judgement or that of their physicians, are at high risk should not be discouraged from having smears more frequently than every 5 years if they request them.

8. Provincial mechanisms that establish young women's independent responsibility for health insurance purposes (usually at or about the age of 19 years) should be used to remind women that if they are sexually active

they should have a cervical smear if they have not already done so.

Reference is made by the Task Force to the value of integrating cytology screening with other screening programmes (e.g. cancer of the breast, large bowel, ovary, lung and endometrium). With respect to the use of colposcopy, this is not recommended as a screening method but as a diagnostic tool for gynaecologists, adequately trained in the technique, for localizing and assessing premalignant disease and early invasive carcinoma of the cervix in women with abnormal smears. The report refers to the need for laboratory staff and for their need to deal with sufficient numbers to develop the necessary expertise. Encouragement is given to ensure quality control; terminology and the registration should be such that data is reported also in a uniform manner. The mass screening programme should ensure the recall of individuals at regular intervals for repeat testing and that action is taken following the discovery of an abnormality. Long-term follow-up is provided for patients who have received treatment following the diagnosis of dysplasia.

Emphasis is also given to the importance of a central registry and in developing compatible data processing systems, as well as the administrative arrangements of the health care system to cope with follow-up necessary, for example, when women may move from one province to another.

In Britain the Committee on Gynaecological Cytology recently (News and Notes (Lancet) 1984) reaffirmed the emphasis previously given to the screening of women over 35 and those who had had three or more pregnancies at five-yearly intervals, particularly for women who had not been screened. For younger women their advice was that screening should take place for any woman who is or has been sexually active on her first presentation for contraceptive advice, or whenever she first requests screening. It was advised that screening should be repeated after that first occasion at the ages of 20, 25, 30 and 35 and not on any other occasion, except that every woman should be screened early in every pregnancy.

Patients attending departments of genito-urinary medicine certainly should have a cervical smear taken with Ayre's spatula for diagnostic exfoliative cytology. Ordinarily the test should be taken at the first visit, although in inflammatory states of the cervix or vagina it may be better first to treat the infection in cases where the patient is unlikely to default. Repeated tests — annually until the age of 35 years and five-yearly or more often after this age in high risk groups — as advocated by the Canadian Task Force (1982) will enable the detection of cervical intra-epithelial neoplasia in the age group in which these lesions are commonest. In patients attending departments of genito-urinary

medicine, an 'at-risk' group, the first cytology smear is carried out as a 'primary benefit' and is reassuring to the individual often made anxious by reading articles in fashionable journals or on the radio or by watching television programmes. Should dysplasia be detected, follow-up can be continued within the department and referral for colposcopy should be readily available. If the patient wishes to be discharged it is good practice to devote effort to persuade her to agree to the sending of reports to her general practitioner. In those without cervical dysplasia or other abnormality they should be encouraged to attend their general practitioner's surgery and join the screening programme available. In those with atypia in their cervical smears the follow-up will be dictated by the 'requirements for diagnosis, surveillance and treatment'. Although recent study has shown that 'flat koilocytosis' of the cervix can only be detected by colposcopy this technique is not yet widely available at clinics and, although desirable, it will be generally on the basis of the discovery of cervical intra-epithelial neoplasia that colposcopy or other gynaecological assessment will be sought. In those without atypia advice will be given to attend their general practitioner, contraceptive clinic or well woman clinic for regular cervical cytology tests. No attempt should be made to categorize women at high risk on the basis of behaviour but appropriate means should be taken to inform patients of their degree of risk.

In educating the patient and public about the possible causal relationship to cancer of the cervix of either their infection, viz. HPV, HSV-2, or some other sexually transmissible agent, or their life style, anxiety can be mitigated by an explanation and reassurance about risks. It can be said that in Britain, for example, the average annual incidence for cervical cancer is about 9–17 per 100 000 for all age groups (Fig. 25.7) and the condition can be mostly recognized and effectively treated long in advance of it becoming invasive. In England and Wales, while there has been an increase in the death rate in the 25–34 year age group (from 11 deaths per million in 1968–1970 groups to 36 per million in 1983), the numbers of deaths at ages below 35 is a small percentage of the total (in 1983 there were 1959 deaths, of which 121 (6.2%) were in those under 35 years of age) (Draper 1982, Roberts 1982, Mortality Statistics 1981–1983 included) (see also Fig. 25.7).

In discussion with the individual patient, encouragement can be given further by reference to the fact that in Iceland, for example, where the policy has been to examine every woman in the age range 25–70 once every 2–3 years, mortality fell by 60% between 1959 and, 1970 and 1975 and 1978 (Draper 1982). It can be further explained that the early lesions of squamous cell carcinoma of the uterine cervix are accessible to examination by routine screening techniques (diagnostic

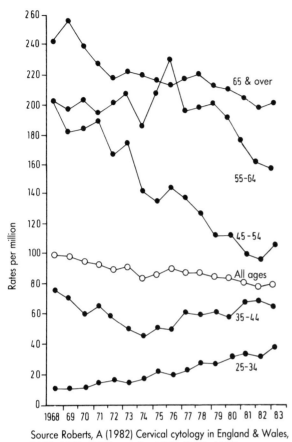

DEATHS FROM CANCER OF THE CERVIX UTERI

Source Roberts, A (1982) Cervical cytology in England & Wales, 1965–1980; OPCS mortality statistics 1981–1983

Fig. 25.7 Cancer of the cervix uteri. Age-specific death rates per million in England and Wales for the years 1968–1983. Data from Roberts (1982) and Mortality Statistics 1981–1983. Estimates of populations based on 1981 census.

exfoliative cytology). At the present time also at colposcopy the magnification of the instrument allows evaluation of the striking changes in the surface pattern of the lesion and biopsy can be obtained from accurately identified areas (Kolstad & Stafl 1983). More positively, laser and other techniques under colposcopic control allow the precise eradication of a focal lesion. The patient selected for this type of management is described as a young woman, desiring future pregnancy, who has a focal colposcopic lesion of a minor grade and columnar epithelium visible in the cervical canal (Coppleson 1977). Such patients will be discovered readily among those who attend departments of genito-urinary medicine. The optimistic and positive explanation of the situation will be of value to the anxious as well as to those attending for follow-up of detectable lesions.

In a critique of cytology screening programmes, Knox (1982) discusses the relative failures and costs in England and Wales. In broad terms Knox credits the present system with 500 deaths saved out of a total of 24 000 deaths over a period of 10 years. He notes the losses of 100 000 cervices excised and 20×10^6 smears examined over the same period. He discusses the difficulties arising from concentrating efforts and expenditure on the young when there is an undiminished death rate in the older age groups. Data based on numbers of people are faulty when hysterectomy rates are high. In 1976 almost 10% had had a hysterectomy by the age of 44 and 18% by the age of 64. Scientific and conceptual questions, also, cannot be isolated from those of resources, service responsibilities and even career structures. Endeavours will have to be made to provide adequately for the young, however, as the situation is dynamic in the population where there is an increasing prevalence of genital HPV infection.

NOTES TO CHAPTER 25

Note 25.1: Definitions

Euploid — of a cell, having each of the different chromosomes of the set present in the same number; therefore with an exact multiple of the haploid chromosome number, e.g. diploid or polyploid.

Polyploid — having three or more times the haploid number of chromosomes.

Aneuploid — having more or less than an integral multiple of the haploid number of chromosomes; therefore genetically unbalanced (Abercrombie et al 1980).

Note 25.2: Cytology of cervix uteri (fixation of smears)

Excellent fixation of smears can be obtained by using a mixture of equal parts of 96% ethanol and diethyl ether (very inflammable). Methylated 96% ethanol or 99% propan-2-ol are satisfactory alternatives. The slide should be immersed for at least 20 minutes.

REFERENCES

Abercrombie M, Hickman C J, Johnson M L 1980 The Penguin Dictionary of biology. Penguin, Harmondsworth

Abou-Daoud K T 1966 Morbidity from cancer in Lebanon. Cancer 19: 1293–1300

Alzate H 1978 Sexual behavior of Columbian female university students. Archives of Sexual Behavior 7: 1: 43–54

Alzate H 1984 Sexual behavior of unmarried Columbian university students: a five-year follow-up. Archives of Sexual Behavior 13: 2: 121–132

Anonymous 1983 Oral contraceptives and neoplasia. Editorial, Lancet ii: 947–948

Aurelian L, Kessley I I, Rosenhein N B, Barbour G 1981 Virus and gynecologic cancers. Herpesvirus protein (ICP 10/AG-4), a cervical tumour antigen that fulfills the criteria for a marker of carcinogenicity. Cancer 48: suppl: 455–471

Baird P J 1983 Serological evidence for the association of papillomavirus and cervical neoplasia. Lancet ii: 17–18

Beaudenon S, Kremsdorf D, Croissant O, Jablonska S, Wain-Hobson S, Orth G 1986 A novel type of human papillomavirus associated with genital neoplasias. Nature 321: 246–249

Beilby J O W, Bourne R, Guillebaud J, Steele S J 1982 Paired cervical smears: a method of reducing the false-negative rate in population screening. Obstetrics and Gynecology 60: 46–49

Beral V 1974 Cancer of the cervix: a sexually transmitted infection. Lancet i: 1037–1039

Bourne R, Beilby J O W 1976 Trial of new cervical spatula. Lancet i: 1330–1331

Canadian Task Force 1982 Cervical cancer screening programs. Canadian Medical Association Journal 127: 581–589

Cedarloff R, Floderus-Myrhed B 1980 Cancer mortality and morbidity among 2300 unselected twin pairs. In: Gelboin H V et al (eds) Genetic and environmental factors in experimental and human cancer. Japan Scientific Societies Press, Tokyo, p 151–160

Clarke E A, Morgan R W, Newman A M 1982 Smoking as a risk factor in cancer of the cervix: additional evidence from a case control study. American Journal of Epidemiology 115: 59–66

Cook G A, Draper G J 1984 Trends in cervical cancer and carcinoma in situ in Great Britain. British Journal of Cancer 50: 367–375

Coppleson M 1977 Colposcopy. In: Stallworthy J, Bourne G (eds) Recent advances in obstetrics and gynaecology. Churchill Livingstone, Edinburgh, p 155

Cross H E, Kennel E E, Lilienfeld A M 1968 Cancer of the cervix in an Amish population. Cancer 21: 102–108

Draper G J 1982 Screening for cervical cancer: revised policy. The recommendations of the DHSS Committee on Gynaecological Cytology. Health Trends 14: 37–40

Draper G J, Cook G A 1983 Changing patterns of cervical cancer rates. British Medical Journal 287: 510–512

Drife J 1983 Which pill? British Medical Journal 287: 1397–1399

Durst M, Gissmann L, Ikenberg H, zur Hausen H A 1983 A papillomavirus DNA from a cervical carcinoma and its prevalence in cancer biopsy samples from different geographic regions (human papillomaviruses/low-stringency hybridization/molecular cloning/genital tumours) Proceedings of the National Academy of Sciences USA 80: 3812–3815

Fletcher S 1983 Histopathology of papilloma virus infection of the cervix uteri: the history, taxonomy, nomenclature and reporting of koilocytic dysplasias. Journal of Clinical Pathology 36: 616–624

Fu Y S, Reagan J W, Richart R M 1981 Definition of 'precursors . Gynecologic Oncology 12: S220–S231

Gissman L, Wolnik L, Ikenberg H, Koldovsky U, Schnurch H G, zur Hausen H 1983 Human papilloma virus types 6 and 11 DNA sequences in genital and laryngeal papillomas and in some cervical cancers. Proceedings of the National Academy of Sciences USA 80: 560–563

Grubb C 1977 Colour atlas of gynaecological cytopathology. H M + M Publishers, Aylesbury

Hakama M 1982 Trends in the incidence of cervical cancer in the Nordic countries In: Magnus K (ed) Trends in cancer incidence. Causes and practical implications. Hemisphere Publishing Corporation, Washington, p 279–292

Hakama M 1983 Cancer of the uterine cervix. In: Bourke G J (ed) The epidemiology of Cancer. Croom Helm, London, The Charles Press, Philadelphia, p 162–175

Hakulinen T, Pukkala E, Hakama M, Lehtonen M, Saxen E, Teppo L 1981 Survival of cancer patients in Finland in 1953–1974. Annals of Clinical Research 13 (suppl.31): 50–52

Hoffken H, Soost H-J 1981 Cervical cytology as a screening

method. In: Dallenbach-Hellweg G (ed) Cervical cancer. Springer Verlag, Berlin, p 21–65

Husain O A N, Watts K C, Fray R E, To A C W 1984 Immunocytochemical markers in cervical screening. Correspondence, Lancet i: 338–339

Knox E G 1982 Cancer of the uterine cervix. In: Magnus K (ed) Trends in cancer incidence. Hemisphere Publishing Corporation, London, p 271–277

Kolstad P, Stafl A 1983 Atlas of colposcopy, 3rd revised edn. Universitetsforslaget, Oslo. University Park Press, Baltimore, Churchill Livingstone, London

Koss L G, Greenbaum E 1983 Precancerous lesions. In: Bourke G J (ed) The epidemiology of cancer. Croom Helm, London, p 31–59

Leading Article 1987 Human papillomaviruses and cervical cancer: a fresh look at the evidence. Lancet i: 725–726

McCance D J, Walker P G, Dyson J L, Coleman D V, Singer A 1983 Presence of human papillomavirus DNA in cervical intraepithelial neoplasia. British Medical Journal 287: 784–788

Macgregor J E, Teper S 1978 Mortality from carcinoma of the cervix uteri in Britain. Lancet ii: 774–776

Meanwell C A, Cox M F, Blackledge G, Maitland N J 1987 HPV 16 DNA in normal and malignant cervical epithelium: implications for the aetiology and behaviour of cervical neoplasia. Lancet i: 703–707

Meisels A, Fortin R 1976 Condylomatous lesions of the cervix and vaginal cytological patterns. Acta Cytologica 20: 505–509

Meisels A, Fortin R, Roy M 1977 Condylomatous lesions of the cervix and vagina II. Cytologic, colposcopic and histopathologic criteria. Acta Cytologica 21: 379–389

Meisels A, Morin C, Casas-Cordero M 1982 Human papillomavirus infection of the uterine cervix. International Journal of Gynaecological Pathology 1: 75–194

Mortality Statistics 1981–1983 Statistics and Research Division DHSS 14 Russell Square London WC1B 5ED

News and Notes 1984 New advice on cervical screening. Lancet i: 1196

Oriel J D 1971 Natural history of genital warts. British Journal of Venereal Diseases 47: 1–13

Osmond C, Gardner M J, Acheson E D 1982 Analysis of trends in cancer mortality in England and Wales during 1951–1980 separating changes associated with period of birth and period of death. British Medical Journal 284: 1005–1008

Osmond C, Gardner M J, Acheson E D, Adelstein A M 1983 Trends in cancer mortality 1951–1980. Analysis by period of birth and death. Office of Population Censuses and Surveys London. HMSO, DH1 No 11 VIII, 38–39

Parkin D M, Stjernsward J, Muir C S 1984 Estimates of the worldwide frequency of twelve major cancers. Bulletin of the World Health Organization 62: 163–182

Pfister H 1984 Biology and biochemistry of papillomaviruses. Reviews of Physiology, Biochemistry and Pharmacology 99: 111–167

Purola E, Savia E 1977 Cytology of gynecologic condyloma acuminatum. Acta Cytologica 21: 21–31

Richart R M 1973 Cervical intraepithelial neoplasia. In: Sommers S C (ed) Pathology Annual: 301–328

Richart R M, Barron B A 1969 A follow-up study of patients with cervical dysplasia. American Journal of Obstetrics and Gynecology 105: 386–393

Roberts A 1982 Cervical cytology in England and Wales, 1965–80. Health Trends 14: 41–43

Robertson M 1983 Oncogenes and multistep carcinogenesis. British Medical Journal 287: 1084–1086

Rotkin I D 1981 Etiology and epidemiology of cervical cancer. Current Topics in Pathology 70: 151–160

Sharp F, Duncan I D, Hare M J et al 1983 Cervical intraepithelial neoplasia. Correspondence. Lancet ii: 515

Singer A, Walker P G, McCance D J 1984 Genital wart virus infections: nuisance or potentially lethal? British Medical Journal 288: 735–737

Skegg D C G, Corwin P A, Paul C, Doll R 1982 Importance of the male factor in cancer of the cervix. Lancet ii: 581–582

Souter W P, Brough A K, Monaghan J M 1984 Cervical screening for younger women. Lancet ii: 745

Trevathan E, Layde P, Webster L A, Adams J B, Benigno B B 1983 Cigarette smoking and dysplasia and carcinoma in situ of the uterine cervix. Journal of the American Medical Association 250: 499–502

Vessey M P, Lawless M, McPherson K, Yeates D 1983 Neoplasia of the cervix uteri and contraception: a possible adverse effect of the pill. Lancet ii: 930–934

Waterhouse J, Muir C, Shanmugaratnam K, Powell J (eds) 1982 Cancer in five continents, vol 4. International Agency for Research on Cancer, Lyon

Zuckerkandl E 1984 Herpes simplex transforming fragments. Nature 311: 418

zur Hausen H 1977 Human papillomaviruses and their possible role in squamous carcinomas. Current Topics in Microbiology and Immunology 78: 1–30

26

Herpes simplex virus infection

HERPES SIMPLEX

Herpes simplex is an acute infectious disease, characterized by a sometimes recurring vesicular eruption, occurring anywhere on the skin, but most often on or near the lips or the genitals. Sometimes the infection involves the eye to cause a conjunctivitis with or without corneal involvement. The causative virus, herpes simplex virus (HSV) can be divided into two types on the basis of certain antigenic, biochemical and biological differences. Type 1 HSV (HSV-1) is usually isolated from lesions round the mouth or eye and transmitted by the direct contact of kissing or by droplet, in cases or from carriers; Type 2 HSV (HSV-2) is responsible for the majority of genital tract infections and is spread by direct contact during sexual intercourse. The very common nature of inapparent infections, whether of HSV-1 or HSV-2, is becoming better appreciated.

HERPES SIMPLEX VIRUS (HSV) (synonym — human alphaherpesvirus, see Ch. 2)

The herpesvirion consists of an electron-opaque *core*; an icosadeltahedral *capsid* (100 nm) enclosing the core; an electron-dense, asymmetrically distributed material abutting the capsid, designated the *tegument*; and an outer membrane or *envelope* which surrounds the capsid tegument. The core of the mature virion contains the viral DNA in the form of a torus (Roizman & Batterson 1985).

Herpes simplex virus is a member of the sub-family Alphaherpesvirinae, which is characterized by the capacity to cause rapid spread of infection in cell culture resulting in mass destruction of susceptible cells (Roizman et al 1981). Its mode of transmission is mainly by contact of mucosal surfaces. The Alphaherpesvirinae (see Ch. 2) discussed in this chapter consist of herpes simolex virus Types 1 and 2; brief reference is made to infection by the other member of this sub-family, varicella-zoster virus.

Virological studies at the University of Chicago have shown that the electrophoretic patterns of HSV-1 and HSV-2 DNA, cut with restriction endonucleases, vary and that epidemiologically unrelated isolates can be identified. The restriction endonuclease patterns therefore can be used as an epidemiological tool to trace the spread of virus in the human population (Buchman et al 1978, Roizman & Tognon 1982) although care is needed in interpretation. DNA restriction endonuclease patterns among virus isolates show two kinds of differences: 1. with respect to the presence or absence of cleavage sites; and 2. with respect to electrophoretic mobility of DNA fragments. The latter is suggestive of variation in the number of specific sequences contained in those fragments. Roizman & Tognon (1982) advise that conclusions should be reached on the presence or absence of known *cleavage sites*. Variability in the restriction endonuclease patterns reflects spontaneous insertions, deletions and substitution of bases at non-lethal sites in the HSV DNA. Such mutations do occur spontaneously in the human population but at a slow rate and although perpetuated, when the mutated virus is transmitted, only a small fraction of the virus population in an individual will exhibit this mutation. With the technique (Note 26.1) it has been possible to 'fingerprint' HSV isolates (Linnemann et al 1978) — for further discussion see Distribution of herpesvirus types, p. 331.

NATURAL HISTORY OF HERPES SIMPLEX

In most virus infections affecting humans the virus rapidly establishes itself in susceptible cells, is replicated, and after a few days it and its progeny are eliminated by host-mediated immunity. In a number of viruses, however, and in particular in herpes simplex virus and varicella-zoster virus, an elegant strategem has been evolved by which, in spite of immunity, the virus can persist in the host for life and also provide for its spread to other hosts. In a discussion on the natural history of herpes simplex virus infection it is necessary first to define and name the various events in infection.

The definitions given below are based on those of Wildy and his Cambridge colleagues (1982) but modified to take into account suggestions made by Rawls (1985); clinical and virological features in herpes genitalis at various stages in its natural history are represented diagrammatically in Figure 26.1.

1. *Primary infection.* This is an infection which may be asymptomatic, remain localized, or become generalized in an individual who has not been previously infected with either type of HSV as shown by a lack of antibodies to herpes viruses.

2. *Initial infection.* This denotes the first infection of

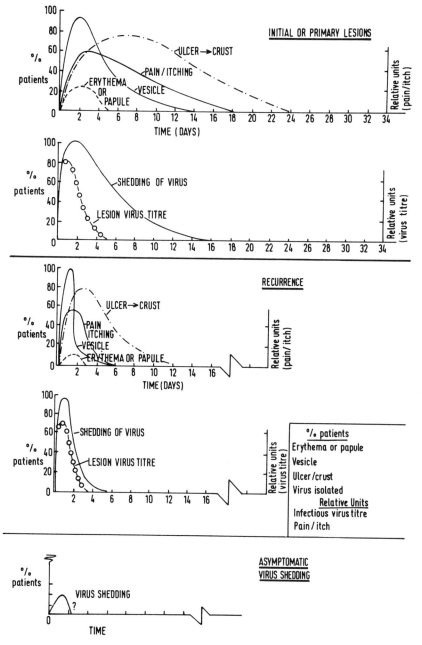

Fig. 26.1 Diagrammatic representation of surface clinical and virological features in herpes genitalis at various stages in its natural history. The patterns evolve during the approximate times shown and latency is indicated by the horizontal axis (based on Wildy et al 1982, Spruance et al 1977, Rawls 1985, and other sources — see text).

a virus type. It may be a *primary infection* in those *without* serological evidence of a previous herpetic infection or a *non-primary* in those *with* evidence of previous infection. Clinically primary and non-primary initial infections may be indistinguishable on physical examination.

3. *Latency*. There is apparent recovery but some virus remains dormant in nervous tissue, particularly in certain sensory ganglion cells; this is latency (latent means hidden).

4. *Reactivation*. Virus may be reawakened spontaneously, or as a result of external stimuli, so that infective virus may once again be found.

5. *Recurrence*. The reactivated virus may on occasion initiate a peripheral lesion in the dermatome relating to the sensory ganglion. The lesion is referred to as a *recurrent lesion* and the phenomenon is *recurrence*. Wildy et al (1982) used the term 'recrudescence' to describe this phenomenon but since the term 'recurrence' is deeply embedded in the literature it is used instead (Rawls 1985).

6. *Axonal transport*. The whole phenomenon requires translation of the virus from the periphery to the sensory ganglion and back again by way of, it is believed, the cytoplasm within the axon. The rate of translocation from the skin to the ganglion lies within the range of 2–10 mm per hour.

7. *Asymptomatic virus shedding*. Sometimes the virus evidently reactivates and passes to a peripheral site but fails to cause a noticeable lesion, although it probably multiplies and can be isolated. The term asymptomatic virus shedding (Rawls 1985) is used in this situation to distinguish this event from *recurrence*.

The cell bodies of the sensory neurones are situated in the dorsal root ganglia, and the axons of these cells pass to the dorsal columns of the spinal cord and peripherally to the skin. Each dorsal root ganglion innervates an area of skin, called the dermatome. The ganglion cell, the sensory nerve and the skin it innervates occupy the area of operation of both herpes simplex virus and varicella-zoster virus and is conveniently called the *neurodermatome*.

Herpes simplex is the commonest virus infection encountered in man, and as a successful parasitic agent herpesvirus has few equals. It is able to infect generally without causing serious disease, it is readily transmitted from person to person and can persist in its host.

Notwithstanding the wide variation in the severity of clinical disease in *primary infection* the majority appear to be asymptomatic. The severity of signs and symptoms in primary infection appears to be age-related; usually asymptomatic infections occur in the 2–3 year age group and symptomatic in the adolescent or young adult. In the majority of cases of clinically apparent disease the lesions are localized to the site of inoculation, the sensory neurons innervating that site, and the lymphatics draining it. Spread to contiguous areas or transfer to more distant sites by auto-inoculation can also occur. Although primary infections can occur at any site, the lesions are characteristically vesicles affecting the mucosa and/or adjacent skin of the mouth or genitals which evolve rapidly into greyish or yellowish painful shallow ulcers.

As the virus diminishes in quantity in the primary lesion at the periphery, so infectious virus, it is believed from laboratory evidence, is to be found in increasing titres in the sensory ganglion within days of the infection. The theory that translation of virus from the periphery to the sensory ganglion occurs by axonal transport is the orthodox view; it may be, however, that the virus migrates to the ganglia by systemic routes and accumulates in neurons by a continuous supply from the site of primary infection. Within a week or two, however, infectious virus cannot be found in the ganglion and the infection becomes latent. Latent virus may also be recoverable from affected autonomic ganglia. During latency virus cannot be recovered from skin or mucosal sites where herpes lesions have previously occurred. The virus may, however, be reactivated as infectious virus under appropriate conditions and travels peripherally along the axon to the epithelial site where replication may give rise to local lesions that may be apparent to the patient (termed recurrence or recurrent lesions) or inapparent (termed asymptomatic virus shedding). Reactivation may be induced by trauma to the affected sensory ganglion, trauma or exposure to UV light to the previously affected epithelial surface site, immunosuppression by drugs or bacterial infections, e.g. pneumococci. Recurrent lesions are less severe than primary. *Non-primary initial infections* with a heterologous type are less severe than *primary initial infections* (Klein 1982, Wildy et al 1982, Rawls 1985).

Asymptomatic virus shedding occurs in between 1 and 5% of adults in their oral secretions. In the case of genital secretions this depends upon age and sexual behaviour. Among groups undergoing cervicovaginal examinations, female university students and pregnant women, levels of 0.5% may be found; in those attending clinics dealing with sexually transmitted disease, virus shedding is found in 1.6–6.9%. Asymptomatic virus shedding is thus a substantial source of virus (Update, World Health Organization 1985a, & b).

The majority of the adult population, including women of childbearing age, particularly in the lower socio-economic groups, carry neutralizing antibody to HSV. This antibody is transferred across the placenta and confers passive immunity to the newborn child, but antibody will have disappeared by the age of six to eight months, when a primary infection can then occur in the non-immune infant. The commonest time at which the infection is acquired, particularly in lower socio-economic groups, is between two and three years of age. Primary infections at this age are HSV-l infections and the vast majority are subclinical; in an important early study, only between 1 and 11% of children showed some manifestation clinically, usually of stomatitis (Spence et al 1954). Following primary infection antibody appears and usually remains at a constant level for a prolonged period, although it may decline until re-infection or reactivation may bring about an increase and stabilization of the titre. As the amounts of virus antigen produced may influence the magnitude of response, in many recurrent infections where virus replication is limited little or no increase in virus antibody may be observed.

DISTRIBUTION OF HERPESVIRUS TYPES

HSV Type 1 may occasionally be recovered from saliva, tears and the genital tract between attacks and regularly from lesions during attacks. In the case of HSV-2, as well as in HSV-l, asymptomatic carriers probably constitute the principal source of infection. The virus may be isolated in such cases from the cervix in the female or from the urethra in the male; symptoms or signs of urethritis may be absent or slight. Transmission occurs by direct or very close contact with a person who is shedding virus with or without a lesion; transmission is probably more likely when there is a lesion producing a high virus titre. A herpetic whitlow — a painful HSV infection of a digit, a recognized occupational hazard of medical, paramedical and dental personnel (Watkinson 1982) — gave rise to an outbreak of herpetic gingivostomatitis among 20 of 46 patients seen in a dental hygiene practice (Manzella et al 1984). In the sexually active age groups spread occurs by sexual intercourse, kissing or direct or indirect orogenital contact.

In the case of genital lesions HSV-1 is less commonly found than HSV-2. In Edinburgh 16% of male patients with genital herpes were infected with HSV-l; in females the proportion of HSV-l isolates from genital lesions was substantially higher (31%) (Smith et al 1973, Peutherer et al 1982). Similar results were obtained from women in Japan (Kawana et al 1976), and in Sweden (Wolontis & Jeansson 1977) about 17% of genital lesions of both sexes were caused by HSV-l. This rate is similar to that found in Edinburgh (21.4%) and both studies emphasize the importance of HSV-1 genital infections in young patients. In the USA, on the other hand, studies have shown a lower recovery of HSV-1 (9.1% for females and 3.4% for males), a finding

perhaps explained by differing social background of patients.

In higher socio-economic groups high proportions (40–90%) may have no antibody to either HSV-1 or HSV-2 whereas the corresponding figure in lower groups is only 20%. HSV-1 is associated with the mouth and stomatitis but genital infection is likely to occur, particularly in populations where 30% of young adults (15–24 years) are without antibody to HSV (Smith et al 1967). Orogenital contact or contact of the genitals with saliva-contaminated fingers may be the means of transmitting the virus. In two male patients simultaneous oral and urethral infections have been observed and in one female both oral and cervical infections. The presence of the virus at these separate sites at the same time in a primary infection suggests simultaneous infection of oral and genital mucosae by one partner. HSV-l was only seen once in a homosexual male.

Recurrent lesions in genital sites are not as frequent in HSV-l infections as in those of HSV-2 (Kawana et al 1976); this could be due to relative inefficiency of HSV-1 in establishing a latent infection of the sensory nerve cells in the sacral ganglia. Prospective studies showed that among patients with a first episode of HSV-1 genital infection only 14% experienced a subsequent recurrence in contrast to 60% of those with a HSV-2 infection (Reeves et al 1981). Recurrent oral lesions are mostly due to HSV-1 whereas recurrent genital lesions are mostly due to HSV-2; such differences may represent selective advantage for establishing latency and reactivation in ganglia innervating oral and genital tissues respectively (Update, World Health Organization 1985a, b).

Complement fixation and neutralization tests can be applied to the serum of patients to determine their antibody status. Complement fixing antibody can be detected before neutralizing antibody, and conversion from absence of antibody to its presence in serum will signify a primary infection, which can occur in the genital area with either Type 1 or Type 2.

Using the restriction endonuclease patterns of HSV DNA to 'fingerprint' the virus isolates on the basis of the presence or absence of known cleavage sites it has been possible to begin to study the spread of the agent in the community (Buchman et al 1978). The possibility of transmission of HSV-l within a nursery for the newborn has been confirmed (Linnemann et al 1978). With the technique it has been shown that in most patients suffering from recurrent lesions of genital herpes, even in those with new partners the symptomatic recurrence of virus at a peripheral mucosal or skin site results from endogenous reactivation of latent virus, and reinfection with new strains was uncommon (Schmidt et al 1984). Insofar as HSV-1 is concerned, the number of variable cleavage sites (e.g. recognition sites for deletions and insertions in the virus genome) appears to be very large (viz. 87) (Chaney et al 1983a, b) and hence there may be very large numbers (87!) of recognizably different subtypes of HSV-l in a community (Note 26.2). In contrast, in HSV-2 the number of variable cleavage sites appears to be much smaller (11) (Chaney et al 1983a) and hence the number of subtypes of HSV-2 in a community will be very much lower in number (of the order of 11!). Restriction endonuclease analysis for epidemiological tracing of HSV-l is useful but because there is only a small number of variable cleavage sites in the HSV-2 genome caution is needed in the extrapolation of the results of HSV-2 analysis to establish proof of the source of an infection (Smith et al 1981, I W Smith — personal communication — 1985).

IMMUNITY IN HSV INFECTION

Herpes simplex virus persists throughout the life of the individual infected and achieves this by mechanisms which enable it to avoid host responses, viz. the ability of the virus to pass from cell to cell by a fusion process circumventing the need to emerge into the extracellular environment; to secure latent infection of a neuronal cell, by a mechanism as yet not precisely known; and to evade natural defence systems of the host, i.e. macrophages, natural killer cells and interferon.

Evidence about humoral immunity can be obtained from the study of infection in man but most of the data on other aspects of its natural history or cell-mediated immunity is obtained from animal studies, particularly in mice, where supplementary evidence indicates that the mouse is a useful model for studying the infection.

Following infection there are both humoral and cell-mediated immune responses lasting many years. HSV-l and HSV-2 possess shared antigenic determinants so that infection with one results in the production of antibodies and lymphocytes which will react with the other.

Primary infection yields a rise in antibody with titres reaching a peak in about 4–6 weeks and remaining stable afterwards. Virus-specific IgM antibodies are produced in the early stages and persist for 6–8 weeks.

In individuals with pre-existing antibodies recurrence is not associated with a marked change in antibody titre; similarly reinfection with the same or different type of virus produces little change. In neither recurrence or reinfection is there an IgM response unless the infection is extensive, when there may be an IgM and an IgG response.

In the newborn passively transferred maternal antibodies are often present but are gradually lost during the first six months of life. HSV-1 antibodies appear in childhood more often in the lower socio-economic groups than in the higher, in whom HSV-1 and HSV-2 are therefore more likely to produce a primary infection during adolescence and early adult life.

At least three immunological responses contribute to the clearance of virus: antibody, specific cytotoxic T-cells and specific delayed hypersensitivity. Antibody hinders the establishment of persisting infection and in high concentration may prevent the invasion of the nervous system. T-cells are essential for protective immunity, but which type is not clear (Wildy & Gell 1985).

The nature of ganglionic latency is enigmatic and what controls the state is unknown.

PATHOLOGY

The basic lesion is one of localized necrosis. The nuclei of affected cells become swollen and the chromatin marginated. A dense basophilic mass fills the whole nucleus and later retracts from the nuclear margin. Finally an eosinophilic intranuclear inclusion appears (the Lipschutz or Cowdry type A inclusion); all stages may be found in any one section.

The lesions of the skin and mucous membrane are characterized by intra-epidermal vesicle formation. The earliest changes can be seen in epithelial cells in the middle epidermal layer. Intracellular and extracellular oedema leads to formation in the epidermis of a vesicle with a thin-walled roof. The inflammatory cells at this stage are mainly mononuclear. With rupture and maceration of the vesicles polymorphonuclear leucocytic infiltration follows. The margins of the vesicles are usually clearly demarcated showing a sudden transformation from normal epithelium to balloon degeneration and multinucleate epithelial cells containing basophilic and eosinophilic inclusions.

The histological characteristics of HSV proctitis include the presence of multinucleate cells, intranuclear inclusions and lymphocytic infiltration around submucosal vessels (Goodell et al 1983).

In severe disseminated infections visceral lesions consist of parenchymal lesions of coagulative necrosis with specific intranuclear changes. In the liver and adrenals, the areas of focal necrosis can be seen with the naked eye. In early encephalitis, necrosis is a marked feature and in the adult form, there is asymmetrical softening with numerous haemorrhages on the surface of affected areas. The temporal lobes and the posterior orbital gyri are most commonly affected (Dudgeon 1970).

CLINICAL FEATURES

The very common nature of inapparent infections, whether by HSV Type 1 or 2, is becoming better appreciated with increasing availability and improvement of isolation techniques. When apparent, the prepatent or incubation period of HSV-1 or HSV-2 infections lies between 3 and 9 days (Update, World Health Organization 1985a).

Primary infections

Primary herpetic gingivostomatitis is the commonest clinical manifestation of primary infection of HSV-1 in children between 1 and 5 years of age. The stomatitis begins with fever, malaise, restlessness and excessive dribbling. Drinking and eating are very painful and the breath is foul. Vesicles containing high titres of virus appear as white plaques on the tongue, pharynx, palate and buccal mucosa. The plaques are followed by ulcers with a yellowing pseudo-membrane. Regional lymph nodes are enlarged and tender (Nagington et al 1986). An identical clinical picture may be seen in adolescents and young adults who escaped infection in childhood but acquired the infection by kissing someone with a 'primary infection': most often a reactivated lesion or 'cold sore' is the source of the virus. The lesions usually heal in 10–14 days. Virus shedding continues for 14–21 days on average after the appearance of lesions caused by a primary infection (Update, World Health Organization 1985a).

The prevalence of antibodies against HSV-1 in young adults of developed countries appears to be declining, indicating that infections in childhood are less common. In this situation primary infections in adolescence become more common and, as in ocular infections (Darougar et al 1985), more severe clinical forms of the disease in this age group will be seen more often.

Herpes genitalis

In the experience of Corey et al (1983a) in Seattle, SA, first episode genital herpes systemic symptoms occurred in 67%; local pain and itching in 98%; dysuria in 63% and tender adenopathy in 80%. Fever, headache, malaise and myalgia tended to last for more than 2 days; to reach a peak in severity at 4 days; and to last longer in the female than in the male: these symptoms were seen in 39% of men and 68% of women with primary HSV-2 infections. Complications such as aseptic meningitis were noted in 8%; sacral autonomic nervous system dysfunction in 2% and the development of extragenital lesions in 20%. The frequency of constitutional symptoms; the number of lesions; and the duration of symptoms were similar for HSV-1 and HSV-2 primary infections. In those with non-primary first episode HSV-2 infections the frequency of constitutional symptoms was lower and their duration shorter. Thus a previous attack of HSV-1 appeared to lessen the severity of first episode genital herpes. Tender inguinal adenopathy appeared during the second and third week and

was often the last sign to resolve; this manifestation tended to last longer in the female than in the male.

Primary herpes genitalis in the female

Signs and symptoms of primary genital herpes tend to be more severe in women than in men and are usually those of vulvovaginitis accompanied by systemic symptoms of fever and malaise; local pain and dysuria can be severe. Difficulty in starting micturition or retention may be the presenting clinical feature. White plaques are present on the red swollen mucosae of the vulva, cervix and occasionally the vagina (4%); scattered vesicles are seen on the labia and these may extend to involve the perianal skin and the skin of the thigh (Fig. 26.2). The regional lymphatic glands are enlarged and tender and there may be a vaginal discharge. Healing tends to take place over a period of 1 or 2 weeks, but new lesions sometimes continue to develop over a period of 6 weeks.

In primary cervicitis there may be only swelling and redness of the mucosa but sometimes there is a necrotic ulceration and friability of the cervix which bleeds

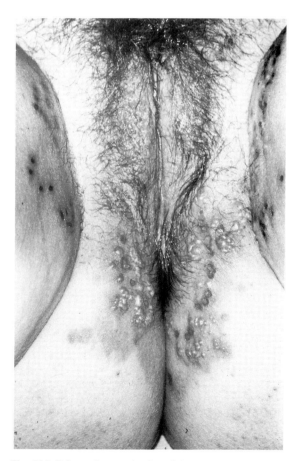

Fig. 26.2 Primary herpes simplex of the vulva.

Table 26.1 Clinical features, treatment and outcome in severe primary herpes simplex virus infection in 9 women in the third trimester of pregnancy.

Reference, year, place	Age (years)	Gestation period weeks	Site of lesions	Main serious manifestations (diagnosis by)	HSV isolations, type when known (anatomical site)	Specific anti-HSV therapy	Outcome Mother	Outcome Fetus
1. Flewett et al 1969, England	24*	28	Mouth, pharynx	HSV hepatitis (biopsy)., Thrombocytopenia	Yes (mouth). Yes (liver biopsy)	None	Recovery	Died (spontaneous abortion, intrauterine death, 31 wks)
2. Anderson & Nicholls 1972, England	19	nr term	Pharynx	HSV encephalitis (biopsy). HSV & necrosis of olfactory bulbs, temporoparietal and hippocampal regions (autopsy).	Microscopy (brain biopsy).	Idoxuridine (i.v.)	Died	Lived (spontaneous delivery)
3. Goyette et al 1974, USA	23	28	Pharynx	HSV hepatitis (autopsy)	Yes, HSV-1 (autopsy material).	None	Died	Died (intrauterine death)
4. Young et al 1976, USA	21*	37	Lower genital tract	HSV hepatitis (biopsy). Pancreatitis (amylase, inspection). Encephalitis (fits, EEG, CSF protein raised). Myocarditis (bradycardia).	Yes, HSV-2 (liver biopsy).	Vidarabine (i.v.)	Recovery	Lived (Caesarean section)
5. Hensleigh et al 1979, USA	19	30	"	HSV hepatitis (autopsy), Coagulopathy (fibrinogen low).	Yes, HSV-2 (lower genital tract blood, ascitic fluid).	None	Died	Lived (Caesarean section, 31 wks)
6. Peacock & Sarubbi 1983, USA	18*	28	"	HSV hepatitis (biopsy). Pancreatitis (amylase)	Yes, HSV-2 (cervix, foot, urine).	Vidarabine (i.v.)	Recovery	Lived (Caesarean section 29 wks. Died after 12 days (hyaline membrane disease, renal failure, subarachnoid haemorrhage)
7. do.	30*	27	"	Hepatitis (plasma enzyme tests). Distant extragenital skin lesions.	Yes, (lower genital tract, liver biopsy).	None	Recovery	Lived (Caesarean section, 32 wks)

8. Grover et al 1985, USA	20*	32	"	Dispersed vesicles on arms, legs, foot, lips, tongue, pharynx, ulcers of cervix uteri.	Yes, HSV-2 (oropharynx, endocervix, arm, thigh).	Acyclovir (i.v.) 2 × 5-day courses	Recovery but recurrence with vesicles (re-treated)	Lived (Caesarean section at term after rupture of membranes)
9. Brown et al** 1985, Scotland	28	34	"	Pyrexia, vomiting, acetonuria, albuminuria, extension of lower genital tract lesions.	Yes, HSV-2 (lower genital tract).	Acyclovir (i.v., 6 doses) (orally, 19 doses of 200 mg)	Recovery	Lived (Caesarean section, 35 wks)

*Cases considered to be primary infection on the basis of HSV serum antibody tests (seroconversion; significant rise in titre; or high titre in the first test, viz. 1:512); the other cases were deemed to be primary on the basis of history and clinical features.
**Unpublished; included with permission of Dr A D G Brown, Department of Obstetrics, Eastern General Hospital, Edinburgh.

easily. The range of clinical effects is wide and asymptomatic cases are common.

Severe primary HSV infection with systemic dissemination of virus in pregnant women

Primary infection with systemic dissemination of HSV appears to be rare in immunocompetent adults but fulminating systemic HSV infection in pregnant women during the last trimester, although rare also, is a recognized and important clinical entity with a high mortality in both mother and fetus. In 7 cases of such maternal infections, traced in the medical literature, there were 3 maternal and 3 fetal or neonatal deaths (Table 26.1: see references in Table). With the advent of acyclovir treatment it is clearly very important that the clinician should be aware of the condition and of the opportunity to halt the infection and to save life. The main manifestations in 9 cases (8 reported in the literature) are summarized in Table 26.1 and the clinical features

detailed in Table 26.2. Figure 26.3 illustrates the important point that there is an initial phase of mild–moderate clinical severity merging into a second phase with severe signs and symptoms. In Cases 1, 3, 4, 5, 6, 7 and possibly in Case 8 the primary infection was characterized by haematogenous dissemination of the virus; in Case 2 necropsy findings of olfactory bulb necrosis together with virus isolation from the temporal lobe supported the hypothesis that the virus spread by the direct neural and not the haematogenous route; in Case 8 haematogenous spread was suspected from the clinical picture. The outcome is not predictable in the individual case and the phase of severe effects may be as short in duration as 16 hours before death. In the cases described and illustrated (Tables 26.1, 26.2; Fig. 26.3) the duration of definite illness varied from 6–20 days with vomiting and pyrexia being the predominant signs of systemic illness in women affected in the third trimester; liver-related plasma enzymes are

Table 26.2 Severe primary herpes simplex virus infection with suspected or actual dissemination in 9 pregnant women in the third trimester. Maternal signs and symptoms are given according to the frequency reported (see also Table 26.1 and Fig. 26.3).

Symptoms	Numbers affected	Signs	Numbers affected
Fever	5	Pyrexia	6*
Vomiting	4	Ulcers/vesicles of lower genital tract	5
Sore throat	3	do. of mouth & pharynx	4*
Vulval pain	3	Stupor, coma	2
Malaise	3	Tachycardia	2
Nausea	2	Anxiety, agitation	2
Anorexia	2	Tonic/clonic seizures	2
Breathlessness	2	Ulcers/vesicles, extragenital	2
Myalgia	2	Adenitis	2
Dysuria	2	Collapse	1
Vaginal discharge	2	Dysphasia	1*
Abdominal pain	2	Bradycardia	1
Sore mouth	1	Hemiparesis	1*
Backache	1	Hyperventilation	1
Cough	1	Cyanosis	1
Constipation	1	Slight jaundice	1
Headache	1	Pale faeces	1
		Hepatomegaly	1
		Splenomegaly	1
Blood/plasma chemistry		*Biopsy/autopsy diagnosis*	
Aspartate aminotransferase raised	4	Hepatitis (liver biopsy/autopsy +	
Alkaline phosphatase raised	3	inclusions + focal necrosis + hepatitis)	3
Alanine aminotransferase raised	2	Encephalitis (biopsy)	1
Lactic dehydrogenase raised	2	*Urine*	
Amylase raised	2	Albuminuria	2
Bilirubin raised	2	Acetonuria	1
Urea raised	1	*CSF*	
Fibrinogen lowered	1	Protein raised	1
ECG abnormalities		*Haematology*	
Myocarditis	2	Primitive leucocytes	6
		Nucleated erythrocytes	2
		Platelets diminished	1

*These features were found in the single case of maternal herpes encephalitis; dysphasia, hemihypaesthesia, hemianopia and deterioration in level of consciousness also developed before death.

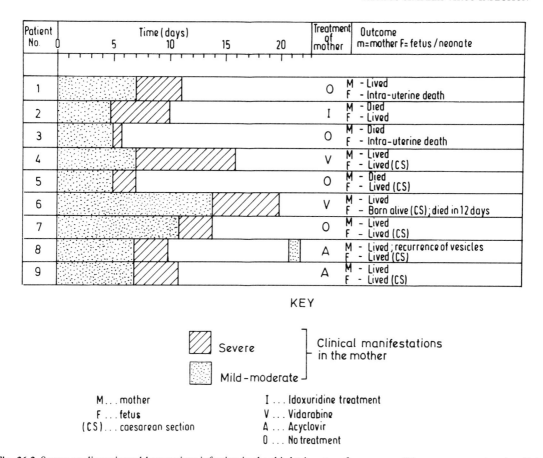

KEY

Severe ⎤
Mild-moderate ⎦ Clinical manifestations in the mother

M ... mother
F ... fetus
(CS) ... caesarean section

I ... Idoxuridine treatment
V ... Vidarabine
A ... Acyclovir
O ... No treatment

Fig. 26.3 Severe or disseminated herpesvirus infection in the third trimester of pregnancy. Diagram representing the clinical course of infection showing the time scale of mild-moderate and severe clinical manifestations. Fuller details are given in Table 26.1 and explanations in the text.

often raised and herpetic hepatitis is common in this serious form of HSV infection. Early diagnosis is very important and the characteristic primary lesions, viz. vesicles or painful ulcers of the vulva with or without involvement of the cervix or of the mouth and pharynx are seen in the majority. It should be emphasized however that the patient may not give a spontaneous history of either genital or throat lesions owing to the predominant systemic symptoms, particularly of fever and vomiting (for discussion on intravenous acyclovir treatment, see p. 342).

Primary herpes genitalis in the male

In primary herpes genitalis in the male the lesions can involve the glans or coronal sulcus and, if severe, there may be a phimosis with accumulation of secondarily infected exudate and occasionally a resulting necrotizing balanitis. In rare instances a necrotizing balanitis (Peutherer et al 1979) may develop without phimosis. In the circumcised, herpes genitalis is less common.

Crops of vesicles may develop on the shaft of the penis, on the anterior aspect of the scrotum and on the skin nearby.

In the homosexual the ano-rectum may be involved. Anorectal pain, constipation, tenesmus, anal pruritus, difficulty in starting micturition, paraesthesia in the sacral area, pain in the back of the thigh, fever and enlargement of the inguinal lymph nodes are more characteristic of proctitis due to HSV than that due to other causes (Goodell et al 1983). Vesicles or shallow ulcers of the perianal or anal region will be seen on examination with the proctoscope. The ulcers are hyperalgesic. There may be friability of the rectal mucosa, and petechiae may form on its surface when touched with a cotton-wool swab. Occasionally there are vesicles or pustules and a diffuse ulceration of the distal 10 cm of the rectal mucosa, very seldom extending to the sigmoid colon (Shah & Scholz 1983).

Herpesvirus may be acquired at other sites by contact, as in herpetic whitlow, seen in patients and medical personnel, as 'scrumpox' in the case of rugby players, or on the trunk among wrestlers. Other forms include *keratoconjunctivitis* and *eczema herpeticum*, where infection has become superimposed on eczematous skin (Kaposi's varicelliform eruption).

The significance of the immune responses becomes clinically evident in a variety of immunodeficiency states in which HSV infection or reactivation may lead to severe local or general disease, e.g. malnutrition, Wiskott-Aldrich syndrome (Note 26.3), lymphoma, immunosuppresive therapy in renal transplantation and in the Acquired Immune Deficiency Syndrome (AIDS) (Ch. 31).

Complicated primary herpes genitalis

Aseptic meningitis

Fever, severe headache, malaise, photophobia, neck rigidity and the presence of Kernig's or Brudzinski's sign indicate meningeal involvement. There is a lymphocyte pleocytosis (5–1000 per mm³) in the CSF which diminishes spontaneously. In the Seattle experience of Corey et al (1983a) this complication may occur within 6–12 days of onset in 36% of women and 13% of men. In 0.5–3.0% HSV-2 has been isolated from the CSF.

Sacral autonomic dysfunction

Sacral anaesthesia, urinary retention, requiring intermittent catheterization, and constipation may occur. The patient may complain of numbness and tingling in the buttocks or of perineal pain and there may be a decrease in perception of fine touch. Urinary retention and constipation may follow. In men impotence is associated with decrease in the bulbocavernosus reflex.

Acute retention

Uncommonly, acute retention may occur and persist for a week or more in association with an attack of anogenital herpes in women particularly, but sometimes also in the homosexual male. Although pain may be responsible, constipation, blunting of sensation over sacral dermatomes and neuralgic pains in the same area and sometimes absence of the bulbocavernosus reflex suggest involvement of sacral nerve roots (Oates & Greenhouse 1978).

Extragenital lesions

Extragenital herpetic lesions may occur nearby, particularly in the buttocks, groin or thighs. Any site may be involved, including the finger (in 8% in the Seattle series of Corey et al 1983a) and conjunctivitis may also occur.

Upper urogenital tract infection

Lower abdominal pain and tenderness of the uterine adnexae accompany involvement of the urogenital tract.

Oesophagitis

Primary herpetic oesophagitis may be encountered as a rarity in the apparently immunocompetent adult without accompanying lesions of the lip or gingivostomatitis. Presenting with severe retrosternal or subxiphoid pain on swallowing, endoscopy of the oesophagus has shown diffuse and sometimes coalescent ulcers, 0.2–1.5 cm in diameter, of the mucosa, which may be haemorrhagic (Owensby & Stammer 1978).

Dissemination

In the rare disseminated infections in adults, HSV Type 2 can be isolated from vesicular or pustular lesions that may appear anywhere on the body. In such cases HSV meningitis or encephalitis does not necessarily occur (see above in section on severe primary HSV infection with systemic dissemination of virus in pregnant women).

Recurrence and recurrent lesions in HSV infection

After the primary or initial infection, whether obvious or inapparent, there may be no further clinical manifestations throughout life. Certain febrile illnesses, such as malaria and pneumonia, provoke attacks in those in whom the disease is latent. Exposure to sunlight, menstruation or emotional stress may have a similar effect.

In the commonest form of herpes of the face, lips or genitals, itching or burning precedes by an hour or two the development of small, closely grouped vesicles on a sometimes slightly raised erythematous base. Ordinarily healing is complete within a week or ten days. The shallow ulcers which develop may be very painful. Recurrent ulcers tend to be in the same region but not precisely on the same site.

In herpes simplex of the genitals, or indeed in any site, recurrences may be heralded by a prodromal sensation of tingling. Mostly several small vesicular lesions appear and may coalesce. Lesions tend to increase in size over the first three days of the episode, remain static for about a week and resolve rapidly thereafter. Constitutional symptoms are infrequent. Symptoms tend to be more severe in the female than in the male.

After a primary genital herpes simplex due to HSV-1 recurrent episodes were reported in 55% of patients compared with 88% of patients with primary genital herpes simplex due to HSV-2. A mean recurrence rate of 0.09 recurrences per month has been reported after primary genital HSV-l infection compared with 0.03 per month in the case of primary genital HSV-2 infections (Corey et al 1983a).

Complications and sequelae

Complications and sequelae are uncommon. On the penis there may be some depigmentation and scarring of the affected site, particularly when there have been multiple recurrences over months or years. In the eye, repeated attacks of ulceration may result in corneal opacity.

Recurrences of herpes genitalis can be more than a temporary annoyance. Virus shedding tends to continue for 3–7 days after the appearance of such lesions (Update, World Health Organization 1985a). The involvement of sexual partners and anxieties, engendered by unpredictable reappearance of lesions, are sometimes heightened by concern over the possible oncogenic effect in relation to carcinoma of the cervix (Ch. 25). Transmission to the fetus and newborn may have serious implications, which are discussed later in this chapter.

DIAGNOSIS

In herpes simplex involving the genitals, it is essential to exclude other sexually transmitted diseases, particularly syphilis, gonorrhoea and chlamydial infection, which may have been acquired concurrently. All genital lesions should be examined carefully to exclude syphilis. It is good practice to carry out at least two dark ground examinations or tests based upon monoclonal antibody (p. 118) on all ulcers unless clearly due to HSV alone. The localized cluster of vesicles on an erythematous base and the exquisite hyperalgesia of herpes simplex ulcer are sufficiently characteristic to permit a diagnosis to be made with a fairly high degree of accuracy by physical examination — in recurrent lesions of the peroral or genital area, in particular. In primary HSV infections of the pharynx shallow ulceration of the pharynx or tonsil will help to differentiate the condition from a bacterial causal infection. Perianal lesions will need careful differentiation from atypical early lesions in syphilis.

Cells from lesions may contain characteristic intranuclear inclusions. Multinucleated giant cells can also be found in scrapings as, for example, in cervical smears. Virus particles may be also found in lesion material by electronmicroscopy, but the different herpesviruses cannot be distinguished by microscopy alone. Viral antigens are detectable in cells using immunofluorescence or enzyme-linked immune techniques. In the case of vesicular lesions diagnosis by tissue culture of lesion

material is more sensitive as infectious virus is usually present. In later ulcers or in crusted lesions where the virus cannot be isolated the diagnosis can be better made by the detection of antigen (Rawls 1985).

Isolations are best made from vesicular fluid, when present, and/or exudate; cellular debris is gently scraped from the lesions with a cotton-wool applicator. The specimen obtained is then agitated in a bijou bottle containing virus transport medium (Cruickshank et al 1975). The virus is isolated in tissue culture of human embryo (lung) cells, which can support a wide range of viruses, including HSV and cytomegalovirus in particular.

In the case of first episode primary herpes genitalis, Corey et al (1983a) record that herpesvirus may be isolated also from the urethra and pharynx of 28% and 7% of men and from the urethra, cervix and pharynx of 82, 88 and 13% respectively of women.

Virus isolates may be characterized in the laboratory by antigenic, biological, or biochemical typing by various methods described below.

Typing herpesvirus isolates

Pock size on the chorio-allantoic membrane
Inoculation of the chorio-allantoic membrane (CAM) of 10–12–day-old embryonated eggs is followed by incubation at 35°C for 7 days, when the CAM is excised, fixed in formol saline, and the diameters of at least six discrete pocks measured. HSV-l produces pocks less than 0.75 mm and HSV-2 pocks of 1.0 mm or greater. With care, this test can be used in typing various isolates, but it has been superseded by other tests.

Cytopathic effect (CPE)
In BHK (baby hamster kidney) and fibroblast cells, HSV-l produces a CPE characterized by the formation of rounded cells, whereas HSV-2 is characterized by the formation of fusiform syncytia in addition to round cells. This method of distinguishing the two types is rapid, 48 hours being sufficient in most cases, and observations can be made on unstained preparations.

Filament production in nuclei
Monolayers of BHK, Vero or Hep-2 (Note 26.4) cells, are inoculated with sufficient virus to give complete cytopathic effect (CPE) in 24 hours. After fixation in glutaraldehyde, post-fixing in osmium tetroxide and embedding in araldite, sections are examined by electronmicroscopy. HSV-2 produces filaments (Smith et al 1973) in the nuclei of infected cells in addition to normal virions. This test, while possible in some laboratories, is time-consuming and unlikely to be applied routinely.

Typing by microneutralization

Virus isolates can be typed by a microneutralization test using rabbit antisera to HSV Type 1 and 2. Neutralizing potency values are established for each virus isolate tested against reference type-specific antisera: the virus can then be allocated to either Type 1 or Type 2. Such procedures are possibly too time-consuming for a diagnostic laboratory.

Immunofluorescent antibody test

As human embryo lung cells may be used for isolation of HSV, and as the CPE is variable in different strains of such cells, isolates of HSV are now typed by an immunofluorescence test. Fluorescein-conjugated monoclonal antibodies which are type-specific are now available.

Restriction-endonuclease analysis

HSV-1 and HSV-2 can be separated unambiguously by restriction-endonuclease analysis and the endonuclease Hpal shows the distinction most clearly (Lonsdale 1979).

The use of restriction endonucleases and of electrophoretic patterns of HSV DNA so treated has already been discussed and the possibilities of tracing the spread of HSV in the community are also considered (see p. 331: Distribution of herpesvirus types).

Serological testing

Blood samples should be taken on first attendance and again after 10–14 days for a complement fixation test to determine whether the lesion is due to a primary or a recurrent infection. Antibody of the IgM class is produced during a primary infection, but is not detected often in recurrent states. Recently it has been shown that antibody to glycoprotein G is apparently type-specific and this has been utilized in measuring the patient's serological response to HSV-1 and HSV-2 (Lee et al 1985).

TREATMENT

Acyclovir

In 1978 the discovery of a new compound with both remarkably good anti-viral activity and extremely low toxicity to the host cell — 9-(2-hydroxyethoxymethyl) guanine — heralded a new era in the chemotherapy of HSV infections. The compound, an acyclic purine nucleoside analogue, first referred to by the name of acycloguanosine, was synthesized and studied by research workers in the Wellcome Research Laboratories who found it to be ten times more active in vitro against a strain of HSV-1 than idoxuridine (Schaeffer et al 1978). This compound, now known as acyclovir, has proved to be a highly potent inhibitor of HSV-1, HSV-2 and V-ZV and has extremely low toxicity for the normal host cells. In man acyclovir is the safest antiherpes agent so far discovered (Keeney et al 1982); its pharmacodynamic and therapeutic efficacy have been fully reviewed by Richards et al 1983). Anti-viral compounds, including acyclovir, may give some temporary relief in recurrent herpes, but ganglionic latency — the source for future recurrent episodes — is not affected by anti-viral drugs. In the treatment of primary mucocutaneous HSV infections, with or without dissemination, or in recurrent herpes in the immunosuppressed, acyclovir is highly effective and can be life saving.

Mechanism of action and selectivity of acyclovir

The high potency and selectivity of acyclovir for herpes simplex viruses can be understood on the basis of a number of differences between cellular and HSV-specified enzymes. Firstly, whereas the HSV-specified thymidine kinase phosphorylates acyclovir to a monophosphate (acyclo-GMP), cellular thymidine kinase does not (normal cells contain an enzyme other than thymidine kinase, and as yet unidentified, capable of phosphorylating acyclovir to a very small extent). The acyclovir monophosphate (acyclo-GMP) is subsequently converted to acyclovir triphosphate (acyclo-GTP) by cellular enzymes. Acyclo-GTP persists in HSV-infected cells for many hours after acyclovir is removed from the medium. The amounts of acyclo-GTP formed in HSV-infected cells are 40–100 times greater than in uninfected vero cells. Acyclo-GTP acts as a more potent inhibitor of the viral DNA polymerases than of the cellular polymerases. The DNA polymerases of HSV-1 and HSV-2 also use acyclo-GTP as a substrate and incorporate acyclo-GMP into the DNA primer template to a much greater extent than do cellular enzymes. The viral DNA polymerase binds strongly to the acyclo-GMP-terminated template and is thereby inactivated (Elion 1982).

Pharmacokinetics of acyclovir

In patients with genital herpes simplex on an oral dose of 200 mg every 4 hours, 5 times a day, the standard oral treatment, peak levels are found 1.5–1.75 hours after the oral dose. Peak plasma acyclovir levels ranged from 1.4–4.0 μM with a mean of 2.5 μM (1 μM = 0.225 $\mu g/ml$) (Blum et al 1982). Acyclovir levels in saliva are well correlated with simultaneous plasma levels, saliva levels being approximately 13% of plasma levels. Simultaneous plasma and vaginal contents levels are poorly correlated; peak levels in vaginal secretions range from 0.5–3.6 μM (Van Dyke et al 1982).

The peak acyclovir concentrations in plasma and vaginal fluid were in the range of the 50% inhibitory dose of 0.5 μM for HSV-1 and 1.62 μM for HSV-2 determined by Crumpacker et al (1979), with saliva levels at the lower end of this range.

With intravenous acyclovir (5.0 mg/kg) given every 8 hours, peak plasma levels of 12.7–43.2 μM (mean 26.1 μM) have been found in 30 patients with herpes genitalis and the estimated half-life of acyclovir to be 3.3 hours (Van Dyke et al 1982)

These authors concluded that inhibitory levels of acyclovir can be achieved in plasma and body secretions with oral therapy without evidence of drug toxicity. Inhibitory levels in secretions may prove useful in controlling mucosal herpes simplex recrudescences and decreasing local spread of the disease. Oral therapy may also have a role in preventing person-to-person transmission of infection by reducing the amount of virus on mucosal surfaces (Van Dyke et al 1982).

Excretion
Acyclovir appears to be excreted by glomerular filtration and renal tubular excretion. Clearance from plasma is relatively rapid and depends primarily on the efficiency of renal secretion. The clearance of acyclovir is substantially higher than estimated creatinine clearance, indicating that not only glomerular filtration but also tubular secretion contributes to the elimination of the drug. If probenecid is given renal clearance falls but it remains twice the value of estimated creatinine clearance (Blum et al 1982).

Because of the route of elimination, the drug has the potential to crystallize out in the kidney tubules; this was noted in early days when acyclovir was given as a bolus injection intravenously and when the patient was not adequately hydrated. Patients should therefore be so hydrated and with slow intravenous infusion over approximately one hour this problem has not recurred. In those with impaired renal function the dosage of acyclovir should also be reduced (Blum et al 1982).

Metabolic elimination
Blum et al also found that 9-carboxymethoxymethyl-guanine is the only significant metabolite of acyclovir, accounting for 8.5–14.1% of the dose. This metabolite has little anti-HSV activity. In those with moderately impaired renal function more drug is eliminated by metabolism as renal function decreases.

Plasma protein binding
At plasma concentrations of acyclovir of 0.4–5.0 μg/ml only small amounts (15.4% ± 4.4%) of drug are protein bound (Blum et al 1982).

Acyclovir tolerance
Among 350 patients with serious and potentially life-threatening HSV infections receiving rapid (bolus) intravenous injections of acyclovir, raised plasma urea

and/or creatinine levels were noted in 23 (10.3%): with local injection-site reactions in 6 (2.7%), these were the only adverse events considered to be due to acyclovir. Overall, in 465 patients given intravenous acyclovir, only 9% showed renal side effects but these can be virtually eliminated when rapid intravenous injections are avoided, attention is paid to careful hydration of patients and other renal damaging influences are controlled.

Unwanted effects
At therapeutic doses about 20% of acyclovir is absorbed from the gastrointestinal tract. Larger doses are absorbed less efficiently, and it is unlikely that serious toxic effects would occur if an entire treatment course of 25 acyclovir tablets were taken at once.

Acyclovir is not a carcinogen to either rats or mice. Results of tests in animals show no evidence of teratogenicity, nor is it carcinogenic, nor does it affect fertility (Wellcome Medical Division 1984). Acyclovir does not appear to have immunosuppressive properties. Acyclovir appears to prevent the establishment of latency in mice when given up to 24 hours after virus inoculation (Brigden et al 1981). Clinical studies suggest that acyclovir can influence the onset of recurrent infections if used prophylactically, but caution is, however, important so that the potential of acyclovir should not be put in jeopardy by promoting resistance (see below).

Reduced sensitivity to acyclovir in herpes simplex virus
Resistance to acyclovir has been shown experimentally to arise by mutations in the gene of the virus specified enzymes and DNA polymerase. 3 cases in man have been described in which immunocompromised patients on courses of intravenous acyclovir therapy (Burns et al 1982, Crumpacker et al 1982) — a protracted course in one case of a 7-year-old boy with agammaglobulinaemia and progressive renal failure (Crumpacker et al 1982) — yielded isolates that had acquired resistance to the drug. In all 3 cases acyclovir resistance was due to selection of an HSV mutant deficient in viral thymidine kinase. Such mutants are less virulent, have reduced ability to be transmitted and a reduced capacity to become latent.

An experimental model has been established for the development of resistance to acyclovir in HSV-infected mice which depends on the use of prolonged suboptimal therapy with oral acyclovir (Field 1982). These and other experiments have demonstrated that resistant HSV can establish latent infections which subsequently may be reactivated (Field & Darby 1980, Darby et al 1981). In some mutants HSV resistance can arise independently of loss of thymidine kinase induction (Field & Derby 1980). Field & Wildy (1982) consider that extreme caution should be applied to the widespread prophylactic use of acyclovir, especially at low dosage. As acyclovir is such a safe and effective systemic anti-viral drug its potential should not be put in jeopardy by inadvertently promoting resistance. In the immuno-compromised patient, where resistant isolates seem mostly to be found, one might expect more persistent viral replication in the skin and other organs in the absence of an effective immune response, leading to a persisting low-grade infection with spontaneously occur-ring acyclovir-resistant mutants (Burns et al 1982).

Acyclovir formulations available

Acyclovir for intravenous infusion. Acyclovir for intra-venous use is available in vials containing 250 mg sterile acyclovir as the freeze-dried sodium salt (Zovirax IV, Wellcome). It is indicated in HSV infections in immuno-compromised patients and is given by slow intrave-nous infusion of 5 mg/kg over one hour every 8 hours in patients with normal renal function. 5 days treatment is usually adequate. Zovirax IV must be reconstituted immediately before use as follows: 10 ml of either Water for Injections BP or Sodium Chloride Intravenous Infu-sion BP (0.9% w/v) should be added to each vial. This reconstituted solution may be infused directly into a vein by a controlled-rate infusion pump or diluted with other infusion solutions. Reconstituted Zovirax IV has a pH of about 11 and should not be given by mouth. Severe inflammation, sometimes leading to ulceration, has resulted from accidental infusion into the tissues extravascularly. Increased plasma liver-related enzymes, decreases in haematological indices, neurological reac-tions and rashes have been reported, but there is no evidence that they are related to the acyclovir therapy. Caution is required in patients with abnormal renal function (Wellcome Medical Division 1984).

Acyclovir for oral use. Acyclovir is available as a pale blue shield-shaped tablet impressed with ZOVIRAX and containing 200 mg acyclovir; a suspension — one 5 ml spoonful equivalent to one Zovirax tablet — may be used to encourage compliance in case of difficulty in taking tablets. The standard dose in adults is 200 mg 5 times daily at approximately 4-hour intervals, omitting the night-time dose. Administration should commence as early as possible during the prodromal period or when the lesions first appear. It is contraindicated in patients known to be hypersensitive to acyclovir.

In patients with severe renal impairment (creatinine clearance less than 10 ml/per minute), a dose of 200 mg every 12 hours is recommended. In pregnancy caution should be exercised in prescribing (Wellcome Medical Division 1984) as very little information is available on Zovirax during human pregnancy. The importance of recognizing clinically severe HSV infections, a rare

occurrence apparently of the third trimester of preg-nancy and the important contribution that acyclovir treatment is likely to make have both been discussed. Both this problem and the evaluation of acyclovir just before term are considered (p. 346) under the heading: Prevention of transmission to the fetus and newborn.

Acyclovir for skin use. Acyclovir 5% w/w in a white aqueous cream base is available as Zovirax Cream (2.0 g or 10.0 g tube) for the treatment of herpes simplex of the skin (this preparation is NOT for eye use), including recurrences of genital and labial herpes. The cream is applied 5 times daily at approximately 4-hour intervals, and this treatment should be continued for 5 days. If healing is not complete treatment may be continued for a further 5 days. Therapy should begin as early as possible after awareness of the lesion and preferably in the prodromal period. Acyclovir cream is contraindicated in patients known to be allergic to acyclovir or propylene glycol. Transient burning or stinging may occur following application. Erythema or mild drying and flaking of the skin has been reported in a small proportion of patients (Wellcome Medical Division 1984).

Acyclovir for eye use Acyclovir 3% w/v in a white soft paraffin base is available for ophthalmic use as Zovirax Ophthalmic Ointment (4.5 g tubes). A 1 cm ribbon of ointment should be placed inside the lower conjunctival sac 5 times daily at approximately 4-hourly intervals. Treatment should continue for at least 5 days after healing is complete. Transient mild stinging immedi-ately following administration occurs in a small pro-portion of patients. Superficial punctate keratopathy has been reported but has not resulted in patients being withdrawn from therapy, and healing has occurred without apparent sequelae (Wellcome Medical Division 1984).

Intravenous acyclovir (Zovirax IV, Wellcome) experi-ence in its use. Since a transient rise in serum urea and creatinine followed the use of a bolus injection of 5 mg/kg body weight, slow injection of this dose over 45–60 minutes by infusion through an in-dwelling intra-venous cannula every 8 hours is advised when the parenteral route of giving acyclovir is preferred.

Using such dosage for 15 doses in a randomized, double-blind, placebo-controlled trial in 30 patients with a first attack of genital herpes it was found that the medians for healing time, duration of vesicles, new lesion formation, virus shedding and all symptoms were significantly shorter than in controls (Mindel et al 1982). Intravenous acyclovir seemed a safe and effective therapy in patients with a first attack of genital herpes.

Only mild, short-lived unwanted effects, e.g. transient rises in the 'liver enzymes' were noted but these did not differ between the 'treatment' and 'control' groups of patients. In half the patients treated with acyclovir all lesions had healed by the 7th day, compared with less than 10% in those who received the placebo. No new lesions occurred 2 days after the commencement of acyclovir treatment. The most dramatic effect was the reduction in the duration of virus-shedding, reported to have ceased by day 5 in all patients treated with acyclovir, whereas placebo-treated patients continued virus-shedding for up to 20 days.

Acyclovir, given intravenously, has given new hope for immunocompromised patients in whom relatively simple local herpes simplex recurrence can otherwise develop into disseminated and sometimes life-threatening conditions. Such patients may be immuno-suppressed by drugs or radiation given as therapy for malignancy or to prevent graft rejection; or they may have impaired immune response — inborn, due to malignancy or seen in the Acquired Immune Deficiency Syndrome (AIDS) (Ch. 31). These serious infections have been effectively treated with oral or intravenous acyclovir (Zovirax) and repeated treatments with oral or intravenous acyclovir are both effective and well-tolerated (Straus et al 1982) Acyclovir intravenously appears to give a fuller protection if given prophylac-tically in such patients (Prentice 1983). Prophylactic oral acyclovir (200 mg 4 times daily) for the duration of remission induction chemotherapy (6 weeks) in patients with non-Hodgkin lymphoma and acute lymphoid leukaemia significantly reduced the incidence of clinical herpetic infection from 60% on placebo to 5% on acyclovir (Anderson et al 1984). Similar oral acyclovir medication (1–4 months duration) was also effective in renal transplant recipients (Griffin et al 1985; Pettersson et al 1985).

In heart transplant patients acyclovir is an effective therapy of mucocutaneous herpes simplex, and prophy-lactic use of acyclovir brings benefit in the immediate post-transplant period when the degree of immuno-suppression is usually greatest (Chou et al 1981). The combination of efficacy and low levels of toxicity has also been commented upon by Saral et al (1981) in patients undergoing immunosuppressive regimens prior to bone marrow transplant. Prophylactically, oral acyclovir prevented symptomatic recurrence of HSV lesions in such patients. The drug can therefore not only save lives in the immunocompromised with HSV infec-tions but can improve the quality of life for many.

Oral acyclovir (Zovirax Tablets, Wellcome) experi-ence in its use. Oral acyclovir (Zovirax) is without doubt the best specific treatment for primary genital herpes simplex providing a similar level of effectiveness

(Nilsen et al 1982) to the intravenous treatment (Mindel et al 1982) without the disadvantages of admission to hospital and the giving of intravenous transfusions. The duration of symptoms may be expected to be reduced by half or more providing treatment is started early enough. In Nilsen's cases all acyclovir (Zovirax) treated patients were culture negative after 5 days of oral treat-ment, whereas over 75% of placebo patients were still shedding virus. For the great majority of patients a 5-day course of treatment is adequate. Occasionally, however, early recurrences occur. If such patients could be identified prospectively they would merit a longer course of treatment.

The same study showed that oral treatment of recur-rent genital herpes with acyclovir reduced the course of the infection even though therapy was delayed for up to 48 hours after onset of symptoms. Since the course of untreated recurrence is relatively short in duration, the effects of acyclovir are not as dramatic as with primary infections. Early initiation of therapy during the prodromal phase of an attack can be expected to yield better results, and in patients with very frequent or easily predictable recurrences prophylaxis might be the most feasible way of achieving maximum benefit (Nilsen et al 1982).

Although acyclovir given in short 5-day courses speeds the rate of healing, shortens the duration and lessens the severity of symptoms, and decreases the duration of virus shedding it does not seem to decrease the likelihood of subsequent recurrences when used to treat patients either during a primary attack or a recur-rence (Corey et al 1982, Bryson et al 1983, Corey et al 1983b, Mindel & Sutherland 1983). Prophylactic oral acyclovir given continuously seems, however, to be effective, although costs of treatment are high. 56 patients with frequently recurring genital herpes were treated in a double-blind trial with oral acyclovir 200 mg 4 times a day or placebo for 12 weeks (Mindel et al 1984). In the placebo-treated patients (27) the mean recurrence rate per month of treatment was 1.4 and in the acyclovir group (29 patients) 0.05. The median time to the first recurrence after commencement of therapy was 14 days in the placebo group compared with 100 days in the acyclovir group. 26 out of 27 placebo-treated patients had a recurrence during the 12-week treatment period compared with only 4 of the 29 in the acyclovir group (p < 0.0001). No important side effects were seen in the study. After the end of treatment the recurrence rate was similar in the two groups.

Breakthrough recurrence may occur for several reasons. Firstly the dosage may be inadequate; secondly the patient may have missed or delayed therapy or the acyclovir-resistant HSV may emerge — acyclovir-resistant HSV isolates have been found in immunocompromised patients given repeated doses of acyclovir (Burns et al 1982, Schnipper et al 1982).

Questions are raised by the study of Mindel et al (1984) — who should receive the drug and for how long, is the drug safe in the long term and, finally, is the treatment cost-effective? As the authors say, a patient with 10 recurrences a year lasting for 2 weeks on each occasion would clearly benefit, whereas a patient with one would not. Only clinical judgement can decide. (A year's supply of acyclovir for a single patient at the time and at dosage used in this trial would have been £1460.)

Acyclovir was given orally in a dosage of 400 mg 8-hourly to 20 severely immunocompromised patients, seropositive for HSV, for 6 weeks, from the day of bone marrow transplant. 5 out of 20 patients developed oropharyngeal herpes simplex and it was thought that the protection given by oral acyclovir was less than the full protection observed with the i.v. drug (Prentice 1983). Better results were reported by Gluckman et al (1983) who gave 200 mg orally 6-hourly from day 8 to day 35 after transplantation.

Acyclovir cream for skin use (Zovirax Cream, Wellcome) experience in its use. A recent double-blind, placebo-controlled trial investigated the value of a 5% acyclovir cream (Zovirax Cream) in both primary and recurrent herpes genitalis. Virus shedding; new lesion formation; time to complete healing of all lesions; duration of pain, itching and all symptoms combined were significantly reduced. Fiddian et al (1983) commented that the formulation seemed suitable for patient-initiated treatment where recurrences are most effectively treated if treatment is initiated at the first indication of recurrence. Good results were obtained by Kinghorn et al (1983) who noted also the important point that acyclovir applied only to the external lesions was associated with a significant reduction of virus shedding and duration of lesions at all sites, including the internal (31 of 36 women had HSV isolated from the cervix and 13 of 15 men had positive urethral swabs for HSV). In recurrent HSV infections early patient-initiated therapy with acyclovir cream appears to be as effective as early oral therapy in recurrent genital herpes (Kinghorn et al 1983). Benefit in recurrent episodes of genital herpes may be difficult to prove, and the clinical importance of only 1 or 2 days reduction in the clinical course of the disease is debatable (Richards et al 1983).

Acyclovir eye ointment (Zovirax Ophthalmic Ointment, Wellcome) experience in its use. Richards et al (1983) have comprehensively reviewed the trial data on the treatment of ocular herpes (herpetic keratitis) with Zovirax Ophthalmic Ointment, which has proved to be superior in comparison with other anti-viral agents for the eye (Collum et al 1980, 1982). Deeper infections are more difficult to treat than epithelial keratitis.

VACCINES FOR HERPES SIMPLEX

Various vaccines for the prevention of herpes simplex are under experiment or trial. Theoretical reasons for advocating the use of live herpes vaccines are based on the importance of cell-mediated immunity in response to herpes infections. White (1984) in discussing HSV vaccine points out, however, that many virologists are wary about the prospect of live herpesvirus vaccines, lest they produce life-long persistent infections with unknown consequences, conceivably cancer.

An experimental 'subunit' HSV-2 vaccine consisting of a formaldehyde-treated viral glycoprotein adsorbed to alum adjuvant is currently under trial. Other types of vaccine under experiment include: 1. HSV-1 glycoproteins incorporated into liposomes, 2. HSV-1 glycoprotein-gD obtained from a gene cloned in *E. coli*, 3. a chimeric protein containing HSV-1 glycoprotein gD and 4. a synthetic HSV peptide (White 1984).

HERPESVIRUS IN NEONATAL INFECTIONS AND ENCEPHALITIS

The very serious and often fatal infections with HSV are rare and occur as neonatal infections, acquired before or at birth, as sporadic encephalitis, acquired later in life, or as disseminated herpes simplex in the immunologically deficient. HSV is a rare cause of the aseptic meningitis syndrome. An understanding of the nature of these conditions is necessary for an appreciation of HSV infection, although this dimension will not be faced in clinics for sexually transmissible disease, except in so far as it may involve those with the Acquired Immune Deficiency Syndrome (AIDS, see Ch. 31).

Vertical transmission of HSV

The importance of transmission by sexual intercourse and timing is illustrated by the case cited by Hanshaw & Dudgeon (1978). The report describes the exposure of a wife, one week before delivery, to her husband, who had an episode of penile herpes genitalis in a recurrent form at the time of intercourse. His wife had a primary genital herpes lesion at the time of delivery and the infant, born by Caesarean section 6 hours after rupture of the membranes, contracted a disseminated infection and died at 8 days of age. Such a clear-cut HSV situation is not, however, typical of the majority of neonatal cases.

NEONATAL INFECTION

Estimates of incidence of neonatal herpes in the United States vary between 1:30 000 and 1:3 500, with a frequency greater in the lower socio-economic groups. In some countries or social groups, a major source of virus to the infant is the mother's genital tract at the time of delivery, and more than 80% of HSV isolated from the newborn belong to Type 2, the common form of genital herpesvirus (Nahmias et al 1970). In the United Kingdom, in Manchester, however, in the period 1969 to 1973, the incidence of neonatal herpes was thought to be 1:30 000 live births; in one-third of the cases infection was acquired from a person other than the mother and in these cases HSV-1 predominated (Tobin 1975). In Canada severe neonatal herpes is estimated to be 1 per million (Update, World Health Organization 1985b).

If viral cultures are taken from the vulva and cervix in women with suspected herpes genitalis in late pregnancy, and Caesarean section carried out if HSV is cultured near the time of delivery, the risk of neonatal infection can be apparently avoided (Boehm et al 1981, Vontver et al 1982). In some 70% of cases of neonatal herpes, however, the mother has had no signs or symptoms of the infection at the time of delivery (Whitley et al 1980) and the shedding of virus during pregnancy but without manifest disease is known to occur (Bolognese et al 1976, Vontver et al 1982). This situation is in keeping with the natural history of the disease where the virus reactivates and passes to a peripheral site but fails to cause a noticeable lesion. Not all infants exposed to HSV at birth become infected. Severe infections appear to be restricted to infants less than 4 weeks of age and prematurity appears to carry greater risk. Risks are higher if the mother's lesion is primary rather than recurrent, and in those born to mothers with recurrent lesions and developing disease the mean titre of neutralizing antibody in their serum is lower than in those remaining asymptomatic (Yeager 1984). The infant may also acquire the infection after delivery from maternal labial herpes or herpes infection in one of the medical or nursing attendants (Francis et al 1975).

Infection in the neonate can produce a wide spectrum of clinical effects from subclinical to disseminated forms or to those localized to the central nervous system, the eye or mouth. Increased application of virus isolation methods has shown that the incidence of subclinical infection is commoner than the serious clinical forms.

Clinical features in neonatal infections

Disseminated forms

The HSV infection affects usually the liver and adrenals, but other organs are commonly involved including the brain, trachea, lungs, oesophagus, stomach, kidneys, spleen, pancreas, heart and bone marrow. Low birth weight or prematurity are more common in this group than that expected in the population at large.

The illness may appear at birth or as long as 21 days afterwards (average 6 days). There are a variety of clinical manifestations in disseminated infection including pyrexia or hypothermia, vomiting, loose stools, lethargy, convulsions, dyspnoea and jaundice. The illness is usually stormy, death occurring on average within 6 days.

Only 6 cases have been described linking HSV to the congenital defects of microcephaly, intracranial calcification, diffuse brain changes, chorioretinitis, retinal dysplasias and microphthalmia associated with vesicular rash at birth. HSV-1 was isolated in 1 case and HSV-2 from the other 5 (Florman et al 1973, Hurley 1978).

Localized forms

Central nervous system. Signs of meningoencephalitis indicate the need for lumbar puncture, which reveals a lymphocyte pleocytosis. In about half the cases, death follows in 1–3 weeks and in the remainder there tend to be sequelae such as microcephaly, porencephaly and varying degrees of psychomotor retardation. Eye effects will also be seen.

Eye. Conjunctivitis and keratitis develop early, and occasionally chorioretinitis develops slowly about a month after birth.

Skin. Isolated vesicular lesions can occur as well as a more generalized rash. The vesicular lesions recur repeatedly up to 2 years after birth, becoming less extensive than the original eruption but tending to be found at the same site.

Although the skin lesions are sometimes benign, central nervous system and ocular sequelae may follow, so a prolonged follow-up is advised.

Oral cavity. Vesicular lesions in the mouth are very rare and appear as a gingivostomatitis or involve the larynx. Diagnosis is dependent on recognition of the lesions and isolation of the HSV.

Treatment of neonates with HSV infection

Acyclovir is so well-tolerated in infants that treatment of all neonates with HSV infection is recommended whether or not there is clinical evidence of systemic involvement. Lack of such evidence does not imply necessarily that the disease is limited to the skin or will remain so, and there are good grounds for believing that for benefit acyclovir should be given early (Gould et al 1982). In the 4 infants with HSV infections whose response could be evaluated, Yeager (1982) recorded that 3 treated within 2 days of onset did well on acyclovir, whereas the fourth, who was not treated until 8 days after the appearance of symptoms, did poorly. Even with anti-viral therapy, whether with acyclovir or adenine arabinoside, the outcome is very variable (Yeager 1984). Earlier identification, diagnosis and treatment, however, is effectively changing the outcome of this disease (Whitley et al 1983).

The intravenous dose of 10 mg per kg body weight, given slowly, 8-hourly for 10 days is suggested for neonates. Since rises on days 2 and 3 may occur, it is wise to monitor the plasma urea and creatinine. For children over one month of age a dose of 250 mg/m^2 8-hourly is safe and effective. Solutions of up to 25 mg per ml of sodium salt in water have been given over a period of 1 hour by an infusion pump, although in older children the drug reconstituted in this way has usually been further diluted with sodium chloride 0.18% w/v and dextrose 4% w/v intravenous infusion BP, to give a concentration of not more than 0.5%. When given in this way, rises in plasma urea/creatinine do not seem to occur (Gould et al 1982).

Prevention of transmission to the fetus and the newborn

Men with penile herpes should be told about the dangers of communicating HSV and advised against intercourse with women who are pregnant. If herpetic penile lesions are present in the partner, the mother's cervix and vaginal secretions should be cultured for HSV in the last month of gestation even if there are no symptoms of infection. If HSV is present, even though inapparent clinically in the last six weeks of pregnancy, Caesarean section should be considered; if actual lesions are present, whether primary or recurrent, vaginal delivery is not advisable. If the membranes have already been ruptured for up to four hours, Caesarean section is not likely to protect the fetus. These recommendations by Hanshaw & Dudgeon (1978) are based on the hypothesis that the principal source of infection for the newborn is exposure to high titres of virus during passage through the birth canal. This approach can be developed further for those with recurrent herpes genitalis. By careful questioning about a past history of genital herpes in the case of the patient or in the case of her present or past partner(s), it is possible to define a high risk group, who may then be monitored closely by questioning and by inspection as well as by virus cultures during the last month of pregnancy. Virus cultures should be taken from the vaginal fornices and endocervix as well as from any visible lesion at weekly intervals during this last month. In this way Jacob et al (1984) identified 8 of 10 women found to be shedding herpes virus among 25 individuals in the high risk group in a study of 215 pregnant women.

Uncertainties remain, as the majority of infants born *per vaginam* to mothers with overt disease do not become clinically ill. In theory hyperimmune-anti HSV-2 gamma globulin, given to the neonate, would be expected to be useful in preventing involvement of an infant delivered vaginally in a woman with genital HSV-2 infection. Acyclovir, however, might well become a more acceptable line of approach in such situations.

In the case of patients who become clinically very ill during the last trimester of pregnancy with a primary HSV infection with actual or suspected dissemination (see Tables 26.1, 26.2, Fig. 26.2 and related text) acyclovir offers an important advance in treatment. In such cases early diagnosis and early institution of treatment is important; mouth, throat, vulva, vagina and cervix should be carefully examined for characteristic vesicular or ulcerative lesions. Virological diagnosis by electronmicroscopy of the roof, base or fluid of any vesicle can be made rapidly but the clinical appearance may be sufficiently characteristic.

In women with less dramatic symptoms or localized lesions a cautious evaluation of the safety, efficacy and pharmacokinetics of acyclovir in the mother just before term is necessary before clear-cut advice can be given. With acyclovir cell multiplication is not inhibited at concentrations 1000 times those which will inhibit HSV replication. The unique feature of acyclovir as an anti-viral agent is its selective capacity to kill the virus in human cells. Dosage with acyclovir is constrained by pharmacokinetic factors rather than any evidence of cellular cytotoxicity. Furthermore two generation reproduction-fertility studies in mice showed no evidence that acyclovir was embryotoxic or impaired reproduction or development processes. In rats or rabbits, also, studies failed to produce evidence of teratogenic or fetal problems (Bell et al 1984).

Exclusion of the infant from a mother with infectious lesions due to HSV-l or HSV-2 until these are healed and the exclusion of the nursery personnel with similar infections are warranted.

Like cytomegalovirus and rubella virus, herpesvirus is able to infect the fetus during the period of organogenesis and induce anomalies such as microcephaly and microphthalmia. It is probable, also, that in utero infection may not be compatible with continued life, and lead to abortion. For these reasons, during critical periods of early pregnancy, women should avoid risk of a primary HSV-2 infection.

SPORADIC HERPES ENCEPHALITIS

A tentative estimate of 25 to 50 cases per year has been made for the United Kingdom, and on the basis of an expected mortality of 60% there will be about 25 deaths per year from this cause (Longson & Bailey 1977).

In a recent Swedish study it was believed that the incidence of herpes simplex encephalitis is 2–3 cases per million inhabitants (Skoldenberg et al 1984).

The patient, who can be of any age, will be admitted to hospital because of a disturbance of affect or consciousness; there may be a loss of memory, mutism or a change in behaviour. Sometimes coma or epilepsy will focus attention on the brain, and admission to a neurosurgical unit on suspicion of a space-occupying lesion is one classical presentation. Brain oedema and raised intracranial pressure are the cardinal problem in herpes encephalitis (Longson & Bailey 1977). Fuller clinical descriptions are given by Oxbury and MacCallum (1973).

ASEPTIC MENINGITIS

In the aseptic (or abacterial) meningitis syndrome characterized by fever, signs of meningeal irritation, an increased leucocyte count in the CSF, but no signs of frank encephalitis, HSV is a very rare cause among the wide array of other viruses which have been implicated in the aetiology of a varying minority of cases (Lennette et al 1961, MacRae 1961).

DIAGNOSIS

An early and incontrovertible diagnosis of HSV encephalitis cannot be made without examination by brain biopsy material. The inferior aspect of the temporal lobe is the site of choice for biopsy in the absence of definite localization; recognition of the virus in brain tissue or firm histopathological evidence of acute necrotizing encephalitis is necessary for diagnosis. Except in HSV-2 infections, infectious virus can rarely be isolated from cerebrospinal fluid, which may be normal or show a lymphocytic pleocytosis. The electroencephalogram is never normal. Neuroradiological techniques such as angiography, technetium brain scans and studies with the EMI scanner provide useful information. Antibody assays in the serum are of limited value by themselves and few patients can be investigated sufficiently early in their illness to determine a proper baseline to their antibody response.

TREATMENT

In herpes encephalitis there is a disastrous and progressive necrosis of the brain. Treatment can be effective only if applied as early as possible during the destructive process. Treatment is based on anti-viral chemotherapy and management of brain oedema with dexamethasone or by surgical decompression. Severe residual neurological crippling may be too high a price to pay for chemotherapeutic success (Longson & Bailey 1977).

Of 53 confirmed cases of herpes simplex encephalitis, 51 were evaluated for analysis of efficacy of treatment with either acyclovir or vidarabine. In a prospective randomized study 27 were treated with acyclovir (10 mg per kg 8-hourly i.v. daily for 10 days) and 24 with vidarabine (15 mg per kg daily for 10 days). The mortality was 19% in the acyclovir-treated group compared with 50% in the vidarabine-treated group (p = 0.04). At 6 months observation 15 (56%) of 27 acyclovir-treated patients had returned to normal life compared with 3 (13%) of the 24 vidarabine-treated patients (p = 0.002); and the numbers who died or had severe sequelae were 9 (33% and 19 (76%), respectively (p = 0.005) (Skoldenberg et al 1984).

The study of herpes simplex encephalitis emphasizes that the level of consciousness influences survival. The more extensive the disease, especially in the presence of coma, the less likely that therapy will alter the ultimate outcome (Whitley et al 1983).

NOTES TO CHAPTER 26

Note 26.1: Restriction enzyme analysis of DNA from Herpes simplex virus

DEFINITION

Restriction endonucleases are enzymes which cleave foreign DNA at the same specific sequences of bases that in the host-cell DNA have been methylated and produce a double-stranded break. Biologically these enzymes protect a given organism from the deleterious effects of foreign DNA introduced into the cell by the bacterial virus (bacteriophage).

Every restriction endonuclease (some of those used are shown in the table below) has a specific name which identifies it uniquely. The first three letters, in italics, indicate the biological source of the enzyme, the first letter being the initial of the genus and the second and third the first two letters of the species name. The restriction enzymes from *Escherichia coli* are thus called *Eco*. Then comes a letter that identifies the strain of bacteria: *Eco* R for strain R — strictly for *E. coli* harbouring a plasmid called R. Finally there is a Roman numeral for the particular enzyme if there is more than one in the strain in question. Thus *Eco* RI represents the first enzyme from *Escherichia coli* R; *Eco* RII for the second (Cherfas 1982). A few examples are given in the table.

SUMMARY OF PROCEDURES (Lonsdale 1979)

1. DNA is labelled by growing virus with carrier free ^{32}P-orthophosphate.
2. The infected cells are lysed by a detergent; the DNA phenol extracted; subsequently precipitated with ethanol; and treated with RNA ase previous to restriction.
3. Sufficient restriction enzyme is added to the DNA and incubated for 3 hours at 37°C.
4. The reaction is stopped by the addition of EDTA:sucrose containing bromophenol blue.

5. The samples are analysed by electrophoresis overnight on appropriate concentrations of agarose at 2 v per cm.
6. Gels are air-dried on glass plates and exposed to film for 12–48 hours.
7. Autoradiographs are examined.

Enzyme	Source organism	Recognition and cleavage site°
*Bam*HI	*Bacillus amyloliquifaciens* H	G°GATCC CCTAG°G
Bgl II	*Bacillus globigii*	A°GATCT TCTAG°A
Eco RI	*Escherichia coli* RY13	G°AATTC CTTAA°G
Hin dIII	*Haemophilus influenzae* R_d	A°AGCTT TTCGA°A
Kpn I	*Klebsiella pneumoniae*	GGTAC°C C°CATGG

Note 26.2

The factorial of a positive integer n, symbol n!, is defined as $n! = (n-1)(n-2) \text{------} \times 3 \times 2 \times 1$ (where $0! = 1$ by definition) (Documenta Geigy).

Note 26.3

Wiskott-Aldrich syndrome, a familial disease, affecting boys, characterized by eczema, bloody diarrhoea, thrombocytopenia and abnormal susceptibility to infection (Soothill 1978).

Note 26.4

Vero — cell line initiated from kidney of a normal adult African Green Monkey (*Cercopithecus aethiops*). Hep-2 — human epithelial cell line (epidermoid carcinoma, larynx) (Shannon & Macy 1972).

REFERENCES

Anderson H, Scarffe J H, Sutton R N, Hickmott E, Brigden D, Burke C 1984 Oral acyclovir prophylaxis against herpes simplex virus infections in non-Hodgkin lymphoma and acute lymphoid leukaemia patients receiving remission induction chemotherapy. British Journal of Cancer 50: 45–49

Anderson J M, Nicholls M W N 1972 Herpes encephalitis in pregnancy. Correspondence, British Medical Journal 1, 632

Bell A M, Kingsley S R, Fiddian A P, Brigden W D 1984 Sexually transmitted diseases in pregnancy, Correspondence, British Medical Journal 288: 1456–1457

Blum M R, Liao S H J, De Miranda P 1982 Overview of acyclovir pharmacokinetic disposition in adults and children. The American Journal of Medicine 73: 186–192

Boehm F H, Estes W, Wright P F, Growdon J F 1981

Management of genital herpes simplex virus infection occurring during pregnancy. American Journal of Obstetrics and Gynecology 141: 735–740

Bolognese R J, Corson S L, Fuccillo D A, Traub R, Moder F, Sever J L 1976 Herpesvirus hominis type II infections in asymptomatic pregnant women. Obstetrics and Gynecology 48: 507–510

Brigden D, Fiddian P, Rosling A E, Ravenscroft T 1981 Acyclovir — a review of the preclinical and early clinical data of a new antiherpes drug. Antiviral Research 1: 203–212

Bryson Y J, Dillon M, Lovett M, et al 1983 Treatment of first episodes of genital herpes simplex virus infection with oral acyclovir. New England Journal of Medicine 308: 916–921

Buchman T G, Roizman B, Adams G, Stover B H 1978 Restriction endonuclease fingerprinting of herpes simplex virus DNA: a novel epidemiological tool applied to a nosocomial outbreak. Journal of Infectious Diseases 138: 488–498

Burns W H, Saral R, Santos G W et al 1982 Isolation and characterisation of resistant herpes simplex virus after acyclovir therapy. Lancet i: 421–423

Chaney S M J, Warren K G, Kettyls J A, Zbitnue A, Subak-Sharpe J H 1983a A comparative analysis of restriction enzyme digests of the DNA of herpes simplex virus isolated from genital and facial lesions. Journal of General Virology 64: 357–371

Chaney S M J, Warren K G, Subak-Sharpe J H 1983b Variable restriction endonuclease sites of herpes simplex virus Type 1 isolates from encephalitic, facial and genital lesions and ganglia. Journal of General Virology 64: 2717–2733

Cherfas J 1982 Man made life; a genetic engineering primer. Blackwell, Oxford, p 55

Chou S, Gallagher J G, Merigan T C 1981 Controlled clinical trial of intravenous acyclovir in heart-transplant patients with mucocutaneous herpes simplex infection. Lancet i: 1391

Collum L M T, Benedict-Smith A, Hillary I B 1980 Randomised double-blind trial of acyclovir and idoxuridine in dendritic corneal ulceration. British Journal of Ophthalmology 64: 766–769

Collum L M T, Logan P, Hillary I B, Ravenscroft T 1982 Acyclovir in herpes keratitis. Acyclovir Symposium. American Journal of Medicine 73: 290–293

Corey L, Nahmias A J, Guinan M E, Benedetti J K, Critchlow C W, Holmes K K 1982 A trial of topical acyclovir in genital herpes simplex virus infection. New England Journal of Medicine 306: 1313–1319

Corey L, Adams H C, Brown Z A, Holmes K K 1983a Genital herpes simplex infections: clinical manifestations, cause and complications. Annals of Internal Medicine 98: 958–972

Corey L, Fife K H, Benedetti J K et al 1983b Intravenous acyclovir for the treatment of primary genital herpes. Annals of Internal Medicine 98: 914–921

Cruickshank R, Duguid J P, Marmion B P, Swain R H A 1975 In: Medical microbiology, 12th edn. Churchill Livingstone, Edinburgh, p 219

Crumpacker C S, Schnipper L E, Zaia J A, Levin M J 1979 Growth inhibition by acycloguanosine of herpesviruses isolated from human infections. Antimicrobial Agents and Chemotherapy 15: 642–645

Crumpacker C S, Schnipper L E, Marlowe S I, Kowalsky P N, Hershey B J, Levin M J 1982 Resistance to antiviral drugs of herpes simplex virus isolated from a patient treated with acyclovir. New England Journal of Medicine 306: 343–346

Darby G, Field H J, Salisbury S A 1981 Altered substrate specificity of herpes simplex virus thymidine kinase confers acyclovir resistance. Nature, London 289: 81–83

Darougar S, Wishart M S, Viswalingam N D 1985 Epidemiological and clinical features of primary herpes simplex virus ocular infection. British Journal of Ophthalmology 69: 2–6

Dudgeon J A 1970 Herpes simplex. In: Heath R B, Waterson A P (eds) Modern trends in medical virology 2. A P Butterworth, London, p 78

Elion G B 1982 Mechanism of action and selectivity of acyclovir. Proceedings of a Symposium on Acyclovir. The American Journal of Medicine 73(1A): 7–13

Fiddian A P, Kinghorn G R, Goldmeier D, Rees E, Rodin R, Thin R N T, de Konig G A J 1983 Topical acyclovir in the treatment of genital herpes: a comparison with systemic therapy. Journal of Antimicrobial Chemotherapy 12 (suppl B) 67–77

Field H J 1982 Development of clinical resistance to acyclovir in herpes simplex virus infected mice receiving oral therapy. Antimicrobial Agents and Chemotherapy 21: 744–752

Field H J, Darby G 1980 Pathogenicity in mice of strains of herpes simplex virus which are resistant to acyclovir in vitro and in vivo. Antimicrobial Agents and Chemotherapy 17: 209–216

Field H J, Wildy P 1982 Clinical response of herpes simplex virus to acyclovir. Correspondence, Lancet i: 1125

Flewett T H, Parker R G F, Philip W M 1969 Acute hepatitis due to herpes simplex virus in an adult. Journal of Clinical Pathology 22: 60–66

Florman A L, Gershon A A, Blackett P R, Nahmias A J 1973 Intrauterine infection with herpes simplex virus. Journal of the American Medical Association 225: 129–132

Francis D P, Herrmann K L, McMahon J R, Chavigny K H, Sanderlin K C 1975 Nosocomial and maternally acquired herpesvirus hominis infections. A report of four fatal cases in neonates. American Journal of Diseases of Children 129: 889–893

Gluckman E, Lotsberg J, Devergie A et al 1983 Oral acyclovir prophylactic treatment of herpes simplex infection after bone marrow transplantation. Journal of Antimicrobial Chemotherapy 12: suppl B, 161–167

Goodell S E, Quinn T C, Mkrtichian E, Schuffler M D, Holmes K K, Corey L 1983 Herpes simplex virus proctitis in homosexual men. The New England Journal of Medicine 308(15): 868–871

Gould J M, Chessells J M, Marshall W C, McKendrick G D W 1982 Acyclovir in herpesvirus infections in children: experience in an open study with particular reference to safety. Journal of Infection 5: 283–289

Goyette R E, Donowho E M Jr, Hieger L R, Plunkett G D 1974 Fulminant Herpesvirus hominis hepatitis during pregnancy. Obstetrics and Gynecology 43: 191–196

Griffin P J A, Colbert J W, Williamson E P M, Sells R A, Hickmott E, Fiddian A P, Salaman J R 1985 Oral acyclovir prophylaxis of herpes infections in renal transplant recipients. Transplant Proceedings XVII: 84–85

Grover L, Kane J, Kravitz J, Cruz A 1985 Systemic acyclovir in pregnancy. Obstetrics and Gynecology 65: 284–287

Hanshaw J B, Dudgeon J A 1978 Viral diseases of the fetus and newborn. In: Schaffer A J, Markowitz M (eds) Major problems in clinical pediatrics, vol XVII. Saunders, Philadelphia, p 153–181

Hensleigh P A, Glover D B, Cannon M 1979 Systemic Herpesvirus hominis in pregnancy. Journal of Reproductive Medicine 22: 171–176

Hurley R 1978 Antenatal infections associated with foetal malformations. In: Scrimgeour J B (ed) Towards the prevention of foetal malformations. Edinburgh University Press, p 101

Jacob A J, Epstein J, Madden D L, Sever J L 1984 Genital herpes infection in pregnant women near term. Obstetrics and Gynecology 63(4): 480–484

Kawana T, Kawaguchi T, Sahamoto S 1976 Clinical and virological studies on genital herpes. Lancet ii: 964

Keeney R E, Kirk L E, Bridgen D 1982 Acyclovir tolerance in humans. Proceedings of a Symposium on Acyclovir. The American Journal of Medicine 73(1A): 176–181

Kinghorn G R, Turner E B, Barton I G, Potter C W, Burke C A, Fiddian A P 1983 Efficacy of topical acyclovir cream in first and recurrent episodes of genital herpes. Antiviral Research 3/5–6: 291–301

Klein R J 1982 The pathogenesis of acute, latent and recurrent herpes simplex virus infections: brief review. Archives of Virology 72: 143–168

Lee F, Pereira L, Coleman R M, Bailey P, Tatsuno M, Griffin C, Nahmias A 1985 New Type-specific antigens for detecting antibodies to herpes simplex viruses Type 1 (HSV-l) and Type 2 (HSV-2). 6th International Meeting, International Society for STD Research, Brighton. (Abstract 58), p 44

Lennette E H, Magoffin R L, Longshore W A, Hollister A C 1961 An etiologic study of seasonal aseptic meningitis and encephalitis in the central valley of California. American Journal of Tropical Medicine and Hygiene 10: 885–896

Linnemann C C, Light I J, Buchman T G, Ballard J L, Roizman B 1978 Transmission of herpes-simplex virus Type 1 in a nursery for the newborn. Identification of viral isolates by DNA 'fingerprinting'. Lancet i: 964–96

Longson M, Bailey A S 1977 Herpes encephalitis. In: Waterson J P (ed) Recent advances in clinical virology. Churchill Livingstone, Edinburgh, p 1–15

Lonsdale D M 1979 A rapid technique for distinguishing herpes-simplex virus Type 1 from Type 2 by restriction-enzyme technology. Lancet i: 849–852

MacRae A D 1961 Viruses as a cause of meningo-encephalitis. In: Wolstenholme G E W, Cameron M P (eds) CIBA Foundation Study Group No 7. Churchill, London, p 7

Manzella J P, McConville J H, Valenti W, Menegus M A, Swierkosz E M, Arens M 1984 An outbreak of herpes simplex virus Type 1 gingivostomatitis in a dental hygiene practice. Journal of the American Medical Association 252(15): 2019–2022

Mindel A, Adler M W, Sutherland S, Fiddian A P 1982 Intravenous acyclovir treatment for primary genital herpes. Lancet i: 697–700

Mindel A, Sutherland S 1983 Genital herpes — the disease and its treatment including acyclovir. Journal of Antimicrobial Chemotherapy 12 (suppl B): 51–59

Mindel A, Weller I V D, Faherty A, Sutherland S, Hindley D, Fiddian A P, Adler M W 1984 Prophylactic oral acyclovir in recurrent genital herpes. Lancet ii: 57–59

Nagington J, Rook A, Highet A S 1986 Herpes simplex. In: Rook A, Wilkinson D S, Ebling F J G, Champion R H, Burton J H (eds) Textbook of dermatology, 4th edn. Blackwell, Oxford, vol 1 p 685–690

Nahmias A J, Alford C A, Koroner S B 1970 Infection of the newborn with Herpesvirus hominis. Advances in Paediatrics 17: 185–226

Nilsen A E, Aasen T, Halsos A M, Kinge B R, Tjøotta E A L, Wikstrom K, Fiddian A P 1982 Efficacy of oral acyclovir in the treatment of initial and recurrent genital herpes. Lancet ii: 571–573

Oates J K, Greenhouse R D H 1978 Retention of urine in anogenital herpetic infection. Lancet i: 691–692

Owensby L C, Stammer J L 1978 Esophagitis associated with herpes simplex infection in an immunocompetent host. Gastroenterology 74: 1305–1306

Oxbury J M, MacCallum F O 1973 Herpes simplex encephalitis. Postgraduate Medical Journal 49: 387–389

Peacock J E, Sarubbi F A 1983 Disseminated herpes simplex virus infection during pregnancy. Obstetrics and Gynecology 61: No 3(suppl) 13s–18s

Pettersson E, Hovi T, Ahonen J et al 1985 Prophylactic oral acyclovir after renal transplantation. Transplantation 39: 279–281

Peutherer J F, Smith I W, Robertson D H H 1979 Necrotising balanitis due to a generalised primary infection with herpes simplex virus type 2. British Journal of Venereal Diseases 55: 48–51

Peutherer J F, Smith Isabel W, Robertson D H H 1982 Genital infection with herpes simplex virus type I. Journal of Infection 4: 33–35

Prentice H G 1983 Use of acyclovir for prophylaxis of herpes infections in severely immunocompromised patients. Journal of Antimicrobial Chemotherapy 12 Suppl B: 153–159

Rawls W E 1985 Herpes simplex virus. In: Fields B N (ed) Virology. Raven Press, New York, ch 26, p 527–561

Reeves W C, Corey L, Adams H G, Vontver L A, Holmes K K 1981 Risk of recurrence after first episode of genital herpes. Relation to HSV type and antibody response. New England Journal of Medicine 305: 315–319

Richards D M, Carmine A A, Brogden R N, Heel R C, Speight T M, Avery G S 1983 Acyclovir. A review of its pharmacodynamic properties and therapeutic efficacy. Drugs 26: 378–438

Roizman B, Batterson W 1985 Herpesviruses and their replication. In: Fields B N (ed) Virology. Raven Press, New York, ch 25, p 497–526

Roizman B, Tognon M 1982 Restriction enzyme analysis of Herpesvirus DNA: Stability of restriction endonuclease patterns. Lancet i: 677

Roizman B, Carmichael L E, Deinhardt G de-The et al 1981 Herpesviridae, definition, provisional nomenclature and taxonomy. Intervirology 16: 201–217

Saral R, Burns W H, Laskin O L, Santos G W, Lietman P S 1981 Acyclovir prophylaxis of herpes simplex virus infections. A randomised, double-blind, controlled trial in bone-marrow transplant recipients. New England Journal of Medicine 305: 63–67

Schaeffer H J, Beauchamp L, de Miranda P, Elion G B, Bauer D J, Collins P 1978 9-(2-Hydroxyethoxymethyl) guanine activity against viruses of the herpes group. Nature 272: 583–585

Schmidt O W, Fife K H, Corey L 1984 Reinfection is an uncommon occurrence in patients with symptomatic recurrent genital herpes. Journal of Infectious Diseases 149: 645–646

Schnipper L E, Crumpacker C S, Marlowe S I, Kowalsky P, Hershey B J, Levin M J 1982 Drug resistant herpes simplex virus in vitro and after treatment in an immunocompromised patient. American Journal of Medicine 73: 387–392

Shah S J, Scholz F J 1983 Anorectal herpes: radiographic findings. Radiology 147: 81–82

Shannon J E, Macy M L 1972 (eds) The American Type Culture Collection. Registry of Animal Cell Lines, 12301 Parklawn Drive, Rockville, Maryland, 20852

Skoldenberg B, Forsgren M, Alestig K et al 1984 Acyclovir versus vidarabine in herpes simplex encephalitis. Randomised multicentre study in consecutive Swedish patients. Lancet ii: 707–711

Smith I W, Peutherer J F, MacCallum F O 1967 The incidence of Herpesvirus hominis antibody in the population. Journal of Hygiene 65: 395–408

Smith I W, Peutherer J F, Robertson D H H 1973 Characterisation of genital strains of Herpesvirus hominis. British Journal of Venereal Diseases 49: 385–390

Smith I W, Maitland N J, Peutherer J F, Robertson D H H

1981 Restriction enzyme analysis of Herpesvirus-2 DNA. Lancet ii: 1424

Soothill J F 1978 Immunodeficiency. In: Forfar J O, Arneil G C (eds) Textbook of paediatrics. Churchill Livingstone, Edinburgh, p 1153

Spence J, Walton W S, Miller F J W, Court S C M 1954 A thousand families in Newcastle-on-Tyne. Oxford University Press, London

Spruance S L, Overall J C Jnr, Kern E R, Krueger G G, Pliam V, Miller W 1977 The natural history of recurrent herpes simplex labialis. New England Journal of Medicine 297: 69–74

Straus S E, Smith H A, Brickman C, de Miranda P, McLaren C, Keeney R E 1982 Acyclovir for chronic mucocutaneous herpes simplex virus infection in immunosuppressed patients. Annals of Internal Medicine 96: 270–277

Tobin J O H 1975 Herpesvirus hominis infection in pregnancy. Proceedings of the Royal Society of Medicine 68: 371–374

Update, World Health Organization 1985a Prevention and control of herpesvirus diseases. Part 1 Clinical and laboratory diagnosis and chemotherapy. Bulletin of the World Health Organization 63(2): 185–201

Update, World Health Organization 1985b Prevention and control of herpesvirus diseases. Part 2 Epidemiology and immunology. Bulletin of the World Health Organization 63(3): 427–444

Van Dyke R B, Connor J D, Wyborny C, Hintz M, Keeney R E 1982 Pharmacokinetics of orally administered acyclovir in patients with herpes progenitalis. The American Journal of Medicine 73: 172–175

Vontver L A, Hickok D E, Brown Z, Reid L, Corey L 1982 Recurrent genital herpes simplex virus infection in pregnancy: infant outcome and frequency of asymptomatic recurrences. American Journal of Obstetrics and Gynecology 143: 75–84

Watkinson A C 1982 Primary herpes simplex in a dentist. British Dental Journal 153: 190–191

Wellcome Medical Division 1984 Zovirax (acyclovir). The Wellcome Foundation, Crewe, Cheshire

White D O 1984 Antiviral chemotherapy, interferons and vaccines. In: Melnick J L (ed) Monographs in virology, vol 16. Karger, Basel, p 72–74

Whitley R J, Nahmias A J, Visintine A M, Fleming C L, Alford C A 1980 The natural history of herpes simplex virus infection of mother and newborn. Pediatrics 66: 489–94

Whitley R J and the NIAID Collaborative Antiviral Study Group 1983 Interim summary of mortality in herpes simplex virus infections: vidarabine versus acyclovir. Journal of Antimicrobial Chemotherapy 12, suppl B. 105–112

Wildy P, Gell P G H 1985 The host response to herpes simplex virus. British Medical Bulletin 41(1): 86–91

Wildy P, Field H J, Nash A A 1982 Classical herpes latency revisited. In: Mahy B W J, Minson A C, Darby G K (eds) Virus persistence. Cambridge University Press, p 133–167

Wolontis S, Jeansson S 1977 Correlation of herpes simplex virus types 1 and 2 with clinical features of infection. Journal of Infectious Diseases 135: 28–33

Yeager A S 1982 Acyclovir pharmacokinetics and tolerance in man: use of acyclovir in premature and term neonates. American Journal of Medicine. Acyclovir Symposium 205–209

Yeager A S 1984 Genital herpes simplex infections: effect of asymptomatic shedding and latency on management of infections in pregnant women and neonates. The Journal of Investigative Dermatology 83: No 1 suppl: 53s–56s

Young E J, Killam A P, Greene J F Jr 1976 Disseminated herpesvirus infection. Association with primary genital herpes in pregnancy. Journal of the American Medical Association 235: 2731–2733

27

Papillomavirus infection and genital warts

GENITAL WARTS

Not only are genital warts due to human papillomavirus unsightly, but their persistence and inconstant response to treatment give rise to anxiety and introspection in the patient as well as the added burden of multiple attendances. Their high prevalence, high infectivity, long prepatent period (average 3 months: range 2 weeks to 8 months) and often poor response to treatment all make effective control by therapy and contact-tracing possible only to a limited extent. Until quite recently genital warts have been regarded virtually as wholly benign growths which regress spontaneously, but human papillomaviruses may not be solely causes of benign tumours of skin and mucosa, but in the longer term and possibly in association with herpesvirus Type 2 and/or other co-factors, such as cigarette smoking, may play a part in the aetiology of cancer, particularly of the cervix uteri. The case against papillomaviruses in regard to cancer of the cervix is, however, not yet proven.

AETIOLOGY

Human papillomavirus (HPV) or, in colloquial terms, the wart virus consists of a heterogeneous group of DNA viruses which were placed until recently in the family of papova viruses (pa = papilloma; po = polyoma; va = vacuolating agent) but now appear not to be related to the two other viruses included in that family, viz. the murine polyomavirus and the vacuolating simian virus 40. The viruses were originally grouped together on the basis of similar structures of their icosahedral capsid (55 nm in size) and nucleic acid (Pfister 1984). Examination of genital warts (condyloma acuminatum) and common skin warts (verruca vulgaris) showed that both lesions contain morphologically identical virus but with the techniques using immune electronmicroscopy, it was clear (Almeida 1976) that the viruses were antigenically distinct.

Since papillomaviruses cannot be propagated in vitro in any cell culture system, progress in research has, until recent years, been difficult and unrewarding. The quantities of wart material in the lesions were so low that their characterization directly from such material was not possible. The extraction of virus DNA from warts and its molecular cloning in bacterial plasmids or in bacteriophage lambda has now enabled the preparation of quantities sufficient to develop methods for the classification of the papillomaviruses from a variety of lesions in a variety of anatomical sites. Papillomavirus DNA is a double-stranded circular molecule which can now be identified in minute traces, as little as one copy per cell, in human tissues. Not only can it be detected but the DNA can be ascribed to a specific subtype even when the presence of virus is undetectable by electron-microscopy or existing immunoassays (Leading Article 1983).

At the present time classification of HPV into separate types is based on nucleic acid hybridization studies; a virus is considered to be a separate type if such DNA studies reveal less than 50% homology with known virus types. Subtypes are those which show more than 50% cross hybridization but differ in their restriction endonuclease cleavage patterns. The classification may be supported by serological data, but in most cases this will be difficult or impossible because of the very limited amounts of antigen (Pfister 1984).

On the basis of these nucleic acid studies, more than 40 types have been reported, of which 7 are specific to the urogenital tract, viz. the common types HPV-6, 11, 16, 18 (Singer et al 1984) and the less common HPV-31, 33 and 35 (Beaudenon et al 1986; for discussion see Meanwell et al 1987). Each type of virus usually produces lesions with distinctive histological features in particular anatomical sites, e.g. HPV-1 causes plantar warts and HPV-6 and HPV-11 cause condyloma acuminatum of the genital tract. Types of viruses and lesions associated with them are shown in Table 27.1.

Skin warts appear to be acquired from environmental sources such as public bathing facilities or in gymnasiums and occur primarily in children, while genital

Table 27.1 Classification of human papillomavirus infections showing their clinical, histological and virological aspects together with tendencies or otherwise of the lesions produced to undergo malignant conversion (Gissmann et al 1982, 1983, Crawford 1984, Pfister 1984, Ikenberg et al 1983, Hauser et al 1985, Beaudenon et al 1986, Coleman et al 1986, Meanwell et al 1987).

Lesion	Anatomical site	Histology	HPV types Main types (others)	Viral particles (numbers)	Incidence mainly	Malignant conversion
a. *Genital*						
Condyloma acumination	Genital and anal mucosa	Acanthosis Papillomatosis	6, 11 (1, 2, 16, 18)	+	Young adult	±
Cervical koilocytosis	Cervix uteri	Acanthosis Koilocytosis	6, 11 (16, 18, 33)	++	Young adult	±
Bowenoid papulosis	Vulva Penis	Carcinoma in situ	6, 16	+	Young adult	±
Invasive carcinoma	Cervix	Carcinoma	16, 18 (6, 11)	−	Adult	Not applicable
b. *Extragenital*						
Respiratory papillomatosis	Larynx, trachea	Acanthosis Koilocytosis	6, 11	+ +	Child (2–5) Adult (20–40)	+ +
Epidermodysplasia verruciformis	Generalized	Hyperkeratosis Hypergranulosis Large clear cells	Flat lesions 3, 10 Pityriasis versicolor-like 5, 8, 9, 12, 14, 15	++	Child	++++
Focal epithelial hyperplasia	Oral mucosa	Acanthosis	13 (1)	+	Child Young adult	−
Verruca vulgaris	Back of hand	Hyperkeratosis Acanthosis	1, 7 (2, 4)	+ to ++	Child Young adult	2 case reports
Verruca plantaris	Soles of feet	Hyperkeratosis Acanthosis Inclusion bodies	1 (2, 4)	+++	Child Young adult	−
Verruca plana	Face, hands	Hyperkeratosis Acanthosis	3, 10	++	Child Young adult	−

warts are acquired mainly by sexual intercourse. The age incidence of genital warts shows a similarity to that of gonorrhoea, with the commonest age of onset being 22 years in the case of men and 19 years in the case of women. The prepatent period varies between 3 weeks and 8 months with an average of about 3 months. About 65% of consorts will be found also to have warts. Vulvar and penile warts are more clearly associated with transmission by sexual intercourse, while anal warts are less certainly associated with anal intercourse, so their origin remains speculative. It has been suggested that wart virus may be a normal inhabitant of the ano-rectum in some patients and that trauma may allow entry of the virus into the epidermis but warts, in fact, are seldom seen in association with anal fissures (Oriel 1971b).

In England and Wales in the period 1972–1980, for example, in the clinics dealing with sexually transmitted diseases there was a substantial increase in new cases of genital warts (increases from about 45.54 to 79.20 per 100 000 (74%) were reported in males and from 23.42 to 43.0 per 100 000 (84%) in females (Chief Medical Officer, DHSS 1983).

BIOLOGY OF HPV INFECTION

Papillomaviruses cause epithelial or fibroepithelial proliferations of the skin or mucosa, but it is in only a few bovine papillomaviruses that fibroblasts are transformed and the virus affects the dermis. In wart lesions there is no direct evidence of papillomavirus DNA in the basal cells of the epidermis. Hybridization studies suggest that viral DNA first occurs in the stratum spinosum (Grussendorf & zur Hausen 1979) where mature virus particles can be seen in association with the nucleoli (Almeida et al 1962). In the stratum granulosum virions are spread throughout the nuclei and appear as paracrystalline arrays. After breakdown of the cell structures, aggregates of virus are seen embedded in the keratin of the stratum corneum. Epidermal cells are therefore non-permissive in the beginning of their differentiation but become more so with increasing differentiation (Pfister 1984). Hybridization studies have shown that HPV DNA is to be found also in apparently normal skin at least 2 cm from the genital wart itself (Ferenczy et al 1985).

Available data on cervical carcinomas and derived cell lines suggest that HPV16 and HPV18 may be integrated in the cell genomes, and integration of HPV33 DNA sequences has been found in one case of vulvar carcinoma in situ (Bowen's disease) (Beaudenon et al 1986). Although integration of HPV types 16 or 18 is a risk factor for the development of cervical cancer conclusions about the biological significance of integration cannot be made. In the case of HPV16 such integration was found to be common in those with cervical cancer and absent in those without, but in this study (Meanwell et al 1987) a number of points were made on HPV-16 DNA:

1. Positive and negative findings were obtained in adjacent areas of the same cervical cancer tumour;

2. HPV-16 occurred as episomal molecules in more than two thirds of these 31 carcinoma cases,

3. The HPV-16 integration, when found, occurred at mostly single host-genome sites but on one occasion at multiple sites;

4. The association of HPV-16 and cervical neoplasia is age-related; the older the patient the more likely is the virus to be found.

IMMUNOLOGY OF PAPILLOMAVIRUS INFECTION

Cottontail rabbit (Shope) papillomavirus (CRPV), immunology.

The immune response in rabbits infected with Shope papillomavirus (CRPV) (Lancaster & Olson 1982) provides a useful model for discussing the process in human papillomavirus infections (Pfister 1984).

Neutralizing antibody

In response to CRPV rabbits form *neutralizing antibody* which protects against reinfection and is demonstrable in animals with regressing (*regressors*) and persisting (*persistors*) papillomas. Neutralizing antibodies do not therefore cause regression, which is dependent on other mechanisms.

In reinfection experiments, where virus inactivation by antibody was avoided by infection of autologous skin in vitro followed by transplantation, papillomas were only induced in *persistors* and not *regressors*. This immunity lasted about 15 months and seemed to be directed against tumour antigens as vaccination with such antigens increased the frequency of regression.

Cellular immunity

In regressing papillomas the mononuclear cell infiltrates suggest cellular immune reaction.

Leucocytes concentrated mostly at the basement membrane of the epithelium suggest lymphokine reaction since cell proliferation is most obvious in the prickle cell layer.

Lymph node cells from *regressors* as well as *persistors* inhibited the formation of colonies of papilloma-derived cells. Serum from *persistors*, however, blocked this effect suggesting a cell-mediated immune response to the surface of tumour cells and that humoral factor can block this effect.

Immunity impairment with steroid treatment (McMichael 1967)

The overall effect on the immune system is shown by the results of impairment by methyl-prednisolone. In the cottontail rabbit infected with the CRPV steroid treatment had no detectable effect on the latent period, papilloma growth rate, virus concentration nor on malignant conversion. Growth in secondary papillomas at sites not directly inoculated and the susceptibility to reinfection with CPRV, however, were both enhanced. Regression of papilloma was diminished (McMichael 1967).

IMMUNOLOGY OF HUMAN PAPILLOMAVIRUS (HPV) INFECTION

The results of immune electronmicroscopy suggest that a one-way antigenic cross exists between the virus of the common skin warts and the virus of genital warts: sera from patients with common warts react with both the common skin and the genital wart virus, while serum from patients with genital warts appears to react only with the homotypic genital wart virus (Almeida, 1976). These studies show that patients with genital warts do produce humoral antibody to the homotypic virus. IgM antibody is the commonest found but IgG is found also, particularly when warts are regressing (Matthews & Shirodaria 1973, Pyrhonen & Johansson 1975). This, however, may not by itself be enough to produce resolution of the lesion, and information on cell-mediated immunity (CMI) is required.

Studies on CMI have been hampered by the lack of a culture technique to obtain sufficient antigen, but modern technology should bring important advances soon. Spontaneous resolution of warts is often associated with infiltration by macrophages and lymphocytes (Oguchi et al 1981). In pregnancy, when CMI is depressed, genital warts may enlarge and extend considerably, although they usually regress during the puerperium. Defective CMI is probably also the reason for florid genital warts which are sometimes seen in patients with Hodgkins disease (Oriel 1976) and occasionally in renal transplant patients. In a renal allograft recipient with an epidermodysplasia-verruciformis-like syndrome, two skin cancers were found to contain

HPV-5 DNA (Lutzner et al 1983), a finding in keeping with the suggestion that both HPV-5 and immunosuppression were factors in oncogenesis.

Langerhans cells, HLA-DR-positive dendritic cells, are to be found in stratified mucosae, including the vagina and cervix, as well as in the thymus, spleen and lymphatics. These cells appear to play a pivotal role in the process of recognition of exogenous antigen (Shelley & Juhlen 1976). The process of T-lymphocyte activation is thought to be initiated by direct cell-to-cell contact between T-lymphocyte and HLA-DR-positive cells which have taken up antigen (e.g. Langerhans cells or macrophages). In response to antigen entry into epithelium, such as that of the cervix, T-effector cells are generated. Those of the T-cytotoxic/suppressor type may migrate into the epithelium while others remain in the stroma. The preponderance of T-helper cells in the stroma may induce B-lymphocyte maturation into immunoglobulin-producing plasma cells at this site: circulation of the antigen-specific cells to regional lymphatics and lymphoid tissue would be important to the development of immunological memory (Morris et al 1983a). In comparison with normal cervical tissue, epithelium infected with wart virus consistently shows a partial depletion or absence of Langerhans cells and T-lymphocytes. The few Langerhans cells which remain show loss of their normal dendritic processes and are confined to the vicinity of the basement membrane. The Langerhans cell depletion may be a direct cytotoxic effect of wart virus (Morris et al 1983b).

HISTOLOGY

In all warts the basal cells (stratum germinativum) are intact and the stratum spinosum is hyperplastic (acanthosis). The stratum granulosum may be many cells thick and the stratum corneum hyperkeratotic or parakeratotic. Dermal papillae are elongated but the underlying dermis is normal. In the stratum granulosum and adjacent prickle cells, large vacuolated cells are seen, known as koilocytes, in which the nuclei are surrounded by an apparently structureless halo; the nuclei are deeply basophilic and are the site of the formation of mature virus (see also Ch. 25). Hyperkeratosis is not a feature of condyloma acuminatum of the genital area where the stratum corneum consists as a rule of only one or two layers of parakeratotic cells. In these warts, acanthosis combined with extensive papillomatosis results in layers of the wart that consist entirely of sheets of hyperplastic prickle cells showing multiple mitotic figures. As the condylomata age hyperkeratosis may develop (Oriel 1983). As a feature hyperkeratosis is more that of plantar or palmar warts rather than plane warts (Table 27.1). In genital condylomata acuminata

wart virus particles are scanty (Dunn & Ogilvie 1968). The association of HPV infection with cervical intraepithelial neoplasia and carcinoma of the cervix uteri is discussed in Chapter 25.

CLINICAL FEATURES

Genital lesions

Various clinical types of wart can be distinguished. In men the fleshy hyperplastic warts (condyloma acuminatum), either one or many, occur most often on the glans penis and on the inner lining of the prepuce. The appearance depends upon the location, although moisture and accompanying inflammation may enhance the size and tendency to coalesce. Those in the terminal urethra have a bright red colour in particular. Hyperplastic warts occur also in women (Fig. 27.1). Genital warts may occur at several sites in the same patient; the distribution, as recorded by Oriel (1971a) was as follows:

In men: fraenum, corona and glans, 52%; prepuce, 33%; urinary meatus, 23%; shaft of penis, 18%; scrotum, 2% and anus, 8%. Genital warts are sometimes very extensive in the uncircumcised male.

In women: posterior part of introitus, 73%; labia minora and clitoris, 32%; labia majora, 31%; urethra,

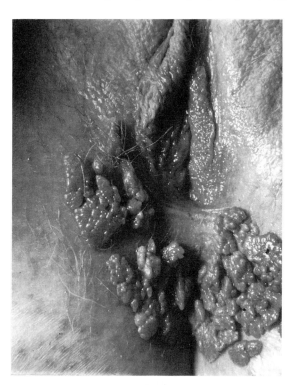

Fig. 27.1 Multiple hyperplastic condylomata acuminata of the vulva and perianal skin (genital warts).

8%; vagina, 15%; cervix, 6% (papillomavirus infection of the cervix uteri is discussed below); perineum, 23% and anus, 18%. Most often warts appeared first at or near the posterior part of the vaginal introitus and on the adjacent labia majora and minora. They tend to cluster at the orifices of the greater vestibular glands.

Other sites include the nipple, urethra and bladder. Urethral condylomata can spread proximally from the common sites of predilection, namely the fossa navicularis and perimeatal portions of the urethra, to involve any part of the urethra and even the bladder. These condylomata have been recognized by a voiding cystourethrography (Pollack et al 1978) following intravenously administered contrast. Although excretory voiding cystourethrography will avoid the need for urethral instrumentation, which itself may contribute to the retrograde spread of condylomata, it carries a recognized risk (a mortality rate of 1/20 000) and therefore is not indicated in the vast majority of cases of urethral meatus warts.

Cervical warts

HPV infection of the cervix frequently does not produce lesions that are recognizable by naked-eye inspection. In visible lesions, thought to be warty and biopsied at colposcopy, about 80% showed changes characteristic of papillomavirus infection using standard histological techniques, and about 35% showed the presence of viral antigen using an immunohistochemical technique (Walker et al 1983). Cervical tissue, however, is only partially permissive for the expression of HPV antigen — as is also the case in vulval condylomata (Kurman et al 1981) — so that not all lesions can be diagnosed even when colposcopy and histology are used together. Modern hybridization techniques, generally available at present only as a research technology, are very sensitive, however, and yield a diagnosis in a much higher proportion of lesions by identifying HPV DNA. McCance et al (1983) have found HPV-6 DNA by these techniques in over half of histologically proved cases of cervical intra-epithelial neoplastic lesions. Different types (e.g. 6, 11, 16 or 18) may also be involved and identified if specific probes are available. A subtype of HPV-6 is the most frequently found papillomavirus in exophytic and vulvar warts in patients in the London area. In Chapter 25 the association of HPV infection with cervical intra-epithelial neoplasia and cancer of the cervix uteri has been discussed. A broad classification into condylomatous koilocytosis and flat koilocytosis has been adopted on histological grounds to cover the lesions of HPV infection of the cervix uteri (Fletcher 1983). With the aid of colposcopy, however, it is possible to assess lesions of the cervix for the surface appearance and to classify them in the following categories (Walker et al 1983).

a. Condyloma acuminatum. Visible exophytic lesions resembling similar condylomata found elsewhere in the female genital tract. These lesions can also be described as condylomatous koilocytosis.

b. Papillary punctation. Patches of individually raised projections of acetowhite (Note 27.1) epithelium which frequently contain a central capillary loop.

c. Coalescent warty atypia. The epithelium of these lesions appears shiny white after washing the cervix with 3% acetic acid and the surface is generally raised and roughened and blood vessels are not prominent. After the application of Lugol's iodine (Schiller's test, Note 27.2) the lesion assumes a speckled appearance.

d. CIN (cervical intra-epithelial neoplasia). This lesion appears as dull acetowhite epithelium that is usually flat and contains the characteristic vessel patterns of punctation or mosaicism from Lugol's solution.

e. Mixed lesions. In certain cases acetowhite epithelium is found in the transformation zone which possesses some of the features of CIN (viz. punctation and/or mosaicism) but the lesion is rough, raised and has a shiny appearance.

Category (c) will be covered by the description 'flat koilocytosis' but the histological examination of the categories (b), (d) and (e) may often reveal koilocytes.

Sessile warts of the genitalia

Sessile warts, resembling plane warts on the non-genital skin, tend to be seen on the shaft of the penis and although often multiple they do not coalesce. Sessile warts do not seem to occur on the vulva. Clear differentiation from the common wart is not always possible. Multiple common skin warts (verruca vulgaris) present as raised lesions; they occur only on the shaft of the penis and occasionally on the vulva and perianal skin.

Oral papilloma

Mouth lesions (lips, tongue, cheek, gingiva, hard palate, floor of mouth) may occasionally occur after orogenital contact with an infected partner. An outbreak of oral 'hairy leukoplakia', associated with HPV and sometimes together with EBV infection, has been described in homosexual males. The white lesions affect the lateral border of the tongue and have a corrugated or 'hairy' appearance due to fine keratin projections. This leukoplakia may presage the Acquired Immune Deficiency Syndrome (Greenspan et al 1984).

Laryngeal papillomata

Papillomata of the larynx may very rarely appear within the first six months of life in babies born to mothers with genital warts at the time of delivery (Cook et al 1973). Hybridization analyses have shown that the papillomaviruses found in laryngeal papillomata are the same as the papillomaviruses found to infect the genital tract. HPV-6 and HPV-11 have been identified respectively in 10 and 3 laryngeal papilloma (Gissman et al 1983). By restriction endonuclease analysis of papillomavirus genomes in laryngeal papillomata, four subtypes of HPV-6 (HPV-6c, HPV-6d, HPV-6e, HPV-6f) have been identified (Mounts & Shah 1984). In juvenile onset disease intrapartum infection is most likely to be the method of transmission of the disease, so Caesarean delivery, prior to the rupture of the membranes, would be expected to provide a high degree of protection against infection. The relative rarity of transmission, however, is to be weighed against the risks of Caesarean section.

In juvenile onset disease (viz. onset of the disease before 16 years) hoarseness is the first symptom in 90% of cases. The larynx is the most common primary site but papillomata can occur in the trachea without involvement of the larynx. The laryngotracheal location presents a threat to the airway and respiratory distress or stridor can occur as a result. Persistent recurrence is a hallmark of the disease. Cases of adult onset disease can be as severe as in juveniles.

DIAGNOSIS

Identification of the virus in the lesion is as yet seldom undertaken for diagnosis owing to the ease of recognizing a wart clinically.

With the new 'high technology' it will be possible to study the epidemiology of the heterogeneous wart viruses and clinicians will expect, for the benefit of patients, to have the facility to recognize HPV types, some of which may have a more serious significance than others. At the present time this depends upon the use of biopsy and, in the case of cervical infection, the colposcope.

Very small lesions cause difficulty and to be certain that a wart has completely disapeared is often a problem, as minor changes in the skin surface often persist at its site.

'Hirsutes papillaris penis' is a title sometimes used for the anatomical state in which filiform papillae are found in parallel rows around the corona of the penis and require to be distinguished from warts. These papillae are anatomical variants (Wigley & Haber 1949) more prominent in some than others.

Skin lesions of secondary syphilis viz. condylomata lata and papular skin eruptions require to be differentiated by dark field microscopy or by tests based on monoclonal antibody (p. 118) for *T. pallidum* and serological tests for syphilis.

Squamous cell carcinoma of the penis, particularly if it is papillary in type, may be difficult to differentiate from condylomata acuminata. Early biopsy of doubtful lesions is essential.

TREATMENT

General considerations

Although ano-genital condylomata acuminata tend to regress spontaneously treatment is important as, in the case of moist hyperplastic warts, spread is sometimes rapid and sepsis can be troublesome. The exclusion, detection and, if required, treatment of other sexually transmissible infections in the affected individual and the sexual contact(s) are essential first steps. The response of warts to treatment diminishes as their duration increases, and early treatment is advised. The presence of genital warts often causes much anxiety in the patient and explanation and encouragement are important. Although there are a wide range of procedures available there is no certain once-only treatment for warts (Bunney 1982).

Before local treatment of genital warts is started it is important to attend to any other local infection, whether sexually transmitted or not, as warts tend to spread more readily in inflamed skin. In the case of men a balanoposthitis should be treated with frequent local saline washes. If necessary, gauze strips (3 × 15 cm) soaked in saline, may be applied 2–4 times daily in such a way as to separate the inflamed inner surface of the prepuce from the glans. The prescription of co-trimoxazole (2 tablets each containing 400 mg sulphamethoxazole and 80 mg trimethoprim twice-daily) by mouth for 5 days is a useful addition to therapy. Alternatively, when anaerobes predominate, metronidazole 200 mg by mouth 8-hourly for 7 days may be used. In the case of women any cause of vaginitis or discharge must be discovered and eradicated, particularly candidiasis or trichomoniasis. Sometimes warts regress after local inflammation has been controlled. Treatment of genital warts is notoriously unsatisfactory and recurrences are common, although when warts are discrete and few, response to treatment may be rapid.

Papillomavirus is frequently present in clinically and histologically normal skin adjacent to the condylomata acuminata. In a recent study 9 of 20 biopsy specimens of clinically normal skin obtained from within 10 mm of the margin of laser-treated lesions showed evidence of papillomavirus DNA sequences. Although recurrence did not occur in all cases these studies (Ferenczy et al 1985) suggest that the latent HPV may be responsible for recurrences so commonly observed following all forms of therapy.

Podophyllin

Podophyllin deserves full consideration because of its

widespread clinical use and its often spectacular initial effects, particularly when applied to hyperplastic condylomata acuminata of the genital skin.

Preparation and content

Podophyllin is an ethanol extract prepared from the dried rhizome and roots of the plant, *Podophyllum* (Greek *podos* — a foot; *phyllon* — a leaf), so-named as the leaf has a fancied resemblance to a webbed foot. The American species, *P. peltatum* (Botanical Magazine, 1816, vol. 43, 1819) grows in moist shady places from New England to Carolina; a second species of therapeutic interest, *P. emodi*, occurs in the Himalaya mountains and Kashmir. In its preparation the syrupy ethanol extract is poured into cold water acidified with hydrochloric acid to form a precipitate which is dried and powdered. Light brown to greenish yellow in colour, it darkens on exposure to light and heat (Windholz 1983). This extract contains, among other compounds, colourless lignans, insoluble in water, which vary quantitatively between the species and from batch to batch, and flavonal pigments. In a study by von Krogh (1978) in the case of *P. peltatum* the lignan content of samples was found to consist of podophyllotoxin, 10% and alpha- and beta-peltatum, 13%: in extracts from *P. emodi*, podophyllotoxin; 40%, and 4'-demethyl-podophyllotoxin 2% were found.

Mode of action

Podophyllotoxin, the main active agent, acts in a manner similar to colchicine and binds specifically at the same (or greatly overlapping) site to tubulin, a component protein of microtubules (Samson 1976) but, in contrast to colchicine, this binding is reversible (Wilson et al 1974). Microtubules form the principal fibrous protein of the mitotic spindle and are an essential component of the biological machinery that moves chromosomes and other cytoplasmic constituents; they act by providing directionality to intracellular movement but not the compelling force. The disintegration of chromatin and arrest of mitosis produced by podophyllin and colchicine (Sullivan & King 1942) are explained by the disassembly of microtubules produced by these compounds (Samson 1976).

The disorder of microtubular function produced by substances which bind to tubulin affects cells generally and is seen, for example, where bidirectional fast axonal transport is blocked by agents which bind to tubulin (Miller & Spencer 1985).

Clinical effects

Topical application of podophyllin in the treatment of genital warts, for many years the practice of urologists of New Orleans, reached the outside world following Kaplan's favourable report in 1942 that condyloma acuminatum rapidly and permanently underwent involution after one or two treatments with a 25% suspension of podophyllum resin (podophyllin) in liquid petrolatum (liquid paraffin) (see review in von Krogh 1981). Later, painful local inflammatory reactions were increasingly recognized and various modifications such as washing off medication 3–24 hours after application and protection of the surrounding epithelial surfaces with inert pastes, creams or ointments were advocated. Intervals between treatments were variously studied and it was generally recommended that a week should elapse between applications. Subsequently Sullivan & King (1947) described in more detail the effects of treatment and preferred to apply 20% podophyllin in 95% alcohol and to allow it to dry to avoid the smearing and spreading effect of the preparation in liquid paraffin. In their studies they recorded that condyloma acuminatum showed first blanching (4–8 hours) and later a drying effect when the pink or red moist warts appeared white, grey and dry; sometimes there was dark brown discoloration. In 4–24 hours the condylomas decreased in size, and in 48 hours there was complete involution. Failures were recorded in chronic perianal condylomas where penetration was prevented by the dry keratinized surface, but as the authors say, condyloma acuminatum undergo involution which 'is remarkable to behold'.

Sullivan & King (1947) recorded also the histological changes and observed the disintegration of the chromatin content and aborted mitoses produced by podophyllin and colchicine. They contrasted these effects with those of salicylic acid (30% in liquid paraffin) in which the superficial skin retained its normal nuclear structure and the subtle cytolytic action of podophyllin was not seen.

Unwanted effects

Unwanted local effects of podophyllin, even with the washing off of the preparation after an interval, vary from local itching, burning, tenderness and erythema to pain, swelling and minor erosions. Balanoposthitis may be severe — associated with phimosis which can, if neglected, lead to a necrotizing balanitis. The skin of the scrotum and vulva may show erythema and scaling. After 1–2 applications apparent cures of the order of 40–70% (von Krogh 1978) may be seen initially, but relapses are frequent and difficult to predict.

When podophyllin has been used aggressively and in quantities beyond that now recommended, systemic ill effects have been recorded including dizziness, lethargy, precoma, nausea, vomiting, abdominal pain, respiratory distress and cold clamminess of the skin. Reversible bone marrow suppression with thrombocytopenia and leucopenia have been recognized (Stoehr et al 1978).

The following case report gives further warning on the dangers of excessively large applications of podophyllin.

Case report

An 18-year-old girl, treated with an estimated 5 ml of 20% podophyllin resin in tincture benzoin for multiple large vulval condylomata acuminata, developed abdominal pain and vomiting after a few hours and became comatose on the following day with loss of reflexes. The coma deepened and by a venovenous shunt her blood was twice perfused through charcoal cannisters. Three hours later she began to recover and by the 6th day she was fully awake. A flaccid paralysis persisted and there was evidence of peripheral neuropathy — difficulty in walking and multiple areas of anaesthesia and paraesthesia. After 4 months she could walk well but still had numbness and tingling of the feet and loss of sensation to pin prick in a glove and stocking distribution (Slater et al 1976).

In pregnancy podophyllin should not be used as it has an antimitotic effect, which although mainly local, is better to avoid. In one case reported in the literature, where a very large amount (7.5 ml) of 25% podophyllin in tincture of benzoin compound was applied to florid vulval warts, the patient developed a severe peripheral neuropathy and intrauterine death of the fetus (32 weeks) occurred (Chamberlain et al 1972).

Recommendations

The present authors recommend dispensing about 0.5 ml quantities to be used for once-only applications given by trained personnel within the clinic; the use of single containers for repeated applications in the clinics is condemned as it may bring risks of cross-infection. Ordinarily, a few warts should be treated at a time, the adjacent skin being protected by yellow or white soft paraffin (BNF), powder, or both. It is good practice to treat, with due regard to any local reaction produced, at frequent intervals (every 3–7 days) with small amounts of 25% podophyllin in liquid paraffin or methylated spirit (not more than 0.3 ml at a time). In the case of the preparation in spirit, time should be given to allow drying. The patient should be instructed to wash off the podophyllin after an interval of about six hours.

Electrocautery

This is an effective treatment in the case of genital warts which are discrete, and especially if they are also pedunculated. A 1% solution of lignocaine is used as a local anaesthetic and the wart removed with the cautery. The aim should be to coagulate the wart down to the basement membrane and cause minimal damage to surrounding skin. In the case of intrameatal warts,

lignocaine gel (20 mg per ml) may be instilled into the terminal urethra and the wart cauterized after 5–10 minutes. Occasionally removal of warts by diathermy or cautery will require general anaesthesia, and circumcision is sometimes required, particularly when there is phimosis.

Scissor excision

Under general anaesthesia the wart-bearing area, in the case of intra-anal warts in particular, is infiltrated with saline adrenaline solution (1/300 000) — quantities of about 20–150 ml are required. The warts are then removed with scissors by cutting at the base of the wart from back to front so that exudate and blood do not obscure progress (Thomson & Grace 1978, Gollock et al 1982).

Cryotherapy

The application of liquid nitrogen (boiling point −195.8°C) to discrete warts is sometimes effective. The aim should be to freeze the wart until a halo of frozen skin is just visible at the base. A cotton-tipped applicator can be immersed in a vacuum flask of liquid nitrogen and then applied to the wart, exposed and immobilized by stretching the skin between the fingers.

Within 30 minutes of freezing, cells begin to show pyknotic nuclei, oedema and other cytoplasmic changes. At the edge of the frozen area cells have eosinophilic cytoplasm and basophilic nuclei. Later changes are those seen in any acutely ischaemic area. The cellular infiltrate is mainly of polymorphonuclear leucocytes, with some lymphocytes and plasma cells most obvious at the edge of the frozen area. Resolution begins within three days and healing usually occurs without scarring (Dawber & Wilkinson 1986).

5-Fluorouracil

Dretler & Klein (1975) reported on the successful use of this substance as a 5% w/w cream in the treatment of intrameatal warts in the male. The cream can be instilled into the anterior urethra with the aid of a nozzle or by using an applicator stick. On 4 occasions daily about 2 ml of cream is instilled after the patient has emptied the bladder. Care is necessary to avoid contaminating the scrotal skin, and treatment should be continued until the wart disappears or an intense inflammation develops (between 6 and 14 days after commencement of treatment). Careful supervision and follow-up with urethroscopy is important. Gentle dilatation of the anterior urethra is advisable after treatment to prevent the development of adhesions. A moderate meatitis after treatment is usual but this tends to settle. In our experience this treatment has been disappointing, as intra-urethral warts recurred in 7 of 8 cases treated, within six weeks to six months after cessation of treatment. The known tendency for warts to regress spontaneously makes assessment of treatment difficult.

Interferons

Interferons are proteins with a broad spectrum of antiviral activity that are released by cells in response to infection or certain other stimuli, are relatively specific, and act indirectly to induce a temporary anti-viral state in uninfected cells and modulate host immune responses. Three types of human interferon are recognized:

1. Interferon-alpha (IFN-α) elaborated mainly by lymphocytes in the peripheral blood and by lymphoid cells elsewhere.
2. Interferon-beta (IFN-β) is produced mainly by fibroblasts.
3. Interferon-gamma (IFN-γ) is produced by lymphocytes in response to antigens and mitogens.

All have different molecular structures and properties, and specific interferons in each group differ in their amino acid composition. To exert their anti-viral activity interferons bind temporarily to receptors on the cell surface and activate cytoplasmic enzymes affecting messenger-RNA translation. The anti-viral state develops after a few hours and may persist for some days. Interferons also have immunoregulatory functions (antibody-synthesis, T-cell mediated cytotoxicity, NK activity and macrophage activation) (Nicholson 1984).

Interferon genes have been cloned into bacterial and yeast plasmids so that large quantities of a single type of specific interferon can be produced. In addition highly purified α-interferons of many different subtypes can be obtained in large quantities from cultured human lymphoblastoid cells (Finter 1984).

Investigations into the use of interferons in the treatment of condylomata acuminata are at an early stage and the experience of Gross and his colleagues in West Germany (1984) indicate the need for caution in its use and precision in diagnosis, including analysis of the papilloma type (see below).

Interferon-alpha (human lymphoblastoid interferon; Hu-IFN-α, Wellcome Foundation). used in an open study in I2 women with longstanding genital warts, produced complete resolution of vaginal warts in all patients and 90–100% clearance in those with vulval or cervical warts. In those with incomplete clearance there was a reduction in number and size of the remaining warts. In those with cervical koilocytosis and an associated dysplasia a reduction in size or complete clearance occurred. The dose used was 4–6 megaunits intramuscularly thrice-weekly for 6 weeks (Alawattegama & Kinghorn 1984).

Interferon-beta (IFN-β), human fibroblast interferon derived from human diploid foreskin cells and prepared as FRONE by Inter Yeda Ltd., Israel, was given by Professor Schonfeld and his group in a double-blind trial of 22 patients (diagnosis made on clinical and histological grounds). In 9/11 of the IFN-β group and 2 in the placebo group the lesions disappeared from about 5 weeks after completion of the course of injections. After 3 months 8 of the non-responders were given a course of IFN-β and all responded to treatment. None of those who responded has had a recurrence, and they have remained free from the disease for 12 months. The dose used was 2×10^6 units IFN-β intramuscularly on 10 consecutive days (Schonfeld et al 1984).

Gross et al found that although HPV-6 DNA or HPV-11 DNA *positive* and HPV-16 DNA *negative* condylomata acuminata responded well to IFN-β without features of dysplasia, in one case after withdrawal of IFN-β there was enhanced proliferation in a case of HPV-ll condylomata acuminata, so that the lesions had to be removed surgically. In addition in one patient, a 28-year-old man with flat condylomata of the prepuce and glans, there was no response to 6 intramuscular injections of 3×10^6 units IFN-β over 15 days. Subsequent intralesional injections of 3×10^6 units IFN-β given 4 times 2 days apart produced flattening and reduction in size of the condylomatous lesions within a few days. After a treatment-free period of 4 weeks very flat papules recurred at the site of the intracutaneous injections and increased rapidly in number and size. Before IFN-β treatment, histologically there was the HPV-associated koilocytosis and structural papillomavirus antigens were detected by the immunoperoxidase technique. After treatment there were histological features of squamous carcinoma in situ (Bowenoid papulosis) and the immunoperoxidase test was negative. Human papillomavirus 16 (HPV-16) DNA sequences were however identified before and after treatment. In Bowenoid papulosis HPV-16 has been demonstrated in 80% cases, and this virus has been demonstrated in 60% of cervical cancers analysed. It may be that IFN-β is papillomavirus-specific (Gross et al 1984).

In the study of Schonfeld and his colleagues (1984) side effects were mild. Of the 19 patients who received IFN-β, 6 had mild fever, lasting for 6 hours after injection, 7 had myalgia, 4 had flu-like syndrome and 3 had headaches for 3–4 hours. Overall the preparation was well tolerated and in no case did treatment have to be interrupted.

PROGNOSIS AND CONTACT-TRACING

Whenever possible it is important to ensure that each partner is examined. Although treatment of warts is far from satisfactory it is important to examine the patient to exclude other sexually transmitted diseases and to relieve anxieties by explanations. In the case of the female contact a cervical smear should be taken for exfoliative cytology examination and an explanation given about the importance of a lifetime follow-up.

MALIGNANT TRANSFORMATION OF ANAL AND GENITAL CONDYLOMATA ACUMINATA

Malignant transformation of anal and genital condylomata acuminata is very rare. Zur Hausen (1977) has reviewed the situation and collected instances in the literature of such conversion. Insofar as the cervix uteri and cervical intra-epithelial neoplasia, including invasive carcinoma of the cervix, are concerned, the possible roles of HPV and HSV in the aetiology have been discussed in Chapter 25. Over the wide range of human papillomavirus infections Table 27.1 details the various clinical types of papilloma, the anatomical sites infected, the individual histological pictures, the HPV types involved, the main age groups infected and the tendency to malignant transformation. In veruccas of the soles of the feet, the face and hands of the young adult or child, malignant conversion is unknown. In the rare condition epidermodysplasia verruciformis (EV) which affects children there is a congenital defect in cell-mediated immunity which makes them prone to infection with certain HPV types. Carcinoma in situ is the usual cancer which appears on average after 24 years interval and affects anatomical sites, such as the the forehead, that are mainly exposed to light. By DNA hybridization the types of papillomavirus involved in the cancer lesions in cases of epidermodysplasia verruciformis were shown to be mostly HPV-5 HPV-8, although HPV-3 has been found. Pfister (1984) suggests that HPV-5 and HPV-8 may be more likely to be cancerigenic than the other types found in EV which were not found in malignant lesions (Table 27.1).

Condylomata acuminata, cervical koilocytosis and respiratory papillomatosis appear all to be linked, in that HPV-6 and HPV-11 are the commonest types seen. Malignant conversion is a rarity, but in respiratory papillomatosis X-irradiation of recurrent laryngeal or tracheal papillomatosis has been followed by carcinoma after intervals between 5 and 40 years.

Carcinoma in situ occurring in one of a group of anal warts has been described in a homosexual; the warts had been recurrent over a two-year period and were shown on electronmicroscopy to contain papillomavirus (Oriel & Whimster 1971). The present authors have seen a case in which recurrent hyperplastic warts became hyperkeratotic and were later replaced by a cutaneous horn near the fraenum, which was found on histological examination to be a well differentiated squamous cell carcinoma. In Africa, particularly in Uganda, carcinoma of the penis is the commonest tumour in males, representing 11% of all tumours — in some tribes the proportion is 40% (Davies 1959, Dodge et al 1973). Carcinoma of the penis is rare in those tribes where circumcision at an early age is practised, but in the uncircumcised, geographical location and genital hygiene may also play a part (Schmauz & Jain 1971). It may be relevant to note that in East Africa, an area of high risk for cancer of the penis, both genital warts and cancer tended to occur 10 years earlier than in Germany or the USA (zur Hausen et al 1978).

In the case of cancer of the cervix conclusions on the relationship of HPV infection cannot yet be made. In South Africa cervical papillomavirus infection has been found in two-thirds of the black women examined, and although this group has also a high risk of cervical cancer, the high frequency of HPV in the normal cervix suggests that there may be other events required to initiate the cancerigenic process in the cervix (Leading Article 1987).

NOTES TO CHAPTER 27

Note 27.1: Colposcopy, acetowhite

Flooding the cervix with an aqueous solution of 3% acetic acid is followed in 15–20 seconds by disappearance of the cervical mucus and a corresponding improvement in the clarity of the colposcopic image the point where many lesions are revealed by this reagent. Differences in cellular density, thickness and keratinization of the mucosa, breaks in the epithelium and even the columnar papillae may be clearly seen after the acetic acid solution has been applied. After two minutes the effect of acetic acid disappears and reapplication becomes necessary. The vascular bed, however, becomes less evident with acetic acid, perhaps due to arteriolar spasm — a green filter over the colposcope lens provides the best visualization of the vascular bed of the cervix (Dexeus et al 1977).

Note 27.2: Colposcopy: Schiller's test

Schiller's test (use of Lugol's solution) is a useful adjunct and makes it possible to define exact limits of a lesion and to study its degree of maturation as well as the extent of regularity of the epithelium. The principle of Schiller's test is that only mature tissues containing stores of glycogen take up iodine; carcinomatous epithelium is iodine-negative (Dexeus et al 1977).

REFERENCES

Alawattegama A B, Kinghorn G R 1984 Letter to editor on human lymphoblastoid interferon (HU IFN-α) in the treatment of genital warts. Lancet i: 1468

Almeida J D 1976 Virological aspects of genital warts. In: Caterall R D, Nicol C S (eds) Sexually transmitted diseases. Academic Press, London, p 179–186

Almeida J D, Howatson A F, Williams M G 1962 Electron microscope study of human warts: sites of virus production and nature of the inclusion bodies. Journal of Investigative Dermatology 38: 337–345

Beaudenon S, Kremsdorf D, Croissant O, Jablonska S, Wain-Hobson S, Orth G 1986 A novel type of human papillomavirus associated with genital neoplasias. Nature 321: 246–249

Bunney M H 1982 Viral warts: their biology and treatment. Oxford University Press, Oxford

Chamberlain M J, Reynolds A L, Yeoman W B 1972 Toxic effect of podophyllum application in pregnancy. British Medical Journal 2: 391–392

Chief Medical Officer, DHSS 1983 Sexually transmitted diseases. Extract from Annual Report of the Chief Medical Officer of the Department of Health and Social Security for the year 1981. British Journal of Venereal Diseases 59: 206–210

Coleman D V, Wickenden C, Malcolm A D B 1986 Association of human papillomavirus with squamous carcinoma of the uterine cervix. In: Papillomaviruses, Ciba Foundation Symposium 120. John Wiley, Chichester, p 175–189

Cook J A, Cohn A M, Brunschwig J P, Butel J S, Rawls W 1973 Wart viruses and laryngeal papillomas. Lancet i: 782

Crawford L 1984 Papilloma viruses and cervical tumours. Nature, London 310: 16

Davies J N P 1959 Cancer in Africa. In: Collins D H (ed) Modern trends in pathology. Butterworth, London p 132–160

Dawber R P R, Wilkinson J D 1986 Physical and surgical procedures. In: Rook A, Wilkinson D S, Ebling F J G, Champion, R H, Burton J L (eds) Textbook of dermatology, 4th edn, vol 3. Blackwells Scientific Publications, Oxford, p 2575–2607

Dexeus S, Carrera J M, Coupez F 1977 Colposcopy, Major problems in Obstetrics and Gynecology, vol 10. W B Saunders, London, p 6–7

Dodge O G, Owor R, Templeton A C 1973 Tumours of the male genitalia. In: Templeton A C (ed) Tumours in a tropical country. A survey of Uganda 1964–1968. William Heinemann Medical Books, p 132–144

Dretler S P, Klein L A 1975 The eradication of intra-urethral condyloma acuminata with 5 per cent 5-fluorouracil cream. Journal of Urology 113: 195–198

Dunn A E G, Ogilvie M M 1968 Intranuclear virus particles in human genital wart tissue: observations on the ultrastructure of the epidermal layer. Journal of Ultrastructure Research 22: 282–295

Ferenczy A, Mitao M, Nagai N, Silverstein S J, Crum C P 1985 Latent papillomavirus and recurring genital warts. New England Journal of Medicine 313: 784–788

Finter N B 1984 Interferons from culture. Lancet ii: 876

Fletcher S 1983 Histopathology of papilloma virus infection of the cervix uteri: the history, taxonomy, nomenclature and reporting of Koilocytic dysplasias. Journal of Clinical Pathology 36: 616–624

Gissmann L, Diehl V, Schultz-Coulson H J, zur Hausen H 1982 Molecular cloning and characterization of human papilloma virus DNA derived from a laryngeal papilloma. Journal of Virology 44: 393–400

Gissmann L, Wolnik L, Ikenberg H, Koldovsky G, Schnurch H G, zur Hausen H 1983 Human papillomavirus types 6 and 11 DNA sequences in genital and laryngeal papillomas and in some cervical cancers. Proceedings of the National Academy of Sciences USA 80: 560–563

Gollock J M, Slatford K, Hunter J M 1982 Scissor excision of anogenital warts. British Journal of Venereal Diseases 58: 400–401

Greenspan D, Greenspan J S, Conant M, Petersen V, Silverman S, de Souza Y 1984 Oral 'hairy' leucoplakia in male homosexuals: evidence of association with both papillomavirus and herpes group virus. Lancet ii: 831–834

Gross G, Ikenberg H, Gissmann L 1984 Bowenoid dysplasia in human papillomavirus-16 DNA positive flat condylomas during interferon-treatment. Correspondence, Lancet i: 1467–1468

Grussendorf E I, zur Hausen H 1979 Localization of viral DNA-replication in sections of human warts by nucleic acid hybridization with complementary RNA of human papilloma virus type 1. Archives of Dermatological Research 264: 55–63

Hauser B, Gross G, Schneider A, de Villiers E-M, Gissmann L, Wagner D 1985 HPV-16-related bowenoid papulosis. Correspondence, Lancet ii: 106

Ikenberg H, Gissman L, Gross G, Grussendorf-Conen E L, zur Hausen H 1983 Human papillomavirus type 16 related DNA in genital Bowen's disease and in bowenoid papulosis. International Journal of Cancer 32: 563–565

Kurman R J, Shah K H, Lancaster W D, Jenson A B 1981 Immunoperoxidase localization of papillomavirus antigens in cervical dysplasia and vulvar condylomas. American Journal of Obstetrics and Gynecology 140: 931–935

Lancaster W D, Olson C 1982 Animal papillomaviruses. Microbiological Reviews 46: 191–207

Leading Article 1983 Human papillomaviruses and neoplasia. Lancet ii: 435–436

Leading Article 1987 Human papillomaviruses and cervical cancer: a fresh look at the evidence. Lancet i: 725–726

Lutzner M A, Orth G, Dutronquay V, Ducasse M-F, Kreis H, Crosnier J 1983 Detection of human papillomavirus type 5 DNA in skin cancers of an immunosuppressed renal allograft recipient. Lancet ii: 422–424

McCance D J, Walker P G, Dyson J L, Coleman D V, Singer A 1983 Presence of human papillomavirus DNA sequences in cervical intraepithelial neoplasia. British Medical Journal 287: 784–788

McMichael H 1967 Inhibition by methylprednisolone of regression of the Shope rabbit papilloma. Journal of the National Cancer Institute 39: 55–65

Matthews R S, Shirodaria P V 1973 Study of regressing warts by immunofluorescence. Lancet i: 681–691

Meanwell C A, Cox M F, Blackledge G, Maitland N J 1987 HPV 16 DNA in normal and malignant cervical epithelium: implications for the aetiology and behaviour of cervical neoplasia. Lancet i: 703–707

Miller M S, Spencer P S 1985 The mechanisms of acrylamide axonopthy. Annual Review of Pharmacology and Toxicology 25: 643–666

Morris H H B, Gatter K C, Stein H, Mason D Y 1983a Langerhans' cells in human cervical epithelium: an immunological study. British Journal of Obstetrics and Gynaecology 90: 400–411

Morris H H B, Gatter K C, Sykes G, Casemore V, Mason D Y 1983b Langerhans cells in human cervical epithelium: effects of wart virus infection and intraepithelial neoplasia. British Journal of Obstetrics and Gynaecology 90: 412–420

Mounts P, Shah K V 1984 Respiratory papillomatosis: Etiological relation to genital tract papillomaviruses. Progress in Medical Virology 29: 90–114

Nicholson K G 1984 Antiviral agents in clinical practice. Properties of antiviral agents. Second of two parts. Lancet ii: 562–564

Oguchi M, Komura J, Tagami H, Ofuji S 1981 Ultrastructural studies of spontaneously regressing plane warts. Macrophages attack verucca epidermal cells. Archives of Dermatological Research 270: 403–411

Oriel J D 1971a Natural history of genital warts. British Journal of Venereal Diseases 47: 1–13

Oriel J D 1971b Anal wart and anal coitus. British Journal of Venereal Diseases 47: 373–376

Oriel J D 1976 Genital warts — the clinical problems. In: Catterall R D, Nicol C S (eds) Sexually transmitted diseases. Academic Press, London, p 186–195

Oriel J D 1983 Condylomata acuminata as a sexually transmitted disease. Dermatologic Clinics 1: 93–102

Oriel J D, Whimster J W 1971 Carcinoma in situ associated with virus-containing anal warts. British Journal of Dermatology 84: 71–73

Pfister H 1984 Biology and biochemistry of papillomaviruses. Review of Physiology, Biochemistry and Pharmacology 9: 111–181

Pollack H M, de Benedictis J J, Marmar J L, Praiss D E 1978 Urethrographic manifestations of venereal warts (condylomata acuminata). Radiology 126: 643–646

Pyrhonen S, Johansson E 1975 Regression of warts. An immunological study. Lancet i: 592–596

Samson F E 1976 Pharmacology of drugs that affect intracellular movement. Annual Review of Pharmacology and Toxicology 16: 143–159

Schmauz R, Jain D K 1971 Geographical variation of carcinoma of the penis in Uganda. British Journal of Cancer 25: 25–32

Schonfeld A, Nitke S, Schattner A et al 1984 Intramuscular interferon — injections in treatment of condylomata acuminata. Lancet i: 1038–1042

Shelley W B, Juhlin L 1976 Langerhans cells form a reticuloepithelial trap for external contact antigens. Nature (Lond.) 261: 46–47

Singer A, Walker P G, McCance D J 1984 Genital wart virus infections; nuisance or potentially lethal. British Medical Journal 288: 735–737

Slater G E, Rumack B H, Peterson R G 1976 Podophyllin poisoning. Systemic toxicity following cutaneous application. Obstetrics and Gynecology: 52–94

Stoehr G P, Peterson A L, Taylor W J 1978 Systemic complications of local podophyllin therapy. Annals of Internal Medicine 89: 362–363

Sullivan M, King L 1947 Effects of resin of podophyllum on normal skin, condylomata acuminata and verrucae vulgaris. Archives of Dermatology and Syphilology 56: 30–47

Thomson J P J, Grace R H 1978 The treatment of perianal and anal condylomata acuminata. Journal of the Royal Society of Medicine 71: 180–185

von Krogh G 1978 Topical treatment of penile condylomata acuminata with podophyllin, podophyllotoxin and colchicine. A comparative study. Acta Dermatovenereologica (Stockholm) 58: 163–168

von Krogh G 1981 Podophyllotoxin for condylomata acuminata eradication. Clinical and experimental comparative studies on Podophyllum lignans, colchicine and 5-fluorouracil. Acta Dermatovenereologica Supplementum 98 (Stockholm)

Walker P G, Singer A, Dyson J L, Shah K V, Wilters J, Coleman D V 1983 Colposcopy in the diagnosis of papillomavirus infection of the uterine cervix. British Journal of Obstetrics and Gynaecology 90: 1082–1086

Wigley J E M, Haber H 1949 Hirsutes papillaris penis. British Journal of Dermatology 61: 427

Wilson L, Bamburg J R, Mizel S B, Grisham L M, Creswell K M 1974 Interaction of drugs with microtubule proteins. Federation Proceedings 33: 158–166

Windholz M (ed) 1983 7418 Podophyllum resin, podophyllin. The Merck Index 10th edition. Merck, Rahway NJ., USA, p 1088–1089

zur Hausen H 1977 Human papillomaviruses and their possible role in squamous cell carcinomas. Current Topics of Microbiology and Immunology 78: 1–30

zur Hausen H, Gissman L, Pfister H, Steiner W, Ojwang S 1978 Papilloma viruses and squamous-cell carcinomas in man. Perspectives in Virology 10: 93–102

28

Cytomegalovirus infection

Cytomegaloviruses are ubiquitous agents widespread among many animals including man and non-human primates such as the owl monkey (*Aotus* spp); spider monkey (*Ateles* spp); marmoset (*Callithrix* spp); capuchin monkey (*Cebus* spp); and African green monkey (*Cercopithecus* spp) (Roizman et al 1981). These viruses are highly species-specific and, as in the case of man, have been closely linked to their natural hosts over aeons of time, and over the generations many, probably thousands, of genetically different strains have emerged to circulate continuously throughout the world. The vast majority of CMV infections are subclinical but there is increased tendency for virulence in the very old, very young, debilitated and immunocompromised persons. As with other herpesviruses, primary CMV infection is often followed by persistence, when reactivation of latent virus may occur; recurrence may, however, also occur as a result of reinfection, probably because of the antigenic diversity of CMV (Alford & Britt 1985).

If transmission is expedited by poor environmental conditions, as in some tropical countries, the acquisition of CMV in infancy or early childhood may confer a measure of protection (Weller 1971). Primary infection, however, may be delayed until in adolescents or young adults, aged 15–35 years, the requirement of close physical contact, such as kissing or sexual intercourse, enables the effective spread of the virus. Although generally asymptomatic, the infection becomes important medically when it occurs as a primary infection during pregnancy, bringing with it a risk of placental passage of virus to the fetus and brain damage (Stern 1977). In the vast majority of cases however, CMV infections are subclinical including those acquired in utero and at, or shortly after, birth. The virus has an oncogenic potential and in vitro transformation can be induced in restrictive infections (see Note 28.1).

CYTOMEGALOVIRUS

Cytomegalovirus (CMV) is one of the slowly growing herpesviruses (Family — Herpesviridae; Sub-family — Betaherpesvirinae; see Ch. 2). On electronmicroscopy the virus particles, after negative staining, are indistinguishable from other members of the Family. When inoculated in vitro into permissive human fibroblasts (Note 28.1). clinical specimens containing human CMV produce a characteristic cytopathic effect — striking cytomegaly with intranuclear inclusions — within hours or weeks following infection. With inocula of high infectivity focal collections of swollen rounded refractile fibroblasts may be detectable in 24–72 hours, whereas with inocula of low infectivity it may take several weeks to produce sparse focal lesions (Weller 1971).

Enveloped virions enter host cells directly by adsorption followed by fusion of the envelope with the plasma membrane or, indirectly, through fusion of the envelope with the membrane phagosome after phagocytosis. Within minutes of entry into the cell the virus is transported towards the nucleus to the region of the Golgi apparatus.

The replicative cycle of cytomegalovirus

CMV has a very large genome, some 50% larger than that of herpes simplex virus, and its massive size suggests that the virus can encode a 'myriad of proteins. The replicative cycle, based on the appearance of different classes of CMV-specific proteins with progressive transcription of the viral genome, can be divided into three time-periods (Alford & Britt 1985).

1. *Immediate-early period* (2–4 hours after infection) characterized by DNA transcription in the absence of either protein synthesis or viral DNA replication. Restricted transcription of specific segments of the genome occurs with the production of what are referred to as '*regulatory immediate-early proteins*' and which may control transcription of early messenger RNA (mRNA).

2. *Early period* (follows (1) and persists through long eclipse phase of CMV multiplication) characterized by DNA replication and the synthesis of a distinct class of infected cell proteins (e.g. DNA polymerase), referred to as *early proteins*.

3. *Late period* (36–48 hours after infection) characterized by continued DNA replication, the formation of

virion structural proteins referred to as *late proteins* and the release of infectious virus about 72 hours after infection. Quantitatively the production of *late proteins* is markedly increased as DNA replication reaches its maximum.

The capability of CMV to stimulate cellular DNA and RNA synthesis is intriguing in view of its oncogenic potential; stimulation of host DNA is a common property of oncogenic viruses.

A 'myriad' of proteins encoded by CMV

Among the 'myriad' of proteins encoded by CMV there are an unknown number of *infected-cell proteins*; and about 33 *structural proteins*, mostly found in small amounts. Of the more abundant proteins there are a major and minor capsid protein; two matrix proteins linking the capsid to the virion envelope; and at least six envelope glycoproteins which are thought to express antibody sites for neutralizing antibodies. Other proteins with as yet an unknown functional and structural role in CMV have been found (Alford & Britt 1985).

Heterogeneity of CMV

As can be shown by (i) DNA-DNA reassociation between strains and (ii) the number and size of fragments produced by restriction enzyme analysis of DNA, CMV isolates vary in base composition of their DNA. There is also some interstrain variation in the composition of the viral proteins which are detectable as slight differences in their 'SDS-PAGE profiles' (see Note 28.2) and antigenicity.

Immunological aspects of cytomegalovirus infection

The differences in the immunological responses of the body at different stages of infection are summarized in Table 28.1; it is convenient to discuss these separately.

During CMV mononucleosis; an event in a CMV primary infection.

During the early acute phase of the illness which is seen almost always in young people after puberty, virus can be cultured from the buffy coat of blood samples and often, but not always, from the urine, saliva and semen. CMV can only rarely be recovered from the peripheral blood leucocytes during convalescence, but both viruria and viraemia are common and often persist for more than two years.

Figure 28.1 illustrates diagrammatically the humoral antibody response during CMV mononucleosis. The IgM and IgG (usually IgG$_1$ and IgG$_3$) antibodies are directed against viral glycoproteins and structural and non-structural viral antigens respectively. Neutralizing and complement-fixing (CF) antibodies are directed primarily against late, structural antigens. The appearance of the former is often delayed with respect to the other antibodies, but neutralizing and CF antibodies persist indefinitely. Antibodies against immediate-early and early antigens are present at high titre during active infection and often, but not always, decline in titre during convalescence.

During the acute phase of the illness various autoantibodies are detectable, probably as the result of the polyclonal B-cell stimulation following exposure to CMV.

In the peripheral blood there is an increased number of lymphocytes of the T8 phenotype. The ability of mononuclear cells to proliferate and produce lymphokines in response to in vitro exposure to various mitogens, including phytohaemagglutin, is impaired. The number of T4 cells is normal. The T8 cells have an increased spontaneous proliferation rate and their inability to produce cytotoxic effector cells may result from re-exposure to antigen that has previously produced memory T8 cells. These abnormalities are

Table 28.1 Immunological findings in individuals infected with cytomegalovirus.

	CMV mononucleosis		Congenitally infected infant	Postnatally infected child	Pregnancy
	Acute	Convalescent			
Isolation of CMV from:					
Blood	+	−	?	?	−
Urine	+	+	++	++	+
Saliva	+	±	+	+	?
Serum immunoglobulin concentration	increased	normal	increased	normal	normal
Activated T8 cells	present	absent	?	?	?
Number of T8 cells	increased	increased	increased	normal	normal
Proliferative responses to mitogens	impaired	impaired	normal	normal	impaired*
Lymphokine production by leucocytes	impaired	?	normal	normal	impaired
Ability to produce cytotoxic effector cells	impaired	?	impaired	impaired	normal
Specific proliferative response of leucocytes to CMV	impaired	normal (late)	impaired	impaired	impaired

*With the exception of the proliferative response to phytohaemagglutinin.

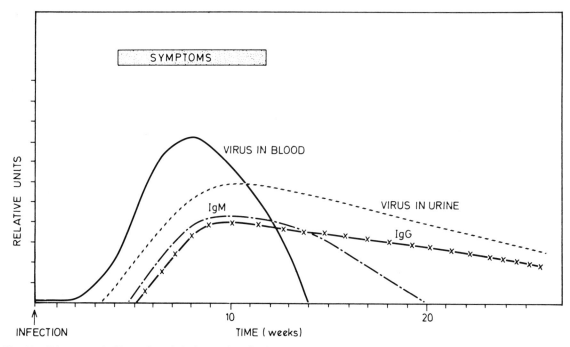

Fig. 28.1 Diagrammatic illustration of the humoral antibody response during CMV mononucleosis.

maximal during the acute phase of the illness, and some resolve during convalescence. Specific *delayed type hypersensitivity* reaction develops as the mitogen-proliferative responses recover.

In congenitally infected infants

IgM against CMV is detectable in the cord blood of most congenitally infected infants. Complement-fixing antibodies are present in the serum at birth and remain detectable at high titre. Antibodies detected by immuno-fluorescence against early and late antigen are found at high titre in the neonate's serum; antibodies against the late antigen persist for years, but against the early diminish and become undetectable generally within three to four years. Immune complexes, present in high concentration in the blood of congenitally infected infants, may play a part in the disease process.

In contrast to CMV mononucleosis, the proliferative response of peripheral blood lymphocytes (PBL) to mitogens other than CMV is normal; specific responses are impaired for at least one year. Immunosuppression in congenital CMV infection lasts much longer than in CMV mononucleosis.

In postnatally infected infants

Although the humoral immune response is similar to that seen in CMV mononucleosis, general cell-mediated immune responses are intact. PBL responses to CMV antigen, however, are impaired and this impairment may persist for years.

During pregnancy

CMV mononucleosis is rare in pregnancy. In seropositive pregnant women CMV-specific PBL proliferative responses become progressively depressed during pregnancy (Gehrz et al 1981). Responses to other mitogens are also depressed. Within four months of delivery, however, the immune suppression has generally resolved. There is no correlation between the suppression of CMV-specific proliferation and excretion of virus. During reactivation of CMV infection there is no specific IgM response.

Transmission

Congenital infection in babies is associated with primary CMV infection in the pregnant mother. It rarely follows reactivation of a latent infection in the mother, where pre-existing circulating antibody effectively prevents placental passage of the virus, although virus is usually cell-associated. Early postnatal infection of the baby tends to be mild, possibly the result of maternally transferred antibodies (Stern 1977).

After a primary infection CMV persists in the body in a latent form, probably for life. Although antibody is present in the serum, virus excretion due to reactivation occurs in pregnancy and in patient on immunosuppressive therapy. CMV has been recovered, for example, from the cervix of 18% of pregnant Chinese in Taiwan; 14% of Navajo women; 5% of Negro; and 4% of Caucasian women in Pittsburg. If recovery of CMV from the cervix is the result of reactivation of a latent infection, then a measure of the reactivation rate within these infected groups is provided by dividing the number with positive cervical cultures for CMV by the number with complement-fixing antibody to CMV (i.e. latent infection) and, when these calculations are applied to the Pittsburg and Navajo populations, the rates are about the same (about 14%). Reactivation occurs more often in the third trimester than in the first or second and more often in the younger and primiparous, than in the older and multiparous patient (Montgomery et al 1972).

The other main mode of transmission to the neonate is by breast feeding. Amongst infants fed infected breast milk, 12% developed neonatal infection (Dworsky et al 1982). The prevalence of serum CMV antibody increases with age, at a rate which varies from country to country and between communities. In developing countries most individuals are seropositive by the age of 5 years, whereas less than 5% of children in developed countries are seropositive by that age. Living under crowded conditions is the most likely reason for this difference in antibody prevalence (Sarov et al 1982).

In clinics for sexually transmitted diseases in Leicester, CMV was isolated from the cervix in about 3% of women, and in Manchester antenatal clinics an isolation rate of 0.7% was obtained (Harris 1975). Handsfield et al (1985) showed that the prevalence of CMV antibodies was greater amongst male contacts of seropositive women than those of seronegative females. They showed further, by DNA restriction typing, that isolates from partners were identical. Sexual intercourse, as a method for the spread of CMV, is supported by the finding of the virus, as extracellular aggregates, in the semen of asymptomatic men convalescent from heterophil-antibody-negative CMV mononucleosis (Lang et al 1974, Oill et al 1977). In one case, virus persisted in the semen for 14 months but, although the specimen was negative for CMV at 2 years, the urine still contained the virus; CMV was also recovered from the uterine cervix of a sexual contact 3 days after the most recent intercourse (Lang & Hanshaw 1969). More than incidental reports of CMV

in the semen have been given by Lang & Kummer (1972), who obtained positive results in 2 of 18 men seeking fertility assessment; in 1 of 10 patients attending a clinic for sexually transmitted disease; and in 3 of 54 young adults. Table 28.2 shows that the prevalence of CMV antibodies amongst young homosexual men is higher than amongst heterosexual men. Up to 15% of homosexual men attending an STD clinic in Copenhagen excreted CMV in the semen (Biggar et al 1983).

Reports on CMV infection amongst homosexual men living in Amsterdam and San Francisco suggest attack rate of 71% and 27% over a 9 and 23 month period respectively (Mintz et al 1983, Coutinho et al 1984). Although comparable studies have not been reported from the UK, these rates are much higher than that of 1.47% over a 7 month period reported amongst British students by university health physicians (University Health Physicians and PHLS Laboratories 1971). Amongst 501 seropositive homosexual men, Coutinho and his colleagues (1984) found a CMV recurrence rate (four-fold increase in titre paired sera) of 6.2% within the 23 month follow-up period.

Persons acquiring a primary infection, perhaps those experiencing reinfection and some with activation of an existing infection may excrete virus in the urine or saliva for months. The urine may contain 10^6 infectious CMV units per ml so that widespread dissemination of infection occurs in closed institutions. Infection rates, in England, as determined serologically, rise appreciably in adolescents. CMV, like infectious mononucleosis due to Epstein-Barr virus, may be a 'kissing disease' (Weller 1971).

CLINICAL FEATURES

A primary CMV infection in adolescents or young adults is almost invariably subclinical. A clinical syndrome may occasionally occur characterized by low-grade fever, diffuse lymphadenopathy, hepatomegaly and pharyngitis; a lymphocytosis develops with atypical lymphocytes in the peripheral blood. Paul-Bunnell-

Table 28.2 Prevalence of CMV antibody in homosexual and heterosexual men attending sexually transmitted diseases clinics.

Locality	Percentage (number tested) of seropositive individuals		Reference
	Homosexual men	Heterosexual men	
San Francisco	94 (139)	54 (70)	Drew et al (1981)
Copenhagen	87 (170)	50 (50)	Melbye et al (1983)
Aarhus	73 (89)	50 (50)	Melbye et al (1983)
Antwerp	71 (191)	57 (95)	Coester et al (1984)
London	93 (152)	56 (108)	Mindel & Sutherland (1984)
Amsterdam	71 (710)	nt	Coutinho et al (1984)
Edinburgh	90 (207)	59 (183)	Edmond et al (unpublished data 1984)

nt = not tested

Davidsohn heterophile antibodies are not produced and the monospot test is therefore negative (Chapter 29).

Primary postnatal infections similarly are usually asymptomatic, but hepatitis with hepatomegaly may occur with abnormalities of liver enzymes. Serious ill effects in previously healthy adults, as for example, chorioretinitis (Chawla et al 1976) or thrombocytopenia (Sahud & Batchelor 1978) are exceedingly rare.

In the post-perfusion syndrome, named for its frequent association with the use of extracorporeal circulation and characterized by splenomegaly and heterophil-antibody-negative CMV mononucleosis, the infection is primary and the virus may be transmitted with fresh blood in the fraction rich in leucocytes (Lang & Hanshaw 1969).

Those with immunological deficiencies, whether due to debilitating disease or due to therapy with suppressive drugs, particularly in organ transplant recipients, are also susceptible to CMV illness (Chatterjee et al 1978) when the infection may be generalized or confined to one organ; interstitial pneumonitis is the most frequent form (Krech et al 1971).

In the United Kingdom 40 to 60% of women enter pregnancy without complement-fixing antibodies to CMV and about 3% of them suffer a primary infection at some time during the course of pregnancy. In about 50% of cases the fetus is infected. About 0.5 to 1% of all babies are congenitally infected and are excreting virus in the throat and urine (Stern 1977). The consequences of fetal infection may range from inapparent infection to the classical syndrome of neonatal cytomegalic inclusion disease (hepatosplenomegaly, purpura, chorioretinitis, uveitis and microcephaly, (Forfar & Arneil 1984). Less severe brain damage may also occur in symptom-free, prenatally infected babies. In a survey of congenital infection in London (Stern 1977), CMV was isolated from urine collected on the day of birth from 16 of 4259 unselected babies screened. 1 of the infected babies died and of the 15 survivors, who were followed for at least 1 year, 3 were mentally retarded (20%); 1 was severely retarded and microcephalic, the other 2 less severely affected. In the United Kingdom, on a national scale, it has been projected that about 2800 infants annually are congenitally infected with CMV and about 500 of them suffer severe brain damage. Possibly double or thrice this figure might suffer brain damage of a lesser degree (Stern 1977). These figures, which compare with an estimated frequency of 200 cases of congenital defects due to rubella in non-epidemic years (Dudgeon 1973), stress the need for prevention of primary infection during pregnancy.

Kaposi's sarcoma, which is possibly associated with CMV infection in the Acquired Immune Deficiency Syndrome (AIDS), is discussed in Chapter 31.

Laboratory diagnosis

Specimens of urine, or mucus from the throat and cervix, collected under sterile conditions, should be sent to the laboratory as soon as possible (as described for herpesvirus, Ch. 26). If storage is required these specimens should be kept at 4°C, but under no circumstances frozen, for isolation of virus (Alford & Britt 1985) in cultures of human embryo lung fibroblasts. On staining the cells with Giemsa, CMV is identified by characteristic intranuclear 'owl's eye' inclusions. Fluorescent antibody staining can also be used to identify CMV in tissue culture. Isolation of CMV from the urine is more likely to occur as a manifestation of primary infection. The CMV complement fixation test can be used to detect previous exposure to infection, although the indirect immunofluorescent antibody test which can also be used for the detection of CMV-IgM, is more sensitive, as is the ELISA technique.

In semen the presence of CMV may be demonstrable only when diluted specimens are inoculated into tissue culture. This fact may reflect toxicity of undiluted semen to the cell culture or may reduce the virus neutralizing capacity of any specific antibody present in the semen (Lang & Kummer 1972).

PREVENTION OF CONGENITAL INFECTION

CMV infection is much more difficult to deal with than rubella. Prevention, based on early diagnosis of primary infection in the pregnant woman, followed by termination, is even less satisfactory than in the case of rubella. The primary CMV infection in the mother is almost always subclinical, making diagnosis difficult. Detection of primary infection would require routine monitoring of women throughout the greater part of pregnancy by complement fixing and CMV-IgM antibody tests. The fetus also can be severely damaged in the second trimester, making termination impracticable. Because of these problems, vaccination of adolescent girls has been proposed by Stern (1977) as a method of preventing primary CMV infection during pregnancy. Increased morbidity and mortality due to fungal and bacterial infections in transplant patients with primary CMV infection are further reasons justifying research into CMV vaccines (Chatterjee et al 1978). Difficulties in matters of attenuation, antigenic differences among human strains of the virus, reactivation of latent infection and the oncogenicity of herpes viruses in general are considered in Stern's (1977) discussion on vaccination, to which the reader is referred. An assessment of the safety and efficiency of one vaccine was disappointing (White 1984).

NOTES TO CHAPTER 28

Note 28.1: Definitions, virus characteristics (Roizman 1985)

a. **Host range.** Type of tissue cells and animal species that virus can infect and multiply.

b. **Susceptibility.** Capacity of tissue cell or animal species to become infected.

c. **Portal of entry.** Cells that become immediately infected are to be found at the portal of entry.

d. **Eclipse phase.** Virus genomes have been exposed to host or viral machinery necessary for their expression but virus production has not yet increased above background.

e. **Maturation phase.** Interval in which progeny virions accumulate in the cell or in the extracellular environment.

f. **Productive infection.*** Characterized by the production of progeny.

g. **Permissive infection.*** Occurs in cells allowing productive infection; cytolytic viruses normally destroy permissive cell.

h. **Abortive infection.** Cell may be susceptible to infection but allow only a few virus genes to be expressed; alternatively virus may be *defective*, lacking full complement of virus genes.

i. **Restrictive (or restringent) infection.*** Cells that are only transiently permissive.

j. **Transformation.** In an infection that is restrictive the virus may injure but not destroy the cell. The consequences may be the expression of host functions which transform the cell from normal to malignant.

k. **Persistence.** Persistence of the viral genomes is an additional consequence of restrictive and abortive infections.

*Productive infection occurs in cells that allow the production of infectious virus — *permissive* cells. Some cells may be transiently permissive, the virus persisting until they become permissive; only a few cells may produce infectious virus at any time. This type of infection is called *restrictive*.

Note 28.2: SDS-PAGE (sodium dodecyl sulphate polyacrylamide gel electrophoresis) profile

By this technique polypeptides are analysed according to their size. Proteins treated by SDS become strongly negatively charged and are then electrophoresed through a polyacrylamide gel which acts as a molecular sieve. Since larger peptides bind more SDS, different peptides have similar charge/size ratios and the rate at which they pass through the gel is dependent solely on their charge. Smaller molecules are retarded to a lesser degree and migrate fastest (Male 1986).

REFERENCES

Alford C A Jr, Britt W J 1985 Cytomegalovirus. In: Fields B N (ed) Virology. Raven Press, New York, ch 29, p 629–660

Biggar R J, Anderson H K, Ebbesen P, Melbye M, Goedert J J, Mann D L, Strong D M 1983 Seminal fluid excretion of cytomegalovirus related to immunosuppression in homosexual men. British Medical Journal 286: 2010–2012

Chatterjee S N, Fiala M, Weiner J, Stewart J A, Stacey B, Warner N 1978 Primary cytomegalovirus and opportunistic infections. Incidence in renal transplant recipients. Journal of the American Medical Association 240: 2446–2449

Chawla H B, Ford M J, Munro J F, Scorgie R E, Watson A R 1976 Ocular involvement in cytomegalovirus infection in a previously healthy adult. British Medical Journal 3: 281–282

Coester C-H, Avonts D, Colaert J, Desmyter J, Piot P 1984 Syphilis, hepatitis A, hepatitis B and cytomegalovirus infection in homosexual men in Antwerp. British Journal of Venereal Diseases 60: 48–51

Coutinho R A, Wertheim-van Dillen P, Albrecht-van Lent P et al 1984 Infection with cytomegalovirus in homosexual men. British Journal of Venereal Diseases 60: 249–252

Drew W L, Mintz R C, Miner L, Sands M, Ketterer B 1981 Prevalence of cytomegalovirus infection in homosexual men. Journal of Infectious Diseases 143: 188–192

Dudgeon J A 1973 Intrauterine infections (CIBA Foundation Symposium 10). Elliott K, Knight J (eds). Elsevier, Amsterdam, p 38

Dworsky M, Yow M, Stagno S, Pass R, Alford C A 1982 Cytomegalovirus (CMV) in breast milk and transmission to the infant. Pediatric Research 16: 239A

Forfar J O, Arneil G C 1984 Textbook of paediatrics, 3rd edn. Churchill Livingstone, Edinburgh, vol 1, p 206–207

Gehrz R C, Christianson W R, Linner K M, Conroy M M, McCue S A, Balfour H H 1981 A longitudinal analysis of lymphocyte proliferative responses to mitogens and antigens during human pregnancy. American Journal of Obstetrics and Gynecology 140: 665–670

Handsfield H H, Chandler S H, Caine V A, Meyers J D, Corey L, Medeiros E, McDougall J K 1985 Cytomegalovirus infection in sex partners: evidence for sexual transmission. Journal of Infectious Diseases 151: 344–348

Harris J R W 1975 Cytomegalovirus infection. In: Morton R S, Harris J R W (eds) Recent advances in sexually transmitted diseases. Churchill Livingstone, Edinburgh, p 361–364

Krech U, Jung M, Jung F 1971 Cytomegalovirus infections of man. S Karger, Basel, p 76

Lang D J, Hanshaw J B 1969 Cytomegalovirus infection and the post perfusion syndrome: recognition of primary infection in four patients. New England Journal of Medicine 280: 1145–1149

Lang D J, Kummer J F 1972 Demonstration of cytomegalovirus in semen. New England Journal of Medicine 287: 756–758

Lang D J, Kummer J F, Hartley D P 1974 Cytomegalovirus

in semen. Persistence and demonstration in extracellular fluids. New England Journal of Medicine 291: 121–123

Male D 1986 Immunology. An illustrated outline. Gower Medical Publishing, London; Churchill Livingstone, Edinburgh, p 715

Melbye M, Biggar R J, Ebbesen P, Andersen H K, Vestergaard B F 1983 Lifestyle and antiviral antibody studies among homosexual men in Denmark. Acta Pathologica Microbiologica Immunologica Scandinavica Sect B 91: 357–364

Mindel A, Sutherland S 1984 Antibodies to cytomegalovirus in homosexual and heterosexual men attending an STD clinic. British Journal of Venereal Diseases 60: 189–192

Mintz L, Drew W L, Minec R C, Braff E H 1983 Cytomegalovirus infections in homosexual men. An epidemiological study. Annals of Internal Medicine 99: 326–329

Montgomery R, Youngblood L, Medearis D N 1972 Recovery of Cytomegalovirus from the cervix of pregnancy. Pediatrics 49: 524–531

Oill P A, Fiala M, Schofferman J, Byfield P E, Guze L B 1977 Cytomegalovirus mononucleosis in a healthy adult. Association with hepatitis, secondary Epstein Barr virus antibody response and immunosuppression. American Journal of Medicine 62: 413–417

Roizman B 1985 Multiplication of viruses: an overview. In: Fields B N (ed) Virology. Raven Press, New York, ch 5, p 69–75

Roizman B, Carmichael L E, Deinhardt F et al 1981 Herpesviridae: definition, provisional nomenclature, and taxonomy. Intervirology 16: 201–217

Sahud M A, Batchelor M McC 1978 Cytomegalovirus-induced thrombocytopenia. Archives of Internal Medicine 138: 1573–1575

Sarov B, Naggan L, Rosenveig R, Katz S, Haskin H, Sarov I 1982 Prevalence of antibodies to human cytomegalovirus in urban, kibbutz and Bedouin children in Southern Israel. Journal of Medical Virology 10: 195–201

Stern H 1977 Cytomegalovirus vaccine. Justification and problems. In: Waterson A P (ed) Recent advances in clinical virology. Churchill Livingstone, Edinburgh, p 117–134

University Health Physicians and PHLS laboratories 1971 Infectious mononucleosis and its relationship to EB virus antibody. British Medical Journal iv: 643–646

Weller T H 1971 The cytomegaloviruses: ubiquitous agents with protean clinical manifestations. New England Journal of Medicine 285: 203–214, 267–274

White D O 1984 Antiviral chemotherapy, interferons and vaccines. In: Melnick J L (ed) Monographs in virology No 16. Karger, Basel, p 73–74

29

Infectious mononucleosis

The aetiological role of the Epstein-Barr virus (EBV) as the causative agent of infectious mononucleosis is established, and its acquisition during adolescence or early adulthood as a result of kissing is an important facet of the epidemiology of this virus infection in the developed countries. The sore throat, the generalized lymph node hyperplasia and the typical blood picture occur in some 50% of primary infections in the 15–25 year age group, in contrast to the generally asymptomatic primary infection in childhood. In developed countries about 75–80% of the population ultimately become infected, whereas in developing countries nearly all children are already infected by about the age of 3 years. The delayed infection is more frequent in privileged classes of western societies, enjoying high standards of hygiene, than in the lower socio-economic groups. The uniformly early age of Epstein-Barr virus infection in developing countries, which leaves no adolescents or young adults susceptible, accounts for the virtual absence of infectious mononucleosis (Epstein 1982). The annual incidence of infectious mononucleosis in the United Kingdom is about 20–60 per 100 000 (Pollock 1969). Whenever infection takes place the infected individual carries the virus for life (Epstein & Achong 1986).

In addition Epstein-Barr virus causes a rare and fatal infectious mononucleosis, Duncan's disease, in individuals with the X-linked recessive genetically determined defect. The ubiquitous virus also has an aetiological role, albeit with co-factors, in the induction of the tumours, endemic Burkitt's lymphoma and undifferentiated nasopharyngeal carcinoma (Leading Article 1982). EBV is thought to be a component in the induction of malignant lymphomas under circumstances in which immunosuppressive therapy is known to cause a profound disturbance of cytotoxic T-cells, which have an important role in EBV surveillance. EBV may also be involved in the development of lymphomas in the Acquired Immune Deficiency Syndrome (AIDS) (Ziegler et al 1982, Epstein & Achong 1986).

THE EPSTEIN-BARR VIRUS

Epstein-Barr virus is so named after the discoverers of the virus particles in cultured lymphoblasts from the unusual malignant tumour, African endemic Burkitt's lymphoma (Burkitt 1958, 1963, Epstein et al 1964). It is a herpesvirus, morphologically identical, but serologically distinct from the three human well-known herpesviruses, viz. herpes simplex, varicella-zoster and cytomegalovirus. By reason of its characteristic feature of replicating in lymphoblastoid cells Epstein-Barr virus has been placed in the sub-family, Gammaherpesvirinae with 'human lymphocryptovirus 4' as its specific name (Ch. 2).

INFECTIOUS MONONUCLEOSIS

The marked tropism of the virus for human B-lymphocytes is accounted for by the presence on the surface membrane of the B-lymphocytes of receptors for EBV (see review on lymphocytes by Calvert et al 1984). The virus grows only in a suspension culture of human lymphoblasts and then only a small proportion of cells tend to produce virions, although all cells carry the viral genome. EBV is the cause of infectious mononucleosis, a self-limiting lymphoproliferative disease with a complex natural history in which virus infects two target cell goups, viz. B-lymphocytes and epithelial cells of the oropharynx or parotid gland.

AFRICAN ENDEMIC BURKITT'S LYMPHOMA

African endemic Burkitt's lymphoma is a truly malignant tumour whose cells contain EBV. Hypotheses have been advanced to explain how hyperendemic malaria, acting as a co-factor, could affect the nature or rate of cell transformation by EBV and how increased division of such cells could predispose to the chromosomal rearrangements described in Burkitt's lymphoma (Leading Article 1982). It has now been demonstrated that EBV-specific T-lymphocyte control is dramatically impaired during acute malarial attacks by *Plasmodium falciparum* (Whittle et al 1984).

An outbreak of Burkitt's-like lymphoma (undifferentiated, monoclonal, B-cell tumours) has been reported in homosexual men (Ziegler et al 1982), a manifestation of the Acquired Immune Deficiency Syndrome (AIDS; see also Ch. 31); these lymphomas may be also aetiologically related to co-existing EBV infection (Epstein & Achong 1986).

UNDIFFERENTIATED NASOPHARYNGEAL CARCINOMA

In nasopharyngeal carcinoma, very common in Chinese people, particularly the southern Chinese, the association with EBV is strong and consistent (Leading Article 1982). Despite the well-established tropism to the virus for human B-lymphocytes, the cell type within the oropharynx capable of allowing EBV replication had not been identified until recently, and the association of EBV with nasopharyngeal carcinoma was puzzling. In recent times, however, Sixbey et al (1984), using in-situ cytohybridization, have demonstrated EB virus DNA in oropharyngeal epithelial cells from 10 of 12 patients with infectious mononucleosis and envisage a complex interaction between EBV and two target cell types.

Sixbey and his colleagues (1983) were able to infect human epithelial cell cultures exposed to 'wild-type' virus from fresh filtered oropharyngeal washings from patients with acute infectious mononucleosis but not from culture supernatant fluids from EBV infected lymphoid cell lines. With epithelial cells thus implicated as a source of EB virus, they suggested that EBV may be carried *latently* in rapidly dividing cells of the basal epithelium and that the virus may actively replicate only on cell differentiation or senescence. The demonstration of EB virus DNA, in large amounts, in exfoliated cells from the oropharynx of patients with infectious mononucleosis is consistent with this view (Sixbey et al 1984). In connection with nasopharyngeal carcinoma Sixbey's group (1983) suggest that the carcinoma represents a clonal expansion of a subset of cells with virus receptors.

There is good epidemiological evidence for an environmental co-factor acting with EBV in the aetiology of undifferentiated nasopharyngeal carcinoma and recent suggestions that phorbol esters in such things as traditional herbal medicines are being investigated further (Epstein & Achong 1986, Ito 1986).

NATURAL HISTORY OF INFECTIOUS MONONUCLEOSIS

Inapparent primary infection with Epstein-Barr virus generally occurs in childhood and is always accompanied by seroconversion and immunity to infectious mononucleosis. If the primary infection is delayed, however, until late adolescence or early adulthood then this event leads to infectious mononucleosis in about 50% of cases. As in herpes simplex virus infections, EB virus is most frequently acquired as a primary infection during childhood, particularly in the lower socio-economic groups and, in developing countries, almost all children are infected before the age of ten, so that very few young adults can develop a primary infection and infectious mononucleosis is therefore virtually unknown. However or whenever infected, the individual will carry EBV for life.

In previously uninfected adolescents, often from privileged classes, large doses of EBV virus are ingested when kissing; this virus is shed into the mouth by seropositive healthy carriers, who themselves have practically never shown signs of their original primary infection. In the case of young children indirect methods of spread probably operate and are responsible for the smaller infecting doses, which seem to play a part in determining inapparent infections without disease. Although infectious mononucleosis tends to occur within the 15–25 year age group, it may occasionally occur in those outside the group.

Once in the mouth of a susceptible person, EB virus gains access to the body by infecting B-lymphocytes, probably in the oropharyngeal ring of lymphoid tissue (Waldeyer's Ring). Only B-lymphocytes have been found to have the receptor for the virus, viz. the C3d receptor CR2 (Fingeroth et al 1984) and can carry the viral genome in vivo. In the oropharynx, after an incubation period varying between 6 and 60 days, a replicative virus cycle is set up and the virus must then be carried throughout the body by the peripheral circulation, either as a viraemia to infect B-lymphocytes everywhere, or alternatively infected B-lymphocytes, involved in the virus replication in the oropharynx, are themselves spread widely to liberate virus and infect other B-cells at distant sites. In the first week of infectious mononucleosis up to 1 in 2000 blood lymphocytes carries the virus, as judged by the ability to infect other lymphocytes in tissue culture. Over ensuing weeks the proportion of infected lymphocytes falls to reach control levels — about 5 in 10^7 cells — three months after the onset (Leading Article 1978).

A virus-determined surface antigen on B-lymphocytes is directly responsible for the disease and especially the haematological manifestations, as it is recognized by helper and suppressor T-cells and eventually by cytotoxic T-cells which are produced in great quantities and are responsible for the clinical features of the disease, viz. hepato-splenomegaly, jaundice, abnormal plasma enzyme tests, tonsillar and adenoidal changes and the typical blood picture. The characteristic mononucleosis and atypical cells have been shown to consist largely of T-lymphocytes which are specifically cytotoxic in vitro for EBV genome positive target cell lines (Royston et al 1975). Tissue necrosis, due to death of cells supporting a full replicative cycle, may also contribute to the sore throat; the pharyngitis may be explained by the ability of EBV to infect oropharyngeal epithelium (Sixbey et al 1984).

Shedding of virus into the buccal fluid occurs as early as 8 days after the onset of symptoms. Virus is regularly detectable in the saliva of infectious mononucleosis patients (Gerber et al 1972) and seropositive healthy persons (Golden et al 1973) The site of virus production was thought to be the B-lymphocytes of the oropharynx because only these cells are known to have EBV receptors. Specialized cells at specific sites, however, might provide suitable conditions for the persistence and low-level production of the virus. The isolation of EBV from cell-free secretions from the efferent duct of the parotid gland and the detection of the virus in the parotid gland are in favour of this hypothesis (Morgan et al 1979, Wolf et al 1984). The capacity of wild-type Epstein-Barr virus to infect and replicate in human epithelial cells cultured in vitro and the discovery of EBV DNA in large amounts in exfoliated epithelial cells from the oropharynx of patients with infectious mononucleosis (Sixbey et al 1983, 1984) are findings also consistent with this view. It has been possible also to detect directly by dot hybridization Epstein-Barr virus DNA in washed exfoliative cells from bronchial washings, and this finding suggests that the respiratory tract is probably the largest site for EBV latency yet reported. Viral antigen was only rarely detected in these cells (Lung et al 1985).

Genital lesions in infectious mononucleosis have rarely been described but the recovery of EBV from ulcerative lesions on the labia minora in a single case has raised interest both in the possible importance of epithelial cells as a source of infecting virus and of lesions occurring in a genital site enabling transmission of the virus by sexual intercourse (Portnoy et al 1984).

EBV has now been detected in cervical secretions, and in situ hybridization methods have shown the presence of EBV-DNA within cervical epithelial cells (Sixbey et al 1986). As the virus was found in cervical secretions from women with infectious mononucleosis and in individuals with serological evidence of past EBV infection, it is possible that the uterine cervix as well as the oropharynx may be a site of EBV replication and chronic viral shedding. This study suggests that EBV can be transmitted sexually, possibly by orogenital contact, but perhaps also from the male genital tract; studies in men are awaited with interest.

LIFE-LONG ASYMPTOMATIC EBV-CARRIER STATE

Studies in vitro suggest that B-lymphocytes alone express the EBV receptor and sustain an experimental infection. The outcome of the infection is not, however, virus replication but immortalization of the cells into lymphoblastoid cell lines which carry the EBV genome but can seldom be induced into a virus productive cycle. Clearly, EBV replication occurs in the throat, not only in the course of the primary infection of infectious mononucleosis, but also as a stable accompaniment of the asymptomatic virus carrier state. The recent work of Sixbey and his colleagues (1983, 1984) favours the suggestion that the epithelial cell of the oropharynx is a significant site for EBV replication (Rickinson 1984).

IMMUNE RESPONSE IN INFECTIOUS MONONUCLEOSIS

Increase of virus-specific antibodies and T-cell mediated responses brings the disease under control. T-cell numbers are reduced as the mass of latently infected B-cells are themselves reduced. The infection of lymphocytes can result in a temporary depression of cell-mediated immunity response, e.g. the tuberculin skin test may become negative during the acute phase of the disease. After convalescence and for the rest of the patient's life virus production continues at a low level with intermittent release of extracellular virus into the mouth.

The serology of Epstein-Barr virus infections and EBV-associated diseases is based on the detection of antibodies (Henle & Henle 1979) to a number of EBV antigens, viz. viral capsid antigen (VCA), early antigen (EA) and EBV nuclear antigen (EBNA) (Ernberg & Klein 1979) (Table 29.1). In infectious mononucleosis, however, diagnosis depends usually, from the practical point of view, upon the detection of the transient heterophil IgM antibody, and specific virological tests for EBV are often omitted. Transient IgM antibodies to a structural component of the virus particle, namely viral capsid antigen (anti-VCA IgM), reach high titres early in the disease; the anti-VCA IgG antibody develops in two weeks and persists throughout life. Virus neutralizing antibodies have been found to reach a peak later and persist also for life. Antibodies to EBV early antigen complex (anti-EA) are present during the acute primary infection but absent during convalescence or in those

Table 29.1 Antibody patterns characteristic for Epstein-Barr virus-associated diseases with the main feature(s) indicated by square(s). Early antigen consists of two components, one designated 'restricted' (R) confined to the cytoplasm, and the other 'diffuse' (D) more finely dispersed and to be found in both nucleus and cytoplasm (Henle & Henle 1979, Leading Article 1985, see text).

	Antibody to: Viral capsid antigen (VCA)			Early antigen (EA)		EBV nuclear antigen (EBNA)
	IgM	IgA	IgG	Diffuse (D)	Restricted (R)	
Infectious mononucleosis	++	0	++	+	0	0
Persistent ill-health after infectious mononucleosis	+*	0	++	0	+	0
Endemic Burkitt's lymphoma	0	0	++	0	++	0
Nasopharyngeal carcinoma	0	++	++	++	0	++
Controls	0	0	+	0	0	+

*(in some)

with a history of a previous attack of infectious mononucleosis. Antibodies to EBV nuclear antigen (anti-EBNA) are absent during the acute attack but develop during convalescence.

None of the antibodies discussed are related to the transient heterophil Paul-Bunnell-Davidsohn type whose association with EB virus is not understood (Epstein & Achong 1977). This IgM antibody is almost always present when the patient develops symptoms and becomes negative within a few weeks or months. This aberrant response may be due to the effect of the virus as a polyclonal B-cell activator since virus-induced transformation of human B-cells in vitro can stimulate the synthesis of a complex variety of antibodies, some of which react with heterophil determinants, but there may be other mechanisms. Similar antibodies may be found transiently, for example, in viral infections which do not have any B-cell activating properties (Rickinson 1986).

A significant proportion of infections in young children are not associated with a positive Paul-Bunnell-Davidsohn test.

CLINICAL MANIFESTATIONS OF INFECTIOUS MONONUCLEOSIS

Infectious mononucleosis consists of an acute illness characterized by certain clinical and haematological criteria together with the presence of Paul-Bunnell-Davidsohn heterophil antibody in the circulation. The incubation period is difficult to determine as evidence in case-to-case infection is rarely clear-cut. Figures are frequently quoted within the range of 6–60 days. The young adult presenting with malaise, fever with tachycardia, sore throat and skin rash, who is found to have lymphadenopathy and splenomegaly, is the classical clinical picture. There may also be headache, dysphagia and anorexia, myalgia, nausea, neck stiffness, photophobia and chest pain, and even a mild jaundice in a few patients. Hyperplasia of the pharyngeal lymph follicles is common and a pharyngeal exudate is seen in about half the patients. In up to one-third of cases there are petechial lesions 0.5–1.00 mm in diameter at the junction of the hard and soft palate near the midline. Discrete slightly tender lymph nodes are noted, especially in the posterior cervical region.

Skin rashes, when present, usually consist of a faint diffuse erythematous or maculopapular eruption, mostly on the trunk and proximal portions of the limbs. The rash is not diagnostic and may have been drug-induced as patients with infectious mononucleosis are particularly prone to hypersensitivity reactions of this kind.

Genital lesions have only rarely been described in infectious mononucleosis. In one such case, a 14-year-old girl developed buccal and labial (vulval) ulceration following oral-genital contact (Brown & Stenchever, 1977). In another case a shallow single punched-out painless subpreputial erosion was found (Lawee & Shaffir 1983). In the case where EB virus was recovered from genital ulcers, Portnoy et al 1984, describe how a 23-year-old patient first saw a bluish-black irregular lesion on the labia minora which was followed later by tender ulcers in this area which remained painful until healing occurred 32 days after the first appearance of the lesions.

Ampicillin will precipitate a rash in about 8% of individuals, but in patients with infectious mononucleosis or lymphatic leukaemia, a rash develops in more than 70% of cases (Cameron & Richmond 1971). This may be due to alteration of the normal immune mechanisms resulting from the abnormal, but immunologically competent lymphocytes. Impurities of high molecular weight in ampicillin play a part and there is clinical support for efforts of manufacturers to remove these from antibiotics (Parker & Richmond 1976).

Other objective signs sometimes found include also hepatomegaly, periorbital oedema, arthropathy, cough and diarrhoea. Most of the unusual symptoms are associated with some rare complication and their undue emphasis tends to distort descriptions of the true clinical picture which, for the most part, is somewhat stereotyped. The most important and characteristic symptom is the sore throat which develops a few days after the onset of the illness (Finch 1969).

Prognosis

The usual pattern is one of mild fever of about two weeks duration. Complications are rare although a wide variety, including haemolytic anaemia and thrombocytopenia, occasionally develop. Fatalities are very rare (less than 1 per 1000 cases) and may be associated with ruptured spleen, neurological complications, asphyxia and 'toxic' effects. A syndrome has been recognized in which an X-chromosome-linked immunological deficiency has led to deaths as a result of primary virus infection (Epstein & Achong 1977). In this condition (often designated XLP syndrome or Duncan's disease) individuals die of fatal infectious mononucleosis in which a genetically determined failure of specific T-cell and other cellular immunological responses lead to a huge uncontrolled proliferation of B-cells infected with EBV (Leading Article 1982).

Some patients with infectious mononucleosis do not fully recover clinically for several months or even years and there are occasional reports of recrudescences. In patients who fail to make a complete recovery, high levels of T-suppressor cells may be found. Although remaining unwell for a year at least, recovery is the rule, when a return to normal of the lymphocyte subsets is seen (Hamblin et al 1983).

Unusually severe, protracted or recurrent illness after heterophil-antibody positive infectious mononucleosis may be accompanied by a serological 'hallmark' viz. anti-EA(R) after the initial anti-EA(D) responses have subsided, with persisting high levels of anti-VCA (usually IgG but IgM in some) (Table 29.1) (Leading Article 1985). Now that techniques using cloned fragments of Epstein-Barr virus DNA have been developed it is possible to measure serological responses to antigens that represent the product of defined regions of the viral genome; such studies may lead to the discovery of new serological tests which will distinguish more clearly between chronic latent and chronic active infection (Niederman 1985).

Haematological manifestations

The haematological features of infectious mononucleosis are characterized by an absolute lymphocytosis, $4500-5000/mm^3$ $(4.5-5.0 \times 10^9/l)$. A relative lymphocytosis of more than 60% of total leucocytes is seen in 95% of cases. The lymphocytosis tends to persist for two weeks unless bacterial infection supervenes. 20% or more of the lymphocytes are atypical and pleomorphic, varying in size, shape and staining qualities of the cytoplasm and chromatin configurations of the nuclei. Many lymphocytes show a tendency to flow round adjacent erythrocytes. Rapid changes in this picture may occur from day to day.

Plasma enzyme tests

Plasma enzyme tests for hepatocellular damage (see Ch. 30; Note 30.1) (alkaline phosphatase, alanine aminotransferase) show increased activity in 85-100% of patients with infectious mononucleosis. Abnormalities increase during the first week and are most pronounced by the middle or end of the second week. They almost invariably return to normal by the third to fifth week of the illness (Finch 1969).

Serological manifestations

Non-specific cardiolipin tests for syphilis, such as the VDRL test and Wassermann reaction may be positive: a great variety of other antibodies, such as rheumatoid and antinuclear factors may also develop (Finch 1969).

Paul-Bunnell-Davidsohn differential test

Sera from patients with many conditions other than infectious mononucleosis may agglutinate sheep red blood cells, but in such cases the heterophil antibodies are of the Forssman type, which can be absorbed by guinea-pig kidney cells. In infectious mononucleosis, however, the heterophil antibodies are not of the Forssman type and are not absorbed by guinea-pig kidney cells, although the antibody is absorbed by ox cells. In the Paul-Bunnell-Davidsohn differential test, these properties are used to make the test highly specific for infectious mononucleosis. The test can also be made more sensitive by using horse erythrocytes. These principles have been used to provide rapid and specific screening tests, e.g. the monospot slide test (Ortho Diagnostics Inc., New Jersey, 08869, USA). In the monospot test, serum is mixed thoroughly with guinea-pig kidney stroma (GPK) on one spot and with beef erythrocyte stroma (BES) on another, and unwashed preserved horse erythrocytes are added immediately, to each spot. If agglutination of erythrocytes on the spot with GPK is stronger than that on the spot with BES, the result of the test is positive. If the agglutination pattern is stronger on the spot with BES, the result is negative. The test is also negative if no agglutination appears on either spot, or if agglutination is equal on both spots.

All cases of infectious mononucleosis characterized by the clinical and haematological criteria described, together with the presence of the Paul-Bunnell-Davidsohn heterophil antibody in the circulation, will be found to have antibodies against the Epstein-Barr virus. The diagnosis may be facilitated by serial laboratory studies; tests for heterophil antibody are readily available but not, however, for antibody to EBV.

There is a significant number of clinically and haematologically typical cases of infectious mononucleosis, which are Paul-Bunnell-Davidsohn antibody negative, but which are due to EBV, as can be demonstrated by the presence of EBV-specific IgM antibodies.

In patients without antibodies to EBV and without Paul-Bunnell-Davidsohn heterophil antibodies, other diseases which may cause fever with lymph node enlargement should be considered in the differential diagnosis (AIDS, cytomegalovirus infection, toxoplasmosis, listeriosis, tuberculosis, secondary syphilis and brucellosis). Viral or streptococcal pharyngitis, diphtheria, Vincent's infection or primary herpes simplex stomatitis may cause sore throat of similar severity to infectious mononucleosis.

A resurgence of heterophil antibody may occur in response to a non-specific respiratory tract infection (Finch 1969) in patients who have had infectious mononucleosis months or years previously.

Specific antibody tests for Epstein-Barr virus infection
The following criteria may be accepted as definite evidence of *recent* EBV infection: 1. the presence of anti-VCA IgM antibody, 2. the seroconversion of anti-VCA IgG antibody from negative to positive in paired sera. Single high or paired IgG antibody titres are not helpful in diagnosing recent EBV infections, but a fourfold or greater rise in IgG antibody titre is regarded as suggestive evidence.

Reference has been made to other tests for antibody, viz. anti-EA antibody and EBV anti-EBNA (see above, immune response in infectious mononucleosis). Antibody patterns characteristic for EBV- associated diseases are shown in Table 29.1. (Henle & Henle 1979, Leading Article 1985, 1986).

TREATMENT

Patients with uncomplicated infectious mononucleosis usually require rest in bed during the acute phase of the illness. Saline gargles and aspirin are useful for the relief of symptoms. As soon as the temperature is within normal range the patient may become ambulant, and full activity is commonly resumed after about a month from the onset. Violent exercise should be avoided for at least three weeks after the spleen is no longer palpable.

Corticosteroids should be reserved for the rare case of a very ill pateint, when there is, for example, significant thrombocytopenia, impending airway obstruction or acute haemolysis (Finch, 1969).

PREVENTION

Arguments for the development of a vaccine capable of preventing Epstein-Barr virus infection have become increasingly cogent as the clinical consequences — endemic Burkitt's lymphoma, undifferentiated nasopharyngeal carcinoma, Duncan's disease and the EBV-carrying lymphomas of patients on prolonged immunosuppressive therapy (Leading Article 1982) have been enumerated. Interest in intervention against EBV has heightened in recent years, particularly in regions where undifferentiated nasopharyngeal carcinoma is the most common cancer in men and the second most common in women (Epstein & Morgan 1986).

REFERENCES

Brown Z A, Stenchever M A 1977 Genital ulceration and infectious mononucleosis: report of a case. American Journal of Obstetrics and Gynecology 127: 673–674

Burkitt D 1958 A sarcoma involving the jaws in African children. British Journal of Surgery 46: 218–223

Burkitt D 1963 A lymphoma syndrome in tropical Africa. International review of experimental pathology, vol 2. Academic Press, New York, 67–138

Calvert J E, Maruyama S, Tedder T F, Webb F C, Cooper M D 1984 Cellular events in the differentiation of antibody-secreting cells. Seminars in Hematology 21(4): 226–243

Cameron S J, Richmond J 1971 Ampicillin hypersensitivity in lymphatic leukaemia. Scottish Medical Journal 10: 425–427

Epstein M A 1982 Persistence of Epstein-Barr virus infections. In: Mahy B W J, Minson A C, Darby G K (eds) Virus persistence. Cambridge University Press, Cambridge, p 169–183

Epstein M A, Achong B G 1977 Pathogenesis of infectious mononucleosis. Lancet ii: 1270–1273

Epstein M A, Achong B G 1986 The Epstein-Barr virus, recent advances. William Heinemann Medical Books, London, p 1–11

Epstein M A, Morgan A J 1986 Progress with subunit vaccines against the virus. In: Epstein M A, Achong B G (eds) The Epstein-Barr virus, recent advances. Heinemann Medical Books, London, p 271–289

Epstein M A, Achong B G, Barr Y M 1964 Virus particles in cultured lymphoblasts from Burkitt's lymphoma. Lancet i: 702–703

Ernberg I, Klein G 1979 EB virus-induced antigens. In: Epstein M A, Achong B G (eds) The Epstein-Barr virus. Springer-Verlag, Berlin, p 39–60

Finch S C 1969 Clinical symptoms and signs of infectious mononucleosis. In: Carter R L, Penman H G (eds) Infectious mononucleosis. Blackwell, Oxford, p 23

Fingeroth J D, Weis J J, Tedder T F, Strominger J L, Biro P A, Fearon D T 1984 Epstein-Barr virus receptor of human B-lymphocytes in the C3d receptor CR2. Proceedings of the National Academy of Sciences USA 81: 4510–4514

Gerber P, Nonoyama M, Lucas S, Perlin E, Goldstein L I 1972 Oral excretion of Epstein-Barr virus by healthy subjects and patients with infectious mononucleosis. Lancet ii: 988–989

Golden H D, Chang R S, Prescott W, Simpson E, Cooper T Y 1973 Leukocyte-transforming agent: prolonged excretion by patients with mononucleosis and excretion by normal individuals. Journal of Infectious Diseases 127: 471–473

Hamblin T J, Hussain J, Akbar A N, Tang Y C, Smith J L, Jones D B 1983 Immunological reason for chronic ill health after infectious mononucleosis. British Medical Journal 287: 85–88

Henle W, Henle G 1979 Seroepidemiology of the virus. In: Epstein M A, Achong B G (eds) The Epstein-Barr virus. Springer-Verlag, Berlin, p 61–78

Ito Y 1986 Vegetable activators of the viral genome and the causation of Burkitt's lymphoma and nasopharyngeal carcinoma. In: Epstein M A, Achong B G (eds) The Epstein-Barr virus, recent advances. Heinemann Medical Books, London, p 207–236

Lawee D, Shaffir M S 1983 Solitary penile ulcer associated with infectious mononucleosis. Canadian Medical Association Journal 129: 146–147

Leading Article 1978 Limited immunodeficiency. Lancet i: 132–133

Leading Article 1982 New clinical manifestations of Epstein Barr virus infection. Lancet ii: 1253–1255

Leading Article 1985 EBV and persistent malaise. Lancet i: 1017–1018

Leading Article 1986 Enervating illness and Epstein-Barr virus. Lancet ii: 141–142

Lung M L, Lam W K, So S Y, Lam W P, Chan K H, Ng M H 1985 Evidence that respiratory tract is major reservoir for Epstein-Barr virus. Lancet i: 889–892

Morgan D G, Miller G, Niedermann J C, Miller G, Smith H W, Dowaliby J M 1979 Site of Epstein-Barr virus replication in the oropharynx. Lancet ii: 1154–1157

Niederman J C 1985 Chronicity of Epstein-Barr virus infection. Editorial, Annals of Internal Medicine 102: 119–121

Parker A C, Richmond J 1976 Reduction in incidence of rash using polymer-free ampicillin. British Medical Journal 1: 998–1000

Pollock T M 1969 Epidemiology of infectious mononucleosis. In: Carter R L, Penman H G (eds) Infectious mononucleosis. Blackwell, Oxford, p 63–81

Portnoy J, Ahronheim G A, Ghiba F, Clecner B, Joncas J H 1984 Recovery of Epstein-Barr virus from genital ulcers. The New England Journal of Medicine 311: 966

Rickinson A 1984 Epstein-Barr virus in epithelium. Nature 310: 99–100

Rickinson A 1986 Cellular immunological responses to the virus infection. In: Epstein M A, Achong B G (eds) The Epstein-Barr virus, recent advances. Heinemann Medical Books, London, p 75–125

Royston I, Sullivan J L, Periman P O, Perlin E 1975 Cell-mediated immunity to Epstein-Barr-virus-transformed lymphoblastoid cells in acute infectious mononucleosis. The New England Journal of Medicine 293(23): 1159–1163

Sixbey J W, Vesterinen E H, Nedrud J G, Raab-Traub N, Walton L A, Pagano J S 1983 Replication of Epstein-Barr virus in human epithelial cells infected in vitro. Nature 306: 480–483

Sixbey J W, Nedrud J G, Raab-Traub N, Hanes R A, Pagano J S 1984 Epstein-Barr virus replication in oropharyngeal epithelial cells. The New England Journal of Medicine 310(19): 1225–1230

Sixbey J W, Lemon S M, Pagano J S 1986 A second site for Epstein-Barr virus shedding: the uterine cervix. Lancet ii: 1122–1124

Whittle H C, Brown J, Marsh K, Greenwood B M, Seidelin P, Tighe H, Wedderburn L 1984 T-cell control of Epstein-Barr virus-infected B cells is lost during P. falciparum malaria Nature (London) 312: 449–450

Wolf H, Haus M, Wilmes E 1984 Persistence of Epstein-Barr virus in parotid gland. Journal of Virology 51: 795–798

Ziegler J L, Drew W L, Miner R C et al 1982 Outbreak of Burkitt's-like lymphoma in homosexual men. Lancet ii: 631–632

30

Viral hepatitis

Viral hepatitis may be caused by any of six viruses: hepatitis A, hepatitis B, hepatitis D (the delta agent, a defective virus associated with hepatitis B virus). epidemic non-A hepatitis, and at least two non-A, non-B viruses (Tabor 1985, Zuckerman 1985) (see also Ch. 2). In addition hepatitis may be seen as a complication of infection with several different viruses e.g. cytomegalovirus, Epstein-Barr virus, herpes simplex virus, varicella-zoster virus, rubella and yellow-fever viruses. The common forms of viral hepatitis are usually hepatitis A and hepatitis B, although in some areas the most common type of hepatitis, occurring after blood transfusion, is clinically similar but antigenically unrelated to either type (World Health Organization 1977) and is called non-A, non-B hepatitis.

It is particularly the virus of hepatitis B that may be spread by sexual intercourse, although the exact mechanism of spread remains uncertain. Viral antigens can be detected in blood and most body secretions and

Table 30.1 Abbreviations and names in full as used in this chapter.

Abbreviation used	Name in full
HBV	Hepatitis B virus
HBsAg	Hepatitis B surface antigen
anti-HBs	Antibody to hepatitis B surface antigen
HBc	Hepatitis B core antigen
anti-HBc	Antibody to hepatitis B core antigen
HBeAg	Hepatitis B 'e' antigen
anti-HBe	Antibody to hepatitis B 'e' antigen
HDAg	Hepatitis D antigen or delta antigen
anti-HD	Antibody to hepatitis D antigen or delta antigen
HAV	Hepatitis A virus
anti-HAV	Antibody to hepatitis A virus
ALT	Alanine aminotransferase
AST	Aspartate aminotransferase
GGT	Gamma glutamyl transferase
IgG	Immunoglobulin G
IgM	Immunoglobulin M
AFP	Alpha-fetoprotein
HCC	Primary hepatocellular carcinoma
HBIG	Hepatitis B immune globulin
RIA	Radioimmunoassay
NANB hepatitis	Non-A, non-B hepatitis

important information about the infectivity or otherwise of patients may be obtained by the detection or exclusion of these antigens or their associated antibodies. As transmission by sexual contact is important in the spread of hepatitis B it is this infection to which most attention is given in this chapter, although consideration is also given to the hepatitis D virus sometimes associated with it, and to hepatitis A and non-A, non-B hepatitis. Viral antigens and antibodies are discussed particularly in relation to the clinical implications of their detection in serum. The names of these antigens and antibodies and their abbreviations are recognized internationally and used constantly in the literature. For ease of reference they are collected together with other abbreviations in Table 30.1.

HEPATITIS A

Hepatitis A is a small RNA-containing virus (25–28 nm) possessing cubic symmetry. Few or no hepatitis A virus (HAV) particles are found in faecal extracts by the time most patients are seen by physicians (Fig. 30.1), and maximum shedding of virus occurs before the onset of jaundice (World Health Organization 1977).

EPIDEMIOLOGY

The virus of hepatitis A (HAV) is transmitted by the faecal-oral route and undetected symptomless cases may be an important source of infection. Faeces of infected persons become infective 2–4 weeks after exposure and remain so for about 3 weeks (Fig. 30.1). Patients are usually not infective when jaundice appears. In developed countries, infections occur at all ages, with about 50% of clinical cases being seen in children less than 15 years old. In tropical and subtropical areas most infections are probably acquired in childhood and the majority are subclinical. The virus is excreted in the faeces and infection is acquired orally under conditions

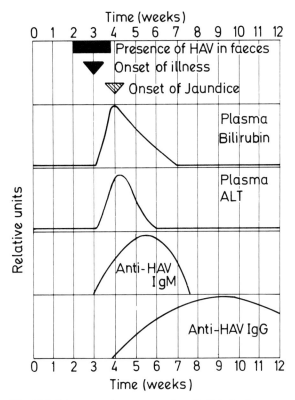

Fig. 30.1 Diagrammatic representation of clinical, plasma enzyme (ALT = alanine aminotransferase) and virological features in symptomatic hepatitis A infection.

of poor hygiene and sanitation and overcrowding, as in childrens' homes and camps.

The prevalence of anti-HAV in the serum can be used to give information about previous exposure to the virus in various populations. In developed countries its prevalence increases with age. In those under 50 years of age the prevalence of anti-HAV is higher in the lower socio-economic groups than in the higher. In those aged 50 years or over, however, these differences are not significant statistically; this finding suggests that all groups were exposed during their youth at a time when hygienic conditions were generally inferior to those of the present day (World Health Organization 1977).

Although the sexual transmission of HAV probably plays a small part in the global epidemiology of hepatitis A, the finding, in Halifax, Nova Scotia, of a higher prevalence of serum anti-HAV amongst STD clinic patients (both male and female) than amongst volunteer blood donors (McFarlane et al 1981), suggests that possibility.

Unlike Corey & Holmes (1980) who reported from Seattle an increased prevalence of serum anti-HAV amongst men who had had homosexual contact, both McFarlane's group in Halifax, Nova Scotia, and Coester

et al (1984) in Antwerp found no significant difference in seropositivity between homo- and heterosexual men. Experience varies geographically: Fawaz & Matloff in Boston, Massachusetts (1981) and Mindel & Tedder in London (1981) recorded that hepatitis A was the most common cause of acute icteric hepatitis in homosexual men attending clinics in their localities. In a prospective study in Amsterdam, Coutinho et al (1983) found that the prevalence of anti-HAV amongst homosexual men correlated with the duration of homosexual activity but was independent of age. In this study 35 of 399 initially seronegative men, followed for up to 23 months, acquired serum HAV antibodies and 28 of these men developed clinical illness. As the numbers of sexual partners increased so the risk of acquiring hepatitis A increased. In relation to sexual practices, too, there is an association between the prevalence of serum anti-HAV or the acquisition of hepatitis A (Corey & Holmes 1980) and the practice of oro-anal contact; as the virus is present in the faeces, transmission by this sexual practice is to be expected.

CLINICAL AND LABORATORY FEATURES

It is likely that the majority of infections with HAV are asymptomatic or produce mild transient and non-specific clinical features. Szmuness et al (1976) found that less than 5% of individuals whose sera contained HAV gave a history of icteric hepatitis.

The clinical and biochemical features of hepatitis A are similar to those of any other viral hepatitis (see below). In general the course of the disease is shorter and less severe than that of hepatitis B, with resolution of both clinical and biochemical abnormalities within one month of the onset of the illness.

As the clinical features in the individual case are not sufficiently specific, the diagnosis of hepatitis A is made by the finding of anti-HAV IgM in the patient's serum (Fig. 30.1).

PREVENTION

Now that hepatitis A virus has been finally cultured unequivocally in vitro the way is open to develop a vaccine against this common and widespread disease (White 1984). Until this vaccine against HAV is available, however, the administration of normal immuno-globulin, prepared from a pool of human plasma, is the only effective means of protection against infection. Passive immunization is offered to individuals prior to travel to areas of the world where the infection is endemic and sanitation poor. The place of immunization in prophylaxis after sexual contact with an infected person is less clear as most individuals will be unaware that they have been at risk. Prophylactic passive immunization of home contacts is recommended.

The dosage of prophylactic normal immunoglobulin injection (HNG) is 0.02–0.04 ml/kg body weight by intramuscular injection; this should give protection for up to three months.

HEPATITIS B

AETIOLOGY

Blumberg (1964) described an antigen in blood, which reacted with serum from patients who had been given many blood transfusions. This antigen was found also most commonly in Australian aborigines and Asians and was termed 'Australia' antigen. The same antigen was subsequently discovered in the serum of patients with serum hepatitis (Blumberg et al 1967). It is now known as the hepatitis B surface antigen (HBsAg).

Later studies have shown that the antigen in the serum consists of three distinct particles, which may be present in variable concentrations:

1. Hepatitis B virus itself (HBV), a large (42 nm) double-shelled spheroidal particle with a central core, approximately 27 nm in diameter, known as the Dane particle (Dane et al 1970).
2. Small spherical particles with average diameter of 22 nm.
3. Tubular forms with a diameter of 22 nm, but varying in length up to 300 nm.

The small spherical particles are always the predominant form. These structures are associated with several antigenic determinants.

The HBsAg is present on the surface of all three types of particle found in the serum of patients, and is the major component of 2 and 3. The HBsAg carries a common antigenic determinant *a* with other type-specific antigens. These are mutually exclusive pairs, named *d* and *y*, and *w* and *r*. Thus the HBsAg can be typed as *adw*, *adr*, *ayw* and *ayr*: these findings are of epidemiological significance and have broad geographical associations. In Europe, the Americas and Australia, *adw* predominates, while in northern and western Africa, the eastern Mediterranean and the Indian subcontinent *ayw* predominates.

Detergent treatment of the HBV or Dane particle removes the outer HBsAg coat to release the core structure. The surface of this particle has a different antigenicity known as the HBcAg. The core also contains a circular piece of double-stranded DNA and a DNA polymerase enzyme.

The core particles can be detected in the nuclei of infected hepatocytes (Huang 1971). whereas the HBsAg is found in the cytoplasm. It is likely that the core particles acquire an outer coat of HBsAg in the cytoplasm. It is not known why the HBsAg is produced in such great excess and released into the serum. Another antigen, the 'e' antigen (HBeAg), is closely associated with hepatitis B infection, and its presence in HBsAg carriers is correlated with a greater risk of transmitting infection.

EPIDEMIOLOGY

The carrier state
The persistent carrier state has been defined as the presence of HBsAg in the serum of the individual for more than six months. In the United Kingdom less than 1% of the population are found to have HBsAg in the serum. The prevalence in apparently healthy adults varies from 0.1% in parts of Europe, North America and Australia to 15% in several tropical countries. Within each country considerable differences in prevalence may exist between different ethnic and socio-economic groups. In homosexual men attending two major clinics for sexually transmitted disease in central London the prevalence of HBsAg was found to be about 5% or about 50 times greater than that in unpaid volunteer blood donors in the United Kingdom (Ellis et al 1979).

The carrier state is more common in males, more likely to follow infections acquired in childhood than those acquired in adult life and more likely in those with natural or acquired immune deficiencies. In countries in which HBV is common, the highest prevalence of HBsAg is found in children 4–8 years old with steadily declining rates among the older age groups. This decline in the HBsAg carriage rates with age suggests that the carrier state is not life-long.

Modes of spread
In areas of low prevalence a major mode of spread continues to be the inoculation of blood and some blood products. Hepatitis B may be transmitted as a result of transfusion or by accidental inoculation of minute quantities of blood as may occur during surgical or dental procedures, intravenous drug abuse, mass immunization, tattooing, acupuncture and laboratory accidents. The sharing of razors, toothbrushes or bath brushes has been implicated as an occasional cause of hepatitis B.

Spread of HBV from carrier mothers to babies appears to be an important factor in some regions, as well as the spread from those with an acute infection. In Taiwan, for example, where the prevalence of HBsAg is 5–20% it was found that, in about 40% of cases, babies born to asymptomatic mothers became antigen positive within the first six months of life (Stevens et al 1975). If an acute infection occurs in the second or third trimester or within two months after delivery there is a substantial risk that the baby will be infected. Women whose serum contains HBeAg will pass on hepatitis B virus to their babies, whereas those with anti-HBe do not (Okada et al 1976). This probably reflects the active viral replication which occurs in 'e' antigen positive individuals. The infection in the baby is usually anicteric and most children infected will become persistent carriers of the virus. Intrauterine infection seems to be rare. Goudeau et al (1983) failed to identify anti-HBc IgM in the serum of neonates born to HBsAg carriers, a finding which argued against the in utero acquisition of HBV.

HBeAg is associated with the acute illness and has been found more commonly in young, rather than adult carriers, while the prevalence of the antibody (anti-HBe) appears to increase with age. Since HBeAg is closely associated with infectivity, young carriers may be more infective.

Jeffries et al (1973) observed that the prevalence of HBsAg in the sera of patients who attended a STD clinic in London was some ten times higher than that in blood donors. They noted that high rates were found in homosexual and non-European patients. Results of other studies, summarized in Table 30.2, have shown clearly the association between homosexual activity and the acquisition of hepatitis B virus; the prevalence of HBV in homosexual men will vary geographically and will be particularly high in countries with high prevalence in the general population.

In flying civil airline personnel (Swissair) hepatitis A immunity (anti-HAV) was found to be similar to that of the blood donor population, but the most outstanding feature was that *male* flight attendants (employees and candidates) significantly more often had anti-HBs and/or anti-HBc antibodies (20–33%) than either flying personnel (1.4–5.6%) or Swiss blood donors (4–8%). Furthermore, the high incidence of manifest hepatitis B cases per 1000 (Swiss population 0.5–0.8 cases per 1000 per year) was mainly among male flight attendants. It was thought that homosexuality associated with a high risk life style was the most realistic explanation for the finding in male cabin attendants (Holdener & Grob 1981).

Several studies have shown that the sera of more than 70% of homosexual men who are persistent carriers of HBsAg contain 'e' antigen (Ellis et al 1979, Lacey et al 1983, Peutherer & McMillan 1984 — unpublished data) suggesting that their sexual contacts would be likely to be at particular risk of infection.

Schreeder et al (1982) noted that sero-positivity for HBV was related to the duration of regular homosexual activity and to the numbers of different sexual partners.

Practices likely to result in mucosal trauma, including genital-anal and oral-anal intercourse and rectal douching, correlated with the presence of HBV serological markers. Reiner et al (1984) studied 22 homosexual men whose serum contained HBsAg (17 sera were HBeAg positive) and found asymptomatic rectal mucosal lesions, in the form of multiple punctate bleeding points in 13 men. HBsAg was detected in specimens taken from the rectal lesions of 10 of these 13 patients and less frequently in material from the normal mucosa and faeces. Such specimens were more likely to give positive results if the serum contained large quantities of HBsAg. Gingival swabs from 20 patients contained HBsAg.

HBsAg positive individuals of either sex may transmit HBV to their sexual contacts (Hersh et al 1971, Heathcote & Sherlock 1973). Szmuness et al (1975) found that 26% of spouses of HBsAg carriers were seropositive for anti-HBs.

In a sample of 293 women, registered as living by prostitution in Athens, there was evidence of hepatitis B infection (HBsAg or anti-HBs) in 61.1% compared with 28.0% of 379 controls; when the prevalence of HBsAg and anti-HBs were related to years in prostitution a substantially higher rate of HBsAg was noted in prostitutes in their first 5 years of prostitution (9.4%), decreasing substantially in those who had been in prostitution for 5 years or more (Papaevangelou et al 1974). De Hoop et al (1984) also noted an increased prevalence of anti-HBs in the sera of female prostitutes who attended a STD clinic in Rotterdam. Sexually promiscuous persons clearly have a higher incidence of seropositivity than the general population in areas of low prevalence.

CLINICAL FEATURES AND COURSE

Acute hepatitis

In the majority of cases, hepatitis, whether type A or B, is asymptomatic and detectable only by biochemical tests for hepatocellular damage. In those who develop clinical manifestations of the disease, following a prepatent period of 30–50 days in the case of type A hepatitis, and 40–160 days in type B, there is a pre-icteric stage (prodrome) during which the symptoms of the disease develop. The patient complains of nausea, malaise, anorexia and discomfort in the upper right abdomen. Tender enlargement of the liver is found in most cases, and in about 20% of patients the spleen is also enlarged. In less than 5% of symptomatic cases manifestations of immune-complex disease appear, consisting of erythematous, maculopapular or urticarial skin rashes, and arthralgia.

Jaundice usually develops within a week of the devel-

Table 30.2 Prevalence of hepatitis B surface antigen (HBsAg) and antibody (anti-HBs) in the sera of homosexual and heterosexual men in various cities. Reference number bracketed after year as follows: Waugh & Hambling 1978 (1); Lim et al 1976 (2); Coleman et al 1977 (3); Coleman et al 1979 (4); Follet & McMillan 1980 (5); Lacey et al 1983 (6); McMillan (unpublished) (7); Szmuness et al 1975 (8); Dietzman et al 1979 (9); Schreeder et al 1982 (10); Coutinho et al 1981 (11); Coester et al 1984 (12). nt = not tested.

Geographical area	Year (ref. no.)	HBsAg						anti-HBs					
		Homosexual			Heterosexual			Homosexual			Heterosexual		
		Nos. tested	Nos. positive	%	Nos. tested	Nos. positive	%	Nos. tested	Nos. positive	%	Nos. tested	Nos. positive	%
UK													
Leeds	1978 (1)	359	12	(3.3)	nt			nt			nt		
London	1976 (2)	71	3	(4.2)	129	0	(0.0)	71	21	(29.6)	129	7	(5.4)
London	1977 (3)	600	31	(5.2)	nt			85	3	(3.5)	nt		
London	1979 (4)	177	11	(6.2)	nt			166	89	(53.6)	nt		
Glasgow	1979 (5)	208	4	(1.9)	124	0	(0.0)	208	65	(31.3)	124	9	(7.3)
Bristol	1983 (6)	599	18	(3.0)	nt			nt			nt		
Edinburgh	1984 (7)	239	8	(3.3)	201	1	(0.5)	239	71	(30.7)	201	7	(3.5)
USA													
New York City	1975 (8)	674	29	(4.3)	597	8	(1.3)	645	295	(45.3)	589	99	(16.8)
Seattle	1979 (9)	144	8	(5.6)	111	1	(0.9)	144	49	(34.0)	111	4	(3.6)
Chicago, Los Angeles, San Francisco, Denver, St Louis	1982 (10)	3816	234	(6.1)	nt			3582	1999	(52.4)	nt		
Netherlands													
Amsterdam	1981 (11)	2946	140	(4.8)	nt			2806	1596	(56.9)	nt		
Belgium													
Antwerp	1984 (12)	195	8	(4.1)	nt			187	58	(31.0)	nt		

opment of the symptoms, and is preceded by the appearance of dark urine and pale stools. The onset of jaundice in hepatitis B may not always be associated with prodromal illness. With the development of jaundice, the patient's condition improves, and within two to four weeks most infections have resolved. Uncommonly, fulminant hepatitis develops, the majority of these patients having hepatitis B infection.

Plasma enzyme tests (PETs) in viral hepatitis and its sequelae

In hepatocellular damage there is a release, particularly, of soluble cytoplasmic enzymes such as *alanine aminotransferase* (ALT) and *aspartate aminotransferase* (AST). Although there are possibly more sensitive indices of liver damage, *aminotransferases* continue to be measured mainly because of their analytical convenience and simplicity (Whitby et al 1984). Plasma ALT measurements are more liver-specific than AST, and increases in ALT are usually greater in early hepatitis. AST has both cytoplasmic and mitochondrial isoenzymes and tends to be released more than ALT in chronic hepatocellular disease.

Gamma-glutamyl transferase (GGT) and *alkaline phosphatase* are enzymes located close to the biliary canaliculi. These tend to be released in small amounts in hepatocellular damage but in much greater amounts when there is cholestasis. GGT is the more sensitive index of cholestasis and is very sensitive in detecting mild cirrhosis.

In the pre-icteric phase of viral hepatitis plasma ALT and AST activities are increased. Urobilinogen is present in the urine, and later bilirubin will be found. By the time jaundice appears aminotransferase activities are usually more than $5 \times$ reference values and sometimes more than $100 \times$ reference values (Note 30.1). Alkaline phosphatase activity is usually only slightly increased ($2 \times$ upper reference value) unless there is a marked cholestatic element.

In chronic disease, which is more likely to follow anicteric hepatitis B than the acute icteric hepatitis B, plasma ALT and AST activities may remain high for many months. Plasma enzyme tests (PETs) and tests for hepatitis B antigens and antibodies are important in the follow-up of HBsAg positive symptomless patients (Fig. 30.2).

Other chemical tests in viral hepatitis and its sequelae

Plasma contains two forms of bilirubin: 1. the unconjugated lipid-soluble form which is transported bound to albumin from the lymphoreticular system to the liver; and 2. the conjugated water-soluble forms which have been regurgitated from the liver to the plasma. Normally most of the bilirubin in the plasma is uncon-

jugated. For most purposes measurement of the total bilirubin is sufficient for clinical purposes when interpreted in relation to the side-room tests and other clinical investigations (e.g. Plasma enzyme tests and tests for hepatitis B antigens and antibodies).

In hepatitis and cirrhosis hepatocellular damage may interfere with the conjugation of bilirubin, or with excretion of conjugated bilirubin into the bile, or with both. This and other abnormalities lead to cholestasis and bring about an increase in plasma bilirubin and bilirubinuria.

Urobilinogen is water-soluble and is formed from degraded bilirubin glucuronide in the colon and is normally excreted in the faeces. Some is reabsorbed and excreted in the urine where it spontaneously oxidizes into a dark brown pigment called urobilin. In hepatitis urobilinogen excess is found in the urine in the pre-icteric stage but as the stools become pale, due to impairment of excretion of bilirubin, urobilinogen disappears from the urine.

Since gross increases in alpha-fetoprotein (AFP) occur in the serum of 50–90% patients with hepatocellular carcinoma (HCC) this investigation may help in the longer-term follow-up of patients who are chronic HBsAg carriers.

The reader is referred to Whitby et al 1984 for fuller discussion of enzyme tests and other chemical analyses in liver disease.

IMMUNE RESPONSE IN ACUTE HEPATITIS B

HBsAg and anti-HBs (hepatitis B surface antigen and its antibody)

HBsAg is found 14 to 120 days following exposure to infection; the interval between exposure and appearance of detectable serum HBsAg is related to the infectivity of the inoculum. A rise in the serum titre of HBsAg occurs gradually, and, after reaching a peak, falls rapidly. The serum ALT level rises after the HBsAg peak, and by the time symptoms develop in uncomplicated cases, the transaminase levels are falling. In most cases, the disappearance of HBsAg and subsequent appearance of anti-HBs signal recovery from infection and the development of immunity to reinfection. Anti-HBs can appear at the time HBsAg disappears (Fig. 30.2). or may not appear for several months. The persistence of HBsAg for more than three months, in some 5–10% of cases, suggests the development of the carrier state. In fulminant hepatitis there is some evidence to suggest that an unusually strong and rapid immune clearance of HBsAg, associated with the early appearance of anti-HBs during the peak of liver damage, may be involved in the pathogenesis of this severe form of infection.

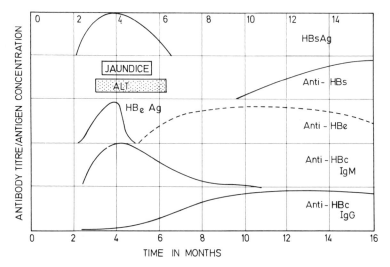

Fig. 30.2 Diagrammatic representation of clinical, plasma enzyme (ALT = alanine aminotransferase) and virological features in symptomatic hepatitis B infection.

Several serological techniques are available for detecting HBsAg and anti-HBs but radioimmunoassay is the most sensitive (World Health Organization 1977). The enzyme-linked immunosorbent assay technique (ELISA) has also been adapted to detect HBsAg: this technique was shown to have a sensitivity similar to that of radioimmunoassay (RIA) and has the advantage of stability, long shelf-life of reagents and simplicity of equipment.

Anti-HBs can be estimated by a radioimmunoassay test. The detection of HBsAg is the main approach in the diagnosis of acute and chronic states. Other antigen and antibody tests are available for some individual cases, especially during the recovery from acute illness and to assess the carrier state.

HBcAg and anti-HBc (hepatitis B core antigen and its antibody)

Although HBcAg has been obtained from HBV-rich plasma and from infected liver tissue, free core antigen has not been detected in circulating blood. However, anti-HBc is found in the serum 2–10 weeks after the appearance of HBsAg and before the appearance of anti-HBs (Fig. 30.2). It often appears during the acute infection while HBsAg is still present and remains detectable for a considerable time after recovery.

Antibody of the IgM class against HBcAg can be detected by radioimmunoassay or ELISA in the sera of almost all patients with acute hepatitis B. This antibody appears about two weeks before the onset of jaundice and generally becomes undetectable within six months (Mortimer et al 1981). In 20% of individuals it is still detectable two years later. Although this antibody can be found in the sera of patients with chronic hepatitis B and carriers, it is present in very low titre and, therefore, the presence of serum anti-HBc IgM can be taken as an indication of acute disease (Gerlich et al 1980, Lemon et al 1981).

Gerlich et al (1980) and Lemon et al (1981) have shown that serum anti-HBc IgM is often found in the sera of patients who have recovered from acute hepatitis but in whom HBsAg is not detected. This test can therefore be used in the diagnosis of recent hepatitis even when the clinical features have resolved.

HBeAg and anti-HBe (hepatitis B 'e' antigen and its antibody)

HBeAg can be detected by ELISA in the sera of all patients with acute hepatitis B. The presence of this antigen and serum-specific DNA polymerase reflects active viral replication. When this ceases, levels of HBeAg in the serum fall and anti-HBe becomes detectable.

Cell-mediated immunity

Cell-mediated immunity may be involved in terminating infection with HBV and, under certain circumstances, in causing hepatocellular damage and creating auto-immunity (World Health Organization 1977). Normal T-cell function may be a prerequisite for the self-limited course of hepatitis; if the function is defective it may favour the development of chronic liver damage, and if it is absent altogether the result may be the asymptomatic carrier state.

CHRONIC HEPATITIS B

Chronic hepatitis may be defined as a primary inflammatory condition of the liver which has persisted without improvement for more than six months.

There are four main consequences of chronic hepatitis B infection.

1. A *chronic carrier state* of the virus with normal plasma enzyme tests and a normal or minimally abnormal histological appearance (de Franchis et al 1980). Randomly distributed ground-glass hepatocytes are found in varying numbers in histological sections. These are enlarged liver cells with a finely granular cytoplasm which contains HBsAg as shown by immunoperoxidase methods (Huang 1975).

2. *Chronic persistent hepatitis.* This is a histological diagnosis as neither clinical features, serological findings nor biochemical tests differentiate this type of chronic hepatitis from chronic active hepatitis. Histologically the lobular architecture is intact, but the portal tracts are enlarged with a dense infiltration of lymphocytes sometimes forming follicles. 'Piecemeal' necrosis is *not* a feature. The prognosis is good, progression to cirrhosis being rare.

3. *Chronic active hepatitis.* This is again a histological diagnosis. The hallmark of this type of chronic hepatitis is 'piecemeal' necrosis which is defined as necrosis of liver cells at the junction of the interface between the liver parenchyma and the connective tissue of the portal tracts or septa of a fibrotic or cirrhotic liver. There is a predominantly lymphocytic infiltration of the portal tracts extending into the hepatic parenchyma. Fibrous tissue septa of varying size surround groups of liver cells. Ground-glass hepatocytes are seen in both chronic active and chronic persistent hepatitis. Although this form of chronic hepatitis may progress to cirrhosis, the prognosis in individual cases is difficult to predict.

4. *Hepatocellular carcinoma* (see p. 387).

Immune response in chronic hepatitis B

Humoral antibody response

In all cases of chronic hepatitis B, serum HBsAg and anti-HBc are detectable: generally anti-HBs is not produced. Although serum anti-HBc-IgM can be detected by sensitive methods this antibody is present in low titre (Gerlich et al 1980). Recent work has shown that the IgM antibody is of low molecular weight (7–8 S) but probably not a breakdown product of 19 S IgM; the source is uncertain (Sjøgren & Lemon 1983).

HBeAg and DNA polymerase activity persists for a variable period after infection is established. These markers indicate active viral replication and the presence of complete virions in the serum; individuals with such markers in their serum are infectious to others through blood contamination or sexual contact. After an indefinite period, many patients show seroconversion from HBeAg to anti-HBe. Such a transition is preceded by a sharp increase in serum transaminase levels which subsequently decline to levels which are significantly lower than those recorded when the patient's serum was HBeAg positive (Perrillo et al 1984). However, seroconversion to anti-HBe is not associated with improvement in the hepatic histology and, indeed, progression to cirrhosis is known to occur in HBsAg positive patients with serum anti-HBe (Realdi et al 1980). Seroconversion to anti-HBe is not always permanent. Perrillo et al (1984) showed spontaneous transient reactivation of HBV in 3 patients who had had documented seroconversion from HBeAg positive to anti-HBe several months previously. Reactivation was associated with a sharp increase in serum transaminase levels. The mechanism or significance of this finding is uncertain.

Cellular immunity

When hepatic cells obtained by needle biopsy from patients with chronic hepatitis B are incubated with peripheral blood lymphocytes from the same individual, there is cytolysis of the hepatocyte mediated through non-T cells and antibody against hepatocyte cell membrane lipoprotein (Mieli-Vergani et al 1982). T-cell cytotoxicity has also been shown in patients with chronic hepatitis B, particularly when the serum contains HBeAg. The blocking of cytotoxicity by anti-HBc suggests that the antigens recognized by the T-cells contain viral nucleocapsid determinants (Mondelli et al 1982). When HBV DNA becomes integrated into the host DNA, HBcAg is not produced and cytotoxicity is less pronounced. This would explain the improvement in plasma hepatic enzyme activity noted during seroconversion, from e-antigenaemia to anti-HBe positivity (Trevisan et al 1982). There have been few studies on T-cell sub-populations in the peripheral blood of patients with chronic hepatitis B, but decreased T4:T8 cell ratios resulting from increased numbers of T8 cells have been reported (Alexander et al 1983).

Delta agent

Delta agent was first discovered in 1977 by Rizzetto and his colleagues. It is an incomplete or defective RNA virus coated in HBsAg which replicates only in patients with acute or chronic HBV infection. Patients with acute or chronic hepatitis B develop a more rapidly progressive disease if they become superinfected with delta agent (Smedile et al 1982, Colombo et al 1983). IgM anti-delta antibodies (anti-HD IgM) are detected by radioimmunoassay in the sera of patients with acute and chronic infection. The prevalence of delta antibodies in HBV carriers varies considerably but is extremely low in European homosexual HBsAg carriers, of whom most are also HBeAg positive (Tedder et al 1982, Weller et al 1983). This somewhat surprising finding may reflect a greater susceptibility of anti-HBe carriers to delta superinfection or to a resistance of HBeAg positive carriers to infection (Thomas 1985). The liberal use of hepatitis B vaccine in special risk groups is clearly worthwhile, both from the point of view of preventing hepatitis B, and hence preventing the spread of hepatitis D virus (Nicholson 1985).

Clinical features and course in chronic hepatitis B

Although chronic disease can follow acute icteric hepatitis B, it seems more likely to be a consequence of anicteric hepatitis (Sherlock 1976). Most patients with chronic disease do not give a past history of jaundice.

The clinical features of chronic hepatitis B vary considerably and often there are no symptoms or signs of the disease, the diagnosis being made after routine testing of the patient's serum for HBsAg. Some patients with chronic active hepatitis and cirrhosis present with clinical evidence of hepatic decompensation with oedema, ascites, or bleeding varices. From time to time patients with chronic hepatitis B develop episodes of acute hepatitis caused by other viruses, including cytomegalovirus (CMV, see Ch. 28), Epstein-Barr virus (EBV, see Ch. 29) and delta agent; diagnosis depends on serological tests for each specific virus. In an individual with acute hepatitis whose serum is found to be HBsAg positive but anti-HBc IgM negative, it is likely that he has chronic hepatitis B with some other super-added viral infection (Lavarini et al 1983).

Plasma enzyme (aminotransferases) tests are abnormal in chronic hepatitis but there is such wide variation in levels of ALT and AST that it is not possible to differentiate between chronic persistent and chronic active hepatitis. Alkaline phosphatase levels are only slightly elevated. Although the presence of 'e' antigen in the sera of patients with chronic hepatitis was considered to indicate progression to cirrhosis, this is no longer considered to be so. During the phase of active viral replication, 'e' antigenaemia occurs early in the course of chronic hepatitis; seroconversion from HBeAg to anti-HBe is frequent, but of no prognostic significance. However, patients whose sera contains anti-HBe are much less infectious to others since, in such individuals, viral replication is considerably reduced and virions (as judged by the absence of specific DNA polymerase activity) are absent from the sera.

Viola et al (1981) conducted a prospective study of 100 patients (77 of whom had had homosexual contact) with persistent hepatitis B surface antigen (HBsAg). In 73 patients plasma enzyme tests were abnormal. Histological abnormalities were found in 66 of these patients in whom liver biopsy had been undertaken: 21 had chronic persistent hepatitis; 29 had chronic active hepatitis, 8 had hepatic cirrhosis and 8 had hepatocellular carcinoma. After a follow-up period of up to 7 years, only 1 of 30 of these patients who had had cirrhosis and developed hepatocellular carcinoma had died. The other patients were alive and at work, indicating a reasonable prognosis in most individuals.

As persistent HBsAg carriers are at greater risk of developing ethanol-induced hepatic disease than individuals whose sera are HBsAg negative, HBV carriers should be advised to abstain or limit their alcohol intake to <20 g per day (Villa et al 1982). Despite initial controversy, it appears that alcoholic liver disease is not more prevalent in individuals who have had previous HBV infection than those who have not (Saunders et al 1983).

Treatment of chronic hepatitis B

Patients will require advice about their health, their infectious state and their alcohol intake. The complex subject of drug therapy has been reviewed in detail by Sherlock & Thomas (1985) and Thomas & Scully (1985). The aims are to eradicate the virus, to reduce infectivity of the patient and to stop progression of the liver disease. Although HBsAg becomes undetectable in the sera of a few patients after treatment, this is a rare event, probably because viral DNA will have already become incorporated in the host cell genome. Seroconversion from HBeAg positivity to anti-HBe positivity has followed treatment of a variable proportion of patients with adenine arabinoside, adenine arabinoside monophosphate or interferon, whether prepared from leucocytes, lymphoblastoid cell lines or by recombinant DNA technology. These drugs have been given as short courses and when treatment has been successful, seroconversion has followed several months later. Although in some patients the inflammatory activity and degree of hepatocyte necrosis have diminished after drug therapy, in others the histology has remained unchanged (Weller et al 1985, Dooley et al 1986).

Although spontaneous seroconversion from HBeAg positivity to anti-HBe positivity and improvement in the hepatic histology both occur, however, it is difficult to assess the results of drug trials, many of which have been open. The results of double-blind studies on larger numbers of patients are awaited with interest. Recent data, however, suggest that homosexual men with chronic hepatitis B are less likely to show seroconversion than heterosexual patients (Novick et al 1984); this may be related to the immune dysfunction associated with a coexistent HIV infection.

HEPATOCELLULAR CARCINOMA (HCC)

Several lines of evidence suggest a causative role for HBV in hepatocellular carcinoma (Szmuness 1978). In geographical areas, especially South East Asia where HBsAg carriers are common, HCC is also frequently found; the converse is also true in that the tumour is rare where the HBsAg carriage rate is low. Case control studies have also shown that the serum of patients with HCC is much more likely to be positive for HBsAg. In a prospective study, Beasley et al (1981a) showed that HBV infection preceded the development of HCC. Further evidence for the association between HCC and HBV comes from DNA hybridization studies. Shafritz & Kew (1981) found integrated HBV-DNA sequences in tumour biopsies from each of 12 patients with serum HBsAg and from 3 of 8 individuals with anti-HBs seropositivity. Although there is now strong evidence for an association between HBV and HCC, other factors must be involved also in its aetiology.

Patients with HCC may present with features of hepatic cirrhosis or with right hypochondrial pain in association with fever, weight loss and a palpable mass. In some cases, the diagnosis is made during routine examination or from the results of liver scanning of patients with chronic liver disease.

Although fluctuating levels of alpha-fetoprotein (AFP) are common in non-malignant liver disease, sustained or high values are strongly suggestive of HCC in non-pregnant patients. Currently a pilot AFP screening programme is being carried out in 20 HBsAg-positive Alaskans from three families at high risk for HCC (Centers for Disease Control 1984a).

SCREENING FOR VIRUS MARKERS IN THE SERUM OF SYMPTOMLESS PATIENTS

Routine screening of serum for HBV markers from men who have had homosexual contact, from intravenous drug abusers and from tattooed individuals is recommended so that appropriate advice with respect to infectivity and the individual's future health can be given. Vaccination of at-risk groups with hepatitis B vaccine deserves active consideration. If the initial tests give negative results in those who are not vaccinated, we recommend repeat serological screening of the first group at a frequency which should be determined by the sexual activity of the individual. If possible, drug addicts should be screened for up to one year after their last intravenous injection.

Figure 30.3 gives, in outline, recommendations on the management of symptomless patients whose sera are found to be HBsAg positive.

The advice given to HBsAg positive individuals is outlined in Note 30.2. Health service personnel are at increased risk of acquisition of HBV from HBsAg carriers and the precautions which should be taken in dealing with blood and other material from these individuals are discussed in Chapter 6.

If a member of staff sustains a prick or cut with an instrument or a needle contaminated with blood, or contaminates a wound or scratch on the skin or mucous membranes of the mouth or eye, then the risk of the recipient acquiring hepatitis B must be assessed promptly. The HBsAg status of the donor must be tested. If the donor is found to be positive, or is known to be positive in a recent test, then the recipient should be given an intramuscular dose of 500 mg of hepatitis B hyperimmune immunoglobulin. The possibility of active/passive immunization with hepatitis B vaccine should be actively considered and would be the procedure to advocate in the previously unvaccinated.

It is normal practice to test the recipient also for HBsAg; if he is already HBsAg positive no serum is given. Passive immunization should be undertaken as soon as possible after exposure and preferably within 24–72 hours. By this means a reduction in the risk of infection can be shown (Final Report of the Veterans Administration Co-operative Study 1978).

It is important to emphasize that hepatitis B virus carriers do present a definite hazard to medical and nursing personnel. However this must not lead to these patients being refused treatment, as it has been established that they can be treated safely provided precautions are taken. Vaccination should be offered to medical and nursing personnel on joining departments with clinical responsibility for the care of patients with sexually transmissible diseases.

HEPATITIS B VACCINE

The development of an effective hepatitis B vaccine as an alum adsorbed inactivated hepatitis B surface antigen, prepared from the pooled plasma of high titre HBsAg human carriers, has been a major advance in the control of this serious disease. In the USA there are 80 000 to 100 000 cases of acute hepatitis B per year, with a fatality rate of 1–2%, and the prevalence of chronic carriers of HBsAg among adults varies between 0.1% and 1%. In South America it is between 1% and 3%; in Russia and southern Europe 3–6%; and in vast areas of Asia and sub-Saharan Africa 10% or more. Szmuness et al (1980) go on to estimate that the total number of carriers is about 0.8 million in the USA and 200 million throughout the world. Although mostly asymptomatic, a substantial proportion do eventually

SAFETY AND PRIORITIES

Two questions remain to be discussed. Firstly, consideration of priorities is required, because the vaccine is costly and will always be in short supply although the new generation of vaccines is becoming available. A list of high risk populations which should be vaccinated is given below (Centers For Disease Control 1982).

- Family contacts of known chronic HBsAg carriers
- Babies born of HBeAg positive mothers
- Patients with diseases requiring frequent transfusions
- Patients and staff of haemodialysis units
- Medical and ancillary personnel in other high risk situations, e.g. blood banks, serology laboratories, dental surgery, surgery, genito-urinary medicine, pathology
- Inmates and staff of homes for the mentally retarded and other custodial institutions
- Immunosuppressed or cancer patients
- Drug addicts
- Male homosexuals, especially 'functionals' or 'open-coupled'
- Prostitutes, male or female

The second question about the safety of the vaccine can be clearly answered. Since the acceptance of the vaccine has been limited by a fear that the AIDS retrovirus could be transmitted in the vaccine, this issue is discussed in detail.

Source and safety of the vaccine

Hepatitis B virus cannot be grown in cell cultures but, since enormous numbers of HBsAg particles circulate in the serum of carriers, they can be extracted from the serum of donors and, after purification and inactivation processes to destroy any possible contaminating live viruses, used as a vaccine (White 1984). Studies of this procedure in the early 1970s by Krugman and his colleagues were followed by the development of a more sophisticated vaccine by Helleman and others at the Merck Institute of Therapeutic Research (Szmuness et al 1980). This vaccine is obtained from pooled plasma collected by regular plasmapheresis of known high titre HBsAg human carriers, negative for infectious virions (Dane particles), DNA polymerase and HBeAg (White 1984). Since some of these carriers are also in high risk groups for the Acquired Immune Deficiency Syndrome (AIDS), concern that the aetiological agent in AIDS might be present in the vaccine and survive the inactivation steps used in its manufacture seriously hindered acceptance of the vaccine both in the United States and later in the United Kingdom. Reluctance to use the vaccine persisted despite the fact that the steps in manufacture were believed to inactivate representative members of all known virus groups. The recent successful identification of the causative retrovirus, however, enabled the direct testing of the effectiveness of the inactivation processes against the AIDS virus (USA isolate known as HTLV-III; see Ch. 2). The techniques used included the search in the vaccine for AIDS virus nucleic acid sequences and the search for markers of AIDS virus in vaccine recipients (Centers for Disease Control 1984b).

Three separate inactivation processes are used in the manufacture of HB vaccine:

1. exposure to pepsin at pH 2 to digest adsorbed plasma or liver proteins,

2. denaturation with 8 molar urea to remove extraneous proteins,

3. treatment with formalin (0.01%) to inactivate any residual virus (Centers for Disease Control 1984b, White 1984).

In tests organized by the Centers for Disease Control (1982), the vaccine manufacturers Merck, Sharp and Dohme and other groups, it was shown that in vaccine to which HTLV-I, HTLV-II and HTLV-III retroviruses had been added no residual virus was detected in samples treated with formalin or urea, while material treated with pepsin did have residual virus present. Tests also failed to detect AIDS virus-related nucleic acid sequences at a sensitivity of 1 picogram of DNA per 20 μg dose at vaccine.

In the third approach to the problem, in 19 vaccinated subjects no antibody to AIDS virus could be detected by means of a highly sensitive and specific ELISA assay (Centers for Disease Control 1984b).

In 700 000 individuals given HB vaccine in the United States 68 AIDS cases have so far been reported; 65 occurred among persons with known risk factors for AIDS, while risk factors for the remaining 3 are under investigation. In summary it is clear that all studies showed that, if virus had been present in the source, it would have been killed by manufacturing procedures. In addition epidemiological monitoring failed to show transmission of AIDS by the vaccine. Clearly, misgivings about possible transmission of the AIDS- associated retrovirus are not justified (Centers for Disease Control 1984b).

NEW HEPATITIS B VACCINES

Advanced chemistry and recombinant DNA technology have opened up new possibilities in vaccine production (Mims & White 1984, White 1984). These rapidly developing advances, as they affect research into hepatitis B vaccine, reviewed fully by Zuckerman (1985), can be considered under four main headings.

1. Natural hepatitis B polypeptides

Two main polypeptides of HBsAg exist, one (p25) with a molecular weight of about 25 000 and the other (gp30) with a molecular weight of about 30 000. Being better defined chemically, they have the added advantage over the plasma vaccine in that they are not likely to contain extraneous contaminating virus or host proteins. Such membrane polypeptides can be prepared as water-soluble protein micelles — aggregates of polypeptides — which elicit a vigorous antibody response.

2. Vaccines derived from recombinant DNA technology

A gene coding for any given viral protein can be isolated and propagated in prokaryotes or yeasts giving expression of that protein. Synthesis of the gene product occurs by transcription of the DNA coding strand in the form of messenger RNA (mRNA) followed by translation of the information carried by the mRNA into an amino acid sequence.

Recombinant DNA techniques have been used for expressing hepatitis B surface antigen in prokaryotic cells (*Escherichia coli* and *Bacillus subtilis*) as well as in eukaryotic cells, particularly in yeast cells (*Saccharomyces cerevisiae*), where important advances have been made in the preparation of effective vaccines. Yeast-derived micelles seem to offer advantages in immunogenic potency.

3. Live hepatitis B vaccines with genetically engineered vaccinia virus

Recombinant DNA technology has made possible the construction of a vaccinia virus containing HBsAg-coding sequences. Although encouraging as a vaccine in experimental animals, there are as yet no generally accepted laboratory markers of attenuation or of virulence of vaccinia virus for man. Research progresses, and the technology makes possible the construction of a single one-off all-purpose vaccine incorporating genes for immunogenic proteins of most human infectious disease.

4. Chemically synthesized hepatitis B vaccines

Vaccines consisting of chemically synthesized polypeptides mimicking viral amino-acid sequences are being investigated as a possible alternative approach to the vaccine problem. Chemical uniformity and safety make possible the replacement of many current vaccines which contain large quantities of irrelevant antigenic material additional to the essential immunogen. Of

many questions to be answered the critical issues are whether the antibodies induced will be protective and whether the protective immunity will persist (Zuckerman 1985).

NON-A, NON-B HEPATITIS

Most cases of post-transfusion hepatitis and about one-fifth of sporadic cases of hepatitis are not associated with HAV, HBV, CMV or EBV infection and are classified as non-A, non-B hepatitis (NANB hepatitis) (Leading Article 1984b). The aetiology of this condition is uncertain, but transmission experiments in chimpanzees suggest a causative role for at least two distinct viruses (Dienstag 1983). Recently Prince et al (1984) cultured a virus from liver cell cultures of a chimpanzee infected with human serum containing the putative agent(s) of NANB hepatitis. The detection of reverse transcriptase activity in the particles contained in the sera of patients who were known to have transmitted the disease through blood transfusion suggests a role for retroviruses in the aetiology of NANB hepatitis (Seto et al 1984).

As there are no serological tests available for NANB hepatitis, the diagnosis is based on the clinical and biochemical findings of hepatitis and the exclusion by serological evidence of recent infection with HBV, HAV, CMV and EBV. Although the acute illness is generally mild, a high proportion of individuals later develop chronic liver disease.

Epidemiological data suggest that the NANB hepatitis agent can be transmitted through transfusion of whole blood or blood products, including factor VIII and gamma globulin prepared by Cohn fractionation of pooled plasma. Sporadic NANB hepatitis has been reported in intravenous drug abusers. The occurrence of the disease in household contacts suggests that close personal contact may be important, but there is little evidence of sexual transmission of the agent. Water-borne epidemics have been described in India, and epidemiological evidence suggests that the aetiological agent differs from that transmitted by the parenteral route. The male:female sex ratio is about 1.4:1, and the peak age group affected is the 20–29 years group (Farrow et al 1981). Descriptive designations have been given to three viruses which may be responsible for NANB hepatitis viz. 'blood-transmitted', 'coagulation-factor transmitted' and 'epidemic water-borne' viruses (Tabor 1985).

NOTES TO CHAPTER 30

Note 30.1: Reference values for plasma enzymes and total bilirubin

	Reference value	CV (range of concentrations)
Alanine aminotransferase	10–40 units/l	12.5% (10–50 units/l) 5% (51–100 units/l) 3% (101–500 units/l)
Alkaline phosphatase	40–100 units/l	3% (up to 150 units/l) 2.5% (over 150 units/l)
Aspartate aminotransferase	10–35 units/l	6% (10–50 units/l) 3.5% (51–100 units/l) 2.5% (101–500 units/l)
Gramma glutamyl transferase	M 10–55 units/l F 5–35 units/l	4% (up to 200 units/l) 2% (201–400 units/l)
Bilirubin, total	2–17 μmol/l	6% (up to 50 μmol/l) 2.5% (51–200 μmol/l)

The term *reference values* (RV) is preferred as a term for the spread of values found in 95% of the healthy population; since about 5% of healthy individuals will by definition fall outside the range, the term 'normal range' is a misnomer. Reference values for various chemical determinations referred to in this chapter and given in the. table are those used currently in Edinburgh Royal Infirmary. As a measure of analytical precision the coefficient of variation (CV) is given. Biological significance should not be attached to any change that is less than 2.8 times the stated analytical precision for the range of concentrations over which the data apply.

In the case of women, up to 40% of those taking oral contraceptives have slight impairment of hepatic anion transport function: plasma bilirubin is usually not increased but alkaline phosphatase may be moderately increased due to induction of the hepatic isoenzyme. Increase of gamma glutamyl transferase (GGT) has also been reported. A small group of women given oral contraceptives may develop overt jaundice of the cholestatic type, the so-called idiosyncratic jaundice. Increases in plasma activities of aspartate aminotransferase (AST) and alanine aminotransferase (ALT) may occur soon after starting treatment with oral contraceptives, but the increases are not marked and levels usually revert to normal although the contraceptive continues to be taken, but otherwise becoming normal again in most women soon after stopping treatment (Whitby et al 1984).

Note 30.2: Advice to HBsAg carrier

1. Your tests have shown that you carry hepatitis B virus.
2. Although you have no symptoms you can transmit the virus to other people. The infection is likely to persist but your health can remain good in the future, although we do not know exactly how you will respond.
3. You will be given information from the doctors about your follow-up tests.
4. You must not donate blood, plasma, your kidney or semen (sperm) for medical purposes.
5. You can infect others by sexual intercourse or from blood. If you use a condom it may reduce the chances of transmission.
6. You must not share your toothbrush or razor with anyone else.
7. If you have an accident and bleed, table tops or similar surfaces contaminated with blood should be cleaned with household bleach freshly diluted; 1 tablespoon with 9 tablespoons water.
8. Any needle used to give injections or to puncture the skin should be safely discarded in a puncture-proof container.
9. When seeking medical, surgical or dental care you must inform the doctor or dentist that you carry hepatitis B virus.
10. If you have troubles or doubts about what to do you should come to the Department here. You will be given information from the doctors about your follow-up tests.

Note 30.3:

$$\text{Protective efficacy rate} = 100 \times \frac{\text{Attack rate in placebo group} - \text{attack rate in treatment group}}{\text{Attack rate in placebo group}}$$

REFERENCES

Alexander G J M, Nouri-Aria K T, Eddleston A L W F, Williams R 1983 Contrasting relations between suppressor-cell function and suppressor-cell number in chronic liver disease. Lancet i: 1291–1293

Barbara J A J, Howell D R, Contreras M et al 1984 Indications for hepatitis B immunoglobulin for neonates of HBsAg carrier mothers. British Medical Journal 289: 880

Beasley R P, Hwang L-Y, Lin C C, Chien C S 1981a Hepatocellular carcinoma and hepatitis B virus. Lancet ii: 1129–1132

Beasley R P, Hwang L-Y, Lin C C, et al 1981b Hepatitis B immune globulin (HBIG) efficacy in the interruption of perinatal transmission of hepatitis B virus carrier state. Lancet ii: 388–393

Beasley R P, Hwang L-Y, Lee G C-Y, Lan C-C, Roan C-H, Huang F-Y, Chen C-L 1983 Prevention of perinatally transmitted hepatitis B virus infections with hepatitis B immune globulin and hepatitis B vaccine. Lancet ii: 1099–1102

Blumberg B S 1964 Polymorphism of serum proteins and the development of isoprecipitins in transfused patients. Bulletin of the New York Academy of Medicine 40: 377–386

Blumberg B S, Garstley B J S, Hungerford D A, London

W J, Suthick A I 1967 A serum antigen (Australia Antigen) in Down's syndrome, leukaemia and hepatitis. Annals of Internal Medicine 66: 924–931

Centers for Disease Control 1982 Inactivated hepatitis B virus vaccine. Morbidity and Mortality Weekly Report 31: 317–328

Centers for Disease Control 1984a Early detection of primary hepatocellular carcinoma. Morbidity and Mortality Weekly Report, US Public Health Service 33(5): 53–54

Centers for Disease Control 1984b Hepatitis B vaccine: evidence confirming lack of AIDS transmission. Morbidity and Mortality Weekly Report, US Public Health Service 33 (49): 685–687

Centers for Disease Control 1985 Suboptimal response to hepatitis B vaccine given by injection into the buttock. Morbidity and Mortality Weekly Report, US Public Health Service 34 (8): 105–108, 113

Coester C-H, Avonts D, Colaert J, Desmyter J, Piot P 1984 Syphilis, hepatitis A, hepatitis B, and cytomegalovirus infection in homosexual men in Antwerp. British Journal of Venereal Diseases 60: 48–51

Coleman J C, Waugh M, Dayton R 1977 Hepatitis B antigen and antibody in a male homosexual population. British Journal of Venereal Diseases 53: 132–134

Coleman J C, Evans B A, Thornton A, Zuckerman A J 1979 Homosexual hepatitis. Journal of Infection 1: 61–66

Colombo A, Cambieri R, Rumi M G et al 1983 Long-term superinfection in HBsAg carriers and its relationship with the course of chronic hepatitis. Gastroenterology 85: 235–239

Corey L, Holmes K K 1980 Sexual transmission of hepatitis A in homosexual men. Incidence and mechanism. New England Journal of Medicine 302: 435–438

Coutinho R A, Schut B J Th, van-Lent W A, Reorink-Brongers E E, Jesdigk L S 1981 Hepatitis B among homosexual men in the Netherlands. Sexually Transmitted Diseases 8: 333–335

Coutinho R A, Lent P A-V, Lelie N, Nagelkerke N, Kuipers H, Rijsdijk T 1983 Prevalence and incidence of hepatitis A among male homosexuals. British Medical Journal 287: 1743–1745

Dane D S, Cameron C H, Briggs M 1970 Virus-like particles in serum of patients with Australia-antigen-associated hepatitis. Lancet i: 695–698

de Franchis R, D'Arminio A, Vecchi M et al 1980 Chronic asymptomatic HBsAg carriers: histologic abnormalities and diagnostic and prognostic value of serologic markers of the HBV. Gastroenterology 79: 521–527

de Hoop D, Anker W J J, Strik Wv, Masurel N, Stolz E 1984 Hepatitis B antigen and antibody in the blood of prostitutes visiting an outpatient venereology department in Rotterdam. British Journal of Venereal Diseases 60: 319–322

Dienstag J L 1983 Non A and non B hepatitis. II. Experimental transmission, putative virus agents and markers and prevention. Gastroenterology 85: 743–768

Dienstag J L, Stevens C E, Bahn A K, Szmuness W 1982 Hepatitis B vaccine administered to chronic carriers of hepatitis B surface antigen. Annals of Internal Medicine 96: 575–579

Dietzman D E, Harnisch J P, Ray C G, Alexander E R, Holmes K K 1979 Hepatitis B surface antigen (HBsAg) and antibody to HBsAg. Prevalence in homosexual and heterosexual men. Journal of the American Medical Association 238: 2625–2626

Dooley J S, Davis G L, Peters M, Waggoner J G, Goodman Z, Hoofnagle J H 1986 Pilot study of recombinant human alpha-interferon for chronic type B hepatitis. Gastroenterology 90: 150–157

Ellis W R, Murray-Lyon I M, Coleman J C et al 1979 Liver disease among homosexual males. Lancet i: 903–905

Farrow L J, Stewart J S, Stern H, Clifford R E, Smith H G, Zuckerman A J 1981 Non-A, non-B hepatitis in West London. Lancet i: 982–984

Fawaz K A, Matloff D S 1981 Viral hepatitis in homosexual men. Gastroenterology 81: 537–538

Final Report of the Veterans Administration Co-operative Study 1978 Type B hepatitis after needle-stick exposure: prevention with hepatitis B immune globulin. Annals of Internal Medicine 88: 285–293

Follett E A C, McMillan A 1980 Homosexuals — a true 'high risk' group for hepatitis B infection. Communicable Diseases in Scotland. CDS Unit, Ruchill Hospital Glasgow, G20 9NB 14: vii–viii

Gerlich W H, Luer W, Thomsen R and the Study Group for Viral Hepatitis of the Deutsche Forschungsgemeiunschaft 1980 Diagnosis of acute and inapparent hepatitis B virus infection by measurement of IgM antibody to hepatitis B core antigen. Journal of Infectious Diseases 142: 95–101

Goudeau A, Yvonnet B, Lesage G et al 1983 Lack of anti-HBcIgM in neonates with HBsAg carrier mothers argues against transplacental transmission of hepatitis B virus infection. Lancet ii: 1103–1104

Heathcote J, Sherlock S 1973 Spread of acute type B hepatitis in London. Lancet i: 1468–1470

Hersh T, Melnick J L, Goyal R K, Hollinger F B 1971 Non-parenteral transmission of viral hepatitis type B Australia antigen-associated hepatitis). New England Journal of Medicine 285: 1363–1364

Holdener F, Grob P J 1981 Hepatitis virus infections in flying air line personnel. Lancet ii: 867–868

Huang S-N 1971 Hepatitis associated antigen hepatitis. An electron microscopic study of virus like particles in liver cells. American Journal of Pathology 64: 483–500

Huang S-N 1975 Immunohistochemical demonstration of hepatitis B core and surface antigens in paraffin sections. Laboratory Investigation 33: 88–95

Jeffries D J, James W H, Jefferiss F J G, MacLeod K G, Willcox R R 1973 Australia (hepatitis-associated) antigen in patients attending a venereal disease clinic. British Medical Journal 1: 455–456

Lacey C J N, Meaden J D, Clarke S K A 1983 Hepatitis B virus infection in homosexual men. British Journal of Venereal Diseases 59: 277–278

Lavarini P, Farci P, Chiaberge E et al 1983 IgM antibody against hepatitis B core antigen (IgM anti-HBc): diagnostic and prognostic significance in acute HBsAg positive hepatitis. British Medical Journal 287: 1254–1256

Leading Article 1984a Prevention of perinatally transmitted hepatitis B infection. Lancet ii: 939–941

Leading Article 1984b Non-A, non-B hepatitis. Lancet ii: 1077–1078

Lemon S M, Gates N L, Simms T E, Bancroft W H 1981 IgM antibody to hepatitis B core antigen as a diagnostic parameter of acute infection with hepatitis B virus. Journal of Infectious Diseases 143: 803–809

Lim K S, Taam V, Fulford K W M, Catterall R D, Briggs M, Dane D S, Simpson P 1976 Australia antigen-positive hepatitis as a sexually transmitted disease. In: Catterall R D, Nicol C S (eds) Sexually transmitted diseases. Academic Press, London, p 197–206

McFarlane E S, Embil J A, Manuel F R, Thiebaux H J 1981 Antibodies to hepatitis A antigen in relation to the number of lifetime sexual partners in patients attending a STD clinic. British Journal of Venereal Diseases 57: 58–61

Maupas P, Chiron J-C, Barin F et al 1981 Efficiency of hepatitis B vaccine in prevention of early HBsAg carrier state in children. Controlled trial in an endemic area (Senegal). Lancet i: 289–292

Mieli-Vergani G, Vergani D, Portmann B et al 1982 Lymphocyte cytotoxicity to autologous hepatocytes — HBsAg positive chronic liver disease. Gut 23: 1029–1036

Mims C A, White D O 1984 Viral pathogenesis and immunology. Blackwell Scientific Publications, Oxford, p 258–260, 296–298

Mindel A, Tedder R 1981 Hepatitis A in homosexuals. British Medical Journal 282: 1666

Mondelli M, Mieli-Vergani G, Alberti A et al 1982 Specificity of T-lymphocyte cytotoxicity to autologous hepatocytes in chronic HBV infection: evidence that T-cells are directed against HBV core antigen expressed on hepatocytes. Journal of Immunology 129: 2773–2778

Mortimer P P, Vandervelde E M, Parry J V, Cohen B J, Tedder R S 1981 The anti-HBeIgM response in the acute and convalescent phases of acute hepatitis. Journal of Infection 3: 339–347

Nicholson K G 1985 Leading article. Hepatitis delta infections. British Medical Journal 290: 1370–1371

Novick D M, Lok A S F, Thomas H C 1984 Diminished responsiveness of homosexual men to antiviral therapy for HBsAg-positive chronic liver disease. Journal of Hepatology 1: 29–35

Okada K, Kamiyama I, Inomata M, Imai M, Miyakawa Y, Mayumi M 1976 e antigen and anti-e in the serum of asymptomatic carrier mothers and indicators of positive and negative transmission of hepatitis B virus to their infants. New England Journal of Medicine 294: 746–749

Papaevangelou G, Trichopoulos D, Kremastinou T, Papoutsahis G 1974 Prevalence of hepatitis B antigen and antibody in prostitutes. British Medical Journal ii: 256–258

Perillo R P, Campbell C R, Sanders G E, Regenstein F G, Bodicky C J 1984 Spontaneous clearance and reactivation of hepatitis B virus infection among male homosexuals with chronic type B hepatitis. Annals of Internal Medicine 100: 43–46

Prince A M, Huima T, Williams B A A, Bardina L, Brotman B 1984 Isolation of a virus from chimpanzee liver cell cultures inoculated with sera containing the agent of non-A, non-B hepatitis. Lancet ii: 1071–1075

Realdi G, Alberti A, Rugge M, Bortolotti F, Rigoli A M, Tremolada F, Ruol A 1980 Seroconversion from hepatitis B 'e' antigen to anti-HBe in chronic hepatitis B virus infection. Gastroenterology 79: 195–199

Reiner W E, Judon F N, Bond W W, Francis D P, Petersen N J 1984 Asymptomatic rectal mucosal lesions and hepatitis B surface antigen at sites of sexual contact in homosexual men with persistent hepatitis B virus infection. Evidence for de facto parenteral transmission. Annals of Internal Medicine 96: 170–173

Saunders J B, Wodak A D, Morgan-Capner P, White Y S, Portmann B, Davis M, Williams R 1983 Importance of markers of hepatitis B virus in alcoholic liver disease. British Medical Journal 286: 1851–1854

Schreeder M T, Thompson S E, Hadler S C et al 1982 Hepatitis B in homosexual men: prevalence of infection and factors related to transmission. Journal of Infectious Diseases 146: 7–15

Seto B, Coleman W G, Iwarson S, Gerety R J 1984 Detection of reverse transcriptase activity in association with the non-A, non-B hepatitis agent(s). Lancet ii: 941–943

Shafritz D A, Kew M C 1981 Identification of integrated hepatitis B virus DNA sequences in human hepatocellular carcinomas. Hepatology 1: 1–8

Sherlock S 1976 Predicting progression of acute type B hepatitis to chronicity. Lancet ii: 354–356

Sherlock S, Thomas H C 1985 Treatment of chronic hepatitis due to hepatitis B. Lancet ii: 1343–1346

Sjøgren M H, Lemon S M 1983 Low molecular weight IgM antibody to hepatitis B core antigen in chronic infections with hepatitis B virus. Journal of Infectious Diseases 148: 445–451

Smedile A, Farci P, Verme G et al 1982 Influence of delta infection on severity of hepatitis B. Lancet ii: 945–947

Stevens C E, Beasley R P, Tsin J 1975 Vertical transmission of hepatitis B antigen in Taiwan. New England Journal of Medicine 292: 771–774

Szmuness W 1978 Hepatocellular carcinoma and hepatitis B virus. Evidence for a causal association. Progress in Medical Virology 24: 40–69

Szmuness W, Much M I, Prince A M, Hoofnagle J H, Cherubin C E, Harley E J, Block G H 1975 On the role of sexual behavior in the spread of hepatitis B infection. Annals of Internal Medicine 83: 489–495

Szmuness W, Dienstag J L, Purcell R H, Harley E J, Stevens C E, Wong D C 1976 Distribution of antibody to hepatitis A antigen in urban adult populations. New England Journal of Medicine 295: 755–759

Szmuness W, Stevens C E, Harley E J et al 1980 Hepatitis B vaccine: demonstration of efficacy in a controlled clinical trial in a high-risk population in the United States. New England Journal of Medicine 303: 833–841

Szmuness W, Stevens C E, Oleszko W R, Godman A 1981a Passive-active immunisation against hepatitis B: immunogenicity studies in adult Americans. Lancet i: 289–292

Szmuness W, Stevens C E, Harley E J, Zang E A, Taylor P E, Alter H J and the Dialysis Vaccine Trial Group 1981b The immune response of healthy adults to a reduced dose of hepatitis B vaccine. Journal of Medical Virology 8: 123–129

Szmuness W, Stevens C E, Oleszko W R, Goodman A 1981c Passive-active immunisation against hepatitis B: immunogenicity studies in adult Americans. The Lancet i: 575–577

Tabor E 1985 The three viruses of non-A, non-B hepatitis. Occasional survey. Lancet i: 742–745

Tedder R S, Briggs M, Howell D R 1982 UK prevalence of delta infection. Lancet ii: 764–765

Thomas H C 1985 The delta agent comes of age. Gut 26: 1–3

Thomas H C, Scully L J 1985 Antiviral therapy in hepatitis B infection. British Medical Bulletin 41: 374–380

Trevisan A, Realdi G, Alberti A et al 1982 Core antigen specific immunoglobulin G bound to the liver cell membrane in chronic hepatitis B. Gastroenterology 82: 218–222

Villa E, Rubbiani L, Barchi T 1982 Susceptibility of chronic symptomless HBsAg carriers to ethanol-induced hepatic disease. Lancet ii: 1243–1244

Viola L A, Barrison I G, Coleman J C, Paradinas F J, Fluker J L, Evans B A, Murray-Lyon I M 1981 Natural history of liver disease in chronic hepatitis B surface antigen carriers. Survey of 100 patients from Great Britain. Lancet ii: 1156–1159

Waugh M A, Hambling M H 1978 Hepatitis B surface antigen in homosexuals. British Journal of Venereal Diseases 54: 352–355

Weller I V D, Karayiannis P, Lok A S F, Montano L,
Bamber M, Thomas H C, Sherlock S 1983 Significance of
delta agent infection in chronic hepatitis B virus infection:
a study of British carriers. Gut 24: 1061–1063

Weller N D, Lok A S F, Mindel A et al 1985 Randomised
controlled trial of adenine arabinoside 5'monophosphate
(ARA-AMP) in chronic hepatitis B virus infection. Gut
26: 745–751

Whitby L G, Percy-Robb I W, Smith A F 1984 Lecture
notes on clinical chemistry, 3rd edn. Blackwell Scientific
Publications, Oxford, p 138–191, 397–417

White D O 1984 Antiviral chemotherapy, interferons and
vaccines. In: Melnick J L (ed) Monographs in virology 16.

Karger, Basel, p 68–72

Wong V C W, Ip H M H, Lelie P N, Reerink-Brongers E E,
Yeung C Y, Ma H K 1984 Prevention of the HBsAg
carrier state in newborn infants of mothers who are chronic
carriers of HBsAg and HBeAg by administration of
hepatitis B vaccine and hepatitis B immunoglobulin.
Double blind randomised placebo-controlled study. Lancet
i: 921–926

World Health Organization 1977 Advances in viral hepatitis.
World Health Organization Technical Report Series
No 602, Geneva

Zuckerman A J 1985 New hepatitis B vaccines. British
Medical Journal 290: 492–496

31

Human immunodeficiency virus infection and the acquired immune deficiency syndrome (AIDS)

The year 1981 saw the start of an epidemic in the USA of a severe acquired immunodeficiency syndrome — AIDS. Up to the middle of February, 1986 over 17,000 cases had been reported from every part of the USA to the Centers for Disease Control, Atlanta and deaths had been recorded in about half of these cases. Increasing numbers of patients with the syndrome have been and continue to be notified from every western European country, Australia, Japan and equatorial Africa. Although it was thought initially to be a disease confined to promiscuous homosexual men — and called the Gay Related Immune Deficiency Syndrome, GRIDS — it soon became apparent that other population groups were at risk and that heterosexual transmission of the infectious agent of AIDS was also possible.

AIDS showed itself first by the appearance of Kaposi's sarcoma (KS) among young white homosexual males, in an age group certainly in which KS had been virtually unknown before. Afterwards it was discovered that the numbers of cases of pneumonia due to *Pneumocystis carinii*, affecting a similar group, had shown a dramatic increase. Hypotheses about the causes were initially numerous but since AIDS began to involve also heterosexuals, particularly those habitually misusing intravenous drugs, recipients of blood transfusions and haemophiliacs, it became clear that an infectious agent was likely to be the cause. Brilliantly conducted research uncovered the cause and characterized the specific retroviruses of which there are many variants; all are now called human immunodeficiency viruses (HIV) (see Ch. 2).

The clinical picture of AIDS is complex. Its pathological and clinical heterogeneity is associated with involvement and profound disturbance of the immune system which is initiated by HIV and partly explained by the fact that the T4 lymphocyte is an important target for the retrovirus HIV. In 1984 Montagnier, in Paris, reported the isolation of a retrovirus from a patient with lymph gland enlargement and named the isolate lymphadenopathy associated virus (LAV); the same year Gallo and his team in Bethesda recorded and named a retrovirus obtained from patients with AIDS

as the human T-lymphotropic virus type III (HTLV-III). Soon afterwards, Levy working in San Francisco isolated retroviruses from AIDS patients and designated these AIDS-associated retrovirus (ARV). All these are considered now to be variants of the same retrovirus and are to be named human immunodeficiency viruses (HIV). To be correct taxonomically now any 'subspecies' of the 'genospecies' HIV should be given a geographically informative letter code and the sequential number of the isolate. In this chapter, however, the term HIV refers to the HIV isolates named as HTLV-III, LAV or ARV. More recent retrovirus isolates mainly obtained from West Africa near to Senegal, viz. HTLV-IV and LAV-2 (Gallo 1987) are excluded from the general discussion as their clinical role is not yet clear.

As clinical experience with AIDS accrued, it became apparent that many affected individuals developed generalized lymph node enlargement in the months before the onset of the fully developed syndrome itself. In an early retrospective analysis of 132 patients with AIDS, 43% of the 71 patients with Kaposi's sarcoma and 23% of 61 patients with opportunistic infections had had antecedent lymphadenopathy (CDC Task Force on Kaposi's Sarcoma and Opportunistic Infections 1982). During the latter half of the 1970s physicians working in clinics in US cities, to which men came as patients, had become aware of an increasing number with unexplained and persistent generalized lymph node enlargement. Pathologists in New York City also observed during the same period an increase in the number of lymph node biopsies showing only hyperplasia obtained chiefly from young men, most (68%) of whom gave a history of homosexual contact.

Although the increased prevalence of persistent generalized lymphadenopathy has paralleled that of AIDS and although many so affected individuals have both immunological abnormalities and serum antibodies against HIV, the relationship between the two conditions is not yet clearly understood. In addition an acute illness resembling infectious mononucleosis has been recognized in early HIV infection. Others at risk of

AIDS have presented with thrombocytopenic purpura and haemolytic anaemia. The prognosis in those infected with HIV can only be regarded as tentative and imprecise until prospective studies in at-risk groups have been completed.

It is only recently that a specific anti-viral agent against HIV, namely 3'-azido-3'-deoxythymidine (zidovudine; trade name — Retrovir, Wellcome), has been discovered and experience in its clinical use is limited. Although human interferon, suramin and ribavirin, suppress retrovirus replication in vitro, clinical trials with these agents have not been encouraging. As the preparation of an effective and safe vaccine appears to be some way off, limiting the spread of the infection within the community will, therefore, be dependent on the modification of sexual behaviour, particularly amongst homosexual men, through health education; the exclusion of homosexual men as blood donors; the heat or chemical treatment of blood products intended for the treatment of conditions such as haemophilia; and the altering of practices among intravenous drug abusers.

The aetiology of the heterogeneous clinical and pathological features of AIDS and its related disorders are extremely complicated. The epidemiology of AIDS and HIV infection; the immunological findings of those infected; and the clinical aspects of these conditions therefore require systematic appraisal and are discussed under the following headings:

A. Aetiology of AIDS and related disorders
   Human immunodeficiency viruses (HIV)
   Immune response to HIV infection
   Other factors in the pathogenesis of AIDS
B. Epidemiology of AIDS and HIV infection
   Definition of the Acquired Immune Deficiency Syndrome AIDS
   Groups at risk of sexually transmissible HIV infection and AIDS
   a. Homosexual males
   b. Heterosexuals
   c. Both sexes in the following groups:
      1. Intravenous drug abusers
      2. Haitians
      3. Recipients of transfusion of blood or blood products or artificial insemination
      4. Infants and children of at-risk groups
      5. Africans mainly from tropical Africa south of the Sahara
C. Immunological findings in those with HIV infection
   Latent HIV infection
   Acute HIV infection
   Persistent generalized lymphadenopathy (PGL) AIDS
D. Laboratory diagnosis of HIV infection

E. Clinical aspects
   Latency
   Acute HIV infection
   Persistent generalized lymphadenopathy (PGL) in adults
      Histopathology of lymph nodes in PGL
      Diagnosis
   Thrombocytopenic purpura
   5. Acquired Immune Deficiency Syndrome (AIDS) in adults
      Kaposi's sarcoma
         Histopathology of Kaposi's sarcoma
         Treatment
      Other neoplasms associated with AIDS
         Non-Hodgkin's lymphomas
      Serious infections in AIDS
      System involvement in AIDS
         Lungs
         Gastrointestinal tract
         Central and peripheral nervous system
         Eye
         Kidneys
         Heart
   AIDS in infants and children
F. Chemotherapy specific for HIV infection
   Anti-retroviral action of drugs
   Drugs under clinical trial in HIV infection
G. Chemotherapy specific for opportunistic virus infections in HIV infection and AIDS
H. Psychosocial phenomena and prevention in HIV infection and AIDS

A. AETIOLOGY OF AIDS AND RELATED DISORDERS

HUMAN IMMUNODEFICIENCY VIRUSES (HIV)

Before the discovery of HIV many hypotheses on the aetiology of AIDS had been put forward including the possible role of the inhalation of volatile nitrites, often used for enhancement of sexual experience by gay men; chronic immunosuppression by spermatozoal antigens; or 'antigenic overload' due to multiple infections caused either by prokaryotes or viruses.

The occurrence of the disease in patients with haemophilia receiving factor VIII prepared from the plasma of many donors supported the view that the infective agent was a virus. The transmission of HIV by sexual intercourse; by the injection or infusion of infected blood; vertically by the pregnant mother to her fetus, and the association of the established disease with the loss of T4 lymphocytes were recognized as a pattern by Robert C Gallo and his colleagues who had isolated in 1978 the first human retrovirus HTLV-I which caused the disease entity known as adult T-cell leukaemia (ATL) as its main effect and also had an affinity for T4 lymphocytes (Gallo, 1987). In 1982 a related but distinct retrovirus, HTLV-II, was isolated from a patient with hairy cell leukaemia (Kalyanaraman et al 1982).

Given the known propensity of HTLV-I and II for T-cells, and the fundamental T-cell abnormalities which occur in AIDS patients, attempts were made to identify retrovirus infection in those affected. Gallo et al (1983), working in Bethesda, USA, isolated retroviruses from three AIDS patients and showed that the isolate from one man was very similar to other HTLV-I strains. In the same issue of the journal 'Science', Montagnier's group in Paris (Barré-Sinoussi et al 1983) reported the culture of a retrovirus (which they called LAV) from a French patient with persistent lymphadenopathy and showed that it was similar, but not identical, to other HTLV-I isolates. Further evidence that suggested a role for retroviruses in the aetiology of AIDS came from the serological studies conducted by Essex and co-workers in Boston (1983). They found antibodies reactive with cell surface glycoprotein (gp61) on HTLV-I infected lymphoid cells in the sera of 19 of 75 patients with AIDS but in only 2 of the 336 control subjects. In the lymphocytes of 2 of 33 AIDS patients examined, Gelmann et al (1983) demonstrated integrated HTLV proviral sequences; both patients had serum antibody against HTLV.

The rarity of AIDS in areas of the world where HTLV-I infections are endemic; the few isolates of the viruses from AIDS patients; the low antibody titres to gp61 protein of HTLV-I; and, in general, absence of antibody to the HTLV structural proteins (p24 and p19) suggested that the known human retroviruses (HTLV-I and II) were not causative.

In the United States and in France, respectively, both Gallo and Montagnier isolated new retroviruses from patients with AIDS and from individuals at risk of the disease. Gallo introduced the term human T-lymphotropic virus type III (HTLV-III) for his isolates and, as his retrovirus isolates were similar to that cultured from the patient with lymphadenopathy referred to above, Montagnier retained the term lymphadenopathy-associated virus (LAV). In San Francisco, Levy et al (1984a) isolated retroviruses with a type D morphology with cytopathic effects on T-lymphocytes from 22 of 45 patients with AIDS. These isolates were termed AIDS associated retroviruses (ARV) and were shown to have immunological similarities to LAV.

As culture methods were perfected, retroviruses could be isolated regularly from patients with AIDS or at risk for AIDS. Gallo et al (1984) isolated HIV from the peripheral lymphocytes from 13 of 43 adults with AIDS

with Kaposi s sarcoma and from 21 adult AIDS patients with opportunistic infection. The virus was also cultured from 18 of 21 patients with 'pre-AIDS' but not from any of 115 heterosexual control subjects. Similar results were reported by Levy et al (1984a) working in San Francisco where they also recovered HIV from 3 of 14 healthy homosexual men who had been the regular sexual partners of men with AIDS; and from 2 of 19 asymptomatic homosexuals not known to have been contacts of anyone infected. A feature of the AIDS-related retroviruses is that the genome of each isolate may differ greatly from another (Alizon et al 1984). Gallo (1987) explains that his HTLV-III comprises a great many variants that form a continuum of related strains. Some pairs of variants differ by as few as 80 nucleotides of the 9 500 making up the genome, whereas others differ by more than 1000 nucleotides.

The various names of retrovirus isolates recovered by the separate research teams and used in abbreviated forms, viz. LAV, HTLV-III and ARV, are explained in Chapter 2. In this chapter the text follows recommendations of the subcommittee of the International Committee on the Taxonomy of Viruses that the retroviruses implicated in 'AIDS' should be designated as human immunodeficiency viruses to be known in the abbreviated form as HIV (Coffin et al 1986). Although 'subspecies' are to be given a geographically informative letter code and a sequential number for the isolate, the abbreviation 'HIV' only is used throughout the text. Differentiation between 'subspecies' is likely to be necessary, however, since a novel retrovirus distantly related to the first HIV isolates (LAV/HTLV-III), has been isolated from 2 patients with AIDS from West Africa (Clavel et al 1986). In AIDS in Africa, HIV have somewhat higher genetic variability, although their antigenic regions are highly conserved in most cases, but the newly described HIV, referred to as LAV-II by Clavel et al, although related, is distinct from them and from a recently described simian retrovirus, STLV-III$_{mac}$, the putative aetiological agent of simian AIDS MAC in captive macaques. A retrovirus HTLV-IV isolated by Essex is apparently apathogenic (Gallo 1987). The situation is complex but it now appears that analysis of the nucleotide sequence of the human retrovirus (HIV-2). associated with AIDS in West Africa, has shown that it is evolutionarily distinct from the retrovirus HIV-I associated with AIDS in the United States and western Europe (Guyader et al 1987).

Serological studies on patients with AIDS and on those at risk of the disease support the view that HIV is aetiologically associated with AIDS. Using sensitive immunoassays, about 90% of patients with AIDS show serological evidence of exposure to HIV. In addition, more than 80% of patients with persistent generalized lymphadenopathy are seropositive for the virus (Cheinsong-Popov et al 1984, Levy et al 1984a, Safai et al 1984, Sarngadharan et al 1985).

The well-recognized feature of T4 lymphocyte depletion in AIDS is explained by the fact that HIV preferentially infect and are cytopathic to T4 lymphocytes. It has been shown that CD4 (T4) antigen is an essential component of the receptor for HIV and so infection is associated mainly with cells which express this antigen (Dalgleish et al 1984, Klatzmann et al 1984). Interestingly, some cells of the macrophage/monocyte system also express CD4 antigen and it is tempting to postulate that macrophage dysfunction in AIDS patients is the result of HIV infection of these cells. EBV-transformed B-lymphoblastoid cell lines can also be infected with HIV (Montagnier et al 1984), as can microglia, astrocytes and probably neurones (Stoler et al 1986).

The infection with HIV is initially latent (hidden) and the carrier apparently well, although some will develop a glandular fever-like illness during seroconversion (Cooper et al 1985). In a short prospective study, Goedert et al (1984) calculated that annually about 7% of HIV subjects seropositive for antibody to HIV develop AIDS. Factors determining progression to this life-threatening condition are not known for sure, but may include repeated viral infections — for example cytomegalovirus can itself produce immunosuppression and is commonly isolated from the urine and semen of homosexual men (see Ch. 28). Repeated exposure of the immune system also to allogeneic spermatozoal antigens (Mavligit et al 1984) may have like effect. These additional antigenic stimuli may help to explain some well-recognized epidemiological features of AIDS (see below).

IMMUNE RESPONSE TO HIV INFECTION

Indirect immunofluorescence for antibody to membrane antigens, the western blot (immunoblot) enzyme-linked immunosorbent and competitive radioimmunoassay methods have been used for the detection of serum antibodies against HIV.

As antigen for the latter two assays, lysates of virus particles concentrated by sucrose gradient centrifugation or infected tissue culture cells are generally used. In the immunofluorescent method, whole virus-infected lymphoid cells are employed. Cheinsong-Popov et al (1984) showed excellent correlation between the results obtained by immunofluorescence and by competitive radioimmunoassay.

The time that may elapse between infection and the appearance of these antibodies to HIV is not well-defined but may be prolonged. In the sera of patients who show seroconversion, IgG against the *gag* gene products, particularly p24, are produced first. Anti-

bodies against p55 *gag* become detectable about 12 weeks from the time of infection and from the 40th week *env* encoded proteins, gp41 and later gp65 are found. Reactivity with the *pol* gene product p33, is noted with increasing frequency from the 12th week following seroconversion (Lange et al 1986a, b). With the onset of AIDS, the antibody titre to p24 declines or becomes negative. T4 cell depletion in those with AIDS may lead to a loss of antibody production by B-cells. In support of this proposition it has been recorded that in a homosexual with lymphadenopathy, his serum initially contained IgG LAV antibody but became seronegative after the development of AIDS when there was profound depletion of T4 cells (Laurence et al 1984). A simplified diagrammatic representation of the results of immunoblot assay of antibodies in HIV infection is given in Fig. 31.1.

IgM reactive with HIV has also been found in the sera of some patients with lymphadenopathy and subjects at risk of infection, suggesting that this represents a primary antibody response to the virus (Ainti et al 1985).

Although the sera of some infected individuals can neutralize HIV in vitro, the prevalence of these antibodies is low. It is also clear that otherwise apparently healthy individuals can harbour the virus but have no detectable serum antibody (Salahuddin et al 1984). These workers found that 4 of 96 individuals from whose blood or saliva HIV could be isolated were seronegative for HIV antibody; in each case the antibody-negative subject was the sexual partner of a patient with AIDS or related disease. The reasons for the failure to detect antibody are not clear, but perhaps this reflects slow multiplication of the virus within the individual's lymphocytes and lack of exposure of its antigens to the humoral immune system. In conditions of antigen excess, the antibody may be bound in immune complexes and not detectable by the methods currently available. In this respect, the record of seroconversion to LAV antibody positive in a homosexual man, 7 months after the development of persistent lymphadenopathy, is relevant (Laurence et al 1984).

OTHER FACTORS IN THE PATHOGENESIS OF AIDS

Although HIV appears to be the prime pathogen in the aetiology of AIDS, it is probable that other factors play a role in the pathogenesis of the disease. For example, Kaposi's sarcoma, common in homosexual men with AIDS but infrequent in others with this disease, has been associated with evidence of cytomegalovirus infection. An increase in prevalence of CMV antibodies in the sera of Europeans and Americans with the classical

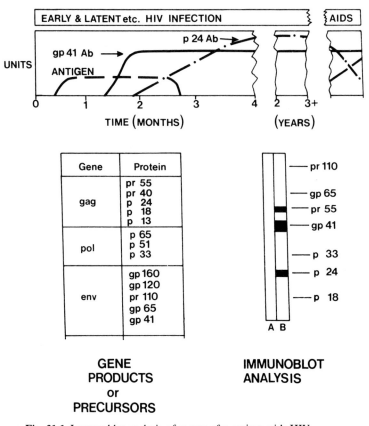

GENE PRODUCTS or PRECURSORS

IMMUNOBLOT ANALYSIS

Fig. 31.1 Immunoblot analysis of serum of a patient with HIV infection about 40 months after seroconversion (B) showing antibodies to p24, pr55 and gp41 (antibodies to p18, p33, gp65 or pr110 are not present in this example); (A) represents absence of antibodies in the serum of an uninfected control. Above is shown a hypothetical time course for the occurrence of specific markers following HIV infection. To the left are listed the proteins, whether gene products or precursors, to which IgG antibodies are directed. See Allain et al 1986, Lange et al 1986a, b, Weber et al 1987. (p = protein; gp = glycoprotein; pr = protein precursor)

neoplasm has been recorded (Giraldo et al 1978). Further studies by the same workers showed the presence of CMV-DNA in 3 of 8 tumour biopsies and CMV-related antigen in 7 of 31 biopsies (Giraldo et al 1980). Virus-specific RNA and CMV-determined nuclear antigens were also found in 5 of 10 tumour tissues (Boldogh et al 1981). Drew et al (1982) also detected CMV-RNA and CMV antigens in biopsies of the sarcoma in homosexual men with AIDS. Cytomegalovirus infection is common in homosexual men (Ch. 28) and it has been postulated that the virus plays a role in the aetiology of Kaposi's sarcoma in AIDS.

Similarly, with respect also to Epstein-Barr virus (EBV), there may be an association between the B-cell lymphomas which occur in homosexual men and the virus as in Burkitt's lymphoma. Abo et al (1982) described a monoclonal malignant lymphoma in a child

with chronic EBV infection and demonstrated nuclear antigen, early antigen and viral capsid antigen in the tumour cells (see Ch. 29). Ziegler et al (1984) detected nuclear antigen in the tumour cells of 2 of 3 homosexual men with Burkitt's-like lymphoma. Interestingly, individuals with a genetically determined failure of specific T-cell and other immunological responses develop uncontrolled proliferation of B-cells infected with EBV (Purtilo et al 1982). A markedly increased frequency of circulating EBV-infected B-cells capable of spontaneous growth in vitro was found in the blood of patients with AIDS (Birx et al 1986), and it was suggested that this resulted from a profound defect of T-cell immunity to EBV.

The majority of opportunistic infections and frequent causes of death observed in patients with AIDS are from the Herpesviridae Family (see Ch. 2); herpes simplex virus type 1 in vitro, it has been shown, can reactivate transcription of HIV (Mosca & Bednarik 1987).

B. EPIDEMIOLOGY OF AIDS

The marked increase in numbers of cases of AIDS in the USA and Europe since the first reports are shown in Figures 3.11 and 3.12. A number of epidemiological and other considerations are discussed in more detail elsewhere (Ch. 3 p. 51–54; Ch. 4 p. 62–65; Ch. 5 e & f).

Of the first 9887 cases of AIDS in adults reported to Communicable Diseases Center (CDC). Atlanta, USA, 49% had died. Precise data on mortality rates are not yet available, but about 35, 55 and 80% of patients are dead within one, two or three years, respectively, of the diagnosis having been made. Although initially recognized in the USA, AIDS has been reported from most western European countries, Australia, Africa and Japan.

DEFINITION OF THE ACQUIRED IMMUNE DEFICIENCY SYNDROME (AIDS)

For the limited purposes of epidemiological surveillance, the CDC (1985a) defined a case of AIDS as a person who has had:

1. a reliably diagnosed disease that is at least moderately indicative of an underlying cellular immune deficiency, but who, at the same time, has had:

2. no known underlying cause of cellular immune deficiency nor any other cause of reduced resistance reported to be associated with that disease.

The definition has been adopted in most countries and is given more fully in Note 31.1. In tropical Africa, south of the Sahara particularly, where laboratory resources are limited or lacking and where there are differences in the clinical presentation of the disease from that seen in North America and Europe an appropriate clinical case definition has been developed following a World Health Organization workshop in Bangui, Central African Republic (Colebunders et al 1987; see also Notes 31.2 and 31.3).

GROUPS AT RISK OF SEXUALLY TRANSMISSIBLE HIV INFECTION AND AIDS

In an analysis of the first 16 137 American cases of AIDS in adult men reported to the Centers for Disease Control, Atlanta, certain high risk groups were identifiable (Table 31.1).

In the first 1129 cases in women, 53% were drug abusers; 16% had had sexual contact with a patient with

Table 31.1 Acquired Immune Deficiency Syndrome (AIDS) in male patients by patient's group up till February 17, 1986.

Patient group	Number	(%)
Homosexual/bisexual	12 689	79
Intravenous drug users	2 340	15
Haemophiliac patients	135	1
Heterosexual contacts of individuals with AIDS or at risk for AIDS	39	0
Transfusion recipients	169	1
Other/unknown*	765	5
Total	16 137	(100)

* Haitian-born AIDS patients have now been placed in this category as current information suggests that both heterosexual contact and exposure to contaminating needles — not associated with i.v. drug abuse — play a role in transmission (Centers for Disease Control 1985a).

AIDS or an individual in a high risk group; 10% had had a recent blood transfusion; and in 21% there was no obvious risk factor. There have been some differences geographically in the patient characteristics; few cases amongst intravenous drug abusers at that time had been described in Europe, and in France and Belgium a high proportion of those with AIDS have been immigrants from equatorial Africa.

a. Homosexual males
Amongst men, AIDS has presented first as a disease of homosexuals, the majority being in the 30–39 year age group, the median age being 37 years. Although the majority of these men in Europe are white, about 28% of homosexuals in the USA are black or Hispanic.

Jaffe et al (1983) conducted a case-control study in four major US cities to identify risk factors for the occurrence of Kaposi's sarcoma (KS) and *Pneumocystis carinii* pneumonia (PCP) in homosexual men. By comparison with healthy homosexuals, patients with KS or PCP had had more sexual partners per year (medians 61 and 27 respectively); were more likely to have had syphilis and non-B hepatitis; were more likely to have regularly used amyl or butyl nitrite inhalants; and to have used drugs such as marijuana. Patients so affected were more likely to have had oral-anal sexual contact and to have participated in 'fisting' (the insertion of a clenched fist into the rectum).

Epidemiologically HIV infection is identical to that of AIDS
The results of serological testing of groups of homosexual men attending STD clinics in different geographical areas are shown in Table 31.2. The prevalence of HIV serum antibody varies considerably from region to region, with high rates in the western USA, particularly in San Francisco. In the UK the prevalence of antibody in patients attending clinics outside London is about

Table 31.2 Prevalence of HIV antibody in the sera of sexually active healthy homosexual men in different geographical areas.

| City (country) | Number of sera containing antibody (%)/number of sera tested | | | | | | Reference |
| | Homosexual men | | | Comparison group | | | |
	Nos. examined	Positive	%	Nos. Examined	Positive	%	
San Francisco (USA)	47	27	(57.5)	56	0	(0.0)	Levy et al 1984a
Paris (France)	44	8	(18.2)	30	0	(0.0)	Brun-Vézinet et al 1984b
Paris (France)	52	13	(25.0)	126	3	(2.3)	Mathez et al 1984
Copenhagen/Aarhus (Denmark)	250	22	(8.8)	69	0	(0.0)	Melbye et al 1984a
London (UK)	308	53	(17.2)	1077	0	(0.0)	Cheinsong-Popov et al 1984
Munich/Cologne (W.Germany)	48	13	(27.1)	18	0	(0.0)	Hehlmann et al 1984
Helsinki (Finland)	200	17	(8.5)	—	—	—	Valle et al 1985

5%. With the introduction into a susceptible population of any infectious agent, however, there is temporal variation in prevalence rates. Mortimer et al (1985a) found that only 5% of 95 homosexual men who attended STD clinics in London were seropositive for antibody to the virus in 1980, but by 1984 the proportion had risen to 34%. There is, however, variability in the specificity of the serological tests presently available (Budiansky 1985), so much care is necessary in the interpretation of results. Of 593 831 units of blood tested during April–May 1985, 0.89% were reported positive for AIDS antibody in the first instance, but only 0.25% of blood samples were positive twice in a row by the test, or 2 times out of 3 if tested 3 times. Persons with certain HLA antibodies appear to react consistently positive to at least one test on the market; the purification process may pick up some HLA antigen found on the human cell membranes. Compared with the ELISA the western blot test is more reliable, but more expensive and difficult from the technical viewpoint.

Amongst homosexual men in Denmark, Melbye et al (1984a) showed a significant association between the prevalence of HIV antibody and sexual contact with individuals from the USA. Both Melbye et al and Goedert et al (1984) identified similar risk factors for the acquisition of the virus, factors which were identical to those for AIDS (see above). Receptive anal intercourse was the most striking risk factor, an observation explained by the presence of HIV both in the semen of patients with AIDS and apparently healthy homosexual men (Zagury et al 1984, Ho et al 1984). Seropositivity for HIV was also strongly associated with large numbers of sexual partners, especially in individuals with the receptive role in anal intercourse. Goedert's group also recognized an association between insertive 'fisting' and seropositivity, a finding which might be attributable to increased risk of infection following gross contamination of the skin with infected faeces and blood.

Further evidence for the sexual transmission of AIDS and HIV has come from the tracing of contacts of homosexual men with AIDS and the AIDS-related complex. In a careful study of sexual contacts of men with AIDS, Auerbach et al (1984) showed a link between 40 cases in 10 US cities, reinforcing the hypothesis that AIDS was caused by a transmissible agent. The prepatent period was estimated as ranging from 7 to 14 months. Gazzard et al (1984) from London reported a clustering of homosexuals with AIDS, the AIDS-related complex or lymphadenopathy linked by sexual contact (Fig. 31.2). As HIV antibody testing was undertaken, this study is of particular interest. Case No. 6 appeared to be the link in both clusters of patients. He had no clinical evidence of AIDS-related disease and his serum did not contain HIV antibodies. It is possible nevertheless that he may have been an infective carrier of the disease.

b. Heterosexuals

In both USA and Europe the sexual transmission of AIDS amongst heterosexuals appears to be less common than amongst homosexual men. In the USA epidemiological data indicate that some 16% of women with AIDS (i.e. about 0.8% of all cases of AIDS) have acquired the disease from sexual contact with a patient with AIDS or a member of a group at high risk for the disease. Harris et al (1983) studied 7 women who were sexual partners of male drug abusers with AIDS. 1 woman had AIDS, 5 had an AIDS-related complex or lymphadenopathy, and the other woman had no clinical evidence of the disease. Further evidence for the sexual transmission of the disease comes from the report of AIDS in the wife of a haemophiliac with the disease (Pitchenik et al 1984). Jarlais et al (1984) studied a group of male drug abusers and showed that although there was a large population of female sexual partners who themselves were not using intravenous drugs the incidence of AIDS amongst these women was small. They postulated that the low risk for AIDS may be related to the less efficient sexual transmission of the virus in heterosexuals or to the lower frequency of exposure to other contributing factors (Guinan et al 1984). Redfield et al (1985), however, studied the wives of 7 men with AIDS or related HIV features and found that 4 women, 3 of

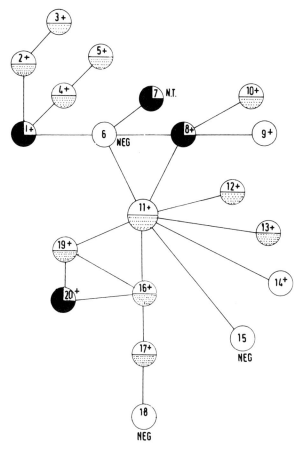

Fig. 31.2 Clustering of homosexual cases linked by sexual contact. Circles represent 20 promiscuous homosexuals linked by a history of ano-genital sexual contact. Cases 1–7 form one cluster and 8–20 the other, with Case 6 apparently linking the two clusters. The men in clusters were resident in central London, none were intravenous drug abusers. Open circles represent symptomless males; circles with light shading represent those with persistent generalized lymphadenopathy and black circles represent those with AIDS (Gazzard et al 1984). + = positive for serum antibody to HIV; NEG = negative for serum antibody to HIV; NT = not tested for serum antibody to HIV.

whom had lymphadenopathy, were seropositive for the virus. In addition, they succeeded in culturing HIV from the peripheral leucocytes of one woman who was clinically well and whose serum did not contain antibody against the virus. The sexual transmission of HIV to the partner of seropositive haemophiliacs was further shown by Kreiss et al (1985) who found that the wives of 2 of 21 men had serum antibody against the virus. HIV can be isolated from the cervical secretions of up to 50% of seropositive women. As filtration of secretions prevents the subsequent culture of HIV, it appears that the virus in these fluids is cell-associated (Vogt et al 1986). Epidemiological data from the USA and Europe,

however, suggest that the female-to-male transmission of HIV during vaginal intercourse is uncommon. This may be explained by the finding of only small quantities of virus in cervico-vaginal secretions (Wofsy et al 1986). In Africa, however, bidirectional sexual transmission of the virus is perhaps important. The sequence of events in the two clusters of AIDS cases in heterosexual African partners described by Piot et al (1984) suggested male-to-female and female-to-male transmission with a much lower male:female ratio (1.1:1) than that reported from the USA. 7 of 25 male clients of prostitutes working in Rwanda were seropositive, and the data presented suggested that the risk of infection increased in relation to the number of different sexual partners per year (Van de Perre et al 1985). Both in Rwanda and Nairobi a high prevalence of HIV antibody has been found in prostitutes who did not misuse drugs (Van de Perre et al 1985; Kreiss et al 1986). Although 6% of 200 prostitutes in Athens were seropositive, anti-HIV was not detected in the sera of women in London, Paris, or Aviano, Italy (Barton et al 1985, Brenky-Faudeux & Fribourg-Blanc 1985, Papaevangelou et al 1985, Tirelli et al 1985).

In the continent of Africa south of the Sahara, Gallo (1987) identifies Congo, Zaire, Zambia, Malawi, Tanzania, Burundi, Rwanda, Uganda and Kenya as areas of high incidence for HIV (HTLV-III); and Gabon, Cameroon, Central Africa, Zimbabwe, Botswana, South Africa, Swaziland and Lesotho as areas of low incidence. Both HIV (HTLV-III) and an apparently non-pathogenic HTLV-IV are seen in Ivory Cost and Upper Volta and HTLV-IV alone in Senegal and Guinea. A further HIV (Clavel et al 1986) designated LAV-II, distantly related to LAV and distinct from the simian retrovirus STLV-III$_{mac}$, the cause of AIDS in macaques, has been isolated from two AIDS patients, one from Guinea Bissau and one from Cape Verde.

Estimates of risk and risk factors for heterosexuals
These will be identified only when large prospective studies on HIV infection in groups at risk have been completed. At present a number of relevant factors can be identified and discussed.

c. Both sexes in the following groups

1. Intravenous drug abusers
About 17% of patients with AIDS in the USA have been intravenous drug abusers; 20% of those patients have been women. About 80% of new cases have occurred in the New York/New Jersey area, but a few cases of AIDS amongst drug abusers have been reported outside the USA. Although some men give a history of homosexual contact, the majority of affected individuals have no other identifiable risk factors, and presumably have

Table 31.3 Prevalence of HIV antibody in the sera of intravenous drug abusers.

Geographical area	Percentage sera containing antibody (number of sera tested)				Reference
	i.v. drug abusers		*Comparison group*		
New York (USA)	8.6	(87)	3	(70)	Spira et al 1984
London (UK)	1.5	(269)	0	(1042)	Cheinsong-Popov et al 1984
The Tyrol (Austria)	44	(34)	NS		Fuchs et al 1985
Valencia (Spain)	37	(112)	0	(95)	Rodrigo et al 1985
Bern (Switzerland)	32	(37)	NS		Mortimer et al 1985b
Bari (Italy)	76	(45)	NS		Angarano et al 1985
California (USA)	1.7	(345)	NS		Levy et al 1986
Edinburgh (UK)	51	(164)	NS		Robertson et al 1986
Glasgow (UK)	4.5	(606)	NS		Follett et al 1986

NS = Not stated

acquired the disease through sharing of contaminated syringes and needles. In general, these patients tend to be of lower socio-economic class than others with AIDS.

Using an ELISA method, Spira et al (1984) identified antibodies against HIV in the sera of 11 (65%) of 17 drug abusers with AIDS. Studies on the prevalence of antibody against HIV in the sera of intravenous drug abusers (Table 31.3) indicate that the virus is spread widely throughout this population group. Most reports indicate a rapid increase in the numbers of seropositive individuals within a two-year period (1984–1985).

2. Haitians

About 4% of cases of AIDS in the USA have been in Haitians living in that country. Viera et al (1983) described 10 Haitian men with AIDS who had migrated from the island to New York on average 2.7 years (range 3 months to 8 years) before the onset of symptoms. These men denied homosexual contact and the previous use of intravenous drugs. How AIDS in this group is acquired is uncertain, but the sexual transmission of the virus may be important. The estimated prevalence of AIDS in Haitian immigrants to the USA is 8 per 1000 of the population aged 24 to 39 years.

Cases of AIDS have also been reported from Haiti, and Pape et al (1983) described the demographic and other characteristics of 61 patients living on that island. 9 of these individuals were women who did not abuse drugs and were not sexually promiscuous. 2 women had had blood transfusions within the preceding 6 years. Although it is difficult to be certain about the veracity of the information obtained, only one patient gave a history of homosexual contact. The median age (32 years) of these patients was similar to that of AIDS patients living in the USA.

3. Recipients of transfusion of blood or blood products or artificial insemination

Just under 1% of cases of AIDS has occurred amongst haemophiliacs and almost always in those with haemophilia A in whom there has been no other identified risk

factor. It has been estimated that the incidence of AIDS in haemophiliacs is 1–2 per 1000 (Bloom 1984). As retroviruses are able to withstand the methods used previously for the preparation of factor VIII concentrate (Levy et al 1984b) it seems likely that haemophiliacs with AIDS have acquired the retrovirus from these concentrates.

Antibodies against HIV have been found in the sera of haemophilia patients with no clinical evidence of AIDS or related diseases. Although it is likely that the initial cases of AIDS in haemophilia patients in Europe have been infected with concentrate imported from the USA (Melbye et al 1984b) it is likely that, as the virus has spread within the continent, others have acquired HIV from blood donated locally.

AIDS has developed in those who have received multiple blood transfusions but in whom no other risk factor has been identified. Of the 17 266 cases of AIDS in adults reported to the Centers for Disease Control in the United States in the period up to February 17, 1986, 277 (1.6%) were considered to have acquired the infection by transfusion of infected blood.

A collaborative study of AIDS associated with transfusion was undertaken by Curran et al (1984) from CDC, Atlanta. They identified 18 patients whose only apparent risk factor had been the receipt of blood transfusions. 6 of the 7 patients, whose donors had been identified, had been exposed to at least one donor from a high risk AIDS group. Although none of these donors had AIDS, all had immunological abnormalities and/or lymphadenopathy. The interval between transfusion and the development of AIDS ranged from 15 to 57 months, with a median of 27.5 months. In general, patients with transfusion-associated AIDS had been given blood from many donors (range 2–48, median 14). The mean age of these patients was 54 years (range 19 to 67 years). In contrast to the relatively small number of cases of transfusion-associated AIDS in adults, 18% of 217 children (1 December, 1985) in the USA have acquired the infection from contaminated blood.

The majority of transfusion-associated AIDS cases in

the USA were reported during the first few years of the recognition of the syndrome. The declining numbers of such cases probably reflect the success of excluding from therapeutic use blood donated by any person known to be at risk of acquiring HIV.

Transmission of HIV as a result of artificial insemination with semen from an infected donor has been recorded (Stewart et al, 1985).

4. Infants and children of at-risk groups

Transfusion-associated AIDS has constituted a small proportion of paediatric cases (Table 31.4). Although some infants developing AIDS have been born to parents of Haitian origin, the majority have had mothers who were drug abusers, sexually promiscuous or known contacts of men with AIDS. Most infants develop features of the syndrome within 3–6 months of delivery. In infants epidemiological evidence suggests transplacental or perinatal transmission. The cultivation of HIV from the thymus, lungs, liver, brain, spleen and kidney of a 20 week fetus of a seropositive mother and the detection by immunofluorescence of HIV antigen in the tissues of a 28 week fetus support the evidence for transplacental transmission of the virus (Jovaisas et al 1985, Lapointe et al 1985). Ziegler et al (1985) reported HIV infection in the child of a mother transfused with infected blood after the delivery of the baby, and postulated transmission via breast milk, a hypothesis strengthened by the isolation of HIV from the breast milk of three healthy but infected individuals (Thiry et al 1985).

Table 31.4 Risk factors associated with AIDS in infants.

Risk factors associated with AIDS in infants	
Parent with AIDS or at increased risk for AIDS	76%
Haemophilia	18%
Transfusion with blood products	
No apparent risk factor	6%

Vilmer et al (1984) described three unrelated families (two Haitian and the other from Zaire) each with an affected infant. HIV was isolated from one infant whose parents and brother were both seropositive for the virus. Antibodies against HIV were also found in the affected child and both parents of the second family. The third child reported had no serological evidence of HIV infection, but HIV-associated reverse transcriptase was found in the supernate of stimulated T-lymphocytes from the mother. In the USA Laurence et al (1984) similarly described 3 infants with AIDS, each born to i.v. drug-abuser mothers, who although clinically well had antibodies against HIV and/or cellular immune dysfunction. 2 of the 2 children were seropositive for HIV, a finding in support of vertical transmission. The

degree of risk of transmission of the virus from mother to fetus cannot be estimated with certainty; in one study of 11 infected women, 4 of the 12 infants were infected (Scott et al 1985). As there was some selection bias in this report, however, the risk of infection of the child may have been overestimated.

5. Africans from Africa south of the Sahara

With the exception of Haitians, the patient characteristics in cases of AIDS in western Europe are similar to those in the USA. The occurrence of AIDS in heterosexual men and women who have emigrated from equatorial Africa (Brunet et al 1983, Clumeck et al 1984), has, however, presented a new problem. Similarly, AIDS in Caucasians who have returned to Europe after living for some time in areas of Central Africa (Bygbjerg 1983, Shiach et al 1984) has raised new questions. Within recent years individuals living in Zambia, Rwanda and Zaire have developed illnesses meeting the CDC diagnostic criteria for AIDS and the number of such cases has risen markedly (Vandepitte et al 1983, Piot et al 1984). In addition the occurrence of lymphadenopathy associated with HIV has been recorded. The male:female ratio of cases of AIDS in Africans (1.1:1) is very much less than that of cases in Americans and Europeans (13.3:1) but similar to that in Haitians with AIDS (1.5:1). Unlike the situation in the USA and Europe, neither homosexuality nor drug abuse are the major risk factors in Africa. The finding of two clusters of cases of AIDS in heterosexual partners has suggested heterosexual transmission of the causative agent.

Ellrodt et al (1984) isolated HIV from the lymphocytes of a married couple from Zaire; the husband had AIDS and the wife prodromal features of the disease. Further evidence of the role of HIV in African AIDS comes from serological studies. Using a radioimmunoprecipitation method, Brun-Vézinet et al (1984a) detected antibodies against HIV in the sera of 35 of 37 patients with AIDS (including patients with disseminated Kaposi's sarcoma) in Kinshasa, Zaire; they also detected antibodies in the sexual partners of 2 patients. In striking contrast to European and American experience, the prevalence of serum antibody in a control group of hospital patients with no evidence of AIDS or related diseases was high (6 of 26 in Kinshasa and 7 of 100 in Ngaliewa), a finding confirmed by the results of another group of workers in Katana, Zaire, who, using an ELISA method, found HIV antibodies in the sera of 12.4% of 250 out-patients with no overt evidence of AIDS (Biggar et al 1984).

The relative rarity of heterosexually-transmitted AIDS in the USA and Europe, and the contrary finding in Africa, suggests either that there are two main strains of the virus, differing in infectivity, in circulation or that other co-factors operate.

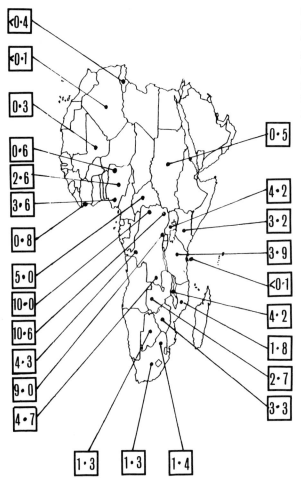

Fig. 31.3 Map showing proportional frequencies of endemic (African) Kaposi's sarcoma (male and female combined) before the appearance of AIDS. Data from Hutt (1984). Sketch map, Arno Peters projection.

Kaposi's sarcoma is endemic in Central Africa (Fig. 31.3) (Hutt 1984) and in many areas accounts for 10% of all malignancies. African KS occurs in young adults (age range 25 to 44) and children under the age of 10 years (the male:female sex ratios being 17.1 and 3.1 respectively) (Hood et al 1982).

The relationship of African KS to AIDS is as yet not clear. Although immunological abnormalities similar to those found in AIDS have been reported in Africans with Kaposi's sarcoma (Downing et al 1984), antibodies against HIV were not found in the sera of 14 patients in Zaire with the disease (Biggar et al 1984). However, KS can be the result of immunosuppression from whatever cause (see below) and it is likely that KS in Africa has a mixed aetiology which includes HIV infection. Since 1980 Bayley (1984) has noted increasing numbers of patients in Lusaka, Zambia, with an aggressive form

of KS resembling that seen in iatrogenic KS. They found HIV antibodies in the sera of 20 of 22 patients with aggressive KS, but only of 4 of 17 individuals with endemic KS (Bayley et al 1985). The low prevalence of antibody in the comparison group of Zambian natives and the recent appearance of this atypical form of KS strongly suggested that the virus had been recently introduced into the area.

C. IMMUNOLOGICAL FINDINGS IN THOSE INFECTED WITH HIV

LATENT HIV INFECTION

Studies conducted in the USA and London before the discovery of HIV showed a high prevalence of immunological abnormalities amongst apparently healthy homosexual men (Kornfeld et al 1982, Pinching et al 1983).

As these results did not take account of the presence or absence of the virus, their relevance is uncertain but it has now been shown that decreased numbers of T4 (CD4$^+$) cells correlate with the presence of antibody to HIV (Lang et al 1987).

ACUTE HIV INFECTION

During acute HIV infection, with seroconversion, there is a transient T-lymphopenia with reduced numbers of T4 and T8 cells. Several weeks afterwards the ratio of T4:T8 is reduced as a result of increased numbers of circulating T8 cells with normal numbers of T4 cells. Some of the peripheral blood mononuclear cells at this stage appear atypical with irregular nuclei with nucleate and deeply basophilic cytoplasm. Mild thrombocytopenia and neutropenia are also features of the acute illness (Cooper et al 1985, Tucker et al 1985).

PERSISTENT GENERALIZED LYMPHADENOPATHY (PGL)

In general in PGL the peripheral blood lymphocyte findings are similar to, but less pronounced than, those in AIDS (see below). Cells with the T4 phenotype are heterogeneous with respect to function, and Nicholson et al (1984) have shown that it is a subset of these cells which is principally affected in patients with persistent generalized lymphadenopathy. Using monoclonal antibodies they found that the subset T4:TQ1$^-$ or T4:Leu-8$^-$ (the major helper subset for B-cell responses) was normally represented in the peripheral blood, but T4:TQ1$^+$ or T4:Leu8$^+$ cells were depressed in numbers. Similarly, T8:TQ1$^-$ or T8:Leu8$^-$ cell numbers were increased and T8:TQ1$^+$ or T8:Leu8$^+$ numbers were normal.

Bacterial infections of the skin are not uncommon in homosexual men with PGL (see below), an occurrence which may be related to the defective polymorphonuclear chemotaxis and diminished release of lysosomal enzymes noted by Valone et al (1984). Murphy et al (1985) noted mild neutropenia in 6 homosexual men with PGL whose sera contained HIV antibodies. Immunoglobulin bound to the surface of the leucocytes from these patients was detected by means of a granulocyte immunofluorescence test. The mechanism of the neutropenia may be similar to that of thrombocytopenia (see paragraph below on 'immune complexes and their attachment to platelets').

AIDS

Immunological findings in patients are summarized in Table 31.5. HIV is a retrovirus which attacks and is cytotoxic for lymphocytes which express the T4 phenotype (see Note 31.4). As the other human retroviruses HTLV-I and HTLV-II are also T4 tropic and interfere with the function of these lymphocytes it is not surprising that it is the cellular branch of the immune system which is primarily affected in HIV infection.

T4 lymphocyte dysfunction
The most profound immunological abnormalities are found in AIDS patients with opportunistic infections. Although sometimes within the normal range, in general

Table 31.5 Immunological findings in patients with AIDS and related diseases.

Immunological findings in patients with AIDS and related diseases	
Lymphocytes in peripheral blood	reduced
Peripheral blood T4 cells (peripheral blood T4:TQ1+ or T4:Leu 8+)	reduced
Peripheral blood T8 cells (peripheral blood T8:Ql− or T8:Leu8−)	normal or increased
Ratio of peripheral blood T4:T8 numbers	reduced
Response of T-lymphocytes to mitogens	defective
Peripheral blood B-lymphocytes count	normal
B-cells (polyclonal activation)	present
Hypergammaglobulinaemia (especially IgG)	present
Cutaneous anergy to recall antigens	present
Natural killer cell activity	reduced
Immune complexes in serum	present
Polymorphonuclear chemotaxis	defective
Autologous mixed lymphocyte reaction	defective
Monocyte chemotaxis	impaired

the total peripheral blood T-lymphocyte count is low (Schroff et al 1983) because the numbers of circulating T4 lymphocytes ('helper cells') are reduced. As the numbers of T8 ('suppressor/cytotoxic') lymphocytes are normal or increased, the ratio of T4:T8 cell numbers is lower than normal. The low numbers of T4 cells in the peripheral blood are paralleled by the T4 depletion and T8 proliferation in lymph nodes from patients with Kaposi's sarcoma observed by Modlin et al (1983) who also showed B-cell proliferation in the nodes. The initiation of a cellular immune response to an antigen is partly dependent on the functional integrity of T4 cells. It is understandable therefore that peripheral lymphocytes from patients with opportunistic infection and some patients with Kaposi's sarcoma show decreased proliferative responses in vitro to a variety of antigens including phytohaemagglutinin, concanavalin A, pokeweed mitogen, *Candida* spp and purified protein derivative of tuberculin (Gottlieb et al 1981). Gupta & Safai (1983) demonstrated poor peripheral T-cell responses in the autologous and allogeneic mixed lymphocyte reaction, a finding which again indicated a functional abnormality of T4 cells.

B-lymphocyte dysfunction
Although the numbers of circulating B-lymphocytes in AIDS patients are normal, in vitro studies have shown marked functional abnormalities (Lane et al 1983). The proliferative response of peripheral blood mononuclear cells from AIDS patients to pokeweed mitogen (a T-cell dependent B-cell mitogen) is significantly reduced in comparison to cells from control subjects. This indicates reduced numbers of circulating, partially activated, B-cells. When B-cells from these patients are incubated with formalinized *Staphylococcus aureus* Cowan Strain I, a selective B-cell mitogen, the proliferative response of these cells is markedly reduced, indicating a lack of resting B-cells in the peripheral blood. However, the peripheral blood B-cells which are spontaneously secreting antibody, as measured by a reverse haemolytic plaque-forming cell assay, are greatly increased in number over that of control B-cells, suggesting increased numbers of circulating fully differentiated B-cells. This polyclonal B-cell activation is reflected in the increased immunoglobulin concentrations found in the sera of many patients with AIDS.

Diminution in specific antibody response
An important finding reported by Lane et al (1983), was the lack of a specific antibody response in vivo to new antigenic stimuli. In healthy individuals, specific IgM and IgG antibodies appear within 10–14 days of immunization with the potent immunogen, key-hole limpet haemocyanin; this response is absent in patients with AIDS. This lack of specific antibody response is

important, as serological tests for the various infectious diseases from which AIDS patients may suffer are of limited value. For example, in immunocompetent individuals the diagnosis of toxoplasmosis is made by the detection of specific IgM in the patients sera, an antibody response usually absent in AIDS patients with toxoplasmosis (Luft et al 1983).

Cutaneous anergy
As T4 cells are important in the initiation of delayed hypersensitivity reactions, cutaneous anergy to a variety of recall antigens is common in patients with AIDS (Gottlieb et al 1981); in the early stage of the disease, however, delayed hypersensitivity reaction may be normal.

Immune complexes and their attachment to platelets
Levels of circulating immune complexes in the sera of AIDS patients are higher than normal (Gottlieb et al 1981). Their attachment to platelets by an Fc receptor and subsequent platelet ingestion by monocytes/macrophages bound to the free Fc domains of attached IgG molecules may be responsible for the thrombocytopenic purpura found in some AIDS patients (Walsh et al 1984).

Natural killer cells
Natural killer cell activity is often reduced (Gerstoft et al 1982) and mononuclear cells from patients with opportunistic infection show impaired production of alpha-interferon in response to HSV-I infected fibroblasts (Lopez et al 1983). Pre-incubation of peripheral blood lymphocytes from patients with AIDS with interleukin-2 has been shown to restore natural killer cell activity to normal levels (Lifson et al 1984). An unusual acid-labile form of human leucocyte interferon-alpha is found in some patients with Kaposi's sarcoma (De Stefano et al 1982); the significance of this finding in relation to the pathogenesis of AIDS is uncertain.

Monocyte chemotaxis
Blood monocyte chemotaxis to various agents (including N-formylmethionyl leucylphenylalanine, lymphocyte-derived chemotactic factor and extract of *G. intestinalis*) is greatly reduced in AIDS patients and to a lesser extent in homosexual men with lymphadenopathy (Smith et al 1984); this may explain why in tissues there is no granuloma formation in response to *M. avium-intracellulare* (variant of *M. avium* infection; see Ch. 2).

Langerhans cells in epidermis
Belsito et al (1984) found reduced numbers of Langerhans cells (antigen-presenting cells of the skin) in the epidermis of each of 24 patients with AIDS; the significance of this finding, however, remains to be elucidated.

Armstrong & Horne (1984) noted expanded follicular dendritic cells (see Note 31.4) in lymph nodes removed from patients with AIDS-related disease.

HLA antigens
Friedman-Kien et al (1982) reported an increased frequency (63%) of HLA-DR5 allele in patients with Kaposi's sarcoma, both in KS associated with AIDS and that of classical disease, compared with 23% of controls — a highly significant difference.

Beta 2 microglobulin
Elevated levels of beta 2 microglobulin are found in almost every patient with AIDS (Francioli et al 1982). Beta 2 microglobulin is a polypeptide, non-covalently linked to the major histocompatibility antigens coded by the HLA-A, -B and -C foci on the surface of all nucleated cells. Increased serum levels are found in acute viral infections, multiple myeloma, collagen diseases and the lymphomas.

Thymus changes
Seemayer et al (1984) reported on the post-mortem appearance of the thymus glands of 6 Haitians who had died from opportunistic infections. In each case there was marked involution without the appearance of a distinct cortex and medulla. Thymocytes were markedly depleted and Hassall's corpuscles were absent; variable plasma cell infiltration was noted. Whether these anatomical findings are or are not related to the elevated levels of alpha-thymosin noted in the sera of AIDS patients (Hersh et al 1983) is not known.

D. LABORATORY DIAGNOSIS OF HIV INFECTION

DIAGNOSIS OF HIV INFECTION BY DETECTION OF ANTIBODY

Enzyme-linked immunosorbent assay (ELISA)
Commercial assays for the detection of antibody to HIV (anti-HIV) are in two main forms:

1. Direct binding assays in which detergent-salt disrupted HIV is bound to microtitre wells and reacted with the test sera. Immune reactivity is detected using an enzyme-labelled second antibody to human immunoglobulins (Sarngadharan et al 1985).

2. Competitive assays in which antibody in the patients serum competes with specific enzyme-labelled anti-HIV to bind to HIV antigens on the solid phase.

Most of the direct binding assays gave occasional 'false-positive' reactions, i.e. some sera gave repeatedly reactive results which could not be confirmed by competitive and immunoblot assays. In some cases these reactions were due to the presence of lymphocyte antigens in the viral antigen preparation. Assays which incorporate an uninfected T-cell extract as a control antigen can show the extent of the cross-reaction with cell components. Newer assays use antigens prepared by cloning and expressing viral genes in *E. coli*.

Immunoblot or western blot assay for antibody to HIV antigens

SDS (sodium dodecyl sulphate) is an anionic detergent which is reacted with HIV antigens to form denatured soluble rodlike protein-SDS complexes. These complexes, under the influence of an electric field, will migrate through a polyacrylamide gel towards the anode, generally at a rate inversely proportional to the logarithm of their molecular weights (mol. wt.).

In the test the lysed HIV is fractionated by electrophoresis on the polyacrylamide gel in the presence of SDS. The protein bands are then electrophoretically transferred (blotted) to a nitrocellulose sheet to which they bind. The patient's serum is then reacted with a strip of the blotted sheet: bound antibody is detected by radioimmune assay or by an ELISA with an anti-human globulin tracer (Allain et al 1986, Lange et al 1986a, Weber et al 1987; see Fig. 31.1). In effect, this procedure is equivalent to the direct binding ELISA tests described above. Occasional false-positive reactions can be found, but it is usually possible to identify them as they occur with proteins of a certain mol. wt. Parallel assay with a cell extract antigen could also be useful.

Diagnosis by the detection of antibody is reliable in well-established infections. There is, however, a gap of some weeks (perhaps months) between exposure to infection and seroconversion. Thus a negative result in the test for antibody to HIV does not exclude infection, unless there has been no recent exposure to infection.

DIAGNOSIS OF HIV INFECTION BY VIRUS ISOLATION

This procedure is not generally available to the clinician as a means of diagnosis. It consists of the following in its essentials:

1. Peripheral blood lymphocytes are co-cultivated with normal human T-lymphocytes in the presence of interleukin-2 (IL-2) and phytohaemagglutinin (PHA); antiserum to alpha-interferon can also be added.

2. Cultures are monitored for reverse transcriptase (RT) activity in the supernate and for the presence of HIV antigens. A cytopathic effect (CPE) may also be seen and consists of multinucleate giant cells and extensive cell lysis. Sections of infected cells when examined by electronmicroscopy show mature virions and budding viral particles. In the HIV isolates, first identified by the research workers and named as

LAV/HTLV-III, spikes on the surface of the virus are *not* always identifiable, whereas in the so-named LAV-2, recently isolated from patients from West Africa (near to Senegal) the surface of the virus always showed such spikes (Clavel et al 1986).

After infection of cultured cells, both a burst of virus production and pronounced CPE are detectable after 1–2 weeks (Sarngadharan et al 1985).

DIAGNOSIS OF HIV INFECTION BY ANTIGEN DETECTION

Assays for HIV antigen detection, based on the detection of p24 antigen, are now available (Du Pont, Abbott Diagnostics). They can be used to detect antigen production during virus isolation studies, or applied directly to serum samples. The role of such a test is not fully evaluated, but viral antigens can be found during the incubation period and may be present in the absence of an antibody response. Antigenaemia declines after seroconversion but may recur later as the infection progresses towards AIDS. This may correlate with a decline in the immunoblot pattern of antibody reactivity to p24 protein (Lange & Goudsmit 1987; see Fig. 31.1).

E. CLINICAL ASPECTS

LATENCY

The clinical manifestations of HIV infection cover a wide spectrum, with AIDS being the most extreme; a few infections are clinically obvious, others are not. Persistent generalized lymphadenopathy is one manifestation of this viral infection, but the factors which determine resolution (if at all) or progression to AIDS are as yet unknown. Since HIV can be cultured from individuals with no apparent evidence of disease the infection may be latent (hidden) from the start.

Mucocutaneous lesions suggestive of immune deficiency in otherwise healthy individuals seropositive for antibody to HIV include HSV infection of the lips or ano-genital region, herpes zoster, warts, candidal infection of the toe web, molluscum contagiosum, hypertrophic pharyngitis, extensive seborrhoeic dermatitis and extensive folliculitis (Valle et al 1985, Walker et al 1987).

ACUTE HIV INFECTION

During a prospective study of homosexual men in Sydney, Australia, Cooper et al (1985) noted that 11 subjects who showed seroconversion during the period of the study had developed a glandular fever-like illness in the interval between tests. The prepatent period was difficult to define accurately, but may have been as short as 6 days from sexual contact. The patients complained of fever with sweating, myalgia, arthralgia, lethargy, malaise, sore throat, anorexia, nausea, vomiting, headache, diarrhoea and the appearance of an erythematous rash on the trunk. Several days after the onset of the illness lymph node and splenic enlargement was found. In general, the illness lasted for about 14 days, but the lymphadenopathy may persist. Acute encephalopathy and meningitis have been described in association with seroconversion for anti-HIV. The onset of encephalopathy is generally preceded by a prodromal period of about 2 weeks characterized by pyrexia, malaise and mood changes (Ho et al 1985b). Epileptiform seizure may also occur (Carne et al 1985). Rapid resolution of the neurological features with no permanent sequelae occurs.

PERSISTENT GENERALIZED LYMPHADENOPATHY (synonyms — persistent diffuse lymphadenopathy; chronic generalized lymphadenopathy; AIDS-related lymphadenopathy; lymphadenopathy syndrome)

Persistent generalized lymphadenopathy (PGL) is the term suggested by the National Institutes of Health AIDS Working Group for the condition of swollen lymph nodes involving *at least two extra-inguinal sites for at least three months duration* in the absence of any intercurrent illness or drug known to cause lymphadenopathy. These nodes are enlarged (diameter >1 cm) firm, discrete and generally not tender. In a study of 70 patients (Abrams et al 1984) the most commonly affected groups of glands were the axillary, inguinal and posterior cervical; in one-third of patients the epitrochlear, femoral, submental, pre- and post-auricular and submandibular glands were involved. Care should be taken in making the diagnosis of persistent generalized lymphadenopathy in intravenous drug abusers since the axillary nodes are frequently enlarged as a result of chronic infection of injection sites. When the nodes are greatly enlarged there may be pressure effects in neighbouring structures, including nerves. In one-third of cases the spleen was enlarged. Although mesenteric and retroperitoneal lymphadenopathy appear to be common, hilar lymph node enlargement is rare.

Systemic features may also be prominent amongst men with lymphadenopathy, the most common being easy fatiguability, night sweats, intermittent fever and muscle pains. Oral candidiasis, recurrent viral-like illnesses, recalcitrant superficial fungal infections, seborrhoeic dermatitis of the face, scalp and trunk,

impetigo of the face and inguinal area, herpes zoster and recurrent skin warts have all been described in this group of patients.

PGL and its clinical course

Metroka et al (1983) from New York, in a prospective study of 90 homosexual men with PGL, found that 15 men developed opportunistic infections, lymphomas, Kaposi's sarcoma or immunoblastic sarcomas after the lymphadenopathy had been present for a median duration of 31 months (range 4–56 months). Spontaneous diminution in size of the nodes was noted in 4 patients, 3 of whom developed opportunistic infections 6–11 months later.

Mathur-Wagh et al (1984) conducted a similar study of homosexual men with unexplained lymphadenopathy. In the first 18 months of surveillance 6 of 42 had developed AIDS; a further 2 men showed features of AIDS within 36 months of entry into the study. The median duration of lymphadenopathy before the development of AIDS was 21 months, with a range of 4–42 months.

Some 75% of patients with lymphadenopathy who develop additional features such as progressive unexplained diarrhoea and weight loss (10% of body weight) easy fatiguability, depression and impotence progress to AIDS.

Histopathology of lymph nodes in PGL

The most common finding is reactive follicular hyperplasia (Guarda et al 1983). The lymph nodes are enlarged and the cut surface shows prominent nodules. Histologically the follicles, sometimes of irregular shape, are enlarged with prominent germinal centres containing large lymphocytes, macrophages, nuclear debris from cell destruction and marked cellular mitoses; the follicles are margined by a rim of small lymphocytes. The interfollicular tissue shows increased vascularity with prominent endothelial cells and contains lymphocytes, plasma cells, large clear cells resembling immunoblasts and occasional multinucleated cells. In addition to mononuclear cells, polymorphonuclear leucocytes are often present in the lymphatic sinuses and scattered throughout the node. There is a marked extension of the centroblasts and centrocytes and in some cases a depletion of T4 cells in the paracortex of the node. Destruction of the follicular dendritic cells is sometimes seen (Janossy et al 1985).

A less common finding is that of lymphocyte depletion of the lymph node cortex. The germinal centres are depleted of cells and many become hyalinized, but the medullary cores are closely infiltrated with plasma cells. Lymph nodes showing these changes have been removed from individuals who have had severe cellular immune dysfunction (Fernandez et al 1983), many of whom subsequently develop Kaposi's sarcoma or lymphoma.

Angioblastic lymphadenopathy (a condition which occurs in middle-aged and elderly individuals and is characterized by lymphadenopathy and polyclonal hypergammaglobulinaemia) has been described in AIDS patients (Blumenfeld & Beckstead 1983). There is diffuse replacement of the lymph nodes with immunoblasts, plasma cells, macrophages and lymphocytes with vascular proliferation.

Diagnosis

Transient generalized lymph node enlargement is a common feature of many infectious diseases and the appropriate diagnostic investigations are indicated in Table 31.6. When a patient presents with lymphadenopathy of short duration, it is sometimes difficult to predict whether this will be transitory or persistent. After appropriate tests outlined (Table 31.6) a period of observation is justified. If there is persistence of the lymphadenopathy for more than three months and serum anti-HIV is not detected, lymph node biopsy is indicated to diagnose or exclude the presence of lymphoma or Kaposi's sarcoma confined to the lymph nodes. In addition, the histological appearance may suggest some other specific cause for the lymphadenopathy such as sarcoidosis.

THROMBOCYTOPENIC PURPURA

Morris et al (1982) described severe thrombocytopenic purpura in 11 homosexual men. However, serological tests for antibody to HIV were not available, and conclusions regarding the association of this phenomenon and the virus cannot yet be reached.

ACQUIRED IMMUNE DEFICIENCY SYNDROME (AIDS) IN ADULTS

In 75% of cases AIDS presents as opportunistic infection or neoplasia, most frequently in the form of Kaposi's sarcoma. As it was the striking occurrence of the latter which first alerted physicians to the problem of immunodeficiency amongst homosexual men, it is appropriate to consider this disorder first.

Kaposi's sarcoma

With the exception of the lymphadenopathic form of the disease in young Africans, the clinical features of KS in AIDS patients do not resemble those found in classical European or African KS ordinarily seen in older age groups. For details on the presentation of KS in these groups the reader is referred to the review by Hood et al (1982).

Table 31.6 Causes of generalized lymph node enlargement.

Cause of lymph node enlargement	Diagnostic tests
Neoplasms	
Lymphomas	Lymph node biopsy
Leukaemias	Bone marrow/blood smear microscopy
Metastases	Lymph node biopsy if primary not apparent
Infections	
Bacterial	
Syphilis	Serological tests
Tuberculosis	Lymph node biopsy. Tuberculin test
Brucellosis	Serology
Salmonellosis	Blood culture. Widal test
Tularaemia	Culture of *Pasteurella tularensis* from aspirate
European and African typhus	Weil-Felix reaction
Q fever	Blood culture; serology
Viral	
EB virus	Monospot
Cytomegalovirus	Serology
Herpes simplex virus	Viral isolation and serology
Rubella	Serology
Measles	Serology
Varicella	Viral isolation and serology
Hepatitis A & B	Serology
Protozoa	
Toxoplasmosis	Serology
Trypanosomiasis	Blood smear examination, lymph node aspiration
Visceral leishmaniasis	Sternal marrow/splenic aspirate examination
Fungi	
Histoplasmosis	Culture
Coccidioidomycosis	Culture
Nematode	
Filariasis	Blood smear examination
Collagen diseases	
Rheumatoid arthritis	Serology for RA factor
Disseminated lupus erythematosus	DNA anti-DNA binding capacity
Drugs	
Hydantoins	
Antibiotics, especially penicillin	History
Nitrofurantoin	
Immunological disorders	
Primary macroglobulinaemia	Plasma protein examination
Storage diseases	
Lipidoses	Biopsy of lymph node
Others	
Sarcoidosis	Kveim test; angiotensin converting enzyme; lymph node biopsy
Whipple's disease	Jejunal biopsy

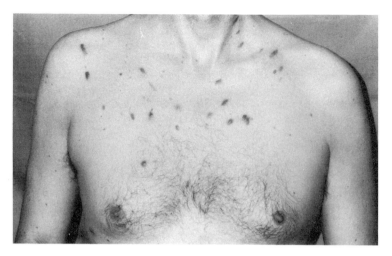

Fig. 31.4 Kaposi's sarcoma of the chest in the acquired immune deficiency syndrome.

The first lesions of Kaposi's sarcoma, as it occurs in AIDS, are generally painless or, at most, mildly pruritic, reddish macules which gradually become purplish papules or nodules (Fig. 31.4). Unlike the lesions of classical KS, as it occurs in middle-aged or elderly Europeans, they are not confined to the extremities but can affect any area of the skin. The papules or nodules are of variable size, ranging from a few millimetres to several centimetres in diameter. In some cases there is a tendency for lesions to coalesce. Although almost any organ can be involved by the sarcoma the clinical manifestations of visceral involvement are usually confined to the oropharynx and lymph nodes. In the mouth the lesions are reddish-purple velvety papules or nodules arising from the gingiva, tongue, buccal mucosa and palate. Multiple lesions of the rectum may be seen at sigmoidoscopy as small telangiectatic macules but generally they produce few symptoms. Pulmonary involvement with Kaposi's sarcoma may produce clinical and radiological features indistinguishable from infection (Ognibene et al 1985). Haemorrhagic lesions of the conjunctiva have been described.

Painless lymph node enlargement is found in about half of patients with cutaneous KS, and biopsy studies have shown that at least half of these individuals have sarcomatous infiltration of the nodes (Finkbeiner et al 1982). The affected lymph nodes are firm, non-tender, discrete and mobile. Sometimes KS of the lymph nodes is found in the absence of skin lesions.

Although survival data are incomplete, the overall two-year survival rate of patients with KS in the USA is about 70%. Prospective studies are necessary before more precise information on mortality rates can be given. Spontaneous resolution of the KS associated with immunosuppression following organ transplantation has been reported following discontinuation of drug therapy, and Maurice et al (1982) noted spontaneous healing of a KS lesion in a homosexual male. In most cases of untreated KS, however, there has been steady progression of the disease, often together with opportunistic infections.

The diagnosis of the lesions requires differentiation from pigmented naevi, insect bite reaction, trauma, pyogenic granuloma, histiocytoma and atypical granuloma annulare. Histological examination of biopsy specimens is essential for the diagnosis of KS.

Histopathology of Kaposi's sarcoma
Histologically (Gottlieb & Ackerman 1982) the early lesions of KS resemble granulation tissue. There are irregularly-shaped, dilated, endothelium-lined channels which grow between bundles of collagen in the dermis. The endothelial cells are flattened and mitotic figures are uncommon. As the macular lesions become papular or plaque-like, spindle-shaped pleomorphic cells intermingle with the vascular channels and there is a mild infiltration of plasma cells and lymphocytes. Commonly erythrocytes are found within slit-like spaces not lined by endothelial cells. Macrophages containing haemosiderin are also common. Necrotic endothelial cells, characterized by pyknotic nuclei and eosinophilic cytoplasm, are seen frequently in biopsies from KS patients with AIDS. In the nodular stage the spindle-shaped cells predominate.

McNutt et al (1983) have described the electron-microscopic appearance of the lesions of Kaposi's sarcoma. They found that the majority of the cells which infiltrate the dermis and line the vascular channels are endothelial. Interruption of the cellular lining of these channels and of the basal lamina is common. Dendritic pericytes are reduced in number and necrotic endothelial cells are often prominent. The authors found that benign lesions with a histology resembling early KS, viz. histiocytoma, stasis eczema, pyogenic granuloma, capillary haemangioma, telangiectasia, angiokeratoma, benign haemangioendothelioma, were altogether different when studied by electronmicroscopy.

Treatment

In localized KS, therapy is not indicated unless the tumour causes clinical problems, as for example, in the mouth when electron beam irradiation is helpful. When KS is disseminated, treatment with alpha interferon or chemotherapeutic agents such as vinblastine is the approach commonly used. As management falls within the province of the oncologist early referral is advised.

Other neoplasms associated with AIDS

Non-Hodgkin's lymphomas

Numerically, Kaposi's sarcoma is the most important of the neoplasms occurring in AIDS. However, increasing numbers of patients with non-Hodgkin's, that is B-cell, lymphomas are being reported — not an unexpected finding as lymphoproliferative disorders have been reported in patients with primary and secondary immunodeficiencies. The most comprehensive study, involving 90 cases of non-Hodgkin's lymphoma in homosexual men, is that of Ziegler et al (1984) and this section summarizes their report.

The 30–39 year age group is the most frequently affected. About one-half of the patients in whom lymphomas develop have prodromal manifestations, most commonly persistent lymphadenopathy. In almost every case the lymphoma is extranodal with lesions developing (in order of frequency) in the central nervous system, bone marrow, gastrointestinal tract, skin or mucosae, liver and lung. The clinical manifestations depend on the location of the tumour and its effect on surrounding structures.

The survival rate of patients with non-Hodgkin's lymphoma correlates well with the histological grade, the median survival times in high and intermediate grades being 6 and 5 months respectively; although patients with low-grade lymphomas are few the prognosis appears to be better. Opportunistic infections account for some half of the deaths in these patients, the others dying from progressive tumour growth.

The diagnosis of lymphoma is made by histological examination of affected lymph nodes or accessible viscera. In the case of cerebral lymphoma, computerized tomography may reveal a space-occupying lesion suggestive of the diagnosis; the wisdom of undertaking biopsy in such a site to confirm the diagnosis may be questionable.

Serious infections in AIDS

As a result of the profound cellular immunodeficiency found in patients with AIDS, their susceptibility and liability to adverse effects of infection with pathogenic and usually commensal viruses, bacteria, fungi and protozoa is greatly increased. Table 31.7 shows the more important infectious agents which have been identified in such cases, the organs affected and therapeutic agents presently available. In the care of extremely sick patients, the physician should consider carefully what benefits the patient is likely to derive from a course of often toxic drugs, not likely to prolong life significantly.

Table 31.8 lists the various chemotherapeutic agents which are used commonly in the serious infections from which AIDS patients suffer. The duration of therapy will vary according to the clinical response and development of side effects. This is particularly so in the case with co-trimoxazole used in the treatment of *Pneumocystis* pneumonia. Patients whose infections have initially responded to co-trimoxazole but who develop side effects can usually be treated successfully with pentamidine; if, however, there has been little response to co-trimoxazole few patients are cured with pentamidine. As *P. carinii* can be found in lung tissue from patients after apparently successful treatment there is probably a place for prophylactic treatment with co-trimoxazole or, in view of the side effects with that drug, pyrimethamine-sulfadoxine. Similarly, patients who have had extensive or disseminated HSV or VZV infection will require prophylactic treatment with acyclovir.

System involvement in AIDS

Lungs

The most common pulmonary condition in AIDS patients is *Pneumocystis carinii* pneumonia. Patients present with increasing dyspnoea, chest pain, nonproductive cough and fever. On auscultation diffuse crepitations may be heard and chest radiographs in the early stages show evidence of perihilar interstitial pneumonia and later diffuse infiltrates in both lung fields; pleural effusion is absent. Other radiographic features may be less typical with lobar consolidation and cavity formation. The chest radiograph may, however, be normal in some cases in *P. carinii* pneumonia. Other infections including CMV, the variant of *M. avium* referred to as *M. avium-intracellulare* (see Ch. 2) and fungi may produce a similar radiographic appearance. Pulmonary function tests in patients with *P. carinii* pneumonia show reduced PaO_2, lowered vital capacity and total lung capacity, impaired DL_{co} and abnormal alveolar arterial oxygen gradients.

Acute diffuse pulmonary infiltrates in AIDS patients may be caused by bacteria, usually *Haemophilus influ-*

Table 31.7 Clinical presentation and treatment of serious infections in AIDS.

Organism	Clinical presentation	Chemotherapeutic agents available	References
Protozoa			
Pneumocystis carinii	Pneumonia	Sulphamethoxazole/ trimethoprim.	Gottlieb et al (1981)
		Pentamidine isothionate	Follansbee et al (1982)
Toxoplasma gondii	Cerebral abscess Meningoencephalitis Retinochoroiditis	Pyrimethamine Sulphadiazine	Luft et al (1983)
Crytosporidium spp	Persistent severe diarrhoea ? Pneumonia	Nil	Soave et al (1984)
Isospora belli	Diarrhoea	Sulphonamides or pyrimethamine	Whiteside et al (1984)
Fungi			
Candida spp	Oropharyngeal candidiasis Oesophageal candidiasis, rarely, cerebral abscess	Amphotericin B lozenge Ketoconazole	Gottlieb et al (1981)
Cryptococcus neoformans	Meningitis; rarely brain abscess Pneumonia	Amphotericin B Flucytosine	Vandepitte et al (1983) Cohen et al (1984)
Histoplasma capsulatum	Pneumonia, lymphadenopathy, hepatic & splenic enlargement with fever, mucocutaneous lesions	Amphotericin B	Bonner et al (1984)
Coccidioides immitis	Diffuse or focal pneumonia. Rarely meningitis, skin lesions, hepatitis	Amphotericin B	Kovacs et al (1984)
Aspergillus spp	Lobar or interstitial pneumonia	Amphotericin B	Cohen et al (1984)
Bacteria			
Mycobacterium avium intracellulare	Disseminated disease. Pyrexia, lymphadenopathy, hepatomegaly, pneumonia	Clofazime, ansamycin but most infections are fatal	Greene et al (1982)
Mycobacterium xenopi	Pyrexia, pneumonia, hepatomegaly		
Mycobacterium tuberculosis	Disseminated form	Standard anti-bacterial chemotherapy	Weinberg et al (1985) de la Loma et al (1985)
Nocardia spp	Septicaemia, pneumonia, lung abscesses brain abscesses	Trimethoprim/ sulphamethoxazole	Bonner et al (1984)
Salmonella spp	Septicaemia	Standard chemotherapy	Profeta et al (1985)
Viruses			
Cytomegalovirus	Lymphadenopathy, retinitis, encephalitis, peripheral neuropathy, colitis, pneumonia, hepatitis.	—	Quinnan et al (1984) Moskowitz et al (1984)
	Retinitis	Dihydropropoxymethylguanine may arrest but not cure	Palestine et al (1986) Harris & Mathalone (1987)
Herpes simplex virus	Extensive mucocutaneous	Acyclovir	Siegal et al (1981)
JC virus	Dementia. Focal neurological signs	—	Miller et al (1982)

enzae; lobar consolidation is a feature of *Streptococcus pneumoniae* infection. Examination of sputum, produced by a cough induced by directing a jet of hypertonic saline (3%) against the posterior pharyngeal wall, may reveal *Pneumocystis* (Bigby et al 1986). As patients with *Pneumocystis* pneumonia have increased pulmonary parenchymal uptake of isotope on gallium lung scans, this procedure may be helpful in establishing a diagnosis

of lung disease even when the chest radiograph and/or blood gases are normal. In many patients with suspected *Pneumocystis* pneumonia, however, fibre optic bronchoscopy and broncho-alveolar lavage and/or transbronchial lung biopsy are indicated: broncho-alveolar lavage is safer, and as sensitive as biopsy, so this procedure should be undertaken initially if the sputum test already described is negative. Broncho-alveolar washings, tissue

Table 31.8 Dosage and toxicity of the chemotherapeutic agents commonly used in the management of AIDS patients with opportunistic infections.

Drug	Dosage	Side effects	References
Acyclovir	Slow i.v. infusion of 5 mg/kg every 8 hours until healed. Prophylaxis with oral preparation 200 mg 6-hourly	Transient elevation of plasma urea and creatinine	Mitchell et al (1981)
Amphotericin B	a. intravenously: 1 mg/kg per day by i.v. infusion to total 1–3 g. b. orally: 100–200 mg 6-hourly	Pyrexia, anorexia, vomiting, hypokalaemia, nephrotoxicity	Armstrong (1981)
Flucytosine	100–150 mg/kg per day in four divided doses for 6 weeks *with* amphotericin B	Neutropenia, thrombocytopenia, vomiting	Armstrong (1981)
Ketoconazole	200–400 mg daily until symptom-free for one week. Antacids reduce absorption. May potentiate coumarins.	Hepatotoxic	Hay (1982)
Pentamidine	4 mg/kg once-daily by intramuscular injection for 10–14 days	Nephrotoxic, leucopenia, thrombocytopenia, hypoglycaemia, hepatitis. Sterile abscesses at site of injection	Gordin et al (1984)
Pyrimethamine (used with sulphadiazine)	100–200 mg as initial oral dose followed by 1 mg/kg per day for at least one month	Leucopenia, thrombocytopenia	Ruskin (1981)
Sulphadiazine	100 mg/kg/day in 6 divided doses	Renal blockage, hypersensitivity reaction; agranulocytosis, haemolytic anaemia in patients with G6-pD deficiency	Ruskin (1981)
Trimethoprim	20 mg/kg per day sulphamethoxazole by i.v. infusion or by mouth. Prophylaxis with co-trimoxazole or pyrimethamine-sulfadoxine	Maculopapular rash and fever Leucopenia, thrombocytopenia, hepatitis	Gordin et al (1984) Gottlieb et al (1984)

G6pD = Glucose 6-phosphate dehydrogenase

impression smears and histological sections can be examined microscopically after staining with silver-methenamine or Giemsa for cysts of *P. carinii*, tachyzoites of *T. gondii*, budding yeasts of *Histoplasma capsulatum*, *Coccidioides immitis*, *Cryptococcus neoformans* and *Aspergillus* spp. Ziehl-Neelsen stained smears may show *Mycobacteria* spp or *Nocardia* spp. Rarely, *Cryptosporidia* spp has infected pulmonary tissue and has been identified in the alveoli by a modified Ziehl-Neelsen stain. Broncho-alveolar washings and lung biopsy specimens should be cultured for *Mycobacteria* spp, fungi and viruses. As the chest radiograph is often normal, bronchoscopy is necessary for the diagnosis of Kaposi's sarcoma of the bronchi.

Gastrointestinal tract
Lesions of Kaposi's sarcoma and plaques of *Candida*

may be seen in the mouth. Extensive herpetic ulceration of the oral cavity is a distressing feature in cases of cellular immunodeficiency, but healing generally occurs rapidly with acyclovir treatment.

Oral hairy leukoplakia presents as painless, white, slightly-elevated lesions of variable size of the tongue and buccal mucosa (Greenspan et al 1984). Histologically there are keratin projections, producing the roughened appearance of the tongue associated with parakeratosis and acanthosis and ballooning changes in the prickle-cell layer. Some pleomorphism of the basal cells is common. Papillomavirus antigen and EB virus have been found in these lesions but their significance aetiologically is uncertain.

Involvement of the oesophagus and pharynx with Kaposi's sarcoma or *Candida* spp usually manifests itself as dysphagia and retrosternal discomfort. A tentative diagnosis may be made by double contrast barium swallow examination. Although oesophagoscopy and biopsy of the lesions is the most definitive means of diagnosis such invasive procedure may not be advisable. The present authors consider a trial of ketoconazole (200 mg as a single oral dose daily until there is resolution of symptoms, i.e. in about 14 days) is justified in a patient with clinical and radiological features suggestive of oesophagopharyngeal candidiasis; failure to respond to such therapy would be an indication for oesophagoscopy.

Kaposi's sarcoma can affect any part of the gastrointestinal tract, but with the exception of the anal region, when it produces painful swellings superficially resembling abscesses, it is usually asymptomatic and found only at endoscopy for some unrelated problem.

Diarrhoea and weight loss are prevalent amongst patients with AIDS. In some cases this is caused by specific organisms such as *Cryptosporidium* spp, *Giardia intestinalis*, *Entamoeba histolytica*, *Salmonella* spp, *Shigella* spp, *Campylobacter* spp, the variant of *Mycobacterium avium* known as *Mycobacterium avium-intracellulare* (see Ch. 2), *Clostridium difficile*, CMV and rotaviruses, but in others no such organisms can be identified. The pathogenesis of this diarrhoeal illness is uncertain but Kotler et al (1984) found partial villous atrophy with crypt hyperplasia and increased numbers of intra-epithelial lymphocytes in jejunal biopsies from 12 homosexual men with AIDS and biochemical evidence of malabsorption. Rectal biopsies from the same patients showed focal cell degeneration at the base of the crypts with mast-cell infiltration of the lamina propria.

The methods used for the diagnosis of *G. intestinalis*, *E. histolytica*, *Cryptosporidium* spp, *Salmonella* spp, *Shigella* spp, *Campylobacter* spp, and rotaviruses have been noted elsewhere (Ch. 38).

Although infection with the variant of *Mycobacterium avium*, known as *Mycobacterium avium-intracellulare* (see Ch. 2), is generally systemic it may cause diarrhoea. The diagnosis of these mycobacterial infections is made by Ziehl-Neelsen staining of tissue sections and faecal smears and culture of material in Lowenstein-Jensen medium.

Cytomegalovirus is common in AIDS, and amongst its many clinical manifestations colitis is frequent. There is diffuse inflammation of the lamina propria of the intestine with the presence of cells containing intranuclear and intracytoplasmic eosinophilic inclusions suggestive of the presence of the virus. The diagnosis is confirmed by culture of rectal biopsy material.

Herpes simplex virus infection of the ano-rectum produces extensive ulceration of that area and proctitis. The diagnosis is made by isolation of the virus in tissue culture cells (Ch. 26).

As the majority of patients with AIDS receive high dosage broad spectrum antimicrobial agents, antibiotic-associated colitis with *Clostridium difficile* is to be anticipated. The diagnosis rests with the finding of enterotoxin-producing organisms.

Central and peripheral nervous system

In AIDS cases the central nervous system can be affected by primary and secondary lymphomas, *Toxoplasma gondii*, cytomegalovirus, JC virus, cryptococcal and mycobacterial infections.

Snider et al (1983) found that the most common neurological abnormality was subacute encephalitis, characterized by malaise, lassitude, withdrawal and impaired libido; the clinical state deteriorated over a period of weeks to months as dementia developed. Electroencephalography is often abnormal in patients with AIDS or persistent generalized lymphadenopathy, with about 50% showing a slow alphabasal activity (Enzensberger et al 1985). CT scans show prominent cortical sulci and enlarged ventricles, indicating cerebral atrophy, a finding confirmed at autopsy. As cerebellar coning may result from lumbar puncture in patients with space-occupying lesions of the cerebrum, CT scanning should always be undertaken before this procedure is considered. Acute hypersensitivity reactions to the contrast medium used in radiological examinations have been reported in patients with persistent generalized lymphadenopathy, and care is required when such injections are being made. CSF changes include increased white cell count (usually lymphocytes), mildly elevated protein and slightly low glucose concentration. The aetiology of this is not known with certainty but is probably the direct result of HIV infection. Non-integrated HIV DNA has been found in cells of the cerebral cortices of patients who had had neurological abnormalities (Shaw et al 1985), and the virus has been cultured from the CSF or neural tissue from the majority of patients with AIDS-related neurological disease (Ho et al 1985b). Further evidence for infection of the CNS by HIV comes from the study reported by Resnick et al (1985) who showed synthesis of specific IgG within the blood-brain barrier in patients with AIDS-related neurological features. Which of the brain cells are infected is unknown.

Epileptic seizures, altered consciousness and focal neurological signs are found in patients with *Toxoplasma* or *Candida* cerebral abscesses, primary or secondary cerebral lymphomas or progressive multifocal leuco-encephalopathy (PML). Contrast-enhancing single or multiple lesions are found on CT scans of cerebral abscesses or lymphomas. Generally patients with PML have lesions which are not contrast-enhancing.

The diagnosis of cerebral toxoplasmosis is difficult. As already emphasized the serological response to any infection in AIDS is of little value in diagnosis. Specific IgM is generally not detectable in those with AIDS and IgGs showing high titres or changes in titres in paired sera are not common. The CSF is often normal, although a definitive diagnosis can be made by the histopathology of biopsy material. The taking of cerebral tissue has a high morbidity rate and cannot be justified on a routine basis. A therapeutic trial of pyrimethamine with sulphadiazine in the case of toxoplasmosis is probably indicated; amphotericin B may be tried if a fungal cause is suspected.

Progressive painful sensorimotor neuropathy and vacuolar myelopathy of uncertain aetiology have been reported in AIDS (Snider et al 1983, Petito et al 1985).

Cryptococcal meningitis diagnosed by the finding of yeasts or cryptococcal antigens in the CSF (Armstrong 1981) is rare in AIDS, as is tuberculous meningitis. Skin lesions in which fungi can be shown may point to a diagnosis of cryptococcal meningitis in patients with fever or altered consciousness but without features of meningitis.

Cerebral haemorrhages as a result of thrombocytopenia are also uncommon CNS manifestations.

Eye

Although Kaposi's sarcoma can involve the conjunctival sac most lesions are within the eye itself (Holland et al 1982). Both *Toxoplasma gondii* and CMV can produce rapidly progressive chorioretinitis. CMV retinitis is characterized by foci of irregular white patches which coalesce and often sheath the retinal vessels, and haemorrhages may also be seen. *Candida* infection produces retinitis with vitreous haemorrhage — resulting in blindness.

Kidneys

Rao et al (1984) described 11 AIDS patients with renal disease; 9 had presented with the nephrotic syndrome and 2 with renal failure. A common histological feature was focal or segmental glomerulosclerosis with segmental glomerular deposition of IgM and C3; the pathogenesis is unknown, and the prognosis poor.

Heart

Clinically inapparent cardiac abnormalities including increased ventricular size, left ventricular hypokinesia and mitral incompetence are common in AIDS patients (Fink et al 1984).

AIDS IN INFANTS AND CHILDREN

Before the discovery of HIV as the retrovirus causing AIDS and the availability of tests for antibody it was convenient to categorize the syndrome in infants and children as paediatric AIDS or PAIDS (Ammann et al 1984). Most children so affected had a mother who either misused intravenous drugs or lived by prostitution; others were offspring of other at-risk groups, and in the early groups a few had received blood transfusions from a donor suspected of or having AIDS. First diagnosed in children in the USA in 1983, by December 1986 there were 394 affected children under the age of 13 years comprising 1.4% of the total 28 098 cases of AIDS (Centers for Disease Control 1986). Of the 394 children 52% were diagnosed with PCP, 47% with other opportunistic diseases and 1% with Kaposi's sarcoma alone. Most (79%) came from families with one or both parents with AIDS or at risk of AIDS, 6% had haemophilia, and 13% had received blood transfusion or blood compound. There continued to be no evidence of nonspecific transmission through casual contact.

In tropical Africa south of the Sahara evidence suggests that HIV infection is widespread. Although in developed countries children under 13 years of age make up less than 3% of cases, in tropical Africa many infants may develop AIDS, as in Kampala, Uganda for example, 14% of the pregnant women studied were infected (see review by Liskin et al 1986).

Before reaching the diagnosis in children it was necessary, before the availability of specific assays of antibody to HIV, to exclude causes of secondary immunodeficiency such as severe malnutrition, malignancy, or the fetal alcohol syndrome as well as rare causes of congenital immunodeficiency such as the DiGeorge syndrome and agammaglobulinaemia. Diagnosis will generally be suspected on the basis that the mother is in an at-risk group or that the child has received blood or its products from a donor suspected or at risk of HIV infection.

Most affected children will show weight loss or failure to thrive; they may have chronic diarrhoea, lymphadenopathy, hepatosplenomegaly, fevers or chronic dermatitis. *Candida* infections are common and affect the mouth or cause oesophagitis. Recurrent bacterial infections are common and include staphylococcal infection of the skin. Infections with Gram-negative organisms may be fulminant and occur before death. *Mycobacterium avium* (*intracellulare*) may cause systemic infection and *Pneumocystis carinii* pneumonia is difficult to treat effectively (Ammann et al 1984). Chronic swelling of the parotid gland is common. Central nervous system abnormalities have been reported in 50–80% of children with AIDS, whereas Kaposi's sarcoma is uncommonly seen. Lymphoid interstitial pneumonia in infants is characteristic of the paediatric syndrome and is only rarely seen in adults with AIDS (Scott et al 1984, Ammann 1985).

A dysmorphic syndrome, believed to be distinct, has

been reported in children born to intravenous drug-abusing women and infected with HIV in utero (Marion et al 1986). This 'AIDS embryopathy' was characterized by the following features: growth retardation (75%); microcephaly (70%); a prominent box-like forehead (75%); hypertelorism (50%); flattened nasal bridge (70%); mild upward or downward obliquity of the eyes (65%); blue sclerae (60%); well-formed philtrum with short columilla (65%) and patulous lips (60%). As distinct from the fetal alcohol syndrome, the more severely affected the child the earlier the onset of immunological dysfunction.

Most infants and children have a polyclonal elevation of immunoglobulins — in some cases six to eight times reference values; decreased helper/suppressor T-cell ratio and functional impairment of T-cell immunity. Mitogen stimulation of lymphocytes has been suggested as the most useful functional assay of T-cell immunity. The first detectable immunological abnormality was an early (at about 2 months of age) elevation of serum IgG and IgM. Abnormalities in T-cells did not show until about 5 months of age. In infants less than 6 months of age the presence of antibody to HIV may represent passive transfer of IgG (Ammann 1985).

Immunodepressed children are at great risk of severe complications from infections such as varicella, cytomegalovirus, tuberculosis, herpes simplex and measles. In varicella prompt use of specific immune globulin following known exposure is advised. The use of live vaccines such as measles/mumps/rubella vaccine may be hazardous in affected children (Centers for Disease Control 1985b).

Since HIV and other infective agents may be present in blood or body fluids, those looking after children should take hygienic precautions to prevent spread, although the chance of such spread is very small. Soiled surfaces should be cleaned promptly with an effective disinfectant (e.g. household bleach — sodium hypochlorite solution — diluted 1 part bleach to 10 parts water — and disposable towels or tissues should be used wherever possible. Those who are doing the cleaning should avoid exposure of open skin lesions or mucous membranes to blood or body fluids (Centers for Disease Control 1985a).

Guidelines for the foster-care and education of HIV-infected children involve complex issues of confidentiality. Difficulties arising from a mostly unjustified fear of infection may bring about social isolation of the child, and therefore those responsible for caring should be sensitive to the need for confidentiality. Detailed recommendations have been made on the subject of care of affected children who should be allowed to attend school or to be fostered in an unrestricted setting (Centers for Disease Control 1985a); those responsible for children should refer to the original text.

F. CHEMOTHERAPY SPECIFIC FOR HIV INFECTION

ANTI-RETROVIRAL ACTION OF DRUGS

The different stages in the replicative cycle of HIV present a variety of possible molecular targets for therapy. After attachment and binding to the CD4 antigen and possibly other receptors, HIV enters the target cell. Losing its envelope coat, the retroviral RNA and the HIV *pol* product, reverse transcriptase, are released into the cell cytoplasm. Reverse transcriptase makes a complementary-strand DNA copy of the RNA genome and then catalyzes the production of a positive-strand DNA copy so that the genetic information is eventually encoded in a double-stranded DNA form. The DNA copy may either remain unintegrated or become integrated into the genome of the host cell to form a provirus through a viral 'integrase'. At some later point the DNA is transcribed to mRNA and to viral genomic RNA by host RNA polymerases and the mRNA is translated to form viral proteins again by biochemical mechanisms of the host cell (Yarchoan & Broder 1987). Therapeutic agents can be conveniently classified into two classes: inhibitors of HIV DNA synthesis (i.e. reverse transcriptase inhibitors and DNA chain terminators) or biological response modifiers (i.e. interferons and double-stranded RNAs) (Mitchell et al 1987).

Inhibitors of HIV DNA synthesis

Reverse transcriptase inhibitors
Suramin, chosen early on for clinical trials and well-known for its great value in early-stage African trypanosomiasis in man, falls within this group since it acts as an inhibitor of reverse transcriptase, but it failed to bring clinical benefit.

DNA chain terminators
The nucleoside analogue, 3'-azido-3'-deoxythymidine (azidothymidine, zidovudine; trade name — Retrovir, Wellcome), however, promises to prolong life and bring other benefits in AIDS; another nucleoside analogue, 2'3'-dideoxycytidine, is currently under trial in patients. In zidovudine the 3'-OH carbon group is modified by an azido (N_3) group and in 2'3'-dideoxycytidine by -H. After phosphorylation in both infected and uninfected cells both substances inhibit HIV replication by acting as chain terminators when incorporated by reverse transcriptase to the end of a growing chain of DNA (Mitsuya & Broder 1987).

The availability for laboratory research of supplies of HIV reverse transcriptase, obtained as a result of its expression in bacteria or yeasts by recombinant DNA technology, should aid in vitro testing and selection of inhibitors. Rapid sensitive in vitro systems also exist for screening substances for action on HIV replication and its cytopathic effect.

Modifiers of the biological response to HIV infection

The octapeptide, Peptide T, acts in vitro by interfering with binding of HIV to the target cell (Pert et al 1986) and the substance 'Ampligen', a non-toxic mismatched polymer of double-stranded RNA which contains uridine in its polycytidylic chain, acts also in vitro at this site (Mitchell et al 1987). Ampligen may have promise in therapy since in vitro the concentration of zidovudine required for virustasis of HIV is reduced five-fold by its presence.

Human interferon alpha, like other interferons, can inhibit the production of viral mRNA, the synthesis of viral proteins or the assembly and release of new particles (Ho et al 1985a); it slows HIV replication in vitro and is now undergoing clinical trials (Hirsch & Kaplan 1987).

Ribavarin is believed to act as a deoxyguanosine analogue that interferes with the 5'-capping of mRNA in other viral systems and may also be useful in retroviral infections (Hirsch & Kaplan 1987).

DRUGS UNDER CLINICAL TRIAL IN HIV INFECTION

Zidovudine

Zidovudine is a thymidine analogue in which the 3'-hydroxy group (OH) is replaced by an azido (N_3) group. The fact that the primary raw material, thymidine, required at first for its manufacture, is usually extracted from herring sperm gave rise to misgivings about possible shortages (Wright 1986) until methods were developed which did not depend on the use of this natural source material. Intracellularly zidovudine is phosphorylated by cellular thymidine kinase to form the monophosphate (zidovudine-MP). by other cellular enzymes to form the diphosphate and ultimately the triphosphate (zidovudine-TP). When zidovudine-TP is incorporated by the action of reverse transcriptase into the growing chain of DNA, no 5'-3' diester linkages can be added because of the 3'-azido (-N_3) substitution, and it is believed that the growing chain of DNA is terminated as a result. HIV reverse transcriptase is 100 times more effective in binding and incorporating zidovudine-TP than is cellular polymerase alpha, and the phosphorylation of zidovudine-MP to zidovudine-TP is limited in human cells (Yarchoan et al 1986, Yarchoan & Broder 1987).

Absorption and fate

Synthesized 20 years ago by Horwitz et al (1964), zidovudine was shown later to inhibit in vitro replication of C-type murine retrovirus but no medical application emerged until its effect in HIV infection was shown. At concentrations of 1–3 μM zidovudine HIV replication is inhibited, and much lower concentrations may also be effective. Well-absorbed orally with a bioavailability of about 60%, zidovudine achieves levels in patients which inhibit replication of HIV; clearance occurs mostly (50–80%) by glucuronidation and to a lesser extent (10–20%) by renal excretion as unchanged drug; the half-life of zidovudine concentration in plasma is about 1 hour. In the cerebrospinal fluid 50–60% of plasma zidovudine levels are attained (Yarchoan et al 1986, Yarchoan & Broder 1987, Data Sheet, Retrovir Capsules, Wellcome, March 1987).

Clinical trials

Zidovudine prolongs life for certain patients with AIDS although uncertainties about the toxic effects and long-term value of this recently introduced drug remain. In the first clinical trials — multicentre, randomized, double-blind, placebo-controlled — only AIDS patients who were within 4 months of their first episode of *Pneumocystis carinii* pneumonia together with those with AIDS-related complex (ARC) (see Note 31.5) were included. A total of 282 patients participated at 12 different centres in the United States; the first patient entered the trial in February 1986 and the last was enrolled at the end of June. Designed to last until December 1986, the trial was terminated prematurely in September since the Data Safety Monitoring Board decided that it would be unethical to withhold the drug from the placebo group. Only 1 patient died out of 145 receiving zidovudine, compared with 16 of the 137 in the placebo group — 11 with AIDS and 5 with ARC. As well as decreasing the mortality rate of patients with *Pneumocystis carinii* pneumonia, zidovudine seemed, at least in the short term, to give them an improved sense of well-being with fewer serious medical complications; in addition they showed also an increase in the numbers of circulating T4 lymphocytes, and those anergic at entry showed a positive delayed type hypersensitivity skin test reaction (Barnes 1986, Yarchoan et al 1986).

The main observations made in the preliminary study (Yarchoan et al 1986) of a 6-week course of treatment with zidovudine were as follows:

1. there was in most an increase in numbers of helper/inducer T lymphocytes (Leu3+ or OKT4+);
2. patients previously showing anergy to skin testing regained a positive skin test (candida extract, purified protein derivative, tetanus toxoid and trichophyton extract);
3. fungal nail-bed infections improved;
4. night sweats or fever improved; and
5. weight gain of 2 kg was noted.

Early experience with zidovudine (Yarchoan et al 1987) showed that certain HIV-associated neurological abnormalities were reversible as a result, possibly, of inhibition of HIV replication in the nervous system or through reduction in the production of a toxic lymphokine. 2 patients with chronic dementia and 1 with both chronic dementia and peripheral neuropathy improved. The fourth patient, with paraplegia, showed no improvement.

Anti-viral effects, observations in patients

HIV core antigen can be detected in the serum of patients with AIDS, and increases in the concentration of this antigen may correlate with clinical deterioration. As part of the multicentre trial of zidovudine 22 patients were studied and randomly assigned to receive zidovudine (250 mg orally every 4 hours) or placebo at the same intervals for 24 weeks; serum samples were obtained at entry and after 4, 8, 11, 20 and 24 weeks of the trial. HIV antigen was detected at the outset in 14 patients whereas in 6 (3 from each group) no antigen was detected at any time. At entry the mean levels were comparable and in those receiving zidovudine, mean HIV antigen levels declined from 278 pg per ml at time of entry to 47 pg per ml at 8 weeks, 91 pg at 16 weeks, and 138 at 20 weeks. In contrast placebo-treated patients had a mean HIV level of 358 pg per ml at entry, 466 at 8 weeks, 788 at 16 weeks, and 870 at 20 weeks. Monitoring HIV core antigen may be an important serological marker of disease progression (Chaisson et al 1986; see also Fig. 31.2).

In the clinical trial of four dose regimens of zidovudine, all were given zidovudine intravenously for 14 days (regimen A — 1 mg/kg/8h; regimen B — 2.5 mg/kg/8h; regimen C — 2.5 mg/kg/4h; and regimen D — 5 mg/kg/4h). For most patients receiving regimen A, B and C virus continued to be detected on culture. For those (4 patients) on regimen D, virus was not detected in cultures established after 2 weeks of therapy (Yarchoan et al 1986).

Toxicity in patients

Haematological effects. Serious haematological toxicity has been observed in patients treated with zidovudine. Anaemia necessitating blood transfusion, leucopenia and, specifically, neutropenia have frequently led to reduction in dosage or discontinuation of the drug. An increase in the red cell mean corpuscular volume, reflecting megaloblastic changes, is often an early sign of these toxic effects. Such bone marrow toxicity does not usually cause thrombocytopenia; some patients even have had increases in circulating platelets during short courses. At the highest dosage, reduction in the numbers of T4 lymphocytes sometimes occurred. Some

patients appear to tolerate long courses (18 months) of zidovudine(Yarchoan & Broder 1987).

Bone marrow suppression is one key side effect of zidovudine, probably a result of a deficiency of normal cellular thymidine triphosphate induced by the drug. Zidovudine is phosphorylated by the same series of cellular enzymes as thymidine. Zidovudine monophosphate interferes with the phosphorylation of thymidine monophosphate by competitive substrate inhibition and this may be a factor that contributes to the toxicity of the drug. Cells exposed to zidovudine may have high levels of thymidine-5′-monophosphate (dTMP) and decreased levels of thymidine-5-triphosphate (dTTP). Patients with folate or vitamin B_{12} deficiency may have decreased production of dTMP by the *de novo* pathway and may therefore be particularly sensitive to zidovudine-induced dTTP depletion unless they receive vitamin replacement therapy (Yarchoan & Broder 1987).

Neurological effects. About half of the recipients of zidovudine report headache, and some show nausea and vomiting. Extreme caution is advised in the use of zidovudine in patients with the late manifestations of AIDS who are very likely to be more susceptible to the toxic side effects of zidovudine because of CNS infection with HIV, or opportunistic pathogens or altered zidovudine metabolism due to liver disease caused by drugs used in their treatment (Hagler & Frame 1986).

In 1 patient with AIDS, zidovudine treatment was associated with Wernicke's encephalopathy (Davtyan & Vinters 1987), developing after 12 doses of zidovudine (Retrovir) (200 mg every 4 hours). Death occurred as a result of septic shock. Autopsy showed symmetrical cortical atrophy and haemorrhages in both mamillary bodies, focal ischaemic changes in the thalamus and bilateral necrotic changes in the pontine tegmentum, all features of acute Wernicke's encephalopathy.

Other effects (Data Sheet, Retrovir Capsules, Wellcome, March 1987). Other frequent adverse events reported in a large placebo-controlled clinical trial included nausea, headache, rash, abdominal pain, fever, myalgia, paraesthesia, vomiting, insomnia and anorexia. Apart from nausea, myalgia and insomnia, which were significantly more common in patients receiving Retrovir capsules, the incidence of these events was only slightly higher than in the placebo recipients.

Less commonly reported and less clearly associated adverse events have included asthenia, malaise, somnolence, diarrhoea, dizziness, paraesthesiae, sweating, dyspnoea, dyspepsia, flatulence, bad taste, chest pain, loss of mental acuity, anxiety, urinary frequency, depression, generalized pain, chills, cough, urticaria, pruritus and influenza-like syndrome. The incidence of these, and other even rarer adverse events, was similar in both Retrovir and placebo-treated patients.

Its weak mutagenic action in some laboratory tests and damaging effect on chromosomes in an in vitro study but not in an in vivo study in rats have no clear clinical significance.

In those using paracetamol chronically, zidovudine treatment is associated with an increased incidence of neutropenia. In those drugs pairing glucuronidation or directly inhibiting hepatic microsomal metabolism *careful thought should be given to the possibilities of drug interactions* if zidovudine is used.

Concomitant therapy with potentially nephrotoxic or myelosuppressive drugs (e.g. co-trimoxazole, dapsone, pyrimethamine, flucytosine, ganciclovar, ribavarin, interferon, vincristine, vinblastine and doxorubicin) may also increase the risk of toxicity with zidovudine.

Probenecid increases the mean half-life and area under the plasma concentration curve of zidovudine, by decreasing renal excretion. Glucuronidation of the drug may also be reduced in the presence of probenecid.

Statement on zidovudine (Retrovir, Wellcome; 3'-azido-3'-deoxythymidine)
Retrovir is indicated for the management of serious manifestations of human immunodeficiency virus (HIV) infections (Data Sheet, Wellcome, March 1987).

Evidence of efficacy has been demonstrated in AIDS patients who have recovered from their first episode of *Pneumocystis carinii* pneumonia within 4 months and others with multiple signs of HIV infection, including mucocutaneous candidiasis, weight loss (more than 10% or 6 kg) lymphadenopathy and unexplained fever.

In adults, for the management of serious manifestations of HIV infections, zidovudine is available for oral use as 100 mg opaque white Retrovir capsules, blue-banded (Wellcome, Crewe, Cheshire, England). Adults are given 200–300 mg every 4 hours, i.e. six times daily, including the night time dose. Dosage may be more accurately calculated as 3.5 mg/kg every 4 hours.

In cases of haematological toxicity, dosage adjustments are required. It is suggested that if the haemoglobin level falls to between 7.5 and 9 g/decilitre or if the neutrophil count to between 0.75 and 1.0 $\times$ 10^9/litre, the recommended dosage should be taken every 8 hours.

If the haemoglobin level falls below 7.5 g/decilitre or the neutrophil count to below 0.75 $\times$ 10^9/litre, therapy with zidovudine should be discontinued. Recovery is usually observed within 2 weeks, after which therapy at a reduced dosage (i.e. recommended dose every 8 hours) may be reinstituted. After a further 2–4 weeks the dosage may be gradually increased, depending upon patient tolerance, until the original dose is reached.

Particular care should be taken in patients with pre-existing bone marrow compromise (e.g., haemoglobin less than 9 g/decilitre or neutrophil count less than 1.0 $\times$ 10^9/litre).

Dosage reduction or cessation of therapy may become necessary whatever form toxicity takes.

No data are available on the use of zidovudine in children and no specific studies have been carried out in the elderly. Special care is needed in the presence of renal impairment, and accumulation is likely to occur in patients with hepatic impairment.

Zidovudine is contraindicated in patients known to be hypersensitive to the drug. It should not be given to those with low neutrophil counts (less than 0.7 $\times$ 10^9/litre) or abnormally low haemoglobin levels (less than 7.5 g/decilitre).

Doses as high as 1250 mg zidovudine taken orally every 4 hours for 4 weeks have been administered to 2 patients. 1 experienced anaemia and neutropenia while the other had no untoward effects. It is not known whether zidovudine is dialysable. Patients should be observed closely for evidence of toxicity.

Peptide T

Peptide T is an octapeptide (Alanine-Serine-Threonine-Threonine-Threonine-Asparagine–Tyrosine–Threonine) which forms a segment of envelope glycoprotein (gp) of HIV. It inhibits HIV in vitro and blocks the binding of the viral envelope to the CD4 receptor (Pert et al 1986). When given to patients with near-to-terminal AIDS, improvements in certain parameters have been noted. At a dose of 1 mg by i.v. infusion twice-daily for 1 week followed by 2 mg by i.v. infusion twice-daily for 3 weeks the lymphocyte count improved and central nervous system involvement, deduced by magnetic resonance imaging, showed a lowering of relaxation times towards normal (Wetterberg et al 1987).

G. CHEMOTHERAPY SPECIFIC FOR OPPORTUNISTIC VIRUS INFECTIONS IN HIV INFECTION AND AIDS

This subject has been considered briefly in relation to each specific infection and discussed earlier in this chapter, but a number of specific matters require mention here.

DIHYDROXYPROPOXYMETHYL GUANINE IN AIDS-RELATED RETINITIS DUE TO CYTOMEGALOVIRUS

The nucleoside 9-(1.3 hydroxy-2-propoxymethyl) guanine (Syntex Corporation) seems to prevent deterioration in AIDS-related retinitis due to CMV (Palestine et al 1986, Harris & Mathalone 1987). Acting by inhibiting DNA polymerase in a manner similar to acyclovir and given orally in adults with this form of retinitis in a dose of 5 mg per kg twice-daily, its long-term efficacy is limited by its toxicity to the bone marrow. The retinitis, if untreated, mostly progresses unremittingly to blindness and, although treatment with the drug dihydroxypropoxymethyl guanine may prevent deterioration, it is effective only if given indefinitely and does not represent a cure.

FOSCARNET (TRISODIUM PHOSPHONOFORMATE)

In vitro studies have shown that trisodium phosphonoformate (Foscarnet) inhibits several viral enzymes including influenza virus RNA polymerase, various retrovirus reverse transcriptases, including those of HIV (Sandstrom et al 1985) and the DNA polymerases of the herpesviruses HSV and CMV. Host cell DNA synthesis is inhibited by concentrations of the drug that are some five to ten times higher than those required for inhibition of viral enzymes, and such cellular effects are reversible.

The drug is of very low toxicity but must be given by intravenous infusion. Although some immunocompromised patients with CMV pneumonia have been treated successfully with Foscarnet (Apperley et al 1985), other studies have given less encouraging results. Preliminary data indicate clinical improvement and return of delayed type hypersensitivity with failure to isolate HIV in some patients with AIDS and related HIV disease treated with Foscarnet (Farthing et al 1986).

ACYCLOVIR

Acyclovir, a drug of low toxicity and available as Zovirax (Wellcome), and potent against herpes simplex virus types 1 and 2 and varicella-zoster virus, has been discussed in Chapter 26. In the immunocompromised patients, as in HIV infection, local lesions may become more extensive and there may be dissemination of infection. Although oral treatment may be effective, acyclovir for intravenous use is available and should be so used when the attack is not controlled. In the case of oral treatment acyclovir is given for HSV infection in adults in a dose of 200 mg 5 times daily for 5 days. For intravenous treatment in adults with normal renal function, the patient should be adequately hydrated and the dose is 5 mg per kg body weight given by slow intravenous infusion over a 1-hour period. Acyclovir given intravenously has been shown to be an effective prophylaxis against HSV infections in severely immunocompromised patients (Hann et al 1983).

In varicella-zoster infections of HIV-infected children aggressive therapy is advised. Intravenous acyclovir therapy has been shown to be effective in immunocompromised children in a dose of 500 mg/m^2/dose over 1 hour, every 8 hours for 7 days and is to be considered the drug of choice (Prober et al 1982). In immunocompromised adults with normal renal function the dose recommended is 10 mg per kg body weight every 8 hours. Each dose is administered by slow intravenous infusion over a 1-hour period. When there is renal impairment dosages are modified and based on the creatinine clearance. Acyclovir (Zovirax) for intravenous use must be reconstituted by the addition of 10 ml of Water for Injections BP or Sodium Chloride Intravenous Infusion BP (0.45 or 0.9% w/v). The required dose/volume should be calculated on the basis of 25 mg per ml of reconstituted solution. After reconstitution the acyclovir (i.v.) may be injected directly into a vein over 1 hour by a controlled rate infusion pump or further diluted for administration with at least 50 ml of infusion fluid (e.g. Sodium Chloride Infusion Fluid BP 0.45 or 0.9% w/v); (ABPI Data Sheet Compendium 1986–1987).

Acyclovir (equal to or greater than 64 μM) has rather weak activity in vitro against HIV, but combined with zidovudine there is a synergistic anti-retroviral effect at a wide range of concentrations without affecting the growth of the tissue culture cells (Mitsuya & Broder 1987). Caution and more experience is required, nevertheless, in using this or indeed any combination of drugs (Bach 1987).

H. PSYCHOSOCIAL PHENOMENA AND PREVENTION IN HIV INFECTION AND AIDS

Since behavioural change is at present the only viable means of halting the spread of HIV infection, every effort is needed to ensure that education and information are available to all who are potentially or actually at risk. Some of these considerations have been touched upon in this book in Chapters 4 and 5 but those involved in counselling will require to know and to be able to explain to others the sexually explicit details needed to promote safety and limit transmission of HIV. A consistent and humane approach to individual patients is essential. When patients request antibody testing precounselling involves making the individual aware of issues relating to testing, and any decision for such testing must be an informed one with patient consent and not as a result of pressure from the physician or any other health staff. In those found to be HIV antibody positive constructive discussion gives hope, but acute anxiety, depression and even suicidal tendencies may develop — hence it is necessary, particularly during the first few days, to ensure that help is available to the individual. It is particularly valuable to give the patient a 'lifeline' — telephone numbers for the counsellors or support group. Patients must be cautioned, however, against revealing their situation to outsiders, whose reaction cannot be predicted. It is necessary for the patient to learn to live with the diagnosis and to involve the lover or spouse of the patient. Confidentiality must be preserved and the patient should be consulted about which information he is prepared to pass on about himself and his condition. Reference has already been made to the importance of at-risk groups attending clinics equipped and staffed to deal with sexually transmitted diseases; it is essential that public policy promotes these principles and avoids deflecting those who need this specialist help. Health personnel are liable to suffer also from the strains of looking after those with HIV infection and need support. Some aspects of the problems from the individual or public health point of view are covered in Chapters 4 and 5 and for fuller consideration of these matters the following sources are recommended: Miller et al 1986, Miller & Green 1987.

NOTES TO CHAPTER 31

Note 31.1: The case definition of AIDS used by CDC for epidemiologic surveillance

For the limited purposes of epidemiologic surveillance, CDC defines a case of 'the Acquired Immune Deficiency Syndrome' (AIDS) as a person who has had:

I. a reliably diagnosed disease that is at least moderately indicative of an underlying cellular immune deficiency, but who, at the same time, has had:
II. no known underlying cause of cellular immune deficiency nor any other cause of reduced resistance reported to be associated with that disease.

This general case definition may be made more explicit by specifying:

I. the particular diseases considered at least moderately indicative of cellular immune deficiency, and
II. the known causes of cellular immune deficiency, or other causes of reduced resistance reported to be associated with particular diseases.

These are detailed below:

I. DISEASES AT LEAST MODERATELY INDICATIVE OF UNDERLYING CELLULAR IMMUNE DEFICIENCY

These are listed below in 5 aetiological categories: A. protozoal and helminthic, B. fungal, C. bacterial, D. viral, and E. cancer. Within each category, the diseases are listed in alphabetical order. 'Disseminated infection' refers to involvement of liver, bone marrow, or multiple organs, not simply involvement of lungs and multiple lymph nodes. The required diagnostic methods with positive results are shown in parentheses.

A. Protozoal and helminthic infections
1. Cryptosporidiosis, intestinal, causing diarrhoea for 1 month, (on histology or stool microscopy);
2. Pneumocystis carinii pneumonia, (on histology, or microscopy of a 'touch' preparation or bronchial washings);
3. Strongyloidosis, causing pneumonia, central nervous system infection, or disseminated infection, (on histology);
4. Toxoplasmosis, causing pneumonia or central nervous system infection (on histology or microscopy of a 'touch' preparation).

B. Fungal infections
1. Aspergillosis, causing central nervous system or disseminated infection (on culture or histology).
2. Candidiasis, causing oesophagitis (on histology, or microscopy of a 'wet' preparation from the oesophagus, or endoscopic findings of white plaques on an erythematous mucosal base);
3. Cryptococcosis, causing pulmonary, central nervous system, or disseminated infection (on culture, antigen detection, histology, or India ink preparation of CSF).

C. Bacterial infections
1. 'Atypical' mycobacteriosis (species other than tuberculosis or lepra), causing disseminated infection (on culture).

D. Viral infections
1. Cytomegalovirus, causing pulmonary, gastrointestinal tract, or central nervous system infection (on histology);
2. Herpes simplex virus, causing chronic mucocutaneous infection with ulcers persisting more than 1 month, or pulmonary, gastrointestinal tract, or disseminated infection (on culture, histology, or cytology).
3. Progressive multifocal leucoencephalopathy (presumed to be caused by Papovavirus) (on histology).

E. Cancer
1. Kaposi's sarcoma (on histology);
2. Lymphoma limited to the brain (on histology).

II. KNOWN CAUSES OF REDUCED RESISTANCE

Known causes of reduced resistance to diseases indicative of immune deficiency are listed in the left column, while the diseases that may be attributable to these causes (rather than to the immune deficiency of AIDS) are listed on the right:

Known causes of reduced resistance	Diseases possibly attributable to the known causes of reduced resistance
1. Systemic corticosteroid or other immunosuppressive or cytotoxic therapy.	Any infection that began during or within one month after such therapy, if the therapy began before signs or symptoms specific for the infected anatomic sites (e.g. dyspnoea for pneumonia, headache for encephalitis, diarrhoea for colitis); or cancer diagnosed during or within 1 month after *more than 4 months* of such therapy, if the therapy began before signs or symptoms specific for the anatomic site of the cancer.
2. Widely spread cancer of lymphoid or histiocytic tissue, such as lymphoma, Hodgkin's disease, lymphocytic leukaemia, or multiple myeloma. (This does not include cancer that is entirely localized to one site, such as primary lymphoma of the brain).	Any other cancer or infection, regardless of whether diagnosed before or after (because a lymphoma may have been present before, even if diagnosed after).
3. Age 60 years or older at diagnosis.	Kaposi's sarcoma.
4. Age under 28 days (neonatal) at diagnosis.	Toxoplasmosis, cytomegalovirus, or herpes simplex virus infections.
5. An immune deficiency atypical of AIDS, such as one involving hypogammaglobulinaemia; or an	Any infection or cancer diagnosed during such immune deficiency.

immune deficiency of which the cause appears to be a genetic or developmental defect (e.g. thymic dysplasia).

III. CASE REPORTING

For the epidemiologic surveillance of AIDS, any patient who has a disease at least moderately indicative of cellular immune deficiency (as listed above in section I). but who has no known cause of reduced resistance to that disease (as listed above in section II), should be reported by clinicians to their state or local public health department. Those agencies should, in turn, report the case to the AIDS Activity, Centers for Disease Control, Atlanta, Georgia 30333. To expedite communication, clinicians may, if they wish, report a case directly to CDC, *in addition* to reporting it to their state or local health department.

Note 31.2: AIDS in Africa

AIDS as it occurs in adults in Africa may be defined by the existence of at least *two of the major signs* in association with *at least one minor sign* in the absence of other known cause of immunosuppression, such a: cancer or severe malnutrition (Colebunders et al 1987).
The major signs are:

1. Weight loss greater than 10% of body weight.
2. Chronic diarrhoea for longer than 1 month.
3. Fever, either intermittent or constant, for longer than a month.

Note: The presence of *disseminated Kaposi's sarcoma* or *cryptococcal meningitis* is sufficient by itself for diagnosis of AIDS.
The minor signs are:

1. Persistent cough for longer than 1 month.
2. General pruritic (papular) dermatitis.
3. Recurrent herpes zoster.
4. Oropharyngeal candidiasis.
5. Chronic progressive and disseminated herpes simplex infection.
6. Generalized lymphadenopathy.

Symptoms and signs of case definition:
Chronic diarrhoea — at least 2 stools of unusually loose consistency per day for at least 30 days during the previous 2 months.
Chronic progressive herpes simplex infection — painful genital ulceration existing for longer than 1 month.
General lymphadenopathy — presence of enlarged lymph nodes > 1 cm in at least two non-contiguous extra-inguinal sites.

The study showed that the clinical case definition had a specificity of 90%; a sensitivity of 59% and a predictive value of 74% for seropositivity. Tuberculosis has many features of HIV infection and is itself strongly associated with HIV infection (33% of 159 patients in a tuberculosis sanatorium in one study) (Colebunders et al 1987).

Note 31.3: Evaluation of case definition

Evaluation of case definition (Colebunders et al 1987) is made as follows:

Numbers of patients meeting criteria	HIV-antibody	
	Positive	*Negative*
Yes	a	c
No	b	d

$$\text{Sensitivity of definition (percentage)} = \frac{a}{a + b} \times 100$$

$$\text{Specificity (percentage)} = \frac{d}{c + d} \times 100$$

$$\text{Positive predictive value} = \frac{a}{a + c} \times 100$$

Note 31.4

Human lymphocyte subsets are defined phenotypically by the binding of monoclonal antibodies to cell surface antigens, although it should be noted that the groups of cells identified by such antibodies may be heterogeneous with regard to function. The monoclonal antibodies are available from several sources, commercial suppliers including Ortho Diagnostics (Denmark House, High Wycombe, Buckinghamshire, UK) and Becton Dickinson (Waldegrave Road, Teddington, Middlesex, UK), each with their own nomenclature. In practice, T-cell surface antigens are often defined by the binding of the monoclonal antibodies provided by Ortho Diagnostics; for example, a monoclonal antibody produced by Ortho which binds to the T-cell receptor is designated OKT3 and this antigen is often referred to as T3. The equivalent antibody from Becton Dickinson is designated Leu 4. To avoid confusion an international workshop on human leucocyte differentiation antigens was established in 1982 to define these antigens and to assign to each a CD (cluster of differentiation) number; the T3 antigen has been designated CD3. A subset of T-cells which bears the CD4 antigen includes those which co-operate with B-cells in the production of antibody (helper/inducer T-cells); these cells are referred to in the text as T4 cells. Antibodies which react with this surface antigen include OKT4 and Leu 3. The CD8 antigen is expressed on cells which include those which suppress antibody production by B-cells, suppress other immune functions mediated by effector T-cells, and are cytotoxic to cells bearing 'foreign' antigens in association with autologous class II MHC-derived (HLA-D) antigens. These are the suppressor/cytotoxic T-cells referred to in the text as T8 cells; monoclonal antibodies reacting with the CD8 antigen include OKT8 and Leu 2.

Follicular dendritic cells are found within both encapsulated (lymph node and spleen) and non-encapsulated (mucosal) lymphoid tissues; they capture and retain antigens and present them to B-cells.

Note 31.5: AIDS-related complex (ARC)

The AIDS-related complex is a combination of symptoms, signs and laboratory abnormalities in the absence of secondary infectious disease or neoplasia. Symptoms include malaise and fatigue. There is persistent intermittent fever and/or night sweats. Persistent diarrhoea (duration more than 1 month) and significant weight loss (10% of body weight) are features. Skin rashes, including eczema, seborrhoeic dermatitis and folliculitis are common. Oral candidiasis and oral hairy leukoplakia may be found. There is almost always persistent generalized lymphadenopathy and the spleen is often palpable. There is lymphopenia (less than $1.5 \times 10^9/1$); thrombocytopenia ($< 150 \times 10^9/1$) and T4 cell depletion ($< 0.4 \times 10^9/1$); proliferative responses to various mitogens are reduced and cutaneous anergy to at least three recall antigens is a feature (test systems usually use as antigens — tuberculin, candida, trichophyton, proteus and group C streptococcal antigens, and tetanus and diphtheria toxoids).

REFERENCES

Abo W, Takada K, Kamada M et al, 1982 Evolution of infectious mononucleosis into Epstein-Barr virus carrying monoclonal malignant lymphoma. Lancet i: 1272–1276

ABPI Data Sheet Compendium 1986–1987 Datapharm Publications, London

Abrams D I, Lewis B J, Beckstead J H, Casavant C A, Drew W L 1984 Persistent diffuse lymphadenopathy in homosexual men: endpoint or prodrome? Annals of Internal Medicine 100: 801–808

Ainti F, Rossi P, Sirianni M C et al 1985 IgM and IgG antibodies to human T-cell lymphotropic retrovirus (HTLV-III) in lymphadenopathy syndrome and subjects at risk for AIDS in Italy. British Medical Journal 291: 165–166

Alizon M, Sonigo P, Barré-Sinoussi F, Chermann J-C, Tiollais P, Montagnier L, Wain-Hobson S 1984 Molecular cloning of lymphadenopathy associated virus. Nature 312: 757–760

Allain J-P, Laurian Y, Paul D A, Sena D 1986 Serological markers in early stages of human immunodeficiency virus infection in haemophiliacs. Lancet ii: 1233–1236

Ammann A J 1985 The acquired immunodeficiency syndrome in infants and children. Annals of Internal Medicine 103(5): 734–737

Ammann A J, Wara D W, Cowan M J 1984 Pediatric acquired immunodeficiency syndrome. Annals of the New York Academy of Sciences 437: 340–349

Angarano G, Pastore G, Monno L, Santantonio T, Luchena N, Schiraldi O 1985 Rapid spread of HTLV-III infection among drug addicts in Italy. Lancet ii: 1302

Apperly J F, Marcus R E, Goldman J M, Wardle D G, Gravett P J, Chanus A 1985 Foscarnet for cytomegalovirus pneumonitis. Lancet i: 1151

Armstrong D 1981 Fungal infections in the compromised host. In: Rubin R H, Young L S (eds) Clinical approach to infection in the compromised host. Plenum Medical Book Company, New York, p 195–228

Armstrong J A, Horne R 1984 Follicular dendritic cells in virus-like particles in AIDS-related lymphadenopathy. Lancet ii: 370–372

Auerbach D M, Darrow W W, Jaffe H W, Curran J W 1984 Cluster of cases of the acquired immune deficiency syndrome. Patients linked by sexual contact. American Journal of Medicine 76: 487–491

Bach M C 1987 Possible drug interaction during therapy with azidothymidine and acyclovir for AIDS. Correspondence, The New England Journal of Medicine 316: 547

Barnes D M 1986 Promising results half trial of anti-AIDS drug. Science 234: 15–16

Barré-Sinoussi F, Chermann J-C, Rey F et al 1983 Isolation of a T-lymphotropic retrovirus from a patient at risk for acquired immune deficiency syndrome (AIDS). Science 220: 868–871

Barton S E, Underhill G S, Gilchrist C, Jeffries D J, Harris J R W 1985 HTLV-III antibody in prostitutes. Lancet ii: 1424

Bayley A C 1984 Aggressive Kaposi's sarcoma in Zambia 1983. Lancet i: 1318–1320

Bayley A C, Downing R G, Cheinsong-Popov R, Tedder R S, Dalgleish A G, Weiss R A 1985 HTLV-III serology distinguishes atypical and endemic Kaposi's sarcoma in Africa. Lancet i: 359–361

Belsito D V, Sanchez M R, Baer R L, Valentine F, Thorbecke G J 1984 Reduced Langerhans' cell Ig antigen and ATP-ase activity in patients with the acquired immune deficiency syndrome. New England Journal of Medicine 310: 1279–1282

Bigby T D, Margolskee D, Curtis J L, Michael P E, Sheppard D, Hadley W K, Hopewell P C 1986 The usefulness of induced sputum in the diagnosis of *Pneumocystis carinii* pneumonia in patients with the acquired immunodeficiency syndrome. Annual Review of Respiratory Diseases 133: 515–518

Biggar R J, Melbye M, Kestems L et al 1984 Kaposi's sarcoma in Zaire is not associated with HTLV-III infection. New England Journal of Medicine 311: 1051

Birx D L, Redfield R R, Tosato G 1986 Defective regulation of Epstein Barr virus infections in patients with acquired immunodeficiency syndrome (AIDS) or AIDS-related disorders. New England Journal of Medicine 314: 874–879

Bloom A L 1984 Acquired immunodeficiency syndrome and other possible immunological disorders in European haemophiliacs. Lancet i: 1452–1455

Blumenfeld W, Beckstead J B 1983 Angioimmunoblastic lymphadenopathy with dysproteinemia in homosexual men with acquired immune deficiency syndrome. Archives of Pathology and Laboratory Medicine 107: 567–569

Boldogh I, Beth E, Huang E-S, Kyalwazi S K, Giraldo G 1981 Kaposi's sarcoma. IV Detection of CMV DNA CMV RNA and CMNA in tumor biopsies. International Journal of Cancer 28: 469–474

Bonner J R, Alexander W J, Dissmakes W E 1984 Disseminated histoplasmosis in patients with the acquired immune deficiency syndrome. Annals of Internal Medicine 144: 2178–2181

Brenky-Faudeux D, Fribourg-Blanc A 1985 HTLV-III antibody in prostitutes. Lancet ii: 1424

Brun-Vézinet F, Rouzioux C, Montagnier L et al 1984a Prevalence of antibodies to lymphadenopathy-associated retrovirus in African patients with AIDS. Science 226: 453–456

Brun-Vézinet F, Rouzioux C, Barré-Sinoussi F et al 1984b Detection of IgG antibodies to lymphadenopathy-associated virus in patients with AIDS or lymphadenopathy syndrome. Lancet i: 1253–1256

Brunet J B, Bouvet E, Leibowitch J et al 1983 Acquired immunodeficiency syndrome in France. Lancet i: 700–701

Budiansky S 1985 AIDS blood test trials inconclusive. News, Nature 316: 96

Bygbjerg I C 1983 AIDS in a Danish surgeon. Lancet i: 925

Carne C A, Tedder R S, Smith A et al 1985 Acute encephalopathy coincident with seroconversion for anti HTLV-III. Lancet ii: 1206–1208

CDC Task Force on Kaposi's Sarcoma and Opportunistic Infections 1982 Epidemiologic aspects of the current outbreak of Kaposi's sarcoma and opportunistic infections. Special Report. New England Journal of Medicine 306(4): 248–252

Centers for Disease Control 1985a Update: acquired immunodeficiency syndrome — United States. Morbidity and Mortality Weekly Report 34, No 18: 246–248

Centers for Disease Control 1985b Education and foster care of children infected with human T-lymphotropic virus type III/lymphadenopathy-associated virus. Morbidity and Mortality Weekly Report 34, No 34: 517–521

Centers for Disease Control 1986 Update: acquired immunodeficiency syndrome — United States. Morbidity and Mortality Weekly Report 35, No 49: 757–760, 765–766

Chaisson R E, Allain J-P, Leuther M, Volberding P A 1986 Significant changes in HIV antigen level in the serum of patients treated with azidothymidine. New England Journal of Medicine 315: 1610–1611

Cheinsong-Popov R, Weiss R A, Dalgleish A et al 1984 Prevalence of antibody to human T-lymphotropic virus type III in AIDS and AIDS-risk patients in Britain. Lancet ii: 477–480

Clavel F, Guétard D, Brun-Vézinet F et al 1986 Isolation of a new human retrovirus from West African patients with AIDS. Science 233: 343–346

Clumeck N, Sonnet J, Taelman H et al 1984 Acquired immunodeficiency syndrome in African patients. New England Journal of Medicine 310: 492–497

Coffin J, Haase A, Levy J A et al 1986 What to call the AIDS virus. Correspondence, Nature 321: 10

Cohen B A, Pomerang S, Rabinowitz J G, Rosen M J, Brain J S, Norton H, Mendelson D S 1984 Pulmonary complications of AIDS: radiologic factors. American Journal of Roentgenology 143: 115–122

Colebunders R, Mann J M, Francis H et al 1987 Evaluation of a clinical case-definition of acquired immunodeficiency syndrome in Africa. Lancet i: 492–494

Cooper D A, Gold J, MacLean P et al 1985 Acute AIDS retrovirus infection. Definition of a clinical illness associated with seroconversion. Lancet i: 537–540

Curran J W, Lawrence D N, Jaffe H et al 1984 Acquired immunodeficiency syndrome (AIDS) associated with transfusions. New England Journal of Medicine 310: 69–75

Dalgleish A G, Beverley P C L, Clapham P R, Crawford D H, Greaves M F, Weiss R A 1984 The CD4 (T4) antigen is an essential component of the receptor for the AIDS retrovirus. Nature 312: 763–767

Davtyan D, Vinters H V 1987 Wernicke's encephalopathy in AIDS patient treated with zidovudine. Correspondence, Lancet i: 917–918

de la Loma A, Manrigue A, Rubio R, Jimenez M S, Alvar J, Palencia E, Najera R 1985 Generalized tuberculosis in a patient with acquired immunodeficiency syndrome. Journal of Infection 10: 57–59

De Stefano E, Friedman R M, Friedman-Kien A E et al 1982 Acid-labile human leukocyte interferon in homosexual men with Kaposi's sarcoma and lymphadenopathy. Journal of Infectious Diseases 146: 451–455

Downing R G, Eglin R P, Bayley A C 1984 African Kaposi's sarcoma in AIDS. Lancet i: 478–480

Drew W L, Conant M A, Miner R C et al 1982 Cytomegalovirus and Kaposi's sarcoma in young homosexual men. Lancet ii: 125–127

Ellrodt A, Barré-Sinoussi F, Le Bras P H et al 1984 Isolation of human T-lymphotropic retrovirus (LAV) from Zairian married couple, one with AIDS, one with prodromes. Lancet i: 1383–1385

Enzensberger W, Fischer P A, Helm E B, Stille W 1985 Value of electroencephalography in AIDS. Lancet i: 1047–1048

Essex M, McLane M F, Lee T H et al 1983 Antibodies to cell membrane antigens associated with human T-cell leukaemia virus in patients with AIDS. Science 220: 859–862

Farthing C F, Dalgleigh A S, Clark A H, Chanas A, McClure M, Gazzara B G 1986 Pilot study on the treatment of AIDS in ARC patients with intravenous Foscarnet. Abstract. International Conference on AIDS, Paris

Fernandez R, Mouradian J, Metroka C, Davis J 1983 The prognostic value of histopathology in persistent generalized lymphadenopathy in homosexual men. New England Journal of Medicine 309: 185–186

Fink L, Reichek N, Sutton M G St J 1984 Cardiac abnormalities in acquired immune deficiency syndrome. American Journal of Cardiology 54: 1161–1163

Finkbeiner W E, Egbert B M, Groundwater J R, Sagebiel R W 1982 Kaposi's sarcoma in young homosexual men. A histopathologic study with particular reference to lymph node involvement. Archives of Pathology and Laboratory Medicine 106: 261–264

Follansbee S E, Busch D F, Wofsy C B et al 1982 An outbreak of *Pneumocystis carinii* pneumonia in homosexual men. Annals of Internal Medicine 96: 705–713

Follett E A C, McIntyre A, O'Donnell B, Clements G B, Desselberger U 1986 HTLV-III antibody in drug abusers in the West of Scotland: the Edinburgh connection. Lancet i: 446–447

Francioli P, Clement F, Vandois C U U 1982 Beta-2 microglobulin and immunodeficiency in a homosexual man. New England Journal of Medicine 307: 1402–1403

Friedman-Kein A E, Lambenstein L J, Rubinstein P et al 1982 Disseminated Kaposi's Sarcoma in homosexual men. Annals of Internal Medicine 96: 693–700

Fuchs D, Blecha H G, Deinhardt F et al 1985 High frequency of HTLV-III antibodies among heterosexual intravenous drug abusers in the Austrian Tyrol. Correspondence, Lancet i: 1506

Gallo R C 1987 The AIDS virus. Scientific American 256(1): 38–48

Gallo R C, Sarin P S, Gelmann E P et al 1983 Isolation of human T-cell leukaemia virus in acquired immune deficiency syndrome (AIDS). Science 220: 865–867

Gallo R C, Salahuddin S Z, Popovic M et al 1984 Frequent detection and isolation of cytopathic retroviruses (HTLV-III) from patients with AIDS and at risk of AIDS. Science 224: 500–503

Gazzard B G, Shanson D C, Farthing C et al 1984 Clinical findings and serological evidence of HTLV-III infection in homosexual contacts of patients with AIDS and persistent generalized lymphadenopathy in London. Lancet ii: 480–483

Gelmann E P, Popovic M, Blayney D, Masur H, Sidhu G, Stahl R E, Gallo R C 1983 Proviral DNA of a retrovirus, human T-cell leukaemia virus in two patients with AIDS. Science 220: 862–865

Gerstoft J, Malchow-Møller A, Bygbjerg I et al 1982 Severe acquired immunodeficiency in European homosexual men. British Medical Journal 285: 17–19

Giraldo G, Beth E, Henle W et al 1978 Antibody patterns to herpesvirus in Kaposi's sarcoma. II Serological association of American Kaposi's sarcoma with cytomegalovirus. International Journal of Cancer 22: 126–131

Giraldo G, Beth E, Huang E-S 1980 Kaposi's sarcoma and its relationship to cytomegalovirus (CMV). III CMV DNA and CMV early antigen in Kaposi's sarcoma. International Journal of Cancer 26: 23–29

Goedert J J, Sarngadharan M G, Biggar R J et al 1984 Determinants of retrovirus (HTLV-III) antibody and immunodeficiency conditions in homosexual men. Lancet ii: 711–716

Gordin F M, Simon G L, Wofsy C B, Mills J 1984 Adverse reactions to trimethoprim-sulfamethoxazole in patients with the acquired immunodeficiency syndrome. Annals of Internal Medicine 100: 495–499

Gottlieb M S, Schroff R, Schahker H M, Weisman J D, Fan P T, Wolf R A, Saxon A 1981 Pneumocystis carinii pneumonia and mucosal candidiasis in previously healthy homosexual men. New England Journal of Medicine 305: 1425–1431

Gottlieb M S, Ackerman A B 1982 Kaposi's sarcoma: an extensively disseminated form in young homosexual men. Human Pathology 13: 882–892

Gottlieb M S, Knight S, Mitsuyasu R, Weisman J, Roth M, Young L S 1984 Prophylaxis of Pneumocystis carinii infection in AIDS with pyrimethamine-sulfadoxine. Lancet ii: 398–399

Greene J B, Sidhu G S, Lewin S et al 1982 Mycobacterium avium-intracellulare: a cause of disseminated life-threatening infection in homosexuals and drug abusers. Annals of Internal Medicine 97: 539–546

Greenspan D, Greenspan J S, Conant M, Petersen V, Silverman S, de Souza Y 1984 Oral 'hairy' leukoplakia in male homosexual: evidence of association with both papillomavirus and a herpes group virus. Lancet ii: 831–834

Guarda L A, Butler J J, Mansell P, Hersh E M, Reuben J, Newell G R 1983 Lymphadenopathy in homosexual men. Morbid anatomy with clinical and immunologic correlations. American Journal of Clinical Pathology 79: 559–568

Guinan M E, Thomas P A, Pinsky P F et al 1984 Heterosexual and homosexual patients with the acquired immunodeficiency syndrome. A comparison of surveillance, interview and laboratory data. New England Journal of Medicine 100: 213–218

Gupta S, Safai B 1983 Deficient autologous mixed lymphocyte reaction in Kaposi's sarcoma associated with deficiency of Leu 3+ responder T-cells. Journal of Clinical Investigation 71: 296–300

Guyader M, Emerman M, Sonigo P, Clavel F, Montagnier L, Alizon M 1987 Genome organization and transactivation of the human immunodeficiency virus type 2. Nature 326: 662–669

Hagler D N, Frame P T 1986 Azidothymidine neurotoxicity. Correspondence, Lancet ii: 1392–1393

Hann I M, Prentice H G, Blacklock H A et al 1983 Acyclovir prophylaxis against herpes virus infections in severely immunocompromised patients: randomised double-blind trial. British Medical Journal 287: 384–388

Harris C, Small C B, Klein R S et al 1983 Immunodeficiency in female sexual partners of men with the acquired immunodeficiency syndrome. New England Journal of Medicine 308: 1181–1184

Harris M L, Mathalone M B R 1987 Dihydroxypropoxymethyl guanine in the treatment of AIDS related retinitis due to cytomegalovirus. British Medical Journal 294: 92

Hay R 1982 Ketaconozole. British Medical Journal 285: 584–585

Hehlmann R, Kreeb G, Erfle V, Piechowiak H, Kruger G, Goebel F D 1984 Antibodies to HTLV-III in patients with acquired immunodeficiency and lymphadenopathy syndrome in West Germany. Lancet ii: 1094

Hersh E M, Reuben J M, Rios A et al 1983 Elevated serum thymosin-alpha 1 levels associated with evidence of immune dysregulation in male homosexuals with a history of infectious diseases or Kaposi's sarcoma. New England Journal of Medicine 308: 45–46

Hirsch M S, Kaplan J C 1987 Antiviral therapy. Scientific American 256(4): 66–75

Ho D D, Schooley R T, Rota T R et al 1984 HTLV-III in the semen and blood of a healthy homosexual man. Science 226: 451–453

Ho D D, Hartshorn K L, Rota J R, Andrews C A, Kaplan J C, Schooley R T, Hirsch M S 1985a Recombinant human interferon alfa-A suppresses HTLV-III replication in vitro. Lancet i: 602–604

Ho D D, Rota T R, Schooley R T et al 1985b Isolation of HTLV-III from cerebrospinal fluid and neural tissues of patients with neurologic syndromes related to the acquired immunodeficiency syndrome. New England Journal of Medicine 313: 1493–1497

Holland G N, Gottlieb M S, Yee R D, Schanker H M, Pettit T H 1982 Ocular disorders associated with a new severe acquired cellular immunodeficiency syndrome. American Journal of Ophthalmology 93: 393–402

Hood A F, Farmer E R, Weiss R A 1982 Kaposi's sarcoma. John Hopkins Medical Journal 151: 222–230

Horwitz J P, Chua J, Noel M 1964 Nucleosides V. The monomesylates of 1-(2'-Deoxy-βa-D-lvxofuranosyl)thymine. Journal of Organic Chemistry 29: 2076–2078

Hutt M S R 1984 Kaposi's sarcoma. British Medical Bulletin 40: 355–358

Jaffe HW, Choi K, Thomas P A et al 1983 National case-control study of Kaposi's sarcoma and Pneumocystis carinii pneumonia in homosexual men. Part 1. Epidemiologic results. Annals of Internal Medicine 99: 145–151

Janossy G, Pinching A J, Bofill M et al 1985 An immunohistological approach to persistent lymphadenopathy and its relevance to AIDS. Clinical and Experimental Immunology 59: 257–266

Jarlais D C Des, Chamberland M E, Yancovitz S R, Weinberg P, Friedman S R 1984 Heterosexual partners: a large risk group for AIDS. Lancet ii: 1346–1347

Jovaisas E, Koch M A, Schafer A, Stanbor M, Lowenthal D 1985 LAV/HTLV-III in 20 week fetus. Lancet ii: 1129

Kalyanaraman V S, Sarngadharan M G, Robert-Guroff M, Miyoshi I, Blayney D, Golde D, Gallo R C 1982 A new subtype of human T-cell leukemia virus (HTLV-II) associated with a T-cell variant of hairy cell leukemia. Science 218: 571–573

Klatzmann D, Champagne E, Chamaret S et al 1984 T-lymphocyte T4 molecule behaves as the receptor for human retrovirus LAV. Nature 312: 767–768

Kornfeld H , Stouwe R A V, Lange M, Reddy M M, Grieco M H 1982 T-lymphocyte subpopulations in homosexual men. New England Journal of Medicine 307: 729–731

Kotler D P, Gaetz H P, Lange M, Klein E B, Holt P R 1984 Enteropathy associated with the acquired immunodeficiency syndrome. Annals of Internal Medicine 101: 421–428

Kovacs A, Forthal D N, Kovacs J A, Overturf G D 1984 Disseminated coccidioidomycosis in a patient with acquired immune deficiency syndrome. Western Journal of Medicine 140: 447–449

Kreiss J K, Kitchen L W, Prince H E, Kasper C K, Essex M 1985 Antibody to human T-lymphotropic virus type III in wives of haemophiliacs: evidence for heterosexual transmission. Annals of Internal Medicine 102: 623–626

Kreiss J K, Koech D, Plummer F A et al 1986 AIDS virus infection in Nairobi prostitutes. Spread of the epidemic to East Africa. New England Journal of Medicine 314: 414–418

Lane H C, Masur H, Edgar L C, Whalen G, Rook A H, Funci A S 1983 Abnormalities of B-cell activation and immunoregulation in patients with the acquired immunodeficiency syndrome. New England Journal of Medicine 309: 453–458

Lang W, Anderson R E, Perkins H et al 1987 Clinical, immunologic, and serologic findings in men at risk for acquired immunodeficiency syndrome. The San Francisco Men's Health Study. Journal of the American Medical Association 257: 326–330

Lange J, Goudsmit J 1987 Decline in antibody reactivity to HIV core protein secondary to increased production of HIV antigen. Correspondence, Lancet i: 448

Lange J M A, Coutinho R A, Krone W J A, Verdonck L F, Danner S A, van der Noordaa J, Goudsmit J 1986a Distinct IgG recognition patterns during progression of subclinical and clinical infection with lymphadenopathy associated virus/human T-lymphotropic virus. British Medical Journal 292: 228–230

Lange J M A, Paul D A, Huisman H G et al 1986b Persistent HIV antigenaemia and decline of HIV core antibodies associated with transition to AIDS. British Medical Journal 293: 1459–1462

Lapointe N, Michaud J, Pekovic D, Chausseau J P, Dupuy J-M 1985 Transplacental transmission of HTLV-III virus. New England Journal of Medicine 312: 1325

Laurence J, Brun-Vézinet F, Schutzer S E et al 1984 Lymphadenopathy-associated viral antibody in AIDS. Immune correlations and definition of a carrier state. New England Journal of Medicine 311: 1269–1273

Levy J A, Hoffman A D, Kramer S M, Landis J A, Shimabukuro J M, Oshiro L S 1984a Isolation of lymphocytopathic retroviruses from San Francisco patients with AIDS. Science 225: 840–842

Levy J A, Mitra G, Mozen M M 1984b Recovery and inactivation of infectious retroviruses added to factor VIII concentrates. Lancet ii: 722–723

Levy N, Carlson J R, Hinrichs S, Lerche N, Schenker M, Gardner M B 1986 The prevalence of HTLV-III/LAV antibodies among intravenous drug users attending treatment programs in California: a preliminary report. New England Journal of Medicine 314: 446

Lifson J D, Benike C J, Mark D G, Koths K, Engleman E G 1984 Human recombinant interleukin-2 partly reconstitutes deficient in vitro immune response of lymphocytes from patients with AIDS. Lancet i: 698–702

Liskin L, Blackburn R, Maier J H 1986 AIDS — a public health crisis. Population reports, issues in world health, population information program, The Johns Hopkins University, Baltimore. Series L No 6, vol XIV, No 3, p L193–L228

Lopez C, Fitzgerald P A, Siegal F P 1983 Severe acquired immune deficiency syndrome in male homosexuals

diminished capacity to make interferon-in vitro associated with severe opportunistic infections. Journal of Infectious Diseases 148: 962–966

Luft B J, Conley F, Remington J S et al 1983 Outbreak of central nervous system toxoplasmosis in Western Europe and North America. Lancet i: 781–784

McNutt N S, Fletcher V, Conant M A 1983 Early lesions of Kaposi's sarcoma in homosexual men. An ultrastructural comparison with other vascular proliferations in skin. American Journal of Pathology 111: 62–77

Marion R, Wiznia A, Hutcheon R G, Rubinstein A 1986 The AIDS embryopathy: a new dysmorphic syndrome in children with acquired immune deficiency syndrome (AIDS) (abstract 1071). Pediatric Research 20(4, pt 2): 339A

Mathez D, Leibowitch J, Matheron S, Saimot A G, Catalan P, Zaguri D 1984 Antibodies to HTLV-III associated antigens in population exposed to AIDS virus in France. Lancet ii: 460

Mathur-Wagh U, Enlow R W, Spigland I et al 1984 Longitudinal study of persistent generalised lymphadenopathy in homosexual men: relation to acquired immunodeficiency syndrome. Lancet i: 1033–1038

Maurice P D L, Smith N P, Pinching A J 1982 Kaposi's sarcoma with benign course in a homosexual. Lancet i: 571

Mavligit G M, Talpaz M, Hsia F T, Wong W, Lichtiger B, Mansell P W A, Mumford D M 1984 Chronic immune stimulation by sperm alloantigens. Support for the hypothesis that spermatozoa induce immune dysregulation in homosexual males. Journal of the American Medical Association 251: 237–241

Melbye M, Biggar R J, Ebbesen P, Sarngadharan M G, Weiss S H, Gallo R C, Blattner W A 1984a Seroepidemiology of HTLV-III antibody in Danish homosexual men: prevalence, transmission and disease outcome. British Medical Journal 289: 573–575

Melbye M, Froebel K S, Madhok R et al 1984b HTLV-III seropositivity in European haemophiliacs exposed to factor VIII concentrate imported from the USA. Lancet ii: 1444–1446

Metroka C E, Cunningham-Rundles S, Pollack M S et al 1983 Generalized lymphadenopathy in homosexual men. Annals of Internal Medicine 99: 585–591

Miller D, Green J 1987 Counselling for HIV infection and AIDS. In: Pinching A J (ed) Clinics in immunology and allergy vol. 6, No 3. W B Saunders, Philadelphia, p 661–683

Miller D, Weber J, Green J (eds) 1986 The management of AIDS patients. MacMillan Press, Basingstoke

Miller J R, Barrett R E, Britton C B et al 1982 Progressive multifocal leukoencephalopathy in a male homosexual with T-cell immune deficiency. New England Journal of Medicine 307: 1436–1438

Mitchell C D, Bean B, Gentry S R, Groth K E, Boen J R, Balfour H H 1981 Acyclovir therapy for mucocutaneous herpes simplex infections in immunocompromised patients. Lancet i: 1389–1392

Mitchell W M, Montefiori D C, Robinson W E, Strayer D R, Carter W A 1987 Mismatched double-stranded RNA (Ampligen) reduces concentration of zidovudine (Azidothymidine) required for in-vitro inhibition of human immunodeficiency virus. Lancet i: 890–892

Mitsuya H, Broder S 1987 Review article. Strategies for antiviral therapy in AIDS. Nature 325: 773–778

Modlin R L, Hofman F M, Meyer P R et al 1983 Altered distribution of B and T lymphocytes and lymph nodes from homosexual men with Kaposi's sarcoma. Lancet ii: 768–771

Montagnier L, Gruest J, Chamaret S et al 1984 Adaptation of lymphadenopathy associated virus (LAV) to replication in EBV-transformed B-lymphoblastoid cell lines. Science 225: 63–66

Morris L, Distenfeld A, Amorosi E, Karpatkins S 1982 Autoimmune thrombocytopenic purpura in homosexual men. Annals of Internal Medicine 96: 714–717

Mortimer P P, Jesson W J, Vandervelde E M, Pereira M J 1985a Prevalence of antibody to human T-lymphotropic virus type III by risk group and area, United Kingdom 1978–1984. British Medical Journal 290: 1176–1178

Mortimer P P, Vandervelde E M, Jesson W J, Pereira M J, Burkhardt F 1985b HTLV-III antibody in Swiss and English intravenous drug abusers. Lancet ii: 449–450

Mosca J D, Bednarik D P 1987 Herpes simplex virus type 1 can reactivate transcription of latent human immunodeficiency virus. Nature 325: 67–73

Moskowitz L B, Gregorios J B, Hensley G T, Berger J R 1984 Cytomegalovirus. Induced demyelination associated with acquired immune deficiency syndrome. Archives of Pathology and Laboratory Medicine 108: 873–877

Murphy M F, Metcalfe P, Waters A H, Linch D C, Cheinsong-Popov R, Carne C, Weller I V D 1985 Immune neutropaenia in homosexual men. Lancet i: 217–218

Nicholson J K A, McDougall J S, Spira T J, Cross G D, Jones B M, Reinberg E L 1984 Immunoregulatory subsets of the T helper and T suppressor cell populations in homosexual men with chronic unexplained lymphadenopathy. Journal of Clinical Investigation 73: 191–201

Ognibene F P, Steis R G, Macher A M et al 1985 Kaposi's sarcoma causing pulmonary infiltrates and respiratory failure in the acquired immunodeficiency syndrome. Annals of Internal Medicine 102: 471–475

Palestine A G, Stevens G Jr, Lane H C et al 1986 Treatment of CMV retinitis with dihydroxy propoxymethyl guanine. American Journal of Ophthalmology 101: 95–101

Papaevangelou G, Roumeliotou-Karayannis A, Kallinikos G, Papoutsakis G 1985 LAV/HTLV-III infection in female prostitutes. Lancet ii: 1108

Pape J W, Liautaud B, Thomas F et al 1983 Characteristics of the acquired immunodeficiency syndrome (AIDS) in Haiti. New England Journal of Medicine 309: 945–950

Pert C B, Hill J M, Ruff M R et al 1986 Octapeptides deduced from the neuropeptide receptor-like pattern of antigen T4 in brain potently inhibit human immunodeficiency virus receptor binding and T-cell infectivity. Proceedings of the National Academy of Sciences USA 83: 9254–9258

Petito C, Navia B A, Cho E-S, Jordan B D, George D C, Price R W 1985 Vacuolar myelopathy pathologically resembling subacute combined degeneration in patients with the acquired immunodeficiency syndrome. New England Journal of Medicine 312: 874–879

Pinching A J, McManus T J, Jeffries D J et al 1983 Studies of cellular immunity in male homosexuals in London. Lancet ii: 126–129

Piot P, Quinn T C, Taelman H et al 1984 Acquired immunodeficiency syndrome in a heterosexual population in Zaire. Lancet ii: 65–69

Pitchenik A E, Shafron R D, Glasser R M, Spira T J 1984 The acquired immunodeficiency syndrome in the wife of a hemophiliac. Annals of Internal Medicine 100: 62–65

Prober C G, Kirk L E, Keeney R E 1982 Acyclovir therapy of chickenpox in immunosuppressed children — a collaborative study. Journal of Pediatrics 101: 622–625

Profeta S, Forrester C, Eng R H K, Liu R, Johnson E, Palinkas R, Smith S M 1985 Salmonella infections in patients with acquired immunodeficiency syndrome. Archives of Internal Medicine 145: 670–672

Purtilo D T, Sakamoto K, Baruabei V et al 1982 Epstein-Barr virus induced diseases in boys with X-linked lymphoproliferative infective syndrome (XLP). American Journal of Medicine 73: 49–56

Quinnan G V, Masur H, Rook A H et al 1984 Herpesvirus infections in the acquired immune deficiency syndrome. Journal of the American Medical Association 252: 72–77

Rao T K S, Filippone E J, Nicastri A D, Landesman S H, Frank E, Chen C K, Friedman E A 1984 Associated focal and segmental glomerulosclerosis in the acquired immunodeficiency syndrome. New England Journal of Medicine 310: 669–673

Redfield R R, Markham P D, Salahuddin S Z et al 1985 Frequent transmission of HTLV-III among spouses of patients with AIDS-related complex and AIDS. Journal of the American Medical Association 253: 1571–1573

Resnick L, di Marzo-Veronese F, Schüpbach J et al 1985 Intra-blood-brain-barrier synthesis of HTLV-III specific IgG in patients with neurologic symptoms associated with AIDS or AIDS related complex. New England Journal of Medicine 313: 1498–1504

Robertson J R, Roberts J J K, Buchnall A B V, Welsby P D, Brettle R P, Inglis J M, Peutherer J F 1986 Epidemic of AIDS-related virus (HTLV-III/LAV) infection among intravenous drug abusers. British Medical Journal 292: 527–529

Rodrigo J M, Serra M A, Aguilar E, del Olmo J A, Gimeno V, Aparisi L 1985 HTLV-III antibodies in drug addicts in Spain. Lancet ii: 156–157

Ruskin J 1981 Parasitic diseases in the compromised host. In: Rubin R H, Young L S (eds) Clinical approach to infection in the compromised host. Plenum Medical Book Company, New York, p 269–334

Safai B, Sarngadharan M G, Groopman J F et al 1984 Seroepidemiological studies of human T-lymphotropic retrovirus type III in acquired immunodeficiency syndrome. Lancet i: 1438–1440

Salahuddin S Z, Groopman J E, Markham P D et al 1984 HTLV-III in symptom free seronegative persons. Lancet ii: 1418–1420

Sandstrom E G, Kaplan J C, Byington R E, Hirsch M S 1985 Inhibition of human T-cell lymphotropic virus type III in vitro by phosphonoformate. Lancet i: 1480–1482

Sarngadharan M F, Markham P D, Gallo R C 1985 Part II: HTLV-III. In: Fields B N, Knipe D M, Chanock R M, Melnick J L, Roizman B, Shope R E (eds) Virology. Raven Press, New York, p 1359–1371

Schroff R W, Gottlieb M S, Prince H E, Chai L L, Fahey J L 1983 Immunological studies of homosexual men with immunodeficiency and Kaposi's sarcoma. Clinical Immunology and Immunopathology 27: 300–314

Scott G B, Buck B E, Leterman J G, Bloom F L, Parks W P 1984 Acquired immunodeficiency syndrome in infants. New England Journal of Medicine 310: 76–81

Scott G B, Fischl M A, Klimas N, Fletcher M A, Dickinson G M, Levine R S, Parks W P 1985 Mothers of infants with the acquired immunodeficiency syndrome. Evidence for both symptomatic and asymptomatic carriers. Journal of the American Medical Association 253: 363–366

Seemayer T A, Laroche A C, Russo P et al 1984 Precocious

thymic involution manifest by epithelial injury in the acquired immune deficiency syndrome. Human Pathology 15: 469–474

Shaw G M, Harper M E, Hahn B H et al 1985 HTLV-III infection in brains of children and adults with AIDS encephalopathy. Science 227: 177–181

Shiach C R, Burt A D, Isles C G, Ball S G 1984 Pyrexia of undetermined origin, diarrhoea and primary cerebral lymphoma associated with acquired immunodeficiency. British Medical Journal 288: 449–450

Siegal F P, Lopez C, Hammer G S et al 1981 Severe acquired immunodeficiency in male homosexuals, manifested by chronic perianal ulcerative herpes simplex lesions. New England Journal of Medicine 305: 1439–1444

Smith P D, Ohura K, Masur H, Lane H P, Fauci A S, Wahl S M 1984 Monocyte function in the acquired immune deficiency syndrome. Defective chemotaxis. Journal of Clinical Investigation 74: 2121–2128

Snider W D, Simpson D M, Nielsen S, Gold J W M, Metroka C E, Posner J B 1983 Neurological complications of acquired immune deficiency syndrome: analysis of 50 patients. Annals of Neurology 14: 403–418

Soave R, Donner R L, Honig C L, Ma P, Hart C C, Nash J, Roberts R B 1984 Cryptosporidiosis in homosexual men. Annals of Internal Medicine 100: 504–511

Spira T J, Des Jarlais D C, Marmor M et al 1984 Prevalence of antibody to lymphadenopathy-associated virus among drug-detoxification patients in New York. Correspondence, New England Journal of Medicine 311: 467–468

Stewart G J, Tyler J P P, Cunningham A L, Barr J A, Driscoll G L, Gold J, Lamont B J 1985 Transmission of human T-cell lymphotropic virus type III (HTLV-III) by artificial insemination by donor. Lancet ii: 581–584

Stoler M H, Eskin T A, Benn S, Angerer R C, Angerer L M 1986 Human T-cell lymphotropic virus type III infection of the central nervous system. A preliminary in situ analysis. Journal of the American Medical Association 256: 2360–2364

Thiry L, Sprecher-Goldberger S, Jonckheer T et al 1985 Isolation of AIDS virus from cell-free breast milk of three healthy virus carriers. Correspondence, Lancet ii: 891–892

Tirelli U, Vaccher E, Carbone A, de Paoli P, Santini G F, Monfardini S 1985 HTLV-III antibody in prostitutes. Lancet ii: 1424

Tucker J, Ludlam C A, Craig A et al 1985 HTLV-III infection associated with glandular fever-like illness in a haemophiliac. Lancet i: 585

Valle S-L, Saxinger C, Ranki A, Antonen J, Suni J, Lahdevirta J, Krohn K 1985 Diversity of clinical spectrum of HTLV-III infection. Lancet i: 301–304

Valone F H, Payan D G, Abrams D I, Goetzl E J 1984 Defective polymorphonuclear leukocyte chemotaxis in homosexual men with persistent lymph node syndrome. Journal of Infectious Diseases 150: 267–271

Van de Perre P, Clumeck N, Carael M et al 1985 Female prostitutes: a risk group for infection with human T-cell lymphotropic virus type III. Lancet ii: 524–526

Vandepitte J, Verwilghen R, Zachee P 1983 AIDS and cryptococcosis (Zaire 1977). Lancet i: 923–924

Viera J, Frank E, Spira T J, Landesman S H 1983 Acquired immune deficiency in Haitians: opportunistic infections in previously healthy Haitian immigrants. New England Journal of Medicine 308: 125–129

Vilmer E, Barré-Sinoussi F, Rouzioux C et al 1984 Isolation of new lymphotropic retrovirus from two siblings with haemophilia B, one with AIDS. Lancet i: 753–757

Vogt M W, Witt D J, Craven D E, Byington R, Crawford D F, Schooley R J, Hirsch M J 1986 Isolation of HTLV-III/LAV from cervical secretions of women at risk for AIDS. Lancet i: 525–527

Walker M M, Griffiths C E M, Weber J et al 1987 Dermatological conditions in HIV infection. British Medical Journal 294: 29–32

Walsh C M, Nardi M A, Karpatkin S 1984 On the mechanism of thrombocytopenia purpura in sexually active homosexual men. New England Journal of Medicine 311: 635–639

Weber J N, Clapham P R, Weiss R A et al 1987 Human immunodeficiency virus infection in two cohorts of homosexual men: neutralising sera and association of anti-gag antibody with prognosis. Lancet i: 119–121

Weinberg J R, Dootson G, Gertner D, Chambers S T, Smith H 1985 Disseminated *Mycobacterium xenopi* infection. Lancet i: 1033–1034

Wetterberg L, Alexius B, Saaf J, Sonnerborg A, Britton S, Pert C 1987 Peptide T in the treatment of AIDS. Correspondence, Lancet i: 159

Whiteside M E, Barkin J S, May R G, Weiss S D, Fischl M A, MacLeod C L 1984 Enteric coccidiosis among patients with the acquired immunodeficiency syndrome. American Journal of Tropical Medicine and Hygiene 33: 1065–1072

Wofsy C, Cohen J, Hauer L et al 1986 Isolation of HYLV-III/LAV from cervical secretions of women at risk for AIDS. Lancet i: 527–529

Wright K 1986 AIDS therapy. First tentative signs of therapeutic promise. Nature 323: 283

Yarchoan R, Broder S 1987 Special report. Development of antiretroviral therapy for the acquired immunodeficiency syndrome and related disorders, a progress report. New England Journal of Medicine 316: 557–564

Yarchoan R, Klecker R W, Weinhould K J et al 1986 Administration of 3′-azido-3′ deoxythymidine, an inhibitor of HYLV-III/LAV replication, to patients with AIDS or AIDS-related complex. Lancet i: 575–580

Yarchoan R, Berg G, Brouwers P et al 1987 Response of human-immunodeficiency-virus-associated neurological disease to 3′-azido-3′-deoxythymidine. Lancet i: 132–135

Zagury D, Bernard J, Leibowitch J et al 1984 HTLV-III in cells cultured from semen of two patients with AIDS. Science 226: 449–451

Ziegler J L, Beckstead J A, Volberding P A et al 1984 Non-Hodgkin's lymphoma in 90 homosexual men. Relation to generalized lymphadenopathy and the acquired immunodeficiency syndrome. New England Journal of Medicine 311: 565–570

Ziegler J B, Cooper D A, Johnson R O, Gold J 1985 Postnatal transmission of AIDS-associated retrovirus from mother to infant. Lancet i: 896–898

32

Molluscum contagiosum

The lesions of molluscum contagiosum are benign virus-induced tumours affecting the human skin and conjunctiva exclusively. The lesions are manifested clinically by discrete papules, waxy in appearance, with a cornified centre which may be umbilicated or project as a plug. Close physical contact, often under moist conditions, appears to be necessary for transmission of the causative organism, a virus of the pox group.

AETIOLOGY

The virus of molluscum contagiosum (MCV), although easily obtained in abundance from the skin lesions, cannot be grown in culture outside the human host. From its size (300 × 200 × 100 nm), shape, fine structure, cytoplasmic site of replication and characteristic inclusion body, the virus is classed as a member of the poxvirus family. In contrast to other DNA viruses, poxviruses lack icosahedral symmetry and have a complex structure (Moss 1985). The genome is a single linear molecule of double-stranded DNA and the virion contains a virus-specified DNA-dependent RNA polymerase (Fenner 1985).

The virus may possibly enter the epidermis not only from the exterior, but also by haematogenous spread from a more distant site or, more probably, by tissue fluid or lymphatic spread from a nearby portal of entry in traumatized skin (Postlethwaite 1970).

The virus cannot be grown in vitro in cell culture. The apparent defectiveness of MCV in mouse embryo cells in vitro may be intrinsic, indicating a need for some complementary host-dependent factor which human epidermal cells in vivo can provide. Alternatively the MCV may be inactivated by prolonged exposure to the temperature of the human skin (Shand et al 1976).

TRANSMISSION

The contagious nature of the disease and its transmission by sexual contact have long been recognized (Henderson 1841, Paterson 1841). In temperate climates (e.g. in Aberdeen, Scotland) it has also been associated with outbreaks amongst those using communal facilities such as a swimming pool, where the virus was thought to have been transmitted by towels. Under these circumstances more boys than girls tended to be affected and there was a peak incidence between 10 and 12 years (Postlethwaite et al 1967). In contrast, in children in moist tropical areas in village settlements such as in Fiji and the West Sepik district of New Guinea, the peak incidence was 2–3 years and over half the cases occurred between the ages of 1 and 5 years (Postlethwaite et al 1967, Stuart et al 1971).

Although not proven, close physical contact — often under moist conditions — appears to be necessary for transmission, as is seen in spread from the external genitalia of one sexual partner to the external genitalia of the other, from masseuse to client and from sibling to sibling (Leading Article 1968, Felman & Nikitas 1983). Infection of the newborn has been reported and raises doubts about the incubation period, ordinarily said to be 14–15 days (Mandel & Lewis 1971). An isolated case has been recorded of the appearance of molluscum contagiosum following professional tattooing, when lesions were localized to the sites inoculated with the carbon pigment (Foulds 1982).

IMMUNOLOGY

Virion antigens are detectable from the time of appearance of the earliest lesion and are found in the stratum spinosum, granular and keratin layers. Virus-specific antibodies are present in the serum in nearly 70% of patients, being of the IgG class in 58%, IgM in 30% and IgA in 10%: the failure to detect antibody in 30% of patients may be due to a lack of sensitivity of the fluorescent antibody technique used or to the fact that virion antigens are released from superficial lesions only after trauma and hence do not induce a humoral immune response. The relatively low incidence of virus-specific IgM in patients' sera, in the presence of virus antigen within the lesion, is in contrast to the findings in wart-virus studies where there was a close correlation between the persistence of wart-virus antigens and wart-specific IgM (Shirodaria & Matthews 1977).

PATHOLOGY

The lesion consists of a localized mass of hypertrophied and hyperplastic epidermis extending down into the underlying dermis, without breaching the limiting basement membrane and projecting above the surface as a papule. Beginning in the lower cells of the stratum spinosum, the intracytoplasmic inclusion bodies, growing larger as the infected cells migrate through the stratum granulosum, ultimately enlarge the host cells, pushing aside their nuclei and assuming dimensions varying between 24–27 microns in width and 30–37 microns in length (Van Rooyen 1938). The core of the lesion consists of degenerating epidermal cells with inclusion bodies and keratin.

CLINICAL FEATURES

In children lesions appear in a generalized distribution or may be localized to the face, forearms or hands, suggesting spread by direct contact. The lesions are pearly, flesh-coloured, raised, firm, umbilicated skin nodules, usually about 2–5 mm in diameter. They may appear in most skin areas, singly or in groups, except for the palms and soles, where they are exceedingly rare. From the central pit, a white curdy material can be expressed. If the lesion is opened with a sterile needle the central core may not be easily detached. This core was described at the turn of the 18th century in Edward Jenner's notebok as a 'white body . . . . . . equal in solidity but not so opaque as the boild crystalline humour of a fishes eye' (Woods 1977).

Where transmission by sexual intercourse is the likely method of spread, lesions are seen on the inner aspect of the thigh and vulva in the case of the female (Wilkin 1977) and on the penis (Fig. 32.1), anterior aspect of the scrotum and pubic area in the male. Lesions often persist for many months or even for a few years, but most resolve spontaneously or following trauma or bacterial infection.

Sometimes molluscum contagiosum may appear in epidemic form. In 1977 it occurred in this way mainly among the young children of the Maasai pastoralists of the Rift valley (70 km west of Nairobi) at a time after famine when the relief diet was different from their normal milk diet. This epidemic, it was suggested, was an example of activation of a suppressed infection in patients being fed after a period of moderate famine.

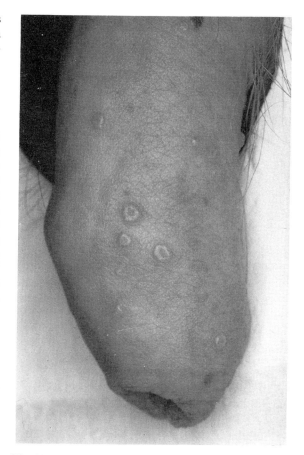

Fig. 32.1 Molluscum contagiosum involving the penis.

The molluscum lesions attained an unusually large size (12 mm). In this epidemic there was also an outbreak of oral or genital herpes, mostly affecting pregnant women within one month of delivery (Murray et al 1980).

DIAGNOSIS

Diagnosis is usually made by the characteristic appearance of the lesion. To identify the virus the surface of the lesion may be opened with the point of a disposable needle and the core extracted with forceps. Fine-toothed ophthalmological forceps are ideal for the purpose (Hoskin Forceps, No.11, Keeler Instruments Ltd., 21–27 Marylebone Lane, London, WIM 6DS). The core is placed on the inner wall of a dry specimen tube and ringed on the outside for ease of identification. In the laboratory after teasing out in saline, an electron-microscope grid is dipped in the suspension. After drying and staining with phosphotungstic acid it is examined by electronmicroscopy.

TREATMENT

Lesions should be treated by destruction. Infiltration of the skin near the lesion with 1% lignocaine and destruction by electrocautery is the preferred method. Complete removal of the lesion does not appear to be necessary as resolution usually follows damage to the core and its opening to the exterior.

REFERENCES

Felman Y M, Nikitas J A 1983 Sexually transmitted molluscum contagiosum. Symposium on Sexually Transmitted Diseases. Dermatologic Clinics 1: 103–110

Fenner F 1985 Poxvirus. In: Fields B N (ed) Virology. Raven Press, New York, p 661–684

Foulds I S 1982 Molluscum contagiosum: an unusual complication of tattooing. British Medical Journal 285: 607

Henderson W 1841 Notice of the molluscum contagiosum. Edinburgh Medical and Surgical Journal 56: 213–218

Leading Article 1968 Molluscum contagiosum. British Medical Journal 1: 459–460

Mandel M J, Lewis R J 1971 Molluscum contagiosum of the newborn. British Journal of Dermatology 84: 370–372

Moss B 1985 Replication of poxvirus. In: Fields B N (ed) Virology. Raven Press, New York, p 685–703

Murray M J, Murray A B, Murray N J, Murray M B, Murray C J 1980 Molluscum contagiosum and herpes simplex in Maasai pastoralists; refeeding activation of virus infection following famine? Transactions of the Royal Society of Tropical Medicine and Hygiene 74(3): 371–374

Paterson R 1841 Cases and observations on molluscum contagiosum of Bateman et al and account of the minute structure of the tumours. Edinburgh Medical and Surgical Journal 56: 279–288

Postlethwaite R 1970 Molluscum contagiosum, a review. Archives of Environmental Health 21: 432–452

Postlethwaite R, Watt J A, Hawley T G, Simpson I, Adam H 1967 Features of molluscum contagiosum in the northeast of Scotland and in Fijian village settlement. Journal of Hygiene (London) 65: 281–291

Shand J H, Gibson P, Gregory D W, Cooper R J, Keir H M, Postlethwaite R 1976 Molluscum contagiosum — a defective poxvirus? Journal of General Virology 33: 281–295

Shirodaria P V, Matthews R S 1977 Observations on the antibody responses in molluscum contagiosum. British Journal of Dermatology 96: 29–34

Stuart R J, Müller H K, Francis G D 1971 Molluscum contagiosum in villages of the West Sepik District of New Guinea. Medical Journal of Australia 2: 751–754

Van Rooyen C E 1938 The micromanipulation and microdissection of the molluscum contagiosum inclusion body. Journal of Pathology and Bacteriology 46: 425–436

Wilkin J K 1977 Molluscum contagiosum in a women's outpatient clinic: a venereally transmitted disease. American Journal of Obstetrics and Gynecology 128: 531–535

Woods B 1977 Edward Jenner and molluscum contagiosum. British Journal of Dermatology 96: 91–93

33

Lymphogranuloma venereum

Lymphogranuloma venereum is a sexually transmissible chlamydial infection and is to be found mainly in warm countries. In the cases seen in temperate climates the infection has been acquired in the tropics. The incubation period is short (2–5 days), after which an evanescent primary lesion develops on the genitals or in the rectum, or, rarely, elsewhere on the body. Two or three weeks after infection the draining lymph nodes enlarge, become matted together, fluctuant and eventually break down and discharge pus. If the disease is untreated the ano-genital region may become scarred and oedematous, and fistulae and strictures may develop. When pelvic nodes, which drain the cervix, upper vagina and rectum, are involved, exudate may be discharged into the pelvic viscera and cause scarring; strictures may develop subsequently.

AETIOLOGY

Lymphogranuloma venereum is caused by *Chlamydia trachomatis biovar lymphogranuloma* (see Ch. 2). The characteristics of chlamydiae have already been discussed in relation to the aetiology of non-gonococcal urethritis (Ch. 17). Inclusion bodies composed of aggregates of the organisms may be identified in scrapings taken from primary lesions, in pus aspirated from buboes, and in histological sections of affected lymph nodes (Jorgensen 1959). Using micro-immunofluorescence techniques, three serovars of *C. trachomatis* (*biovar lymphogranuloma*), viz. L-1, L-2 and L-3, have been identified (Wang & Grayston 1970; see Ch. 2).

Lymphogranuloma venereum is mainly acquired during sexual intercourse with an infected partner. Accidental infections, for example in doctors, are rare. Exudate from the primary lesion, discharging sinuses and the anus are infectious, as may be material from lesions which have persisted for years untreated.

EPIDEMIOLOGY

Lymphogranuloma venereum (LGV) has a worldwide distribution; it is common in tropical and subtropical areas, but rare in temperate climates. In England in 1983, for example, only 40 cases were recorded (30 males and 10 females). Infections diagnosed in the United Kingdom have almost always been acquired abroad; seamen and other travellers are most frequently affected (Alergant 1957). In tropical countries, prostitutes serve as an important source of infection. It seems that the global incidence of the disease is falling. LGV may be associated with other sexually transmitted diseases in the same patient.

PATHOLOGY AND PATHOGENESIS

The histological appearance of the primary genital lesion, a flat base of granulation tissue, surrounded by a narrow zone of necrosis, is not specific. The margins of the ulcer are undermined, and the adjacent epithelium may show pseudo-epitheliomatous hyperplasia. Lymphocytes and plasma cells infiltrate the underlying corium, where there may be necrotic foci.

The micro-organisms spread from the site of the initial lesion to the regional lymph nodes. Multiple necrotic foci appear within the parenchyma of the gland, followed by infiltration — initially with polymorphonuclear leucocytes, and later plasma cells. Marked hyperplasia of the germinal centres occurs.

With the enlargement and coalescence of necrotic areas, abscesses develop. The gland capsule becomes inflamed early in the disease and perinodal tissues, including skin, become involved in this inflammatory process. Penetration of the abscess through the skin results in the formation of multiple sinuses.

In the female, inguinal lymphadenitis is less common than in the male. This is probably because lymphatic fluid from the upper vagina and cervix drains to the external and internal iliac nodes. The disease in females usually presents at a later stage by chronic vulvar ulceration and oedema of the labia, the latter resulting from obstruction of lymphatic vessels by fibrous tissue in the vulva and in the lymph nodes. Evidence of continuing inflammation is manifest as areas of granulomatous tissue in the genitalia (Koteen 1945, Smith & Custer 1950). The name esthiomène, from the Greek meaning 'eaten away', has been applied to the disease at the stages when there has been marked destruction of tissue.

Rectal involvement, consisting essentially of ulceration of the mucosa with penetration of the muscular layer by inflammatory cells and subsequent stricture formation, although seen mainly in women, occurs also in homosexual men who have had anal intercourse. Proctitis associated with LGV serovars is discussed in Chapter 38.

CLINICAL FEATURES

The interval between exposure to infection and the appearance of the primary lesion, if this develops, is usually 2–5 days; longer intervals of up to 5 weeks have been described. A further interval of 1–6 weeks usually elapses before regional lymph node enlargement is detected. Untreated, the disease usually runs a course of between 6 and 8 weeks and may resolve completely. In many cases (at least 70%) there remain changes due to lymphatic obstruction; intermittent recrudescence of disease can occur. In the early stages, LGV may conveniently be divided from the clinical point of view into two syndromes, viz. the inguinal and the genito-anorecta (Abrams 1968).

Inguinal syndrome
This is the most frequent manifestation in the male; it is uncommon in females as the primary lesion is not commonly found in the lower vagina, or on the vulva. There are primary genital lesions, regional lymph node enlargement, and constitutional disturbances.

A history of a primary genital lesion, rare in females, is obtained in 20–50% of male cases. The lesion, usually a painless papulovesicle, tends to occur anywhere on the penis and heals within a few days. Rarely a sore within the urethral meatus may mimic a non-gonococcal urethritis. Extragenital lesions are rare, although oral infections are known to occur.

There is regional lymph node enlargement within 1–4 weeks of the appearance of the primary lesion. In most cases (at least 75%), there is unilateral involvement of the inguinal and/or femoral lymph nodes. The nodes are painful, tender, and although initially discrete, become matted together as a result of periadenitis. Occasionally, multilocular abscesses develop and coalesce within the lymph nodes, which become fluc-

tuant (bubo formation). Although, if untreated, buboes may resolve spontaneously within a few weeks, abscesses may rupture through the overlying adherent skin, producing multiple sinuses. Enlargement of lymph nodes, above and below the inguinal ligament, produces a grooved appearance in the groin, 'sign of the groove', a sign almost pathognomonic of LGV. Healing with scarring eventually occurs, although there may be recurrent sinus formation.

In women the inguinal syndrome is uncommon unless the primary lesion is on the vulva or in the lower vagina, since lymphatic drainage from these sites is to the inguinal nodes which may show the changes already described. Lymphatic drainage from lesions in the middle and upper vagina and the cervix is to the external and internal iliac and the sacral lymph nodes; inflammation of these glands may produce backache or symptoms of peritonitis. More commonly, there may be few symptoms in the early stage of the disease, which shows itself with later manifestations such as esthiomène. Although symptoms and signs of iliac lymph node involvement are rare, the efects of inflammatory reaction in the lumbar glands can be shown by lymphography (Osoba & Beetlestone 1976).

Constitutional symptoms occur more commonly in the inguinal syndrome than in the genito-anorectal syndrome. Pyrexia, malaise, nausea, arthralgia and headache are frequent. Less commonly (respectively about 10% in the female and 2% in the male) erythema nodosum or erythema multiforme may be seen.

Genito-anorectal syndrome
The clinical features of this syndrome are seen predominantly in women and in homosexual men. Extension of the inflammatory process by the lymphatic vessels of the rectovaginal septum, to the submucous tissues of the rectum is thought to be the principal factor involved in the production of the syndrome in females when the primary lesion has been in the vagina (King 1964).

The patient usually complains of bleeding from the anus and later a purulent anal discharge. On proctoscopy, the rectal mucosa is found to be inflamed with multiple punctate haemorrhages and there is a mucopurulent discharge. There may be superficial ulceration and polypoid growths. Histological examination of rectal biopsy material shows a non-specific granulomatous inflammatory reaction (Miles 1959, Quinn et al 1983). Although the rectum is most severely affected, a more generalized colitis often co-exists and can be demonstrated by barium enema examination (Annamunthodo & Marryatt 1961).

In the later stages of both syndromes, if the disease is untreated, lymphoedema may affect the genitalia of both sexes. The interval between the appearance of the early manifestations of the disease and the development of the later features varies between one and 20 years. Women may develop considerable oedema (elephantiasis) of the vulva with the formation of polypoid growths, fistulae, ulceration and scarring (esthiomène). Elephantiasis less frequently affects males, but obstruction of the lymphatic drainage of the external genitalia may led to oedema of the penis or scrotum and later to distortion of the penis. Strictures of the male and female urethra, with the formation of fistulae, are rare late complications.

In the genito-anorectal syndrome late complications include tubular rectal stricture, with or without proctitis and colitis, perianal abscesses, perineal and rectovaginal fistulae. Intestinal obstruction may result from stricture formation, and carcinoma may develop on a chronic rectal stricture (Morson 1964).

DIAGNOSIS

Diagnosis is based on the history, clinical features of the disease backed by bacteriological and serological tests; intradermal tests such as the Frei test are obsolete.

Culture of the organism

Giemsa-stained smears of scrapings from a suspected primary lesion and pus aspirated from a lymph node may be examined by microscopy for inclusions. Attempts should be made to isolate the organism on tissue culture. Material, sent to the laboratory as quickly as possible on suitable transport medium, should be cultured on McCoy cells (see Ch. 17). After incubation, cell cultures are stained with iodine, Giemsa, or by immunofluorescence and examined microscopically for inclusions. Chlamydia are isolated only in about 30% of cases.

Demonstration of chlamydial antigen in tissue biopsies

Using immunofluorescent and immunoperoxidase methods Alacoque et al (1984) have detected chlamydial antigens within the macrophages of biopsy specimens of the granulation tissue from a patient with long-standing LGV and have suggested that such immunological methods may be useful in diagnosis.

Serological tests

Lymphogranuloma venereum complement fixation test (LGVCFT)
The chlamydial group antigen used in this test is prepared from the organism causing enzootic abortion of ewes. This test generally becomes positive during the initial 4 weeks of infection and the titre rises during this period in the untreated patient. Titres of 1 : 16 are

regarded as significant, but as 3–4% of the normal population will give a positive test at this titre, it should be repeated in doubtful cases after 2–3 weeks, to detect a rising titre.

In early LGV the LGVCFT titres fall after treatment and the test usually becomes negative after a variable period of months to several years. Treatment of chronic LGV rarely results in any change in the titre, which may remain high for the rest of the patient's life. If untreated, complement-fixing antibodies may persist for years at high titre; there is a tendency, however, for these titres to diminish, and the results of the test sometimes become negative spontaneously.

In infections with other serotypes of *Chlamydia trachomatis* or *Chlamydia psittaci* cross-reactions occur, but titres of the LGVCFT are usually low.

Micro-immunofluorescence typing (micro-IF test) (Wang & Grayston 1970)
Using this technique, anti-chlamydial type-specific antibody can be detected in the serum and the particular serovar (L-1, L-2, or L-3) of the infecting organism identified. The latter test is available only in a few specialist centres.

Intradermal test (Frei test)
The Frei test is not used, because it not only has the disadvantage of a delayed hypersensitivity test in the evaluation of acute illness but also may be associated with false-positive and false-negative reactions (Schachter et al 1969). The antigen for this test used to be prepared commercially from a growth of chlamydiae in the yolk sacs of chick embryos.

Other laboratory tests
During the course of untreated LGV, the erythrocyte sedimentation rate is usually elevated, particularly in chronic cases. This presumably reflects changes in the levels of plasma proteins. The gamma globulin fraction of the serum is usually elevated, the albumin being normal or low. The total white cell count in the blood is often increased, with a relative lymphocytosis or monocytosis.

Differential diagnosis

Genital ulceration due to LGV must be carefully differentiated from syphilis by appropriate tests (Ch. 8). Other causes of genital ulceration may need to be excluded (Ch. 37).

Lymph node enlargement may occur in syphilis, herpes genitalis, granuloma inguinale, infectious mononucleosis, and in the reticuloses. Usually the onset of the glandular swelling in these cases is less acute and less painful, except in herpes genitalis.

Pyogenic infection, cat-scratch disease and tuberculosis may produce painful swollen inguinal lymph nodes with, or without, a history of a preceding lesion on the genitals.

TREATMENT

The aim of treatment is to eradicate the infecting organism, as far as possible to prevent further damage, and correct any deformities caused by the disease. It is important to examine, if possible, sexual contacts of people with LGV.

To eradicate the organism, sulphonamides and tetracyclines have been most commonly used. The sulphonamides have the advantage of not interfering with the diagnosis of syphilis, particularly in the incubation period of this disease. Sulphadimidine 1 g orally 4 times daily for at least 16 days may be used.

Oxytetracycline in a dosage of 500 mg orally 4 times per day for at least 14 days is usually satisfactory for the treatment of early-stage LGV. Therapy is guided by resolution of suppurating lymph nodes, reduction in size of the nodes, healing of sinuses, and improvement in the patient's general condition.

Response to antibiotic treatment is better in LGV in the early stage than in the late, when repeated prolonged courses may be required. At this stage improvement may not occur.

Buboes should be aspirated with aseptic precautions through a wide bore needle (No. 19 SWG) before they rupture spontaneously. Fluctuant glands should not be incised, as this delays healing. Clean surgical removal of the affected glands appears to be an effective treatment.

Surgical treatment, with simultaneous antibiotic therapy, is often required in the management of late LGV. Polypoid growths on the vulva require excision, and fistulae need surgical repair. Rectal strictures will require regular dilatation, or excision and a colostomy. A stricture may cause acute intestinal obstruction.

REFERENCES

Abrams A J 1968 Lymphogranuloma venereum. Journal of the American Medical Association 205: 199–202

Alacoque B, Cloppet H, Dumontel C, Moulin G 1984 Histological, immunofluorescent, and ultrastructural features of lymphogranuloma venereum. British Journal of Venereal Diseases 60: 390–395

Alergant C D 1957 Lymphogranuloma inguinale in the male in Liverpool, England, 1947 to 1954. British Journal of Venereal Diseases 33: 47–51

Annamunthodo H, Marryatt J 196I Barium studies in intestinal lymphogranuloma venereum. British Journal of Radiology 34: 53–57

Jorgensen L 1959 Lymphogranuloma venereum. A study of the pathology and pathogenetic problems based on observation of eight cases examined post-mortem. Acta Pathologica et Microbiologica Scandinavica 47: 113–139

King A J 1964 Lymphogranuloma venereum. In: Recent advances in venereology. Churchill, London, p 311

Koteen H 1945 'Lymphogranuloma venereum'. Medicine 24: 1–69

Miles R P M 1959 Rectal lymphogranuloma venereum. Postgraduate Medical Journal 35: 92–96

Morson B C 1964 Anorectal venereal disease. Proceedings of the Royal Society of Medicine, London 57: 179–180

Osoba A O, Beetlestone C A 1976 Lymphographic studies in acute lymphogranuloma venereum infection. British Journal of Venereal Diseases 52: 399–403

Quinn T C, Stamm W E, Goodell S E et al 1983 The polymicrobial origin of intestinal infections in homosexual men. New England Journal of Medicine 309: 576–582

Schachter J, Smith D E, Dawson C R 1969 Lymphogranuloma venereum. I. Comparison of the Frei test, complement fixation test, and isolation of the agent. Journal of Infectious Diseases 120: 372–375

Smith E B, Custer P 1950 'The histopathology of lymphogranuloma venereum'. Journal of Urology 63: 546–563

Wang S-P, Grayston J T 1970 Immunological relationship between genital TRIC, lymphogranuloma venereum and related organisms in a new microtiter, indirect immunofluorescent test. American Journal of Ophthalmology 70: 367–374

34

Chancroid

Chancroid is a sexually transmissible disease caused by infection with the bacterium *Haemophilus ducreyi*. There is a high incidence in tropical countries, particularly in areas where living standards are low. Prostitutes constitute an important reservoir of infection. Chancroid may also occur in temperate climates as evidenced by recent outbreaks.

After a prepatent period, usually less than one week, one or more ulcers develop on the genitalia, and are associated, in about half of cases, with inguinal lymphadenitis. Untreated, an abscess develops in the affected lymph nodes and this may rupture through the skin, producing a sinus. Extensive tissue destruction is a distressing complication of the disease.

In the past a diagnosis of chancroid was generally based on clinical findings and exclusion of other conditions. This is no longer acceptable, and a definitive diagnosis of chancroid should be made only where *H. ducreyi* is recovered from genital ulcers.

Resistance to both sulphonamides and tetracyclines is common, and the recommended treatment is erythromycin or co-trimoxazole.

AETIOLOGY

Haemophilus ducreyi

Morphological and cultural characteristics
The causative organism *H. ducreyi* was first described in 1889 by Ducrey (1890): it is a small Gram-negative cocco-bacillus which tends to occur in clumps or chains. In smears made from lesions, or material aspirated from swollen regional lymph glands, intracellular as well as extracellular bacteria may be noted. Typically *H. ducreyi* is seen as short rods in a mucous matrix forming a 'railroad track' or 'shoal of fish' pattern. A similar characteristic pattern is obtained when growth is taken from solid media, crushed on a slide and Gram-stained (Oberhofer & Back 1982).

H. ducreyi is a fastidious organism: a humid atmosphere enriched with 5–10% CO_2, incubation at 33–35°C, and a pH of 6.5 to 7.0 are required for optimum growth. For primary isolation culture, methods with liquid/clotted-blood media have been superseded by solid selective media containing vancomycin. Rabbit, sheep or human blood may be used for enrichment, but horse blood should be avoided as few isolates of *H. ducreyi* will grow on horse blood agar (Nobre 1982).

Taxonomy and biochemical characterization
Our knowledge of the taxonomy of *H. ducreyi* is meagre. Kilian (1976) examined 9 strains of *H. ducreyi* in the course of his impressive study of 426 strains of the genus *Haemophilus*. There were differences between the strains of *H. ducreyi*, all of which were originally isolated from cases of chancroid: he divided them into 2 strains which he felt were acceptable as members of the *Haemophilus* genus, and 7 that were unacceptable. However, as he was unable to judge which of the two groups agreed with Ducrey's original description, he recorded all 9 strains as *H. ducreyi*.

Although new isolation and identification procedures have been developed, some properties of the species are still not clearly defined and its nutritional requirements, biochemical reactions and colony characteristics are still debated (Nobre 1982). For example, *H. ducreyi* has been considered oxidase-negative (Kilian 1976) and oxidase-positive (Sottnek et al 1980). However, Nobre (1982) noted that the oxidase test was positive with the tetramethyl-p-phenylenediamine dihydrochloride but negative with the dimethyl compound.

By definition the genus *Haemophilus* requires X factor (haemin or certain other porphyrins) or V factor (nicotinamide adenine dinucleotide) or both for growth. Although there have been reports that *H. ducreyi* does not require X factor, this is most likely a reflection of the culture medium and the strength of the discs used in the test. Hammond et al (1978c) found that *H. ducreyi* requires a greater haemin concentration for growth than do other *Haemophilus* spp.

The need for exogenous haemin was confirmed by a negative porphyrin test thus demonstrating the lack of enzymic capability of *H. ducreyi* to synthesize haemin from amino-laevulinic acid.

H. ducreyi tends to be inert in biochemical tests. Most investigators have reported little active carbohydrate fermentation, although Sng et al (1982) reported glucose, fructose and mannose utilization. Nitrate reduction is a useful positive character. However, depending on the test conditions, isolates may be nitrate-negative (Oberhofer & Back 1982). Alkaline phosphatase activity is another useful positive identification feature. Nitrate reduction and phosphatase activity form the basis of the rapid identification of *H. ducreyi* in a commercially available system (Hannah & Greenwood 1982); lack of biochemical activity apart from nitrate reduction and phosphatase activity allowed differentiation between *H. ducreyi*, *H. influenzae*, *H. parainfluenzae* and *H. aphrophilus*.

Plasmid-mediated β-lactamase production
The first reports of β-lactamase activity in *H. ducreyi* were published in 1978 soon after the advent of β-lactamase production in *N. gonorrhoeae*. Hammond et al (1978a) examined the antibiotic susceptibility of 19 strains of *H. ducreyi* isolated during an outbreak of chancroid in Winnipeg, Manitoba, Canada. They found that 3 strains were resistant to ampicillin (MIC >128 μg/ml) and produced β-lactamase. Later the β-lactamase activity of these strains was shown to be mediated by a 6.0×10^6 daltons (6 Megadalton; 6 Mdal) non-conjugative plasmid (Brunton et al 1979). Further characterization (MacLean et al 1980) suggested that the β-lactamase produced by *H. ducreyi* was a TEM-1 β-lactamase coded for by a plasmid containing a Tn2 type transposon. Although the Tn2 type transposon is possibly of enteric origin, it has been transposed into a small non-self-transmissible plasmid shared by members of the genera *Haemophilus* and *Neisseria*. Ampicillin resistance plasmids in *H. ducreyi* can be transferred by conjugation to *Haemophilus* recipients, provided that the donor cell also harbours a 23.5 Mdal plasmid with the ability to mobilize the smaller resistance plasmid (Deneer et al 1982).

Handsfield et al (1981) studied plasmids from *H. ducreyi* isolated in Seattle, USA. All strains had an ampicillin resistance plasmid with a mol.wt. of either 7.3, 5.7 or 3.6 Mdal. Plasmid mol.wts were identical for isolates from epidemiologically linked cases and differed according to the geographical origins of the strains.

Although there are varying size estimates of plasmids reported by different authors, there are clear similarities between the plasmids of *H. ducreyi* and those of *N. gonorrhoeae*. The 5.7 (or 6.0) Mdal *H. ducreyi* plasmid carries the entire sequence of pFA7, the 3.2 Mdal β-lactamase-specifying plasmid found in isolates of *N. gonorrhoeae* epidemiologically linked to

West Africa. Plasmids of 7.0 (or 7.3) Mdal carry the entire sequence of pFA3, the 4.4 Mdal β-lactamase-specifying plasmid found in Far Eastern isolates of *N. gonorrhoeae* (Brunton et al 1982). The 3.2 (or 3.6) Mdalton *H. ducreyi* plasmid has also been shown to be the same as that found in gonococci (Anderson et al 1984). β-lactamase production is common among *H. ducreyi* isolates from diverse geographical areas, e.g. Orange County, California, USA (Anderson et al 1984), Singapore (Sng et al 1982), Johannesburg, South Africa (Mauff et al 1983) and Nairobi, Kenya (Fast et al 1982). Isolates of *H. ducreyi* from patients in Sheffield, England (Kinghorn et al 1982a) differ from strains isolated from patients with clinical chancroid in the above areas in being β-lactamase negative. In Sheffield, *H. ducreyi* was most commonly isolated as a secondary pathogen in herpetic lesions.

Virulence and pathogenicity
Virulence of *H. ducreyi* is determined by the intradermal injection of *H. ducreyi* into rabbits. the extent of induration and necrosis are graded according to the criteria outlined by Hammond et al (1978a). Virulent strains produce 0.5 cm of induration with a central inflammatory response at 4 days progressing to an eschar by 11 days. The rabbit intradermal test for virulence was positive for all 19 isolates from the chancroid epidemic in Winnipeg (Hammond et al 1978a). 4 reference strains of *H. ducreyi* gave negative virulence tests. The 'non-virulent' reference strains were inhibited by lower minimum inhibitory concentrations (MICs) of a range of antibiotics than were the virulent strains. Although β-lactamase negative strains associated with genital ulcers in Sheffield gave positive results in the rabbit virulence test (Kinghorn et al 1982a) their sensitivity to antibiotics was similar to non-virulent strains.

Virulent strains as defined by the rabbit virulence test are resistant to serum, to phagocytosis and to killing by human polymorphonuclear leucocytes (PMNLs) (Odumeru et al 1984). Non-virulent strains are sensitive to normal human serum and are readily killed by PMNLs. This association suggests that these factors may mediate the pathogenicity of *H. ducreyi*.

EPIDEMIOLOGY

On a global scale chancroid is a more important cause of genital ulceration than syphilis (Leading Article 1982). The incidence of chancroid is highest in tropical and subtropical countries. Cases reported in temperate climates are usually in patients who have acquired their infection in the tropics (and their subsequent contacts). In recent years there have been outbreaks of chancroid in Greenland (Lykke-Olesen et al 1979), Canada

(Hammond et al 1980), the United States (Carpenter et al 1981), and the Netherlands (Nayyar et al 1979).

The epidemiology of chancroid is poorly understood, but it is hoped that the advent of reliable culture methods for *M. ducreyi* will lead to a better understanding. It has long been considered, however, that there is an association between chancroid, poverty and poor standards of hygiene. Its incidence decreases as the standard of living improves. Chancroid is more prevalent in war-time, and prostitutes are thought to constitute an important reservoir of infection. Among American troops in the Korean war it was 14 to 21 times as common as gonorrhoea (Asin 1952) while in the Vietnam conflict chancroid was second to gonorrhoea among venereal diseases (Kerber et al 1969). Over a 12-month period Hart (1975) reported 269 cases of gonorrhoea, 253 of non-gonococcal urethritis, 163 of chancroid, 5 of syphilis and 62 of herpes genitalis among Australian troops in Vietnam. Unfortunately the diagnosis of chancroid was not made by isolation of *H. ducreyi* but by the appearance of the penile lesion, the presence of Gram-negative cocco-bacilli on Gram-stained smears, a negative dark ground examination, negative serological tests for syphilis and the lack of other demonstrable pathogens.

Recent cultural studies carried out in Nairobi, Kenya, have shown a good correlation between isolation of *H. ducreyi* and genital ulceration (Nsanze et al 1981). *H. ducreyi* was isolated from 60 (62%) of 97 patients with genital ulcers attending a special treatment clinic. No aetiological agent was isolated from 23 patients in whom a clinical diagnosis of chancroid was made. In Johannesberg, South Africa, *H. ducreyi* was isolated from 23 (74%) of 31 white men with genital ulcers (Mauff et al 1983).

Prostitutes are an important reservoir of infection (Plummer et al 1983). In a study of 300 men in Nairobi with culture-proven chancroid, 57% had acquired their infection from prostitutes. There was geographical clustering of areas of acquisition of infection in the city centre and several poorer residential areas, suggesting geographical and social integrity of high-frequency transmission groups. 39 contact pairs in whom the male partner had positive cultures were examined. In 10 pairs the woman was designated the source contact. 8 of the 10 women had symptomatic chancroid and 6 were culture positive. These findings suggest that most female transmitters of *H. ducreyi* have genital ulcers.

Of 29 women who were considered to be secondary contacts, 16 had symptomatic ulcers, 1 a symptomless ulcer and 12 no ulcers. 10 of the 17 women with ulcers had positive cultures. 3 of the 12 women with no evidence of genital ulceration on clinical examination had positive cervical cultures. In nearly half of the women in whom chancroid developed after exposure to the index man, sexual exposure occurred only while the man was incubating chancroid. The infectivity of *H. ducreyi* for women was 63% — secondary contacts who were infected with *H. ducreyi* or had genital ulcers with one exposure to an infected man. *H. ducreyi* infection in women was highly pathogenic; 10 of 13 infected had genital ulcers.

Among prostitute populations implicated in the transmission of chancroid, genital ulcers were detected in 10% and symptomless genital carriage of *H. ducreyi* in 4%. These women could either be transient or persistent carriers of *H. ducreyi* or could be incubating chancroid. Genital ulcers were less common in prostitutes not implicated in chancroid transmission and *H. ducreyi* carriage was not found in such women.

Studies from Sheffield, UK (Kinghorn et al 1982a) suggest that *H. ducreyi* may frequently occur as a secondary invader of damaged genital skin and mucosa. *H. ducreyi* was the most common bacterial pathogen in 161 patients with genital ulcers: it was isolated in 24 (30.8%) of 78 patients with primary herpes, 14 (26.9%) of 52 patients with recurrent herpes, and 8 (25.8%) of 31 patients with non-herpetic ulceration. *T. pallidum* was the cause of genital ulceration in only 1 patient.

These observations suggest a pool of infection amongst patients in Sheffield, the great majority of whom are not infected abroad. No such pool of infection occurs in Seattle, USA, where chancroid is rare and associated with clearly marked importations. Likewise, chancroid has not persisted in the locality following the chancroid outbreak in Greenland in 1977. Sheffield also appears to be atypical of the UK. There is a low incidence of *H. ducreyi* in genital ulcers in Manchester (Mallard et al 1983) and London (Forster et al 1983), with infection usually acquired abroad.

Piot et al (1983) in Antwerp, Belgium, isolated *H. ducreyi* from 3 of 68 consecutive patients with genital ulceration. All 3 men had been infected in chancroid endemic aeas. Genital herpes was diagnosed in 32 (47%) but was not accompanied by *H. ducreyi* infection in any patients. It was concluded that the lack of β-lactamase production by the Sheffield *H. ducreyi* strains suggests that these isolates may be different from *H. ducreyi*. Kinghorn et al (1982a) acknowledge that the Sheffield strains may have a lower pathogenicity in humans than have isolates from the tropics. However, the Sheffield isolates are pathogenic in rabbits and, apart from lack of β-lactamase production, are indistinguishable from strains isolated in Seattle and Manitoba (McEntegart et al 1982).

CLINICAL FEATURES

The prepatent period of chancroid is short, usually 2–3

days, although it may vary from as little as 24 hours to longer than 5 days (Harkness 1950).

The earliest lesion is a papule which soon becomes a pustule and ulcerates as a result of thrombotic occlusion of underlying dermal blood vessels. Characteristically, the superficial ulcer so formed is painful and tender. A grey membrane covers its floor and removal of this membrane reveals glistening granulation tissue which bleeds easily. The edges are ragged and undermined, and a narrow zone of erythema surrounds the ulcer. Unlike the primary lesion of syphilis, the lesions of chancroid are not indurated. The size of the individual ulcers varies from 3 to about 20 mm in diameter.

As a result of auto-inoculation of surrounding tissues, multiple ulcers are often produced and lesions at various stages of development are commonly seen in the same patient. Although single ulcers may occur, multiple ulcers are more common.

In the male, the lesions of chancroid most commonly occur at the preputial orifice, the resulting inflammation producing phimosis and commonly a paraphimosis. A suppurative balanoposthitis may result from the phimosis so produced and necessitate surgical drainage of the preputial sac by a dorsal slit. Less frequently ulceration may occur on the glans penis, the shaft of the penis or the distal urethra. Chancroid of the anal region may occur in male homosexuals, and auto-inoculation from penile lesions may produce lesions of the scrotum and thighs.

The labia majora, introitus, vagina and perianal region are most commonly affected in the female. Rarely, cervical lesions have been described.

Extragenital lesions of chancroid are rare, and disseminated *H. ducreyi* infection is unknown.

In at least 60% of patients with chancroid, inguinal lymph nodes become enlarged on one or both sides within days to weeks of the appearance of the genital lesions. Initially the nodes are discrete and not tender. In about half of those who develop lymphadenopathy, suppuration occurs in the nodes, which become tender, matted together and show evidence of unilocular abscess formation (bubo). The overlying skin, to which the inflamed glands adhere, becomes erythematous and if the inflammatory process continues, the bubo ruptures through the skin, forming a sinus. Bubo and sinus formation are usually unilateral (Kerber et al 1969).

Occasionally, ulceration becomes extensive, with considerable tissue destruction. In such cases, secondary bacterial infection, particularly with *Treponema vincentii*, *Fusobacterium nucleatum* and *Leptotrichia buccalis* (see Ch. 2), probably plays an important role in the destructive process.

In some cases ulceration may be more superficial, but cover a considerable area. Tissue destruction is minimal but healing is slow, with months or years elapsing before resolution is complete. Recurrent chancroid, although described, is a rarity.

It has been suggested that *H. ducreyi* may vary in virulence (McEntegart et al 1982). Apart from the classical clinical features of chancroid, certain strains may be less pathogenic and give rise to asymptomatic infections which may only be diagnosed when they subsequently infect already damaged tissue as secondary invaders. Once established in damaged tissue the organisms contribute to the persistence of lesions until specific treatment is given.

DIAGNOSIS

In the past diagnosis has often been made by exclusion of other causes of genital ulceration. A definitive dignosis of chancroid, however, should only be made when *H. ducreyi* is isolated from genital ulcers. Microscopy may give a rapid presumptive diagnosis.

Microscopy

A presumptive diagnosis may be made by finding organisms morphologically resembling *H. ducreyi* in stained smears prepared from material aspirated from a bubo or taken from the undermined edge of the ulcer: the lesions should be cleansed first with normal saline. Several staining methods can be used, such as Gram's or Giemsa. In preparing a smear, the swab should be rolled through 180° in one direction only, never back and forth, to maintain the arrangement of the organisms. Typically *H. ducreyi* is seen as short rods in a mucous matrix forming a 'rail-road track' or 'shoal of fish' pattern. The bacteria may exhibit bipolar staining.

Many cases previously diagnosed as chancroid have probably been examples of herpes genitalis, perhaps with secondary bacterial infection. Giemsa's stain may be helpful in identifying the giant balloon cells, frequently multinucleate, and the eosinophilic intracellular inclusion bodies characteristic of herpesvirus infections. Improvements in cultural diagnosis have shown that direct microscopy may lack sensitivity: in patients in whom no characteristic Gram-negative rods were seen, over 50% (22/41) of cultures grew *H. ducreyi* (Nsanze et al 1981).

Monoclonal antibodies

In future, suitable monoclonal antibody reagents should improve immediate diagnosis (Hansen & Loftus 1984). A monoclonal antibody against *H. ducreyi* has been evaluated by direct immunofluorescence against a panel of cultured *Haemophilus* spp and other bacteria found in the genital tract (Greenblatt et al 1985). The antibody gave strong fluorescence against 10 isolates of *H. ducreyi* originating from Kenya, South Asia and Canada.

Although 9 isolates of *H. influenzae*, including types B, C, D, E and F and 3 non-typable isolates, were non-reactive, 1 of 4 *H. parainfluenzae* isolates of vaginal origin gave moderately strong fluorescence. Suitable monoclonal antibodies would seem to have potential for the rapid diagnosis of *H. ducreyi* in patients with genital ulcer disease.

Culture

Material from the base of the ulcer is best inoculated directly on to suitable media. Culture plates should be transported to the laboratory as soon as possible and incubated at 35°C in a moist carbon dioxide-enriched atmosphere. Plates should be incubated for at least 72 hours. *H. ducreyi* colonies have a characteristic coherence and can be moved as an entire colony across the plate with an inoculating loop. The identity of the organisms may be confirmed by a negative porphyrin test (Hammond et al 1978c) and positive tests for alkaline phosphatase and nitrate reduction.

Media

For primary isolation, culture methods with liquid/clotted-blood media have been superseded by solid selective media containing vancomycin (3 μg/ml). Hammond et al (1978b), using a gonococcal agar base supplemented with 1% bovine haemoglobin, 1% Isovitalex enrichment and vancomycin (3 μg/ml), isolated *H. ducreyi* from 8 of 16 genital ulcers in Winnipeg, Canada. Addition of fetal calf serum to agar media improves the rates of isolation (Sottnek et al 1980). However, fetal calf serum is expensive and 5% sheep serum may be an acceptable alternative (Nsanze et al 1981).

Although Kinghorn et al (1982b) found that a modified haemin-containing medium worked well in Sheffield, it gave poor results in Nairobi. Piot et al (1983) isolated *H. ducreyi* from only 1 of 50 genital ulcer specimens plated on the Sheffield medium, compared with 35 positive isolates on a gonococcal agar base supplemented with 2% bovine haemoglobin, 5% fetal calf serum, 1% CVA enrichment (Gibco) and vancomycin (3 μg/ml).

As yet no single medium provides an optimal rate of isolation of *H. ducreyi* from genital ulcers. Nsanze et al (1984) compared Mueller-Minton agar base containing 5% chocolated horse blood (MH-HB) with a gonococcal agar base supplemented with 2% bovine haemoglobin and 5% fetal calf serum (GC-HgS): vancomycin (3 μg/ml) and 1% CVA enrichment (Gibco) were added to both media.

GC-HgS medium yielded positive cultures for *H. ducreyi* from 183 (71%) of 201 patients with clinical chancroid, in comparison with 142 (61%) positive cultures with MH-HB medium. 41 patients gave positive cultures only on GC-HgS medium, while 20 were positive only on MH-HB medium. The combination of both media increased the yield of positive cultures to 81%. It was concluded that the use of both media on a single split plate would optimize the detection of *H. ducreyi*.

Immunological diagnosis

Immunological techniques are no longer used in the diagnosis of chancroid. The Ito-Reenstierna skin test involved the intradermal inoculation of a suspension of killed *H. ducreyi* into one site and a control suspension alone at another site. The value of the test was limited due to cross-reaction with other bacteria.

Biopsy

Beneath the ulcerated surface of the lesion there are one or two deeper layers recognizable histologically. The deep zone shows a dense infiltration of plasma cells and lymphocytes, above which there is a marked endothelial proliferation, palisading of blood vessels, degeneration of their walls and occasional thrombosis (Sheldon & Heyman 1946). Routine biopsy, however, is not justifiable as a diagnostic method.

Differential diagnosis

Other conditions which produce ulceration of the genitalia (Ch. 37) must be considered in the differential diagnosis of chancroid, and syphilis must be excluded in all cases, as these diseases may co-exist in the individual patient. Details regarding the tests required to exclude syphilis are to be found in Chapter 8, but it is important to stress the need for searching for *T. pallidum* by dark ground microscopic examination of serum squeezed gently from the depth of lesions. *T. pallidum* may be identified in such serum specimens after drying, fixation in acetone and the application of tests based on monoclonal antibody (p. 118).

Infection with herpes simplex virus produces superficial multiple tender ulcers, which are not indurated, and this condition must be carefully excluded. In the absence of suitable laboratory facilities, it may be impossible to differentiate between the two diseases.

It is possible that some chancroid-like ulcers may be a non-specific host reaction to a variety of organisms rather than a single entity. Lymphogranuloma venereum may co-exist with chancroid, as may other sexually transmitted diseases.

TREATMENT

Chemotherapy

Resistance to sulphonamides and tetracyclines, the

traditional treatments for chancroid, is now common in Africa and the Far East. Some strains of *H. ducreyi* contain a 4.9 Mdal sulphonamide resistance plasmid (Fast et al 1983). Most clinical isolates also produce a β-lactamase of the TEM type mediated by small non-conjugative plasmids (p. 192).

The currently recommended drug treatments include either erythromycin 500 mg 4 times daily for 14 days (Duncan et al 1983) or co-trimoxazole (800 mg sulphamethoxazole with 160 mg trimethoprim) twice-daily for 7 days (Fast et al 1983).

A 7-day course of the combination of amoxycillin (250 mg) and clavulanic acid (125 mg) at a dosage equivalent to 2 tablets 3 times a day was highly effective in eradicating *H. ducreyi* (Fast et al 1982). Limited data also suggest adequate cure rate with single-dose regimens such as 2 g spectinomycin intramuscularly, or 250 mg ceftriaxone intramuscularly. These newer treatments, however, are costly. Streptomycin given intramuscularly in a dose of 1 g daily for 7–14 days remains a reasonably effective alternative.

Local treatment

Local treatment of chancroid consists of frequently repeated application of saline dressings to the ulcerated area to reduce the risk of development of secondary infection. A strip of gauze soaked in saline may be applied to separate inflamed surfaces. When a phimosis is present, and a balanoposthitis develops, the preputial sac should be gently irrigated with normal saline at hourly intervals. In more severe cases, to secure drainage and to prevent phagedaenic ulceration of the glans, a slit should be made, extending dorsally along the prepuce from its orifice (dorsal slit) under general anaesthesia. Such surgical procedures are preferably delayed until after ulcer healing to avoid secondary chancroidal ulcers at the line of incision (Leading Article 1982).

Buboes should be aspirated before commencing treatment with antimicrobial drugs. The efficacy of antimicrobial therapy on the inguinal adenitis of chancroid has been equivocal, and buboes have been reported to develop during antimicrobial therapy despite ulcer healing (Marmar 1972).

REFERENCES

Anderson B, Albritton W L, Biddle J, Johnson S R 1984 Common Beta-lactamase specifying plasmid in *Haemophilus ducreyi* and *Neisseria gonorrhoeae*. Antimicrobial Agents and Chemotherapy 25: 296–297

Asin J 1952 Chancroid. American Journal of Syphilis, Gonorrhea and Venereal Diseases 36: 483–487

Brunton J L, Maclean I, Ronald A R, Albritton W L 1979 Plasmid-mediated ampicillin resistance in *Haemophilus ducreyi*. Antimicrobial Agents and Chemotherapy 15: 294–299

Brunton J, Meier M, Ehrman N, Maclean I, Sloney L, Albritton W L 1982 Molecular epidemiology of beta-lactamase-specifying plasmids of *Haemophilus ducreyi*. Antimicrobial Agents and Chemotherapy 21: 857–862

Carpenter J L, Back A, Gehle D, Oberhoffer T 1981 Treatment of chancroid with erythromycin. Sexually Transmitted Diseases 8: 192–197

Deneer H G, Sloney L, Maclean F W, Albritton W L 1982 Mobilization of non-conjugative antibiotic resistance plasmids in *Haemophilus ducrei*. Journal of Bacteriology 149: 726–732

Ducrey A 1890 Recherches expérimentales sur la nature intime du principe contagieux du chancre mou. Annales de Dermatologie et de Syphiligraphie 1: 56–57

Duncan M O, Bilgeri Y R, Fehler M G, Ballard R C 1983 Treatment of chancroid with erythromycin. A clinical and microbiological appraisal. British Journal of Venereal Diseases 59: 265–268

Fast M, Nsanze H, D'Costa L, Plummer F A, Karasira P, Maclean I W, Ronald A R 1982 Treatment of chancroid by clavulanic acid with amoxycillin in patients with Betalactamase-positive *Haemophilus ducreyi* infection. Lancet ii: 509–511

Fast M V, Nsanze H, Plummer F A, D'Costa L J, Maclean I W, Ronald A R 1983 Treatment of chancroid. A comparison of sulphamethoxazole and trimethoprim-sulphamethoxazole. British Journal of Venereal Diseases 59: 320–324

Forster G E, Karim Q N, White K B, Harris J R W 1983. Isolating *Haemophilus ducreyi*. Correspondence, Lancet ii: 910

Greenblatt R M, Hansen E J, Lukehart S A 1985 Specificity of monoclonal antibody to *Haemophilus ducreyi*. Abstract. 6th International Meeting of the International Society STD Research, Brighton, England

Hammond G W, Lian C-J, Wilt J C, Ronald A R 1978a Antimicrobial susceptibility of *Haemophilus ducreyi*. Antimicrobial agents and Chemotherapy 13: 608–612

Hammond G W, Lian C-J, Wilt J C, Ronald A R 1978b Comparison of specimen collection and laboratory techniques for isolation of *Haemophilus ducreyi*. Journal of Clinical Microbiology 7: 39–43

Hammond G W, Lian F-J, Wilt J C, Albritton W L, Ronald A R 1978c Determination of the hemin requirement of *Haemophilus ducreyi*: evaluation of the porphyrin test and media used in the satellite growth test. Journal of Clinical Microbiology 7: 243–246

Hammond G W, Slutchuk M, Scotliff J, Sherman E, Wilt J C, Ronald A R 1980 Clinical, epidemiological, laboratory and therapeutic features of an urban outbreak of chancroid in North America. Review of Infectious Diseases 2: 867–879

Handsfield H H, Totten P A, Fennel C L, Falkow S, Holmes K K 1981 Molecular epidemiology of *Haemophilus ducreyi* infections. Annals of Internal Medicine 95: 315–318

Hannah P, Greenwood J R 1982 Isolation and rapid identification of *Haemophilus ducreyi*. Journal of Clinical Microbiology 16: 861–864

Hansen E J, Loftus T A 1984 Monoclonal antibodies reactive with all strains of *Haemophilus ducreyi*. Infection and Immunity 44: 196–198

Harkness A H 1950 Chancroid. In: Non-gonococcal urethritis. Livingstone, Edinburgh, p 182

Hart G 1975 Venereal disease in a war environment. Incidence and management. Medical Journal of Australia 1: 808–810

Kerber R E, Rowe C E, Gilbert K R 1969 Treatment of chancroid. A comparison of tetracycline and sulfisoxazole. Archives of Dermatology 100: 604–607

Kilian M 1976 A taxonomic study of the genus Haemophilus, with the proposal of a new species. Journal of General Microbiology 93: 9–62

Kinghorn G W, Hafiz S, McEntegart M C 1982a Pathogenic microbial flora of genital ulcers in Sheffield with particular reference to herpes simplex virus and *H. ducreyi*. British Journal of Venereal Diseases 58: 377–380

Kinghorn G W, Hafiz S, McEntegart M C 1982b Modified haemin-containing medium for isolation of *Haemophilus ducreyi*. Lancet i: 393–394

Leading Article 1982 Chancroid. Lancet ii: 747–748

Lykke-Oleson L, Larsen L, Pedersen T G, Gäarslev K 1979 Epidemic of chancroid in Greenland 1977–1978. Lancet i: 654–665

McEntegart M G, Hafiz S, Kinghorn G R 1982 *Haemophilus ducreyi* infections — time for reappraisal. Journal of Hygiene 39: 467–468

MacLean I W, Bowden E H W, Albritton W L 1980 TEM-type beta-lactamase production in *Haemophilus ducreyi*. Antimicrobial Agents and Chemotherapy 17: 897–900

Mallard R H, Macaulay M E, Riordan T, Chowdhury F H, Chandiok S, Bhattacharyya M N 1983 *Haemophilus ducreyi* infection in Manchester. Correspondence, Lancet ii: 283

Marmar J L 1972 The management of resistant chancroid in Vietnam. Journal of Urology 107: 807–808

Mauff A G, Ballard R C, Bilgreri Y R, Koomhof H J 1983 Isolation of *Haemophilus ducreyi* from genital ulcerations in white men in Johannesburg. South African Medical Journal 63: 236–237

Nayyar K C, Stolz E, Michel M F 1979 Rising incidence of chancroid in Rotterdam. British Journal of Venereal Diseases 55: 439–441

Nobre G N 1982 Isolation of *Haemophilus ducreyi* in the clinical laboratory. Journal of Medical Microbiology 15: 243–246

Nsanze H, Fast M V, D'Costa L J, Tukei P, Curran J, Ronald A 1981 Genital ulcers in Kenya: clinical and laboratory study. British Journal of Venereal Diseases 57: 378–381

Nsanze H, Plummer F A, Maggwa A B N, Maitha G, Dylewski J, Piot P, Ronald A R 1984 Comparison of four media for the primary isolation of *Haemophilus ducreyi*. Sexually Transmitted Diseases 11: 6–9

Oberhofer T R, Back A E 1982 Isolation and cultivation of *Haemophilus ducreyi*. Journal of Clinical Microbiology 15: 625–629

Odumeru J A, Wiseman G M, Ronald A R 1984 Virulence factors of *Haemophilus ducreyi*. Infection and Immunity 43: 607–611

Piot P, Slootmans L, Nsanze H, Ronald R 1983 Isolating *Haemophilus ducreyi*. Correspondence, Lancet ii: 909–910

Plummer F A, D'Costa L J, Nsanze H, Dylewski J, Karasira P, Ronald A R 1983 Epidemiology of chancroid and *Haemophilus ducreyi* in Nairobi, Kenya. Lancet ii: 1293–1295

Sheldon W H, Heyman A 1946 Studies on chancroid I. Observations on the histology with an evaluation of biopsy as a diagnostic procedure. American Journal of Pathology 22: 415–425

Sng E H, Lim A L, Rajan V S, Goh A J 1982 Characteristics of *Haemophilus ducreyi*. British Journal of Venereal Diseases 58: 239–242

Sottnek F O, Biddle J W, Kraus S J, Weaver R E, Stewart J A 1980 Isolation and identification of *Haemophilus ducreyi* in a clinical study. Journal of Clinical Microbiology 12: 170–174

35

Granuloma inguinale (donovanosis)

Granuloma inguinale is a chronic granulomatous infection caused by the bacterium *Calymmatobacterium granulomatis* (*Donovania granulomatis*). The clinical effects are mainly in the ano-genital region and less commonly elsewhere. Most cases occur in tropical and subtropical countries, but in the United Kingdom it may be occasionally seen in immigrants and merchant seamen.

The mode of transmission is not clear, although in many cases sexual intercourse, whether heterosexual or homosexual, probably plays a major role.

After a variable prepatent period, an ulcer develops and slowly increases in size over the course of several months or even years until a considerable area of skin may become affected. The duration of the untreated disease varies from about a month to over 30 years; healing generally occurs, however, within 2–3 years. Recurrences after apparent healing are common, and deformities of the ano-genital region may result. Granuloma inguinale may be associated with carcinoma of the skin.

AETIOLOGY

In 1905, In India, Major Donovan noted the constant presence of intracellular bodies in smears from the ulcerated lesions of patients with granuloma inguinale. These bodies, which he described as 'gigantic bacilli with rounded ends', are usually referred to as Donovan bodies. Following successful culture of the causative organism on chick yolk sac, it was evident that the Donovan bodies were bacterial in origin and the name *Donovania granulomatis* was proposed (Anderson 1943, Anderson et al 1945). If, however, the bacteria failed to adapt by losing their associated capsular material, further passages were not possible. The organism can be grown in a synthetic medium, but it is fastidious and requires a low oxidation-reduction potential and a substance, probably a peptide, present in an enzymic digest of bovine albumin or soya meal (Goldberg 1959).

Due to the problems associated with culture, complete characterization of the organism, which is now classified as *Calymmatobacterium granulomatis*, has not been accomplished, nor have Koch's postulates been fulfilled (Davis & Collins 1969). Clinical disease is not produced by injecting cultured organisms into man or by injecting animals with either cultures or tissue from lesions; injection of material from pseudo-buboes or suspensions of infected tissue, however, can produce clinical disease in men. The inability of cultured organisms to produce disease in man may be related to loss of virulence associated with loss of capsular material. Disease cannot be produced in laboratory animals (Davis & Collins 1969).

C. granulomatis is a pleomorphic Gram-negative bacillus surrounded by a well-defined capsule which can be demonstrated by Wright's stain. The bacteria are intracellular parasites of the large mononuclear tissue cells: occasionally they are found inside polymorphonuclear leucocytes. In smears stained with Leishman or Giemsa stain the organisms usually appear as capsulate ovoid or bean-shaped bodies, varying in size from 1 μ to 1.5 μ in length and from 0.5 μm to 0.7 μm in thickness. A well-defined dense capsular material, pinkish in colour, surrounds the body of the organism, which shows bipolar staining of chromatin material. The bipolar staining gives the organism the appearance of a closed 'safety-pin'. The capsule of *C. granulomatis* shares antigens with various members of the genus *Klebsiella* (Packer & Goldberg 1950). Since bacteriophage material has been found in association with the organism in material from granuloma inguinale lesions, it is possible that *C. granulomatis* is a phage-modified bacterium.

The lack of an animal host and the inability to consistently culture organisms with complete capsular material have severely hampered more complete bacterial studies on this organism (Davis & Collins 1969).

EPIDEMIOLOGY

Granuloma inguinale is found in tropical and subtropical countries; in temperate climates its importation by immigrants or seafarers may occasionally occur. In 1954 it was considered to be endemic along the eastern seaboard of southern India, southern China, the East Indies, northern Australia, West and Central Africa, some countries of Central, South and North America and the West Indies (Rajam & Rangiah 1954). The disease exhibits a male:female ratio of approximately 2:1 and appears to be also related to low socio-economic status and poor hygiene.

In 1980 there were 51 cases of granuloma inguinale reported in the United States, giving a rate of less than 0.05 per 100 000 population (United States Public Health Service 1982). The disease is rare in Europe; only 20 cases were reported in the clinics of the United Kingdom in 1982.

The popular view that granuloma inguinale is usually sexually transmitted has been questioned (Goldberg 1964). The reported incidence of concomitant infection in sexual partners varies from infrequently (Goldberg 1964) to over 50% (Lal & Nicholas 1970). The main points presented in favour of sexual transmission of granuloma inguinale include: history of sexual exposure before the appearance of the lesion; increased incidence of the disease in age groups in which sexual activity is highest; lesions found on internal genitalia, such as the cervix, without any other lesions; lesions found only around the anus in passive homosexuals; and the genital or perigenital location of lesions. The occurrence of the disease in very young children and sexually inactive persons; its rarity in those engaged in prostitution; and the rarity of the disease in the sexual partners of patients with open lesions are cited as evidence against sexual transmission (Goldberg 1964).

As an alternative to sexual transmission it has been suggested that C. granulomatis occurs in the intestine and in conditions of poor hygiene; auto-inoculation of faecal material could establish it on skin made susceptible to trauma or bacterial inflammation — an organism resembling C. granulomatis has been isolated from faeces (Goldberg 1962).

Our lack of knowledge about the organism and its interaction with its host and the environment make it impossible to be certain about the way it is transmitted. Transmission could occur by both sexual and non-sexual means: perineal contamination with faecal organisms might precede transfer by sexual means.

CLINICAL FEATURES

As the mode of transmission is uncertain, the prepatent period is not known. In cases considered to have been acquired sexually, the period between exposure to infection and the appearance of the initial lesion has varied from 3 days to 6 months, but occurring between 7 and 30 days in more than two-thirds of patients (Lal & Nicholas 1970).

The disease has a predilection for the moist stratified epithelium of the skin and the mucous membranes of the genital, anal, inguinal and oral regions. In more than 90% of cases reported the initial, primary lesion is in the ano-genital area (Rajam & Rangiah 1954).

In the male the prepuce, fraenum and glans are the usual sites in which the initial lesions develops. In the female the labia minora, mons veneris and the fourchette are the most commonly affected sites.

The earliest lesion may be a papule, a subcutaneous nodule or an ulcer. Such lesions are often intensely pruritic. The papule' which is usually between 5 and 15 mm in diameter, is elevated above the surrounding skin, flat-topped and covered by skin or mucous membrane; within a few days ulceration occurs.

Less commonly the initial lesion may be nodular. This subcutaneous nodule, of varying size, is at first firm, but as the inflammatory process progresses, softening occurs with the production of an abscess. After several days the abscess ruptures through the skin, resulting in the formation of a granulomatous ulcer.

The lesion most frequently seen in clinical practice is the ulcer. It is of variable size, soft, velvety, bright pink in colour and has a serpiginous edge. The base of the ulcer is covered by a serosanguineous exudate or a thin transparent membrane. Despite the appearance, the ulcer is generally painless unless there is secondary bacterial infection.

The disease spreads slowly along skin folds, taking months to involve a considerable area. In the female, the ulcerative process progresses posteriorly and downwards to involve the perineum and anal region. In Papua, New Guinea, Sengupta & Das (1984) found that 10% of 351 women with granuloma inguinale had cervical involvement, with or without external ano-genital lesions, which often resembled malignant disease. These authors also noted involvement of the endometrium and supporting structures of the uterus in the disease process. There is a tendency in the male for the disease to spread unwards and laterally to the inguinal region. Primary perianal lesions of granuloma inguinale most commonly occur in homosexual males (Davis 1970)

Extragenital lesions have been described, usually secondary to longstanding genital disease. Most commonly these lesions are found in or around the oral cavity, but may occur anywhere in the body (King 1964).

As the disease develops from the initial lesion, the base of the ulcer becomes elevated above the surface of the surrounding skin and the edge becomes thickened and greyish in colour. This hypertrophic type of disease is slow to progress and may remain stationary for years.

In some patients, most commonly female, there is a tendency early in the disease to extensive fibrous tissue formation. This often results in gross deformities.

Occasionally, in patients with longstanding disease, acute inflammation develops, which results in necrosis and destruction of extensive areas of skin and subcutaneous tissue. This uncommon event may be fatal.

Even in extensive granuloma inguinale, the regional lymph nodes are not enlarged, painful or tender. Histological examination of these glands shows only non-specific changes of endothelial hyperplasia and focal collections of mononuclear cells. Donovan bodies are not found (Rajam & Rangiah 1954). Should the regional lymph nodes be enlarged, the possible co-existence of other diseases such as malignant metastases, syphilis, lymphogranuloma venereum or secondary bacterial infection must be considered.

Systemic spread of infection from the primary site is said to be rare, although liver, spleen and bone may be affected (Rajam & Rangiah 1954).

The course of the disease is usually prolonged. Although in a few patients healing apparently takes place within a few weeks the mean duration of the disease is about 18 months. There is a tendency for the disease to recur after apparent healing. Unless there is some concomitant disease such as pulmonary tuberculosis, the patient is otherwise generally well.

Complications

As a result of involvement of lymphatic vessels in the fibrosis associated with the disease, oedema of the genitalia may occur in 15–20% of patients. Females are more commonly affected than males. In longstanding cases, genital deformities may occur; in the sclerotic forms of the disease there may be stenosis of the urethral, vaginal and anal orifices.

Malignancy has been reported in association with granuloma inguinale (Goldberg & Annamunthodo 1966, Davis 1970) and either basal cell or squamous cell carcinoma may occur. As the pseudo-epitheliomatous hyperplasia associated with granuloma inguinale may be difficult to differentiate from early carcinoma, care is required in interpreting histological reports (Beerman & Sonck 1952).

In the aetiology of carcinoma of the vulva or penis the role of *C. granulomatis*, as a predisposing factor, is suspected but not proven.

DIAGNOSIS

The difficulties associated with the growth of the organism exclude culture as a routine diagnostic procedure. A diagnosis of granuloma inguinale is based on the microscopic demonstration of the causative bacterium in tissue smears taken from the lesions. The lesions should be thoroughly and repeatedly cleansed with saline-soaked gauze, followed by gentle wiping with dry gauze. Since *C. granulomatis* is an intracellular parasite, granulation tissue must be examined: this is obtained either by biopsy punch from deep in the ulcer or from the edge of the lesion by means of a curette or scalpel. The tissue is spread between two slides and the resultant smear stained with Leishman, Giemsa or Wright's stain. In 90–95% of lesions of granuloma inguinale, organisms with intense polar staining, resembling closed safety pins, can be seen within mononuclear leucocytes (Rajam & Rangiah 1954). It may be difficult to demonstrate *C. granulomatis* in grossly infected lesions contaminated by other organisms. Repeated examinations are often necessary.

In the diagnosis of granuloma inguinale, biopsy of the ulcer may be helpful (Sehgal et al 1984). After infiltration of the base of the ulcer with lignocaine hydrochloride (1% w/v), a wedge-shaped excision biopsy which includes the margin of the lesion is taken. Microscopically the deeper layers of the dermis are densely infiltrated with plasma cells and macrophages with smaller numbers of polymorphonuclear leucocytes, including eosinophils. The superficial layers of the base of the ulcer contain many polymorphs. At the margins of the ulcer the epidermis may show marked acanthotic changes, with elongation of the rete pegs, a pattern which may be mistaken for squamous cell carcinoma. This pseudo-epitheliomatous appearance was found in sections, however, from only 4 of 42 patients studied by Sehgal et al (1984).

In the deep layers of the dermis, large macrophages, up to 90 μm in diameter, with pyknotic nuclei and cyst-like vacuoles containing *Calymmatobacterium granulomatis* (Greenblatt cells), are found. For the recognition of Donovan bodies in tissue sections, Giemsa-stained preparations are recommended (Sehgal et al 1984).

Biopsy may be helpful in distinguishing the lesions from those of lymphogranuloma venereum; the ulcers of granuloma inguinale show a more subacute type of inflammation (Stewart 1964). Skin tests and a complement fixation serological test have also been applied to the diagnosis of granuloma inguinale, although their use is limited due to lack of specificity and sensitivity and the limited availability of suitable antigen (Willcox 1975).

Since granuloma inguinale is associated with chancroid, syphilis and lymphogranuloma venereum, either alone or in combination in 10–20% of cases (Rajan & Rangiah 1954) it is important to take serological tests and to carry out dark ground or monoclonal antibody

(p. 118) investigation of the lesions for *Treponema pallidum* to exclude syphilis, and to examine a Giemsa-stained smear for *Haemophilus ducreyi*. Granuloma inguinale differs clinically from lymphogranuloma venereum; the latter diagnosis is usually supported by a serological test (Ch. 33).

TREATMENT

Although tetracyclines are said to be of value in the treatment of granuloma inguinale (Willcox 1975), this was not the experience of physicians working in Vietnam (Breschi et al 1975) who found that this drug was not effective. In that locality, ampicillin in a dosage of 500 mg orally 6-hourly for at least 2 weeks was effective in over 90% of cases, complete healing occurring within one month of commencing treatment. Other workers have used ampicillin with good results (Thew et al 1969), but Davis (1970) did not find it useful in the treatment of two of his patients.

Streptomycin, given in doses of 1 g daily by intramuscular injection for at least 20 days, results in healing in about 85% of cases. Higher and more frequent doses have been used, but ototoxicity as a complication of therapy must be borne in mind.

Lincomycin has recently been used as an alternative to ampicillin in patients hypersensitive to penicillins (Breschi et al 1975). This drug has been given orally in a dosage of 500 mg 6-hourly for 2 weeks. Only small numbers of cases have been treated with this agent and, on account of the risk of antibiotic-associated colitis, it should not be used as a routine. However, there may be a place for lincomycin, possibly in combination with erythromycin in the treatment of pregnant women with granuloma inguinale (Ashdown & Kilvert 1979). Co-trimoxazole in an oral dosage of 2 tablets twice-daily for 10 to 15 days has proved valuable in the treatment of donovanosis (Lal & Garg 1980). As with other treatment regimens, the duration of therapy will depend on the clinical response, but healing has usually occurred within 14 days of initiation of treatment.

In infections that are damaging, the problem of masking syphilis by treatment should not cause concern, provided sensitive and specific serological tests are carried out over a three month follow-up period and endeavours are made to ensure the examination of contacts.

REFERENCES

Anderson K 1943 Cultivation from granuloma inguinale of microorganisms having characteristics of Donovan bodies in yolk sac of chick embryos. Science 97: 560–561

Anderson K, DeMonbreun W, Goodpasture E 1945 An etiologic consideration of *Donovania granulomatis* cultivated from granuloma inguinale (three cases) in embryonic yolk. Journal of Experimental Medicine 81: 25–40

Ashdown L R, Kilvert G T 1979 Granuloma inguinale in Northern Queensland. Medical Journal of Australia 1: 146–148

Beerman H, Sonck C E 1952 The epithelial changes in granuloma inguinale. American Journal of Syphilis, Gonorrhoea and Venereal Diseases 36: 501–510

Breschi L C, Goldman G, Shapiro S R 1975 Granuloma inguinale in Vietnam: successful therapy with ampicillin and lincomycin. Journal of the American Venereal Disease Association 1: 118–120

Davis C M 1970 Granuloma inguinale. A clinical histological and ultrastructural study. Journal of the American Medical Association 211: 632–636

Davis C M, Collins C 1969 Granuloma inguinale: an ultrastructural study of *Calymmatobacterium granulomatis*. The Journal of Investigative Dermatology 53: 315–321

Donovan C 1905 Ulcerating granuloma of the pudenda. Indian Medical Gazette 40: 414

Goldberg J 1959 Studies on granuloma inguinale IV. Growth requirements of *Donovania granulomatis* and its relationship to the natural habitat of the organism. British Journal of Venereal Diseases 35: 266–268

Goldberg J 1962 Studies on granuloma inguinale V. Isolation of a bacterium resembling *Donovania granulomatis* from the faeces of a patient with granuloma inguinale. British Journal of Venereal Diseases 38: 99–102

Goldberg J 1964 Studies on granuloma inguinale VII. Some epidemiological considerations of the disease. British Journal of Venereal Diseases 40: 140–145

Goldberg J, Annamunthodo H 1966 Studies on granuloma inguinale VIII. Serological reactivity of sera from patients with carcinoma of penis when tested with Donovania agents. British Journal of Venereal Diseases 42: 205–209

King A 1964 Granuloma inguinale. Recent advances in venereology. J & A Churchill, London, p 334–351

Lal S, Garg B R 1980 Further evidence of the efficacy of cotrimoxazole in granuloma venereum. British Journal of Venereal Diseases 56: 412–413

Lal S, Nicholas C 1970 Epidemiological and clinical features in 165 cases of granuloma inguinale. British Journal of Venereal Diseases 46: 461–462

Packer H, Goldberg J 1950 Studies of the antigenic relationship of *D. granulomatis* to members of the tribe Escherichiae. American Journal of Syphilis, Gonorrhoea and Venereal Diseases 34: 342

Rajam R V, Rangiah P N 1954 Donovanosis (granuloma inguinale; granuloma venereum). World Health Organization, Monograph Series No 24, Geneva

Sehgal V N, Shyamprasad A L, Beohar R 1984 The histopathological diagnosis of donovanosis. British Journal of Venereal Diseases 60: 45–47

Sengupta S K, Das N 1984 Donovanosis affecting cervix,

uterus and adnexae. American Journal of Tropical
Medicine and Hygiene 33: 632–636

Stewart D B 1964 The gynecological lesions of
lymphogranuloma venereum and granuloma inguinale. The
Medical Clinics of North America 48: 773–786

Thew M A, Swift J T, Heaton C L 1969 Ampicillin in
treatment of granuloma inguinale. Journal of the American
Medical Association 210: 866–867

United States Public Health Service 1982 Sexually
transmitted disease (STD) statistical letter; calendar year
1980. U.S. Department of Health and Human Services,
Atlanta, Georgia 30333

Willcox R R 1975 Granuloma inguinale (donovanosis). In:
Morton R S, Harris J R W (eds) Recent advances in
sexually transmitted diseases. Churchill Livingstone,
Edinburgh p 194–197

36

Arthropod infestations

SCABIES

The condition known as scabies or 'the itch' is caused by the invasion of the stratum corneum of man by the mite *Sarcoptes scabiei var hominis*. Although promiscuous sexual behaviour may contribute to its spread among adolescents and young adults in some social circumstances, in most cases it is not spread by this means, and domestic outbreaks within a household or family are more important within the community. Control may be achieved by early diagnosis and correct treatment of the patient and all members of the household, whether sharing beds or not. Individuals harbouring very large numbers of *Sarcoptes* may play an important part in the maintenance and spread of the disease in the community, and waxing and waning of herd immunity may contribute to fluctuations in its incidence.

AETIOLOGY

Morphology and life cycle of the mite

The mite, *Sarcoptes scabiei* var *hominis*, is translucent and hemispherical, measuring 0.4×0.3 mm in the case of the female and about half of this in the male. Transverse corrugations are seen on its body, and spines and bristles on its dorsal surface; the adult has eight legs. Fuller morphological details are given by Mellanby in the important monograph on his original work (1972), and fine anatomical detail is provided beautifully by Heilesen (1946).

Mites can move rapidly on the warm skin (at a rate of about 2.5 cm per minute). The female, when fertilized, reaches its adult size and exercises some selection of the site into which it excavates a burrow in the stratum corneum. The capitulum ('head') dips into the nucleated cellular layer of the stratum granulosum to obtain nourishment and fluids (Shelley & Shelley 1983). It extends the burrow daily by 2 mm, lays 1–3 eggs each day, and dies after 25 or more have been laid. Six-

legged larvae emerge after 3–4 days and shelter in hair follicles where they undergo a moult to form an eight-legged nymph, which possibly moults again to form a second nymph. After another moult a mature adult male or an immature female is formed.

Mites are to be found in burrows at certain anatomical sites not influenced by the site of the initial infestation. The majority of mites (63%) are found on the hands and wrists; the next most favoured site is the extensor aspect of the elbow, where about 11% of the acari are found; the feet and genitals each may harbour about 9%, the buttocks 4%, the axillae 2%, and on the whole remaining surface of the body only 2% of the mite population can be found (Mellanby 1972). The total population of mites is generally only about a dozen, but in 3% of patients there may be over 500. In the case of crusted scabies (Norwegian scabies) there may be very high counts, both on the patient and in the scale from the skin; in one such patient, washings from pyjamas and bed linen over a 48-hour period yielded 7640 mites (Carslaw et al 1975).

EPIDEMIOLOGY

In Britain there appear to have been three epidemics, the first during the 1914–1918 War, the second beginning a few years before the Second World War and reaching a peak in 1943 and the third commencing about 1957. Peterkin & Grant (1959), for example, recorded that 153 cases of scabies were seen in the Department of Dermatology at Edinburgh Royal Infirmary in 1932 and that the numbers increased to 306 in 1938, reaching a peak of 849 in 1941 and steadily declining to 31 in 1951. In the third epidemic, by 1967 scabies had increased seven-fold in Sheffield and three-fold in London. From a study in Sheffield, where notification had been introduced in 1975, it was concluded that spread by sexual contact plays only a small part in the spread of the disease (Church & Knowelden 1978). Infestation is introduced to households mainly by schoolchildren and teenagers, especially girls. The commonest sources are friends and relatives outside the home, and schools do not play an appreciable part in spread. The high incidence in teenage girls is attributed to their greater contact with younger children and their habit of holding hands; girls too may share a bed more often than boys (Christophersen 1978). In Sheffield, notification and contact-tracing led to the detection of cases of scabies in 17% of the 873 contacts examined, but, although effective in this way, incidence of the disease in the community was not reduced (Church & Knowelden 1978).

It is thought that about 15 years of widespread infestation is followed by a similar period when the disease becomes rare, although the cycle does not appear to be clear-cut (Orkin 1971). Some degree of immunity is induced by *Sarcoptes* and epidemics may be related to resurgence of the disease when 'herd immunity' had declined during a period of low incidence (Mellanby, 1972). An increased frequency of HLA-A11 (36.7%) was found in a non-atopic group of patients with scabies, compared to a frequency of 10.4% in a healthy Norwegian population; the Relative Risk (RR — see Note 19.1 for definition etc.) for scabies in those who carry HLA-A11 is about 4. If this tendency holds true for other populations it would support the view that genetic differences in hosts may play some role in defence (Falk & Thorsby 1981). Normally in scabies there is an immune response up to the third month, in which there is a marked reduction in parasite numbers. This is a delayed hypersensitivity due to a cell-mediated immunity response, probably with some skin IgE (Burgess 1973). The persistence of the acarus in asymptomatic patients and in cases of undiagnosed Norwegian scabies will form important sources of infection. Within hospital ward epidemics, isolation of the individual with crusted scabies (Norwegian scabies) may require environmental followed by personal disinfestation, because cuticular fragments containing mites are abundant in the environment nearby in such cases (Carslaw et al 1975). In scabies treated with topical steroids or immunosuppressants, patients sometimes carry large numbers of acari (MacMillan 1972).

Although family outbreaks are important in most communities, it is important to take a sexual history and exclude other sexually transmissible disease when scabies is found in an adolescent or young adult. Scabies is seen not uncommonly in STD clinics; in Edinburgh (1979–1983), for example, the diagnosis has been made about once in males for every 13 cases of gonorrhoea and in females once for every 39 cases. Gonorrhoea and syphilis are transmissible by brief sexual contact, whereas scabies may require more prolonged skin contact than occurs in a casual intercourse.

IMMUNOLOGY OF SCABIES

The morbidity of scabies depends to a very large extent on the inflammation and intense itch which accompanies the host response. Although the attribution of individual immunological responses to specific antigens in or on the surface of the mite is not yet possible, it is useful to consider briefly some of the assembled evidence (Dahl 1983) for the 'classical' types of reaction by which an individual 'sensitized' by previous experiences of the antigen(s) may react and, if the reaction is intense enough, suffer as a result of the allergic state (Coombs & Gell 1976) (Note 36.2).

Type I reactions are 'wheal and flare' responses — with the development of burrows, antigen probably diffuses down gradually through the epidermis and produces interaction with specific IgE on the mast cell surface in a way so insidious or sporadic that sudden whealing does not occur. Although anaphylaxis has not been reported, sometimes there is a generalized urticaria. Among the changes seen in Type I reaction the following have been noted: 1. IgE antibody levels are elevated in infected patients and fall after successful treatment; 2. intracutaneous tests with extract of adult female mites cause wheal reactions in those who have had scabies but not in those who have not; 3. this reaction can be passively transferred by a factor in the serum (Prausnitz-Kustner); 4. serum from a patient with crusted scabies caused histamine release using a basophil degranulation test; 5. in crusted scabies serum IgE levels may be very high; 6. antigen-specific IgE in serum is elevated using crude scabies antigens; and, 7. IgE antibodies cross-react with antigens from a common house mite, *Dermatophagoides pteronyssinus* (Dahl 1983).

Type II reactions are cytotoxic reactions generated by a combination of IgG or IgM antibodies with antigens. High levels of IgG or IgM are sometimes present in some patients with scabies, but it is not known if these are specific or non-specific or are caused by the associated pyogenic infection.

Serum levels of IgA are sometimes decreased during infestation and rise after treatment. The reason for decreased levels is not known.

Levels of complement components C3 and C4 are usually normal. IgM and C3 have been found at the dermal and epidermal junction of affected skin by direct immunofluorescence techniques, but this could be secondary to inflammation or non-specific.

Type III reactions are caused by immune complexes which have been found in the serum of patients with crusted scabies and ordinary scabies before and after treatment. Generalized cutaneous vasculitis has been associated with scabies infections (Hay 1974) and vasculitis with blood vessel necrosis has been seen in biopsy specimens (Ackerman 1977).

Type IV reactions are cell-mediated immune reactions. Cell-mediated immunity is the probable explanation in the production of itchy papules. The evidence for this includes: 1. non-reactivity in the unexposed individual; 2. the latent period between infestation and rash; 3. the clinical appearance of the papules; and, 4. the life of the papules from 2 days–2 weeks. The histopathology of the papules shows a superficial and deep perivascular mixed inflammatory cell infiltrate composed of lymphocytes (mostly T-cells), histiocytes and eosinophils, and is compatible with cell-mediated immune reactions.

In the patient the pattern seen is complex and may involve not one but several of the pathways. Patients with sensory defects who do not sense itch, do not scratch, and thus mites may be allowed to reproduce *ad libidum*. In the immunodeficient and in those applying topical corticosteroids, crusted scabies has occurred; such evidence supports an immunological basis for this form of scabies, at least in some patients.

CLINICAL FEATURES

The presenting symptom is itching, which is worse at night. This appears to be due to sensitization and tends to develop about five weeks after a first infection, but earlier in the second and subsequent attacks. The reaction tends to be most intense on the genitals and buttocks where the acari may be destroyed by scratching.

Burrows and vesicles associated directly with the presence of the mite

The pathognomonic lesions are the burrows, appearing as serpiginous greyish ridges, 5–15 mm in length, which may be difficult to find if hygiene is good. The mite is visible in the burrow as a raised whitish oval with dark pigmentation anteriorly.

Sarcoptes can be found mainly in burrows at specific sites, namely, on the anterior aspect of the wrist, along the ulnar border of the hand, between the fingers, on the extensor aspects of the elbows, around the nipples in the female and in the natal cleft. Mellanby (1977) lists the frequency with which the different sites were affected in 886 cases (given as percentages): hands and wrists, 85; extensor aspect of the elbows, 41; feet and ankles, 37; penis and scrotum, 36; buttocks, 16; axillae, 15; knee, 6; umbilicus, 3; and hip, thigh, abdomen, arm, chest, nipples, back and neck as other sites less commonly affected.

Vesicles occur at the end of burrows and also separately from them, especially at the sides of the fingers. In infants bullae may form, particularly on the palms and soles (Rook 1986).

Urticarial papules not associated directly with the presence of the mite

Although papular lesions occur near the mite, an erythematous rash with urticarial papules is often most prominent in areas where mites are not necessarily found. Mellanby (1972) has mapped these areas (Fig. 36.1). Scratch marks, often with pin-point blood crusts at the apices of follicles, may be numerous. Papules may ulcerate as a result of scratching but could be due to a Type III reaction with local formation of immune complexes (Arthus reaction) (Dahl 1983). In 30% of patients there are penile and scrotal lesions (Rook 1986).

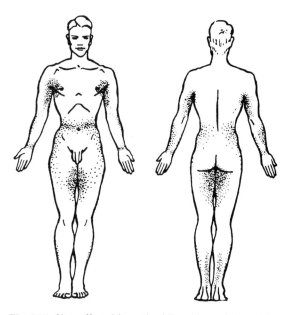

Fig. 36.1 Sites affected by urticarial papular rash in scabies. Note that the rash does not correspond with the sites of election of the acari — see text (Mellanby 1972).

Indurated nodules

In about 7% of cases itchy indurated nodules may be found. The commonest sites have been recorded as: axillae (50%), scrotum (40%), abdomen, sides of chest, groins (each about 30%) and on the penis (about 20%). The nodules may persist after treatment, but in only 20% of cases do they persist for longer than three months (Bagnal & Rook 1977). Nodules may result from persisting antigen although parts of the mite are not usually to be seen after the first month (Dahl 1983).

Other changes seen in scabies

Eczematous changes may follow scratching, and secondary bacterial infection may cause pustular lesions or even pyoderma. Colonization of scabetic lesions with alpha-haemolytic streptococci is common; when these are nephritogenic acute glomerulonephritis may result, as in Trinidad in 1971, where the attack rate for acute glomerulonephritis reached 5.2 per 1000 children of 5–9 years of age (Potter et al 1977).

Crusted scabies or Norwegian scabies, associated with vast numbers of mites, tends to be seen in cases of mental defect, as in Down's syndrome and senile dementia; in cases of debility as in leukaemia, beriberi, tuberculosis, bacillary dysentery and rheumatoid arthritis; and in cases where there is lack of cutaneous sensibility as in leprosy, syringomyelia and tabes dorsalis. Crusted scabies occurs also when there is lack of hypersensitivity due to a failure of sensitization, acquisition of tolerance or to the use of corticosteroid or immunosuppressive drugs (Paterson et al 1973, Epsy & Jolly 1976). It has also been suggested that low IgE levels may predispose to scabies (Hancock & Ward 1974).

DIAGNOSIS

The mite can best be found by means of an illuminated magnifier and can be secured from a burrow on the point of a needle; it may be examined on a dry slide without mounting fluid. The burrows are pathognomonic lesions of scabies, but identification of the mite is desirable to secure accuracy in diagnosis. If scrapings are to be examined, because an individual mite cannot be found, it has been suggested that a drop of liquid paraffin should be placed over the suspected site and the lesion scraped with a scalpel blade. The suspended material can then be examined microscopically as an oily film covered by a cover-slip (Muller 1977).

In scabies of animal origin the clinical presentation is 'scabies without burrows'. Irritable papules or papulovesicles, appearing at sites of close contact with the family pet, may be due to *Sarcoptes scabiei* var *canis*. Its feline counterpart, *Notoedres cati*, is rare in Britain but not uncommon in Czechoslovakia or Japan (Bagnal & Rook 1977).

TREATMENT

Lindane (gamma benzene hexachloride)

Since the successful use of a 1% gamma benzene hexachloride (lindane) cream in the treatment of scabies, recorded by Wooldridge (1948), this insecticide has been regarded as the most effective, safe and least irritant form of treatment. The preferred preparation is lindane, 1% in a water-dispersible base (Quellada Lotion, Stafford Miller — 100 ml). Although ill effects, apart from eczema on rare occasions, have not been found to occur clinically with the one or two applications required in treatment of the individual case, and although such treatment cannot be equated with risks in more intense or prolonged exposure, theoretical considerations of toxicity have led to the advocacy, in the medical literature of the USA particularly, of more caution in its use (Solomon et al 1977).

In the treatment of scabies with lindane lotion, according to Solomon et al there are 'rare anecdotal communications' of toxicity (headache, nausea, transient seizures) which resemble the more serious effects of exposure to a very high dosage. Brief consideration of the subject of toxicity is therefore justified here. Lindane can be absorbed percutaneously, and the scrotal skin, for example, poses virtually no barrier to its penetration (Feldman & Maibach 1974). Early experimental work showed that, although metabolized by the liver and stored in depot fat and other lipophilic tissues, the gamma isomer of benzene hexachloride (lindane) was eliminated very rapidly and disappeared from fat depots in rats, for example, within 3 weeks (Davidow & Frawley 1951); there are, however, no data of this kind for man.

A study of pesticide workers in Hungary (Czegledi-Janko & Avar 1970), showed a correlation between blood concentrations about 0.02 ppm and EEG abnormalities in 15 of 17 subjects; additional toxic effects such as depressed liver function and cardiac arrhythmia have been referred to by Solomon et al (1977) in those suffering from chronic exposure. Although ill effects of a systemic nature resulting from the topical application of the 1% lindane lotion in the limited manner used in the treatment of scabies, have not been recorded in the literature, Solomon et al make certain observations regarding its use. Because percutaneous absorption may well be greater in those whose skin has been damaged by excoriation, or in infants, it is suggested that it might be better to apply the agent to the dry cool skin, or to allow the skin to dry and cool after any cleansing bath is taken, rather than to prescribe the bath with hot soapy water originally advised by Wooldridge (1948). Cannon & McRae (1948) found the application to be quite effective without bathing. Other suggestions of Solomon et al (1977) included a view that to leave the application on the skin for 24 hours before washing it off may be unnecessarily long, and that a shorter contact time might be as effective; similarly the 1% concentration might also be more than required. The substance should be avoided, Solomon et al (1977) suggest, in pregnancy, very small infants and those with marked excoriation. Retreatment, it is also advised, should not take place before 8 days and only if living acari are found.

Although the minimum dose needed to effect a cure in scabies has not been found, extensive clinical experience has shown that lindane 1% is an effective sarcopticide, even when as many as 10% of cases may be also secondarily infected (James 1972). The authors consider that it should be avoided in pregnant women during the organogenetic period within the first trimester, and in infants treatment should consist of one application only. Hospital staff should avoid regular contact with the substance.

Benzyl benzoate application

Benzyl Benzoate Application, a 25% w/v emulsion (British National Formulary 1986, No.11), is effective and suitable for adolescents or adults when there is little excoriation. It is rather sticky to use and irritant to excoriated skins. As it causes stinging in children it should not be used for them.

Crotamiton lotion

Crotamiton lotion, 10% w/v (Eurax Lotion, Geigy Pharmaceuticals — 150 ml; Eurax Cream is an alternative) is effective as a sarcopticide and may relieve pruritus. Its use near the eyes must be avoided. It is not to be used in infants or if there is excoriation of the skin. The secret of success is that the sarcopticide selected should be applied to the whole body surface from the chin to the soles of the feet. It is better to give the patient written instructions and for the nurse to give an explanation carefully. Details given below are suitable for the otherwise healthy adult; in the case of infants or in those with marked excoriation one application may suffice, and there is a case for avoiding unnecessary exposure to the insecticide (Solomon et al 1977).

Instructions for treatment of scabies

Lindane (1% lotion)
1. Have a warm bath and scrub your skin gently but thoroughly; dry yourself with a towel and allow the skin to cool.
2. Apply the lotion to all the skin from below the neck to, and including, the soles of the feet, and allow it to dry.
3. Dress, but retain the same clothing. (If you wash your hands again re-apply the lotion).
4. After 12 hours have a second bath.
5. After an interval of 3 days apply the lotion again to all the skin from below the neck to the soles of the feet for the second and last time and allow to dry.
6. Change your clothing and bed linen.
7. After 12 hours have a third bath.

If benzyl benzoate application or crotamiton lotion is to be used, the instructions may be modified to allow these scabiecides to act for longer. After applying as described, the medicament should be left for 48 hours before being washed off, when a second and last application is made and allowed to act for 48 hours once again. The patient should be told that although itching will diminish rapidly, it may not be completely relieved for some days or weeks.

Where the skin of the patient shows excoriation, and in infants, one application of lindane as a 1% lotion may suffice. In infants or children the skin should not be scrubbed. All members of the household should be treated as well as the sexual contact and an attempt made to find the primary or source case. Ordinary laundering of clothes and bed linen will destroy the mites.

PEDICULOSIS

The human louse, *Pediculus humanus*, is found in two forms, the head louse and the body louse, which can be considered as unstable environmental subspecies of the one species. The morphological differences between them are slight and variable and many specimens cannot be assigned to one or other subspecies (Clay 1973). The two forms are interfertile, with no evidence of type-specific mating choice (Busvine 1977). The pubic louse is a different species, *Pthirus pubis*. All are obligate parasites of man and have mouth-parts adapted for piercing the skin and sucking blood (Clay 1973).

PEDICULUS HUMANUS AS THE BODY LOUSE

The adult female is a greyish-white insect 3–4 mm long, and the male a little smaller. The legs are adapted for grasping hairs. Both sexes suck blood and inject saliva while doing so. During a lifespan of about a month the female lays 7–10 eggs per day. Eggs hatch in 8 days and the nymphs require a further 8 days to reach maturity. The eggs are oval-lidded capsules, firmly cemented to a hair or to a thread, particularly along the inside of seams. Lice survive more than 10 days away from their hosts, but eggs may survive in garments for a month.

Epidemiology

The infestation is occasionally seen in vagrants or mentally handicapped individuals who may attend clinics. The insects are spread by clothing or bedding, but the lice can travel short distances from the host.

The dimension to be faced in areas where a high proportion of the population carry *P. humanus* and where louse-borne typhus is endemic or epidemic, is quite different to that faced by doctors treating a single patient (Gratz 1977).

Clinical features

In previously unexposed individuals the bite provokes only pin-point red macules. After 7 days, small weals or more persistent papules develop as pruritus becomes more troublesome.

Treatment

The resistance of body lice to insecticides has been widely reported and may be determined by the use of the WHO standard test method. Where resistance has been found, various alternative dusting powders may have to be used (e.g. 1% lindane, 1% malathion, 2% temephos, 5% carbaryl and 1% propoxur) (Gratz 1977). Malathion-resistant body lice have occurred in Africa, and resistance ultimately threatens all types of control by conventional insecticides (Busvine 1977).

When a vacuum steam disinfestor is not available, as in overcrowded camps, the infested clothing may be treated with a fumigant, such as ethyl formate, by personnel trained in its use (Davies & Bassett 1977, Gratz 1977). In hospitals, or where a large number of clothes have to be disinfested, the clothes are placed in a cotton bag and disinfested by a vacuum steam method. An ordinary tumble dryer is effective and kills the lice and eggs on dry clothing, after which they may be sent quite safely to a conventional laundry, if desired.

PEDICULUS HUMANUS AS THE HEAD LOUSE

Head lice are almost confined to the scalp, but may be found on hairs in other parts of the body. Long fine hair and infrequent washing increase the chance of infestation.

Epidemiology

The incidence of head louse infestation in the United Kingdom was high in school children before 1939, but by 1960 it had been greatly reduced, until in 1969 it was again found that in some cities 10% of school entrants were infested (Bagnal and Rook 1977). It is occasionally seen in clinics in female patients, although long-haired men may also be infested. Morley (1977) noted that in Teesside 23% of children in areas of poor and over-crowded housing were infested, compared with 0.4% in suburban areas; areas of local authority housing occupied an intermediate position with infestation rates of 13.4%. The lowest infestation rates were in those under 5 years of age, and the highest in teenagers.

Clinical features

Pruritus is most severe around the back and sides of the scalp. Pruritus depends on hypersensitivity to the salivary antigens of the louse, and in heavy infestation there may be no itching. Later the hair may become matted with pus. Impetigo of the scalp of the nape of the neck may accompany the infection.

Treatment

Lice resistant to lindane are common, and the treatment of choice in this infestation is with malathion or carbaryl (British National Formulary 1986, No.12). Malathion Scalp Application (0.5% in an alcoholic base; caution — flammable) is supplied as Prioderm, Napp Laboratories (55 ml is sufficient for five treatments). Sufficient should be sprinkled on the scalp and rubbed well into the hair, *avoiding the eyes*. It is allowed to dry and to remain untouched for 12 hours. After a shampoo the hair should be combed with a fine comb to remove the dead lice and egg cases. The treatment should be repeated in one week. If there is doubt about a patient's capacity to carry out instructions, treatment should be given by a nurse, who should wear rubber gloves when applying malathion.

Carbaryl (0.5%) in an alcoholic base (caution flammable) as a lotion is also available as a treatment of choice in pediculosis (British National Formulary 1986, No.12) and is supplied as Carylderm, Napp Laboratories.

Contacts should be examined where possible, as in some cities 20% of children may be infested (Garretts 1972). Malathion resistance in head lice is as yet unknown. In a study over 44 generations of laboratory colonies of body lice, resistance to malathion did not develop (Cole et al 1969). The potential, however, remains, since resistance to malathion has been recorded in a strain of body lice from Burundi (Cole et al 1973). In practice, at present, malathion is very effective (Taplin et al 1982) but it should be used in conjunction with clearly thought out educational and social measures to prevent, or at least limit, reinfection.

PTHIRIASIS PUBIS

The crab louse (*Pthirus pubis*) (see also Ch. 2 and, at the end of this chapter, Note 36.1). is greyish-white; it measures about 1.2–2 mm in length and is nearly as broad as it is long. There are three spiracles on its first abdominal segment (Clay 1973). It remains almost immobile on its host, the hind legs grasping two hairs. In this position it continues to feed intermittently for hours or days, rarely removing its mouth-parts from their position in the host. The claws on the last two pairs of legs are adapted for grasping the widely spaced pubic hairs (Busvine 1977). As it feeds it defaecates frequently, voiding blood and faeces intermixed. Defaecation is frequent and much more localized on the skin than in *P. corporis* and since feeding is virtually continuous, there is more obvious 'dirtiness' (Nuttall 1918).

Mating takes place on the host and some 26 eggs may

be laid in 12 days. After a week the eggs hatch and the nymph attaches within a few hours. Three moults occur within 17 days. The nymphs and adults cannot survive more than two days when removed from their host (Matheson 1950).

The blue 'spots' induced by the bites of *Pthirus pubis* in the skin are known as *maculae coeruleae* and are caused by an enzyme from its salivary glands. These consist of *bean-shaped* and *horse-shoe shaped* glands and it was established by Pavlovsky & Stein (1924), working in Petrograd, that it is the enzyme specifically from the bean-shaped glands, apparently acting on the haemoglobin, which causes the diffuse bluish discoloration.

EPIDEMIOLOGY

This louse is usually transferred by sexual contact, but it can be spread by clothing. Pubic lice are a common infestation seen at clinics (Fisher & Morton 1970) and in Edinburgh, for example, in the years 1979–1983, a case was seen for every 4 cases of gonorrhoea in males and for every 10 cases in females.

The louse is mainly confined to the hairs of the pubic and perianal regions, but they may be found attached to the hairs of the abdomen, thighs and axillae. Very rarely they may be seen on the margin of the scalp, the eyebrows and eyelashes. In infants they may have reached such sites from the breast hairs of the mother.

CLINICAL FEATURES

Intense irritation is often the only symptom. The blue-grey macules (*maculae coeruleae*) induced by the bite of the insect may be seen sometimes on the abdominal wall and upper thighs. In some patients irritation is minimal and the numbers of lice or eggs to be found are few.

TREATMENT

As treatment of choice for pubic lice, malathion or carbaryl 1% w/v as a shampoo (e.g. respectively Prioderm Shampoo, Napp or Carylderm Shampoo, Napp; ABPI Data Sheet Compendium 1986–1987) is effective. The shampoo should be used as follows:

1. Wet area and apply shampoo directly to the pubic hair and the hair of the axilla and between the legs and around the anus. Apply also to body hair elsewhere below the neck.

2. Cover the skin and hair, particularly in pubic, axillary and perianal regions.

3. Work up a lather and leave for at least five minutes.

4. Rinse thoroughly.

5. Repeat the procedure. A fine toothed 'Napp' comb may be used to remove dead lice and eggs if necessary. Avoid contaminating the eyes or eyelids.

Malathion and carbaryl are persistent and ovicidal so that a single treatment is usually sufficient. Both malathion and carbaryl are effective as a lotion (0.5% in an alcoholic base — flammable) but the lotions may cause transient stinging due to the alcohol content. The lotion should be rubbed into the hair (pubic, perianal and axillary and all hairy parts below the neck), allowed to dry, and after 12 hours washed off.

Lindane (1% in a lotion base, e.g. Quellada, Stafford-Miller; ABPI Data Sheet Compendium 1986–1987) is effective in treatment of pubic lice infestations. The lotion should be rubbed into the pubic, perianal, axillary and all other hairy parts below the neck and allowed to dry. The patient may have a bath after 24 hours. As the preparation is not ovicidal a second application after one week is advised.

There are no reports of insecticide resistance in *Pthirus pubis*, but in view of the increased incidence of the infestation and increased use of lindane, malathion and carbaryl, the future development of resistance cannot be excluded.

In eyelash infestations individual lice may be removed with forceps; an application of yellow soft paraffin may kill the lice by occlusion of its spiracles. Other sites should be treated simultaneously with carbaryl or malathion.

Alexander (1984) refers to the anticholinesterase effect of a 0.75% physostigmine ophthalmic ointment which is toxic to lice as an effective treatment, but advises consultation with an ophthalmologist before prescribing it.

NOTES TO CHAPTER 36

Note 36.1: The correct name for the crab louse is *Pthirus pubis* (Phthirus is a widely dispersed error) (Busvine 1977).

Note 36.2

Type I reactions. Exposure — usually repeated — to an antigen, stimulates an antibody response, including the production of IgE. The latter binds to a receptor on the surface of basophils or mast cells and within a few minutes of further exposure to the same antigen, cross-linkage of IgE molecules and receptors occurs and results in the release from the cells of histamine and other vasoactive amines.

Type II reactions. These are cytotoxic in character. IgG and IgM combine with antigenic determinants on the cell membrane, and the fixation of complement results in cell damage.

Type III reactions. These reactions result from the localization of antigen-antibody complexes in tissue. After complement fixation there is chemotaxis of leucocytes, platelet damage and the release of vasoactive amines, ingestion of immune complexes by polymorphonuclear leucocytes and the subsequent release of lysosomal enzymes, resulting in tissue damage.

Type IV reactions. These cell-mediated immune reactions result from interaction between sensitized lymphocytes and specific antigens. Complement or antibody are not involved. Antigen is bound to specific antigen-receptive T-lymphocytes. Activated lymphocytes release lymphokines: (i) that result in the recruitment of other T- and B-lymphocytes; (ii) induce mitogenesis; (iii) are chemotactic for polymorphonuclear leucocytes and (iv) activate macrophages.

REFERENCES

Ackerman A B 1977 Histopathology of human scabies. In: Orkin & Maibach (eds) Scabies and pediculosis. J B Lippincott, Philadelphia, p 88–95

Alexander J O 1984 *Pthirus pubis*. In: Arthropods and human skin. Springer Verlag, Berlin, p 50–55

Bagnal B, Rook A 1977 Arthropods and the skin. In: Rook A (ed) Recent advances in dermatology. Churchill Livingstone, Edinburgh, p 59–90

Burgess I 1973 Unusual features of scabies associated with topical fluorinated steroids. British Journal of Dermatology 87: 519–520

Busvine J R 1977 Pediculosis: biology of the parasites. In: Orkin M, Maibach H I, Parish L C, Schwartzman R M (eds) Scabies and pediculosis. J B Lippincott, Philadelphia, p 143–152

Cannon A B, McRae M E 1948 Treatment of scabies. Journal of the American Medical Association 138: 557–560

Carslaw E W, Dobson R M, Hood A J K, Taylor R N 1975 Mites in the environment of cases of Norwegian scabies. British Journal of Dermatology 92: 333–337

Christophersen J 1978 The epidemiology of scabies in Denmark, 1900–1975. Archives of Dermatology 114: 747–750

Church R E, Knowelden J 1978 Scabies in Sheffield, a family infestation. British Medical Journal 1: 761–763

Clay T 1973 In: Smith K G V(ed) Insects and other arthropods of medical importance. British Museum, London, p 9

Cole M M, Clark P H, Weidhaas D E 1969 Failure of laboratory colonies of body lice to develop resistance to malathion. Journal of Economic Entomology 62: 568–570

Cole M M, Clark P H, Washington F, Ellerbe W, Van Natta D L 1973 Resistance to malathion in a strain of body lice from Burundi. Journal of Economic Entomology 66: 118–119

Coombs R R A, Gell P G H 1976 Classification of allergic reactions responsible for clinical hypersensitivity and disease. In: Gell P G H, Coombs R R A (eds) Clinical aspects of immunology, 3rd edn. Blackwell Scientific Publications, Oxford, p 761

Czegledi-Janko G, Avar P 1970 Occupational exposure to lindane — clinical and laboratory findings. British Journal of Industrial Medicine 27: 283–286

Dahl M V 1983 Immunology of scabies: a review. Annals of Allergy 51: 560–565

Davidow B, Frawley J P 1951 Tissue distribution, accumulation and elimination of the isomers of benzene hexachloride. Proceedings of the Society of Experimental Biology and Medicine 776: 780–783

Davies F G, Bassett W H 1977 Clay's Public Health Inspectors Handbook, 14th edn. Lewis, London, p 493

Epsy P D, Jolly H W 1976 Norwegian scabies, occurrence in a patient undergoing immunosuppression. Archives of Dermatology 112: 193–196

Falk E S, Thorsby E 1981 HLA antigens in patients with scabies. British Journal of Dermatology 104: 317–320

Feldman R J, Maibach H I 1974 Percutaneous penetration of some pesticides and herbicides in man. Toxicology and Applied Pharmacology 28: 126–132

Fisher I, Morton R S 1970 Pthirus pubis infestation. British Journal of Venereal Diseases 46: 326–329

Gratz N G 1977 In: Orkin M, Maibach H I, Parish L C, Schwartzman R M (eds) Scabies and pediculosis. J B Lippincott, Philadelphia, p 179–190

Hancock B W, Ward A N 1974 Serum immunoglobulins in scabies. Journal of Investigative Dermatology 63: 482–484

Hay R J 1974 Norwegian scabies in a patient with cutaneous vasculitis. Guy's Hospital Reports 123: 77

Heilesen B 1946 Studies on *Acarus scabiei* and scabies. Acta Dermatologica, Suppl 14, 86–138

James B H E 1972 Gamma benzene hexachloride as a scabicide. British Medical Journal 1: 178–179

MacMillan A L 1972 Unusual features of scabies associated with topical fluorinated steroids. British Journal of

Dermatology 87: 496–497

Matheson R 1950 Medical Entomology. Constable, London, p 194–217

Mellanby K 1972 Scabies. Classey, Faringdon

Mellanby K 1977 Biology of the parasite (*S. scabiei*). In: Orkin M, Maibach H I, Parish L C, Schwartzman R M (eds) Scabies and pediculosis. J B Lippincott, Philadelphia, p 8–14

Morley W N 1977 Body infestations. Scottish Medical Journal 22: 211–216

Muller G H 1977 Laboratory diagnosis of scabies. In: Orkin M, Maibach H I, Parish L C, Schwartzman R M (eds) Scabies and pediculosis. J B Lippincott, Philadelphia, p 99–104

Nuttall G H F 1918 The biology of *Phthirus pubis*. Parasitology 10: 383–405

Orkin M 1971 Resurgence of scabies. Journal of the American Medical Association 217: 593–597

Paterson W D, Allen B R, Beveridge G W 1973 Norwegian scabies during immunosuppressive therapy. British Medical Journal 4: 211–212

Pavlovsky E N, Stein A K 1924 *Maculae coeruleae* and *Phthirus pubis*. Parasitology 16: 145–149

Peterkin G A Grant 1959 The changing pattern of dermatology. Archives of Dermatology 80: 1–14

Potter E V, Mayon-White R, Svartman M, Abidh S, Poon-King T, Earle D T 1977 Secondary infections in scabies and their complications. In: Orkin M, Maibach H I, Parish L C, Schwartzman R M (eds) Scabies and pediculosis. J B Lippincott, Philadelphia, p 39–50

Rook A 1986 Human scabies. In: Rook A, Wilkinson D S, Ebling F J G, Champion R H, Burton J L (eds) Textbook of dermatology, 4th edn. Blackwell, Oxford, vol 2, p 1060–1066

Shelley W B, Shelley D 1983 Scanning electron microscopy of the scabies burrow and its contents with special reference to the *Sarcoptes scabiei* egg. Journal of the American Academy of Dermatology 9: 673–679

Solomon L M, Fahrner L, West D P 1977 Gamma benzene hexachloride toxicity. Archives of Dermatology 113: 353–357

Taplin D, Castillero P M, Spiegel J, Mercer S, Rivera A A, Schachner L 1982 Malathion for treatment of *Pediculus humanus* var *capitis* infestation. Journal of the American Medical Association 247(22): 3103–3105

Wooldridge W E 1948 Gamma isomer of hexachloro cyclohexone in the treatment of scabies. Journal of Investigative Dermatology 10: 363–366

37

Ulcers and other conditions of the external genitalia

In this chapter it is necessary to include a number of clinical topics related only on account of the anatomical site involved.

1. Ulcers of the external genitalia
2. The prepuce and the development of the preputial sac
3. Balanoposthitis
4. Some non-infective conditions: erythema multiforme, psoriasis, lichen simplex and lichen planus. Minor conditions sometimes causing anxiety: trichomycosis axillaris, coronal papillae, sebaceous glands — Fordyce's spots.
5. Tinea cruris
6. Erythrasma
7. Balanitis xerotica obliterans (BXO) (penile lichen sclerosis et atrophicus)
8. Erythroplasia of Queyrat
9. Peyronie's disease
10. Lymphocoele and localized oedema of the penis
11. Behçet's syndrome
12. Vulval intra-epithelial neoplasia (VIN)
13. Bowenoid papulosis of the male genitalia

1. ULCERS OF THE EXTERNAL GENITALIA

Acute ulcers

In the differential diagnosis of an acute genital ulcer, the cause to be considered first must be a sexually transmissible agent, particularly *Treponema pallidum*: within this group, ulcers found elsewhere, particularly in the oral and anal regions, must be included also for consideration. In the context of general practice patients should be referred to clinics, where facilities for the necessary procedures are at hand. Antibiotics, which may obscure an important diagnosis, should not be prescribed blindly.

In all cases of a genital ulcer the first objective will be to diagnose or exclude early-stage contagious syphilis and to take steps to trace sexual contacts. Exclusion of other sexually transmissible diseases, particularly

gonorrhoea and herpes genitalis, is also necessary. In warmer climates, or in patients returning from them, possibilities of lymphogranuloma venereum, chancroid and, rarely, donovanosis will require consideration, although in lymphogranuloma venereum the ulcer itself tends to be transitory and herpetiform.

The chancre of primary syphilis may often be a painless indurated ulcer with enlarged indurated non-tender lymph nodes, but its tendency to heal and to be modified by injudicious (e.g. topical steroid applications) and inadequate treatments makes it improper to base a diagnosis on clinical appearance alone. The importance of repeating serological tests for syphilis for a three month follow-up period has been discussed (p. 126).

In secondary syphilis, moist eroded papules are seen in the mouth, on the genitalia or around the anus, but the larger hypertrophic papules (condylomata lata) tend to be most obvious on the vulva in the female and in the anal region of both sexes.

Although chancroid (soft sore) is rare in the United Kingdom and western Europe but common in the tropics and subtropics, it is important to exclude syphilis by dark-ground or monoclonal antibody examinations and serological tests over a period of three months, and to treat with a sulphonamide (e.g. sulphadimidine) or co-trimoxazole to avoid masking the treponemal infection if it is present.

In the diagnosis of granuloma inguinale a small biopsy should be taken from the edge of the lesion and a tissue smear prepared and stained with Giemsa or Leishman stains to demonstrate the capsulate pleomorphic bacillus with bipolar staining.

Among other ulcers caused by infective agents are superficial herpetiform erosions at the introitus, associated with *Trichomonas vaginalis* vaginitis. Some erosions, particularly at the fraenum in the male and at the fourchette in the female, may be traumatic from intercourse.

In *Candida* infection there may be erosions under the exudate in the vagina and fissuring, particularly of the fourchette. In the male contact a small proportion may show balanoposthitis with superficial ulceration of the glans and occasionally with fissures at the preputial orifice and a phimosis. *Candida* tends sometimes to flourish in the vagina in pregnancy, diabetes mellitus and in some patients taking contraceptive pills. Whenever there is a pruritus a search should also be made for pubic lice on the vulva, tinea in the groin in the male, and threadworms (*Enterobius vermicularis*) or their ova if the itch is perianal.

Non-gonococcal urethritis, and the perhaps equivalent non-specific genital infection in the female, is another possibility. In the male with non-gonococcal urethritis, superficial fissuring is sometimes seen in the fraenal and orifice portions of the prepuce. In Reiter's disease there is a circinate balanitis in 21–43% of cases, and in the uncircumcised these lesions on the glans may show maceration.

Molluscum contagiosum, with its small pearl-like and often umbilicated lesions, may be found on the penis in the male and on the vulva and inner aspect of the thighs in the female as well as elsewhere on the skin.

Condylomata acuminata are very common and neglect, co-existent vaginitis, urethritis or herpes infection may cause genital ulceration.

In scabies, indurated papules, sometimes with pustulation and impetiginization, are common on the shaft of the penis. The diagnosis rests on the history of pruritus, finding burrows and the recognition of *Sarcoptes scabiei*.

Even when furuncles and other pyogenic lesions are recognized, exclusion of syphilis remains a first consideration.

Chronic ulcers

Patients with oral aphthous ulcers have a 1 in 5 chance of having some haematological deficiency or malabsorption syndrome (Wray et al 1975). so it is wise to extend the investigations (serum ferritin, serum folate, whole blood folate and serum B_{12}) to cases with recurrent genital or orogenital aphthous ulcers.

In balanitis xerotica obliterans (BXO), described later in this chapter, fibrotic, ivory-white areas are found on the margin of the prepuce, which shows fissuring and adhesion to the glans. This condition may affect the urethral meatus and lead to stenosis with a distinctive white periurethral collar. Ulceration can occur in chronic balanitis in the elderly which may resemble BXO clinically. BXO may be equivalent to lichen sclerosus et atrophicus, essentially a disease of women, in which ivory papules and violaceous tissue-paper skin may be seen in the ano-genital area. In the very rare Behçet's syndrome, considered also in this chapter, there is also recurrent orogenital ulceration associated with iritis. Tuberculosis is now a rare cause of genital ulceration (Sigal et al 1985).

Crohn's disease (regional enteritis) can involve the anal region alone without apparent involvement of other parts of the gastrointestinal tract, presenting clinically as anal ulceration, anorectal fistulae or oedematous anal skin tags. Ulceration of the skin, separated from other areas of ulceration by normal skin, can occur and has been seen on the penis and on the vulva, as well as elsewhere. Spreading ulceration of the skin of the perineum with linear extension into the groins and genitalia may occur after surgical treatment of an anal lesion (Morson 1976). Pyoderma gangrenosum, which may be associated with inflammatory bowel disease or rheumatoid arthritis, can produce extensive ulceration of the vulva. A rare cause of granulomatous ulceration is eosinophilic granuloma.

In cases of chronic ulceration, malignant disease must also be excluded — particularly in erythroplasia of Queyrat, in which there is a raised bright-red, well-demarcated plaque with a velvety surface to be seen on the glans, and in which a biopsy is necessary. Squamous cell carcinoma of the penis is uncommon and, in the circumcised, extremely rare. The neoplasm develops within the preputial sac and it is usually wart-like rather than ulcerative. Other malignant tumours are very rare. Squamous cell carcinoma of the scrotum is associated with contamination of the skin with mineral oil and other carcinogens.

The characteristic symptom of vulvar intra-epithelial neoplasia (VIN), considered in more detail later in this chapter, is intense and persistent itch. Thickened white plaques tend to develop on the vulva, particularly around the clitoris, sometimes extending back to the anus; they do not encroach on the vestibule or vagina. VIN has a tendency to occur in middle age, but an increasing proportion of younger women are being affected. Squamous carcinoma appears as a hard indurated swelling or an ulcerating lesion in the vulva with lymph node enlargement. In cases with pre-existing leukoplakia there is a long history of vulvar irritation.

2. THE PREPUCE AND THE DEVELOPMENT OF THE PREPUTIAL SAC

The development of the prepuce starts when the human embryo is about 65 mm (13 weeks) and it covers the glans when the fetus is 100 mm (end of the 3rd month — 50 g). The inner surface of the prepuce and the surface of the glans receive a common squamous epithelium which separates at about the time of birth gradually and spontaneously as a normal biological process.

Separation of the epithelium common to the glans and prepuce occurs by a process of desquamation. In places the squamous cells arrange themselves into whorls, forming epithelial cell nests, or epithelial 'pearls' which

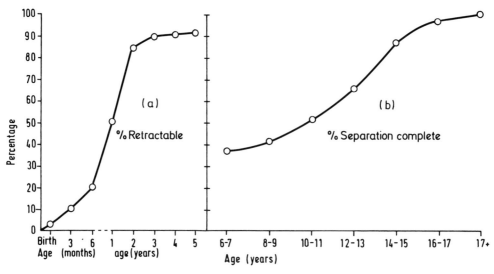

Fig. 37.1 (a) Proportion of boys from birth–5 years in whom prepuce has become spontaneously retractable (Gairdner 1949). (b) Proportion of boys from 6–17 years in whom separation of prepuce and glans was complete (Øster 1968).

contain a laminated mass of keratin. The centres of these nests degenerate to form spaces which increase in size and link up and finally form a continuous preputial sac (Deibert 1933). The prepuce is in the course of developing at the time of birth, and by the age of 3 years the prepuce is still non-retractable in 10%. Spontaneous retractability of the prepuce appeared in Gairdner's study (1949) to be possible by the age of 3 years (Fig. 37.1a) in 90% but Øster (1968) showed in a study of an unselected group of Danish schoolboys that complete separation of the preputial sac may not in fact be completed until the age uf 17 years (Fig. 37.1b); so called 'adhesions' (non-separation) diminish with age gradually and spontaneously. This normal biological process is probably androgen-dependent (Burrows 1944) and the process is known to be arrested by castration.

In mice the glans penis and prepuce are not separable until about 46 days after birth, and this process is prevented by the removal of the testes. Separation of the adherent prepuce, whether brought about naturally through testicular activity or artificially by the administration of androgen in the castrated animal, is caused by keratinization of the hitherto embryonic cells composing the adherent epithelia (Burrows 1944).

Forcible retraction of the prepuce in boys is painful and may lead to overstretching of the preputial orifice and consequent phimosis. The procedure can also cause paraphimosis, and bleeding points may also be seen where the stretching has damaged areas where separation has been incomplete. Very gentle retraction and washing is all that is generally required. Retraction under anaesthesia, whether general (Cooper et al 1983) or local (Griffiths & Freeman 1984), should rarely be necessary (Esscher 1984, Pfaff & Bolkenius 1984).

The predicted lifetime risk for cancer of the penis in the uncircumcised male in the United States is 166 per 100 000, or one in 600, and the estimated median age is 67 years. Since this neoplasm is virtually unknown in those who have undergone circumcision at an early age, the issue has been put forward as a factor to be considered in discussions on the advisability or otherwise of neonatal circumcision (Kochen 1980). Although Kochen (1980) thought that mortality in the USA from circumcision was rare and found only 2 reports in the literature since 1953, adequate statistical records on mortality due to this cause did not seem to be available. In Gairdner's paper (1949) 10–19 deaths in those under 5 years of age were recorded annually between 1942 and 1947 in England and Wales.

The origins of male circumcision are unknown; it is a very ancient practice, with evidence of it in some of the earliest Egyptian mummies. Even in recent years there have been many attempts to justify the operation in western countries on medical grounds (Short 1980).

3. BALANOPOSTHITIS

The terms balanitis and posthitis refer respectively to inflammation of the glans and mucosal surface of the prepuce. As these conditions will ordinarily co-exist, the term balanoposthitis is strictly more correct than the commonly used shorter word balanitis. Acute and chronic forms may be due to traumatic, irritant or infective causes.

Aetiology

Within the moist preputial sac an accumulation of smegma resulting from poor hygiene is an obvious predisposing factor in the aetiology of balanoposthitis. Irritation may also be due to friction of clothes, the unwise application of antiseptics or previous contact during sexual intercourse with pathogenic or opportunistic organisms within the vagina. Bacteria, yeasts or trichomonads may flourish in the moist environment, but sometimes balanitis may develop after intercourse, possibly as a result of sensitivity to a vaginal discharge containing yeasts such as *Candida albicans*, or substances derived from it. With the restricting effect of phimosis, whether primary or secondary and due to inflammation, discharge may accumulate under pressure and, if neglected, may be associated with a necrotizing ulceration of the glans (phagedaena). Under these circumstances anaerobes may be secondary invaders. Although anaerobes are isolated infrequently from the subpreputial sac of healthy men, at least three-quarters of patients with balanoposthitis are infected at that site with anaerobic bacteria, especially *Bacteroides* spp (Masfari et al 1983). In one study (Kinghorn et al 1982), *Gardnerella vaginalis*, usually in association with anaerobes, was cultured from the subpreputial sac of 9 of 39 men with balanoposthitis. Herpes simplex virus may be isolated from erosions.

Balanoposthitis may be associated with diabetes, and occurs with debilitating disease, particularly in the elderly and in urinary infections.

Clinical features

In infective forms of balanitis there is erythema of the glans, coronal sulcus and inner surface of the prepuce. It can be insidious in onset and pass unnoticed, but sometimes erythema and oedema are pronounced, and a resulting phimosis may make inspection of the glans difficult or impossible. In the uncircumcised the affected surfaces become macerated, and a purulent exudate accumulates rapidly, becoming malodorous. Erosion and ulceration may be painful.

In Reiter's disease a recurring circinate balanitis develops in 25% of cases on the glans penis and mucous surface of the prepuce. In balanitis associated with, or due to diabetes or candidiasis, there may be fissuring of the prepuce, particularly at its orifice.

In middle-aged or elderly men a chronic localized balanitis may develop and, as there is a marked plasma cell infiltration of the dermis, this is referred to as plasma cell balanitis of Zoon. The surface of the plaque of balanitis is moist, shiny and often finely speckled. Biopsy is essential to distinguish this condition from erythroplasia of Queyrat (see below).

All forms of balanitis may become chronic or relapse frequently, particularly in the elderly, when fibrotic changes may resemble those seen in balanitis xerotica obliterans.

Treatment

Mild forms of balanitis are cleared readily by retracting the prepuce and bathing with physiological saline. This treatment should be repeated twice- or thrice-daily and, if inflammation is more than trivial, a strip of gauze (2.5 cm × 15 cm) soaked in saline should be applied to the glans and coronal sulcus in such a way that, on bringing the prepuce forward, the skin surfaces of the glans and the inner aspect of the prepuce are separated by gauze. The prescription of co-trimoxazole (2 tablets each containing 400 mg sulphamethoxazole and 80 mg trimethroprim twice-daily) is useful when inflammation is pronounced and when local wide-spectrum antibacterial agents are to be avoided, particularly when the diagnosis of early syphilis is to be considered.

When inflammation is more chronic or unresponsive to the treatment outlined, a rapid response may follow the short-term (2–3 weeks) local application of a topical corticosteroid with an anti-infective agent (e.g. betamethasone valerate 0.1% cream with 3% clioquinol as Betnovate C Cream, Glaxo) which has both antibacterial and anti-candidal activity. A small quantity should be applied gently to the affected area two or three times daily for a few days and then reduced to once-daily for a limited period of 7–10 days. Betnovate C Cream may stain hair, skin or fabric (ABPI, Data Sheet Compendium 1988–1989, p. 540–541). Alternatively, hydrocortisone and clioquinol ointment may be used. Topical steroid applications should not be used in herpes genitalis.

When phimosis is present, subpreputial lavage with saline three- to six hourly is often sufficient to promote drainage and healing. As inflammation subsides the prepuce may become retractable and any ulcer inspected. When a necrotizing ulceration of the glans develops, rapid local destruction can occur. A swab of the subpreputial discharge should be examined microbiologically, and if anaerobes are discovered antibacterial agents, such as metronidazole, may be prescribed. Subpreputial lavage with 0.9% saline may be carried out with a disposable hypodermic syringe. Should this be unsuccessful in securing resolution, the antibiotic or chemotherapeutic agent, effective against the organism isolated, may be given. When there is a dusky erythema of the penile skin with persistent phimosis and the inflammation is unrelieved by the saline lavage described and supplemented by the antibiotic, surgical exposure of the glans by a dorsal slit is necessary to secure the drainage of a necrotizing ulcer.

4. SOME NON-INFECTIVE CONDITIONS (Rook et al 1986)

Erythema multiforme

Erythema multiforme is a condition of unknown aetiology that can be precipitated by many agents including viruses, particularly herpes simplex virus; bacteria, especially mycoplasmas; fungi, especially *Histoplasma capsulatum*; drugs, especially sulphonamides; sarcoidosis; polyarteritis nodosa and malignant neoplasms. In almost 50% of cases, however, precipitating factors cannot be identified.

The skin lesions are dull red, flat maculopapules that often reach one to two centimetres in diameter. As the lesion increases in size the centre becomes purplish and the periphery remains red. Cropping of lesions occurs over a few days and generally the lesions fade within two weeks. Classically the affected sites are the dorsa of the hands, palms, wrists, forearms and feet, elbows and knees.

In the severe bullous form of the disease (Stevens-Johnson syndrome) there is a sudden onset of a bullous eruption of the mouth and lips; these bullae rupture to show the floor of the erosion covered by a greyish white membrane. Haemorrhagic crusting is characteristic. Severe conjunctivitis is often associated with corneal ulceration, genital ulceration and, in about 80% of cases, skin lesions that are similar to those described above or bullous. New crops of lesions develop over a period of about 10 days. Systemic features including fever, malaise and anorexia present for two to three weeks. Renal failure has been reported rarely.

In mild cases of localized bullous erythema multiforme symptomatic treatment is all that is required, but in severe illness, steroids such as prednisolone may be indicated. When there is severe ocular involvement, the advice of an ophthalmologist should be sought.

Psoriasis, lichen simplex, lichen planus

Psoriasis produces scaly lesions on the penis, perianal region or vulva. On the glans of the uncircumcised male, the lesions are bright red and sharply marginated. Psoriatic lesions will occur elsewhere and pits may be found in the fingernails. Lichen simplex with erythema, lichenification and fissuring in the ano-genital lesions is associated with pruritus and affects a 'trigger-zone'. Lichen planus produces annular papular lesions which are pink or violet in colour and sometimes restricted to the genitals and mouth in young men. The surface of the lesions shows a network of fine lines.

Minor conditions sometimes causing anxiety in patients

Trichomycosis axillaris

Trichomycosis axillaris is a superficial infection of the axillary and pubic hairs with the formation of adherent yellow, black or red nodules on the hair shaft. These concretions consist of tightly packed bacteria, which may grow within the cells of the cuticle; the organism is named *Corynebacterium tenuis*.

Coronal papillae

Coronal papillae are dome-shaped or hair-like papules involving the corona of the penis, which may be mistaken for warts. The papillae are a normal variant.

Sebaceous glands

Small yellow papules (about 0.2 mm) may be seen sometimes in clusters on the inner surface of the prepuce; these are seen also on the buccal mucosa and consist of sebaceous glands. Sometimes referred to as Fordyce's spots, they are normal sebaceous glands, which increase in number at puberty and continue to do so in adult life.

5. TINEA CRURIS

Tinea cruris is an infection of the groins by filamentous fungi, known as dermatophytes, which live only in the fully keratinized layers of the skin and, when established, may cause only minimal disturbance to their host. Although a variety of lesions occur, dermatophytes have been found in apparently healthy skin (Noble & Somerville 1974).

Aetiology

In groin infections *Trichophyton rubrum* and *Epidermophyton floccosum* are usually implicated, although *T. mentagrophytes* var *interdigitale* may be detected on occasions. In Denmark it was found that in 17% of *T. rubrum* infections in men, both the groin and feet were involved: this fungus species has become the most common dermatophyte in western Europe since the Second World War (Rosman 1966).

Transmission takes place as a result of sharing towels and communal facilities. Tinea cruris is rare in females.

Clinical features

Itching is a predominant feature whatever species is involved. Initially the lesions are erythematous plaques, arciform with sharp margins extending from the groin towards the thighs. There is little tendency to central clearing and the surface is scaly, sometimes sufficient to mask the underlying erythema. Vesiculation is rare but dermal nodules may be found in older lesions. Lesions due to *E. floccosum* are typically acute in onset and inflammatory. In *T. rubrum* infections, lesions are classically chronic and perhaps more nodular; the rare *T. mentagrophytes* var *interdigitale* infections may be vesicular and inflammatory (Roberts & Mackenzie 1986). Involvement of the scrotal skin by the dermatophyte is common, but the cutaneous reaction is often inconspicuous (La Touche 1967). In one survey of air force recruits in the United States, 9% yielded dermatophytes from the inguinal region or natal cleft (Davis et al 1972), although the skin was apparently normal.

Diagnosis

Material for mycological study may be taken by scraping outwards from the edge of the lesions; for the laboratory it is best to collect the specimens on to a folded slip of black paper. Alternatively, particles of keratin may be stripped from the skin with a vinyl adhesive tape (Scotch tape type 68), affixed to a microscope slide for transfer to the laboratory for culture (Milne & Barnetson 1971).

For routine diagnosis, microscopic examination is most easily carried out by mounting skin scrapings in potassium hydroxide fluid (distilled water 80 ml, potassium hydroxide 20 g, glycerine 10 ml). The process may be hastened by gentle heating. Alternatively the mounting fluid may be prepared with dimethylsulphoxide (40 ml), potassium hydroxide (20 g) and distilled water (60 ml). Fungal elements can then be detected by microscopic examination of the unstained potassium hydroxide preparation covered by a cover-slip (Rebell & Taplin 1970).

Dermatophytes grow well on Sabouraud's medium and are distinguished principally by the nature of the spores. In addition to the species already named, *Microsporus gypseum* is a cause of tinea cruris worldwide and *Trichophyton simiae* a cause in Brazil, Guinea and India (Frey et al 1979). Keys to their identification may be found in Rebell & Taplin (1970) and in an atlas by Frey et al (1979) which provides pleasing visual and textual information.

Treatment

Imidazole derivatives (Sawyer et al 1975a, b) are a new generation of antifungal agents, which are effective as topical agents in the treatment of infections due to dermatophytes as well as in candidosis. Among many possible derivatives, clotrimazole, miconazole and econazole are effective in topical treatment. Used as a cream the various preparations should be applied 2–3 times daily as a thin film to the affected area and rubbed in gently (e.g. econazole nitrate 1% as a cream — Ecostatin, Squibb; miconazole nitrate 2% as a cream — Dermonistat, Ortho-Cilag; clotrimazole as a 1% cream

— Canesten Bayer). Improvement occurs within 10–14 days and treatment may continue for 2–8 weeks and preferably for 2 weeks after disappearance of cutaneous signs. On occasions, reddening of the skin and pruritus may occur, but this is seldom severe enough for the patient to stop treatment. Eradication of the infection may not be achieved by topical agents, although clinical effects are controlled.

Griseofulvin may be used orally in more severe cases, but accurate diagnosis by microscopy and cultures is most desirable. It is taken up by keratin-forming cells and hair shafts, thus coming into intimate contact with the infecting dermatophyte (Cartwright 1975). In tinea of the groin, treatment may be required for a period of 3–4 weeks, to be followed by careful re-examination and, if apparently clear, a follow-up after a month is desirable (Roberts & Mackenzie 1986). It is prescribed as tablets (Griseofulvin Tablets BNF 125 mg; 500 mg); the adult dose is 0.5 g, which may be sufficient if taken once daily-after a meal.

6. ERYTHRASMA

Erythrasma is a mild chronic superficial infection of the skin, characterized by well-demarcated flat lesions caused by a group of closely related aerobic coryneform bacteria usually known as *Corynebacterium minutissimum* (Roberts & Highet 1986).

Aetiology

C. minutissium is a name which covers a complex of fluorescent diphtheroids, which may also be found on normal skin but which appear to be causative in erythrasma. The incidence is higher in boarding schools and in hospitals for the mentally handicapped (Somerville et al 1970).

Clinical features

Smooth and well-demarcated from the surrounding skin, the lesion is initially red in colour. Scaling develops and as the lesion ages it becomes brown. Commonly it involves the toe clefts, but the groin is frequently affected, and the axilla or elsewhere occasionally. Usually there are no symptoms but, particularly in the groins, there may be mild pruritus.

Diagnosis

Under Wood's light erythrasma shows a characteristic coral-red fluorescence which is attributable to coproporphyrin III (Roberts & Highet 1986). Skin scales from the margin of the lesion should be examined, mounted in potassium hydroxide solution (see previous section) to exclude tinea cruris. Exclusion of tinea from the diagnosis should, preferably, include culture of skin scales as well as examination by microscopy. Skin scrapings may be stained with Giemsa to detect the rods and filaments of *C. minutissimum* and cultured to confirm the diagnosis.

Treatment

Without treatment the condition persists indefinitely with exacerbations and remissions. *C. minutissimum* is sensitive to sodium fusidate in vitro and, in one small series, 2 weeks topical treatment with 2% sodium fusidate ointment (Fucidin Ointment, Leo Laboratories Ltd.) was curative (Macmillan & Sarkany 1970). Relapse appears to be more common when the toe web is affected.

Clotrimazole cream is effective in erythrasma and in tinea cruris (Clayton & Connor 1973), although tendency to relapse is a characteristic of both conditions.

7. BALANITIS XEROTICA OBLITERANS (BXO)
(penile lichen sclerosus et atrophicus)

Balanitis xerotica obliterans (BXO), as a term, has tended to be used to describe a naked-eye appearance of the glans penis with individual or confluent ivory white papules. There is sometimes involvement of the urethral meatus and sometimes fissuring and fibrosis of the prepuce (Ive & Wilkinson 1986, Rowell 1986). As this macroscopic appearance can be brought about by different processes it is better to restrict the use of the term to those cases with the characteristic histological picture (Bainbridge et al 1971). It resembles lichen sclerosus et atrophicus and may be a localized form of this condition, although other than penile lesions may be found in less than 20% of cases.

Pathology

The diagnostic histological feature is oedema and homogenization of the dermal collagen, which occurs immediately beneath the epidermis in small islands or in a band of varying thickness. In these areas there is marked loss of elastic fibres. Similar changes occur in the dermal blood vessels. Immediately superficial to the altered collagen, the epidermis shows hyperkeratosis and atrophy of the stratum malpighii, resulting in flattening or absence of the rete pegs. Deep to the abnormal collagen there is a variable band of chronic inflammatory cells, mostly lymphocytes (Bainbridge et al 1971). The histological picture is more fully described in Rowell (1986).

Clinical features

The condition occurs mainly in those of 30–50 years of age, but it has been described between the ages of 11 and 83 years (Mikat et al 1973). Patients may present with symptoms of a non-retractile prepuce, urinary obstruction, haematuria, pain and irritation of the penis or a subpreputial discharge (Bainbridge et al 1971).

Clinically the lesions of BXO are characteristic ivory white macules or confluent plaques on the surface of the glans and prepuce, usually occurring around the corona and extending a short way into the urethral meatus. The glans and prepuce, which may not be retractable, are thickened and fibrous. Involvement of the urethra is usually limited to the meatus and squamous epithelium of the fossa navicularis; in such cases there is a smooth white contracted meatal orifice and an atrophic meatal collar. Although lesions are usually restricted to the penis, unmistakable achromic papules of lichen sclerosus et atrophicus may on occasions be found elsewhere on the body as recorded by Laymon & Freeman (1944) in 4 of 24 cases of BXO. Patients may be alarmed at haemorrhagic bullae developing after intercourse and blood stained urine if these lesions are at the meatus (Ive & Wilkinson 1986).

Differential diagnosis

Diagnosis should be based on histological examination, because the macroscopic appearance may be similar to balanitis chronica circumscripta or due to non-specific inflammation. BXO usually occurs without skin lesions elsewhere, although on histological grounds particularly it is similar to lichen sclerosus et atrophicus, a skin condition most often seen in women (Laymon & Freeman 1944, Ridley 1975).

As in any penile lesion, it is important to exclude syphilis and other sexually transmitted organisms which may cause balanitis and/or a urethritis.

Treatment

Anxiety about sexually transmitted disease may be relieved by satisfactory results in the tests taken to exclude such infections.

When lesions are localized, attempts may be made to control non-specific inflammation of the glans and preputial sac. Short-term applications of 0.1% betamethasone valerate and clioquinol cream or hydrocortisone 0.1% and clioquinol 1% over a period of 6 weeks, with gradual reduction in the number of applications, sometimes produces improvement.

When lesions are extensive the diagnosis should be confirmed histologically and an assessment made at the time by a urologist. Circumcision may be needed when the prepuce is involved and retraction difficult.

If meatal stenosis causes urethral obstruction and the meatal lesion shows only non-specific inflammatory change on histological examination, then regular dilatation by urethral bouginage may be sufficient treatment. If the navicular fossa and urethral meatus, however, show the changes characteristic of BXO then meatotomy or meatoplasty by a urologist may be necessary.

In lichen sclerosus et atrophicus, lesions may extend to involve the site of meatotomy, but this seldom appears to be a cause of further urinary obstruction.

Prognosis

Balanitis xerotica obliterans tends to progress, but sometimes this is at very slow rate. Circumcision will only reduce the added effects of inflammation in the subpreputial sac, and dilatation or meatotomy the effects of recurrent urinary obstruction. Carcinoma of the penis has been reported in some cases of BXO (Laymon & Freeman 1944).

8. ERYTHROPLASIA OF QUEYRAT

This is a premalignant condition of the penis of unknown aetiology, presenting most commonly between the ages of 50 and 60 years; it is rare in those circumcised in infancy.

Clinical features

The condition appears as either single or multiple well-defined red plaques on the glans penis or on the mucosal surface of the prepuce. The lesions have a velvety, shiny appearance, and may occasionally ulcerate; commonly without symptoms, they may on rare occasions cause pruritus or discomfort. The disease is slowly progressive, invasive change being manifest as induration, ulceration or warty growth.

Diagnosis

Psoriasis, lichen planus, fixed drug eruption, fungal lesions, syphilis and balanitis xerotica obliterans need to be carefully excluded in differential diagnosis. Histological examination is essential for diagnosis.

The appearance on microscopy is characteristic: the epidermis is acanthotic with focal parakeratosis, atypical epithelial cells with hyperchromatic nuclei, and dyskaryotic cells. Mitosis is obvious in cells in the upper Malpighian layer. The dermis is infiltrated with lymphocytes and plasma cells.

Treatment

Topical application of antimitotic agents such as 5-fluorouracil or the use of liquid nitrogen spray has produced excellent results in treatment. The subject of erythroplasia of Queyrat and its treatment has been reviewed by Goette (1976)

9. PEYRONIE'S DISEASE (plastic induration of the penis)

In Peyronie's disease a chronic localized fibrous induration involves the intercavernous septa of the penis, causing an angulation or curvature of the penis on erection. The disease, of unknown aetiology, was first described by Francois de la Peyronie, court physician to Louis XIV. In the majority of cases it occurs in the fourth and fifth decades of life, although patients from 18 to 80 years of age have been affected (Billig et al 1975).

Aetiology

The unpredictable occurrence of Peyronie's disease in patients who had been treated for 18 months or more with beta-adrenoceptor blocking agents, such as propranolol (Osborne 1977, Wallis et al 1977) or metoprolol (Yudkin 1977), suggested that Peyronie's disease might have an association with other fibrous tissue abnormalities such as retroperitoneal fibrosis, which can occur with these drugs. Peyronie's disease has also been reported in a patient with an unusual group of multisystem disorders (sclerosing cholangiitis, portal cirrhosis and retroperitoneal fibrosis) who had also a serum α-1-antitrypsin deficiency (Palmer et al 1978). In the carcinoid syndrome, where there is an increase in serotonin, Peyronie's disease has also been described (Zarafonetis & Horrax 1959). More recently, in a scrutiny of the detailed drug and medical histories in 98 men with Peyronie's disease, Pryor & Castle (1982) recorded that 61 of these patients had taken drugs of some sort but only 5 had taken beta-blockers during the previous 10 years. On the other hand, 11 patients were reported as being hypertensive, 8 gave a history of ischaemic heart disease, 5 had diabetes, and there were other cases of circulatory disease as well. In 14 additional cases, hypertension was noted without the patient being aware of it. Pryor & Castle's findings (1982) suggest strongly that Peyronie's disease is indeed associated with chronic degenerative arterial disease rather than with beta-blockade. The condition is known to be more prone to occur in the presence of atherosclerosis, so the link with beta-blockers may be purely coincidental (Laake 1983). Urethritis, sexual problems and trauma have all been postulated as causative but as yet no definitive cause has been discovered.

Clinical features

The symptoms of this disorder are pain and curvature on erection; the sensation of a cord within the penis; the palpation of a lump in the penis; decreased erection distal to the plaque; interference with coitus; and gradual impotence. Curvature of the penis is directed towards the lesion and a dorsal curvature is the most common.

The fibrotic plaque may range in size from a few millimetres to involvement of the entire dorsum of the penis. The plaque is usually located on the dorsum of the penis (about 70%); the lateral aspect (about 20%); and occasionally on the ventrum (about 7%). Plaques may begin as multiple lesions and become confluent. There may be calcification on radiological examination in 20%. The fibrosis tends to be self-limiting and capable of spontaneous remission (Billig et al 1975).

Treatment

In the usual case, in which the lesion is an isolated finding, spontaneous remission may occur in half the cases over a period of a few years.

Although the association with beta-adrenoceptor blocking agents is likely to be coincidental, an alternative therapy may be considered.

X-ray radiation, diathermy, ultrasound, vitamin E, potassium para-aminobenzoate, dimethylsulphoxide, have all been used without proof of value. Intralesional steroids have been popular, but there is often great difficulty in getting the fluid into the hard plaque, and the effectiveness of this treatment is uncertain (Billig et al 1975). Surgical intervention is unjustified.

10. LYMPHOCOELE AND LOCALIZED OEDEMA OF THE PENIS (sclerosing lymphangitis of the penis)

This is a benign, transitory condition, first described in a patient with gonorrhoea (Hoffman 1923). The aetiology is unknown, although trauma, in the form of frequent or prolonged sexual intercourse, frequently antedates the appearance of the lesion by an interval varying between a few hours and several weeks.

Histological examination shows dilated lymphatic vessels with thickening of the wall due to hyperplasia of the smooth muscle cells and production of collagen and ground substance by fibroblasts (Marsch & Stuttgen 1981). Fibrin thrombi occlude the lumen of the vessel and recanalization may be seen in older lesions.

Characteristically there is a worm-like swelling in the coronal sulcus, parallel to the corona of the glans penis, sometimes completely encircling the penis, and on occasion involving the dorsal lymphatic vessels of the shaft. Oedema of the prepuce may also be found. The swelling is neither painful nor tender, and on palpation it has a cartilaginous consistency. Within three weeks of its appearance, the lesion has usually resolved completely, and no treatment other than reassurance is required.

It is probable that there is wide variation in the presentation of this condition, varying between mild preputial oedema, and the 'classical' lesion described (Fiumara 1975). A similar condition may affect the vulva (Stolz et al 1974).

11. BEHÇET'S SYNDROME

Behcet's syndrome is a multisystem illness characterized by the triad of oral, genital and eye lesions, and by its tendency to exacerbation and remission of unpredictable duration. Taking its name from the Turkish physician, who described in 1937 the triad of relapsing iridocyclitis with recurrent oral and genital ulceration, it affects males predominantly and although it shows its highest prevalence in the Eastern Mediterranean basin and in Japan (Lehner & Barnes 1979) cases are also to be found in mainland China, Middle Eastern countries and North Africa (Barnes 1984). A vasculitis appears to be the common histological lesion, and clinical features — present in most patients and considered to be diagnostic — are oral and genital ulcers, uveitis and a variety of skin lesions. Clinical manifestations of the syndrome are protean but include particularly arthritis, thrombophlebitis and various neurological states (Chajek & Fainaru 1975).

The strength of the association of Behcet's syndrome (Svejgaard et al 1983) with HLA-B5 — one of at least 10 loci within the major histocompatibility complex (MHC) — calculated as the Relative Risk, is given as 6.3. The 'Etiologic Factor' (EF) indicating how much of the disease is 'due to' the disease-associated factor HLA-B5, is given as 0.34 (for ankylosing spondylitis in connection with HLA-B27 the RR is 87.4 and the EF 0.89; see also Table 19.1 and Note 19.1). It has been suggested that HLA-B5 is particularly related to ocular involvement, and it is well-recognized that there is a very high incidence of ocular disease in Japanese and Turkish patients where the incidence of HLA-B5 (Bw51 split) is higher in the general population than in the United Kingdom (Barnes 1984).

Clinical features

Four common clinical patterns can be discerned: the *mucocutaneous* (MC) type, there are oral and genital lesions with or without skin manifestations which may be present also in all other types; the *arthritic* type; the *neurological* type with brain involvement; and the *ocular* type (Lehner & Barnes 1979).

Painful recurrent oral ulcers 2–10 mm in diameter occur in half to three-quarters of all patients and are the most frequent initial manifestation. The ulcers are shallow or deep with a central yellowish necrotic base and they occur as single lesions or in crops affecting the mucosa anywhere from the lips to the larynx. The ulcers tend to persist for one to two weeks and recur after intervals of several days to several months.

Genital ulcers resemble those of the mouth both in appearance and in their tendency to persist, heal and recur. They are located on the scrotum or the penis in men and on the vulva or vagina in women. The ulcers are painful and disturbing to men but less troublesome to women. In the mouth or genitalia, fibrosis and scarring at sites of healed lesions produce a characteristic mottled appearance on naked-eye examination or with magnification, described as 'splash fibrosis'. Scarring and tissue loss develop particularly after scrotal ulceration (Dunlop 1979).

Recurrent inflammation of the anterior segment of the eye usually shows itself as iridocyclitis and hypopyon. Posterior segment involvement may be found in about two-thirds of patients with lesions such as choroiditis, phlebitis, arteritis and optic papillitis. Serious sequelae with blindness may result. It is important to exclude syphilis by means of the necessary tests (Ch. 8), otherwise it may be overlooked.

A variety of skin lesions also occur; these include particularly ulceration, erythema nodosum and pustules, but erythema multiforme and thrombophlebitis migrans also occur (Lehner & Barnes 1979). Arthritis with synovial changes, which appear to be characteristic histologically (Vernon-Roberts et al 1978), develops in about 40%. Neurological complications occur after some years and include intracranial nerve palsy, cerebellar and spinal cord lesions and meningoencephalitis, all conditions which tend to regress over several months.

Diagnosis

Diagnosis may be made in those with the 'complete' syndrome where three or four of the major features are present (oral and genital ulceration, ocular and skin lesions). Diagnosis in those with the 'incomplete' syndrome is often debatable (Lehner & Barnes 1979).

In Behcet's syndrome the diagnostic usefulness of the 'pathergy' test has been reported in patients from Turkey and Japan but not in those from Britain. This test is based on a curious phenomenon, almost unique to Behçet's syndrome in some geographical localities, characterized by hyperreactivity of the skin to needle-prick. In recording the result of the test an assessment is made 48 hours after a single or ten needle-pricks in different sites: for needle mark(s) only, 0; for a papule +; for a small pustule 2+; and for a large pustule 3+ (Yazici et al 1984).

In the individual case the value in diagnosis of a test for HLA-Bs is limited — see paragraph on strength of the association; as in Reiter's disease, what is needed is a specific molecular marker.

It is clearly important to exclude by appropriate tests a sexually transmitted infection, including syphilis, not only because of the lesion in mucosal sites but also because the patient is often anxious about such possibilities.

Treatment

Evaluation of treatment is difficult because of the unpredictable natural course of the disease (Chajek & Fainaru 1975). Corticosteroid therapy forms the basis of treatment for all manifestations (James 1979). In those with very severe manifestations the use of 'immuno-suppressive' drugs, with or without corticosteroids, is likely to be of most value (Barnes 1984). Local disease of the mouth or genitalia is not an indication for treatment with systemic corticosteroids, but the local application of corticosteroids — with added antimicrobial agents for the genital tract — has greatly improved the quality of life of those with Behçet's syndrome. As each ulcer is preceded by the development of a painful tender nodule under the mucous membrane or the skin, and under the mucosal surfaces lasts for one or two days before ulcerating, it may be aborted by local corticosteroids. In the mouth it may be felt with the tongue and identified by the patient and aborted or minimized by the local application of triamcinolone 0.1% in an adhesive oral paste (e.g. Adcortyl in Orabase, Squibb) after meals and last thing at night. On the genitalia hydrocortisone 0.5% (with nystatin 100 000 units per g, chlorhexidine hydrochloride 1%) in a water miscible base (e.g. Nystaform-HC, Bayer) may be applied and secondary infection minimized by the use of vaginal antiseptic pessaries (e.g. hydragarphen 1.25 mg white pessary — Penotrane WBP — 2 to be inserted high into the vagina nightly for 15 nights; not to be used with copper IUD, PVC ring pessaries or in the absence of vaginal secretions.) (Dunlop 1979).

12. VULVAR INTRA-EPITHELIAL NEOPLASIA

The term vulval intra-epithelial neoplasia (VIN) encompasses all cases of intra-epithelial squamous cellular atypia which has been referred as 'mild atypia', 'moderate atypia' and 'carcinoma in situ' (Crum 1982). The aetiology of VIN is uncertain, but its association in 20–30% of cases with cervical intra-epithelial neoplasia suggests a common factor. The role of human papilloma virus (HPV) in the causation of cervical carcinoma is discussed in Chapter 27 and it is interesting to note that about 20% of patients with VIN have been treated previously for genital warts. Using DNA hybridization methods, HPV-DNA has been found in biopsies from patients with VIN (Ikenberg et al 1983). Although in many cases of VIN the histology is identical to that of classical Bowen's disease and the disease tends to be multifocal, the patients are younger, (Ikenberg et al 1983). They usually complain of pruritus vulvae with soreness but others have noticed an abnormal swelling (Bernstein et al 1983). The most common finding is a slightly elevated irregular white lesion sharply demarcated from the surrounding tissues and measuring on average 2.5 cm (Andreasson & Bock 1985). In patients under the age of 40 years the lesions are usually multiple whereas in older women single lesions are more common. Less frequently, the lesions are red or brown and sometimes eroded.

Although most VIN lesions are detectable on close naked-eye examination, the use of the colposcope is sometimes useful in defining the extent of an individual lesion. In some cases, only areas of hyperkeratosis with normal surrounding tissues are visible with the colposcope, but in others there are sharply defined punctate or mosaic changes.

Although cytological examination is useful in the detection of cervical intra-epithelial neoplasia, its value in VIN is more limited as the exfoliation of underlying cells may be prevented by an area of hyperkeratosis. In areas of the skin in which punctation or mosaicism can be detected with the colposcope, cytological examination may be helpful. Histological examination of biopsy specimens, however, is essential for diagnosis.

Two basic patterns of atypia are seen: 1. when atypical cells of the basal or parabasal type extend to a varying degree into the upper layers of the epidermis; and 2. when premature cellular maturation occurs. In both forms, mitotic figures are common; there is a high nuclear:cytoplasmic ratio; and there may be hyper- or parakeratosis (Buckley et al 1984). In many cases the histology is identical to that of Bowen's disease.

Little is known about the natural history of VIN, but progression to invasive squamuus cell carcinoma is uncommon (Crum et al 1982) and more likely to occur in the elderly and immunocompromised. Spontaneous regression of the lesions in untreated women has also been described (Friedrich et al 1980, Bernstein et al

1983) but the mechanisms are uncertain. In Friedrich's series 4 of the 5 women whose lesions regressed spontaneously had been pregnant at the time of diagnosis and in these cases it is likely that cell-mediated immune responses played some role.

For small localized lesions, simple excision is the treatment of choice, but for more extensive disease a partial or complete skinning vulvectomy is commonly undertaken. Cryotherapy and CO_2 laser treatment may have some place in the management of localized disease, but too few patients have been treated by these methods to allow firm conclusions to be drawn. Recurrence after local excision is common (about 30% of cases) and most likely to occur if the edges of the excised tissue show, histologically, intra-epithelial neoplasia (Andreasson & Bock 1985).

As about 30% of patients with VIN have concomitant cervical intra-epithelial neoplasia or lower genital tract malignancy, in each patient a thorough gynaecological examination is essential.

13. BOWENOID PAPULOSIS OF THE MALE GENITALIA (synonyms — pigmented penile papules, multicentric pigmented Bowen's disease)

The subject has been reviewed by Kimura (1982). Bowenoid papulosis, a disease of young men, presents clinically as multiple brownish-red raised lesions about 2×10 mm in diameter, usually on the shaft of the penis. Histologically the lesions resemble those of vulvar intra-epithelial neoplasia (Katz et al 1978).

The aetiology of the condition is uncertain, but as patients often give a previous history of genital warts and as in 80% of cases HPV-DNA type 16 has been shown in biopsy specimens, the papillomavirus may play a causative role (Hauser et al 1985).

Spontaneous regression of the lesions has occasionally been described (Berger & Hori 1978), but cryotherapy and local excision have been used successfully in the treatment of this condition.

REFERENCES

1. ULCERS OF THE EXTERNAL GENITALIA
Morson B C 1976 Regional enteritis (Crohn's disease). In: Bockus H L (ed) Gastroenterology, vol 2. H L Saunders, Philadelphia, p 550
Sigal M, Aitken G, Crickx B, de la Charriere O, Blanc F, Belaich S 1985 Chancre tuberculieux primitif de la veze avec dissemination cutanee verruqueuse. Annales de Dermatologie et de Venereologie 112: 459–462
Wray D, Ferguson M M, Mason D K, Hutcheon A W, Dagg J H 1975 Recurrent aphthae: treatment with vitamin B12, folic acid and iron. British Medical Journal 2: 490–493

2. THE PREPUCE AND THE DEVELOPMENT OF THE PREPUTIAL SAC
Burrows H 1944 The union and separation of living tissues influenced by cellular differentiation. Yale Journal of Biological Medicine 17: 397–402
Cooper G G, Thomson G J L, Raine P A 1983 Therapeutic

retraction of the foreskin in childhood. British Medical Journal 286: 186–187

Deibert G A 1933 The separation of the prepuce in the human penis. Anatomical Record 57: 387–399

Esscher T 1984 Why not let preputial adhesions alone? Correspondence, Lancet ii: 581–582

Gairdner D 1949 The fate of the foreskin; a study of circumcision. British Medical Journal 2: 1433–1437

Griffiths D M, Freeman N V 1984 Non-surgical separation of the preputial adhesions. Correspondence, Lancet ii: 344

Kochen M 1980 Circumcision and the risk of cancer of the penis. A lifetime-table analysis. American Journal of Diseases of Childhood 184: 484–486

Øster J 1968 Further fate of the foreskin. Archives of the Diseases of Childhood 43: 200–203

Pfaff G, Bolkenius M 1984 Hands off the prepuce. Correspondence, Lancet ii: 874–875

Short R V 1980 The origins of human sexuality. In: Austin C R, Short R V (eds) Reproduction in mammals, vol 8. Human sexuality. Cambridge University Press, p 19

3. BALANOPOSTHITIS

Kinghorn G R, Jones B M, Chowdhury F H, Geary I 1982 Balanoposthitis associated with Gardnerella vaginalis infection in men. British Journal of Venereal Diseases 58: 127–129

Masfari A N, Kinghorn G R, Duerden B I 1983 Anaerobes in genitourinary infections in men. British Journal of Venereal Diseases 59: 255–259

4. SOME NON-INFECTIVE CONDITIONS

Rook A, Wilkinson D S, Ebling F J G, Champion R H, Burton J L (eds) 1986 Textbook of dermatology, 4th edn. Blackwell Scientific Publications, Oxford, vol 1, 2 & 3

5. TINEA CRURIS

Cartwright R Y 1975 Antifungal drugs. Journal of Antimicrobial Chemotherapy 1: 141–162

Davis C M, Garcia R L, Riordon J P, Taplin D 1972 Dermatophytes in military recruits. Archives of Dermatology 105: 558–560

Frey D, Oldfield R J, Bridges R C 1979 A colour atlas of pathogenic fungi. Wolfe Medical Publications, London, p 32, 50, 61, 71

La Touche C J 1967 Scrotal dermatophytosis. An insufficiently documented aspect of tinea cruris. British Journal of Dermatology 79: 339–344

Milne L J R, Barnetson R St C 1971 Diagnosis of dermatophytoses using vinyl adhesive tape. Sabouraudia 12: 162–165

Noble W C, Somerville D A 1974 Microbiology of human skin. Saunders, London, p 214

Rebell G, Taplin D 1970 Dermatophytes: their recognition and identification. 2nd edn. University of Miami Press, Coral Gables, Florida p 85–86, 110–115

Roberts S O B, Mackenzie D W R 1986 Tinea cruris. In: Rook A, Wilkinson D S, Ebling F J G, Champion R H, Burton J L (eds) Textbook of dermatology, 4th edn. Blackwell Scientific Publications, Oxford, vol 1, p 921–923

Rosman N 1966 Infections with Trichophyton rubrum. British Journal of Dermatology 78: 208–212

Sawyer P R, Brogden R N, Pinder R M, Speight T M, Avery G S 1975a Miconazole: a review of its antifungal activity and therapeutic efficiency. Drugs 9: 406–423

Sawyer P R, Brogden R N, Pinder R M, Speight T M, Avery G S 1975b Clotrimazole: A review of its antifungal activity and therapeutic efficiency. Drugs 9: 424–447

6. ERYTHRASMA

Clayton Y M, Connor B L 1973 Comparison of clotrimazole cream, Whitfield's ointment and nystatin ointment for the topical treatment of ringworm infections, pityriasis versicolor, erythrasma and candidiasis. British Journal of Dermatology 89: 297–303

Macmillan A L, Sarkany I 1970 Specific topical therapy for erythrasma. British Journal of Dermatology 82: 507–509

Roberts S O B, Highet A S 1986 Bacterial infections: erythrasma. In: Rook A, Wilkinson D S, Ebling F J G, Champion R H, Burton J L (ed) Textbook of dermatology, 4th edn. Blackwell Scientific Publications, Oxford, vol 1, p 759–761

Somerville D A, Seville R H, Cunningham R C, Noble W C, Savin J A 1970 Erythrasma in a hospital for the mentally subnormal. British Journal of Dermatology 82: 355–360

7. BALANITIS XEROTICA OBLITERANS (BXO)

Bainbridge D R, Whitaker R H, Shepheard B G F 1971 Balanitis xerotica obliterans and urinary obstruction. British Journal of Urology 43: 487–491

Ive F A, Wilkinson D S 1986 Diseases of the umbilical, perianal and genital regions; lichen sclerosus et atrophicus, syn. balanitis xerotica obliterans. In: Rook A, Wilkinson D S, Ebling F J G, Champion R H, Burton J L (eda) Textbook of dermatology, 4th edn. Blackwell Scientific Publications, Oxford, vol 3, ch 59, p 2190–2192

Laymon C W, Freeman C 1944 Relationship of balanitis xerotica obliterans to lichen sclerosus et atrophicus. Archives of Dermatology and Syphilology 49: 57–59

Mikat D M, Ackerman H R, Mikat K W 1973 Balanitis xerotica obliterans: report of a case in an 11 year old and a review of the literature. Paediatrics 52: 25–41

Ridley C M 1975 The vulva. Saunders, London, p 172

Rowell N R 1986 Lupus erythematosus, scleroderma and dermatomyositis. The 'collagen or connective-tissue diseases' sections on lichen sclerosus syn. lichen sclerosus et atrophicus etc. In: Rook A, Wilkinson D S, Ebling F J G, Champion R H, Burton J L (eds) Textbook of dermatology, 4th edn. Blackwell Scientific Publications, Oxford, vol 2, ch 35, p 1368–1374

8. ERYTHROPLASIA OF QUEYRAT

Goette D K 1976 Review of erythroplasia of Queyrat and its treatment. Urology 8: 311–315

9. PEYRONIE'S DISEASE

Billig R, Baker R, Immergut M, Maxted W 1975 Peyronie's disease. Urology 6: 409–411

Laake K 1983 In: Dukes M N G (ed) Side effects of drugs annual 7 1983. Excerpta Medica, Amsterdam, p 217

Osborne D R 1977 Propranolol and Peyronie's disease. Correspondence, Lancet i: 1111

Palmer P E, Wolfe H J, Kostas C I 1978 Multisystem fibrosis in alpha l-antitrypsin deficiency. Correspondence. Lancet ii: 22

Pryor J P, Castle W 1982 Peyronie's disease associated with chronic degenerative arterial disease and not with beta-adrenoceptor blocking agents. Correspondence, Lancet i: 917

Wallis A A, Bell R, Sutherland P W 1977 Propranolol and Peyronie's disease. Correspondence, Lancet ii: 980

Yudkin J S 1977 Peyronie's disease in association with metoprolol. Correspondence, Lancet ii: 1355

Zarafonetis C J D, Horrax T M 1959 Treatment of Peyronie's disease with potassium para-aminobenzoate (Potaba). Journal of Urology 81: 770–772

10. LYMPHOCOELE AND LOCALIZED OEDEMA OF THE PENIS

Fiumara N J 1975 Nonvenereal sclerosing lymphangitis of the penis. Archives of Dermatology III: 902–903

Hoffman E 1923 Vortanschung primarer Syphilis durch gonorrhoische Lymphangitis (gonorrhoischer Pseudoprimaraffekt). Munchener Medizinische Wochenschrift 70: 1167–1168

Marsch W Ch, Stuttgen G 1981 Sclerosing lymphangitis of the penis: a lymphangiofibrosis thrombotica occlusiva. British Journal of Dermatology 104: 687–695

Stolz E, van Kampen W J, Vuzevski V 1974 Sklerosiesende Lymphangitis des Penis, der Oberlippe und des Labium minus. Hautarzt 25: 231–237

11. BEHÇET'S SYNDROME

Barnes C G 1984 Behcet's syndrome. Journal of the Royal Society of Medicine 77: 816–819

Chajek T, Fainaru M 1975 Behcet's disease: report of 41 cases and a review of the literature. Medicine, Baltimore 54: 179–196

Dunlop E M C 1979 Genital and other manifestations of Behcet's disease seen in venereological practice. In: Lehner T, Barnes C G (eds) Behcet's syndrome. Clinical and immunological features. Academic Press, London, p 159–175

James Geraint J 1979 Behcet's syndrome. Leading Article, New England Journal of Medicine 301: 431–432

Lehner T, Barnes C G 1979 Criteria for diagnosis and classification of Behcet's syndrome. In: Lehner T, Barnes C G (eds) Behcet's syndrome, clinical and immunological features. Academic Press, London, p 1–9

Svejgaard A, Platz P, Ryder L P 1983 HLA and disease 1982 — a survey. Immunological Reviews 70: 193–218

Vernon-Roberts B, Barnes C G, Revell P A 1978 Synovial pathology in Behcet's syndrome. Annals of the Rheumatic Diseases 37: 139–145

Yazici H, Chamberlain M A, Juzun Y, Yurdakul S, Muftuoglu — 1984 A comparative study of the pathergy reaction amongst Turkish and British patients with Behcet's disease. Annals of the Rheumatic Diseases 43: 74–75

12. VULVAL INTRA-EPITHELIAL NEOPLASIA

Andreasson B, Bock J E 1985 Intraepithelial neoplasia in the vulvar region. Gynecologic Oncology 21: 300–305

Bernstein S G, Kovacs B R, Townsend D E, Morrow P 1983 Vulvar carcinoma in situ. Obstetrics and Gynecology 61: 304–307

Buckley C H, Butler E B, Fox H 1984 Vulvar intraepithelial neoplasia and microinvasive carcinoma of the vulva. Journal of Clinical Pathology 37: 1201–1211

Crum C P 1982 Vulvar intraepithelial neoplasia: the concept and its application. Human Pathology 13: 187–189

Crum C P, Fu Y S, Levine R V, Richart R M, Townsend D E, Fenoglio C M 1982 Intraepithelial squamous lesions of the vulva: biologic and histologic criteria for the distinction of condyloma from vulvar intraepithelial neoplasia. Americal Journal of Obstetrics and Gynecology 144: 77–83

Friedrich E G, Wilkinson E J, Fu Y S 1980 Carcinoma in situ of the vulva: a continuing challenge. American Journal of Obstetrics and Gynecology 136: 830–838

Ikenberg H, Gissmann L, Gross G, Grussendorf-Conen E T, zur Hausen H 1983 Human papillomavirus type 16 related DNA in genital Bowen's disease and Bowenoid papules. International Journal of Cancer 32: 563–565

13. BOWENOID PAPULOSIS OF THE MALE GENITALIA

Berger B W, Hori Y 1978 Multicentric Bowen's disease of the genitalia. Spontaneous regression of lesion. Archives of Dermatology 114: 1698–1699

Hauser B, Grosse G, Schneider A, De Villiers E. Gissmann L, Wagner D 1985 HPV-16 related Bowenoid papulosis. Correspondence, Lancet ii: 106

Katz H I, Posalaky Z, McGinley D 1978 Pigmented penile papules with carcinoma in situ changes. British Journal of Dermatology 99: 155–162

Kimura S 1982 Bowenoid papulosis of the genitalia. International Journal of Dermatology 21: 432–436

38

Intestinal and anorectal disorders in homosexual men

I. INFECTIONS

During sexual contact amongst homosexual men the transmission of viruses, bacteria, protozoa and nematodes which infect the intestinal tract may take place, and is well-recognized as important. In the case of certain infective agents or organisms, these are acquired directly as a result of penetration of the rectum in anorectal intercourse, but in the case of others, their habitat is intestinal and transmission occurs by ingestion of faecal material during oro-anal or orogenital contact. Extensive faecal contamination of the skin surface that occurs during anal sexual intercourse facilitates transmission of enteric organisms. With respect to intestinal protozoa, in geographical localities where overall prevalence is high, prevalence of intestinal protozoa among homosexual males may be expected to be very high; in areas of low prevalence, the prevalence among homosexual males will be higher than in the general population.

PROCTOCOLITIS

This a common disorder amongst men who have had homosexual contact. Although proctitis can result from a wide variety of insults including irradiation, chemicals and drug therapy, most cases amongst homosexual men are associated with infection. It should be remembered, however, that men with idiopathic inflammatory bowel disease may present to a STD clinic in the belief that their symptoms are related to anal intercourse.

Aetiology
Proctitis may result from infection with organisms or agents acquired either directly through anal intercourse or alternatively through the faecal-oral route. The first group includes *T. pallidum*, *N. gonorrhoeae*, *C. trachomatis* and herpes simplex virus. The second group consists of enteric organisms such as *E. histolytica*, *Shigella spp*, *Campylobacter spp* and *Cryptosporidium*. Infection with two or more organisms is common, Quinn et al (1983);

in his study 22 out of 119 men with proctitis were infected with two or more organisms or agents. The characteristic of intestinal infection with these organisms, their role in the aetiology of proctitis and their diagnosis and treatment are discussed separately elsewhere in this chapter. There is also a group of patients with clinical features of proctitis but in whom no specific cause can be identified (non-specific proctitis). In some cases an infective cause may not have been identified and in others repeated rectal trauma may be the cause.

Pathology
In the early stages (0–4 days after the onset of symptoms) of *acute infective proctitis* (Kumar et al 1982) there is mucosal oedema, with infiltration of the lamina propria with neutrophils and, to a much lesser extent, with lymphocytes and plasma cells. Polymorphs migrating between the epithelial cells of the mucosal surface and crypts, which may be eroded, are common and crypt abscesses may be a feature.

As the acute inflammatory response resolves, the mucosal oedema becomes less pronounced and there is regeneration of the surface and crypt epithelium, the goblet cells of which show mucus depletion. The neutrophil content of the lamina propria is less pronounced, but there is a moderate increase in the numbers of lymphocytes, plasma cells and eosinophils.

Generally these histological findings are not specific for any particular organism, but in both syphilis and chlamydial infections with LGV immunovars granulomas may be formed, and in herpetic proctitis intranuclear inclusions are to be seen.

Certain histological features usually help to differentiate an acute, self-limiting proctocolitis from ulcerative colitis and Crohn's disease: 1. the lack of distortion of the crypt architecture, 2. lack of marked mucus depletion of the goblet cells in the acute stage, and 3. only moderate increase in numbers of mononuclear cells in the lamina propria (Mandal et al 1982). Occasionally, however, differentiation between the two conditions is not possible.

Clinical features

The most common clinical features of *acute proctocolitis* are mucopurulent anal discharge or, in mild cases, mucus-streaking of the stool, diarrhoea, anorectal bleeding, perianal pain and a sensation of incomplete defaecation. Lower abdominal pain and tenderness over the colon are features more characteristic of colitis. At sigmoidoscopy there is often mucopus on the mucosa, which usually shows loss of the normal ramifying vascular pattern, oedema, contact bleeding and sometimes ulceration. It should be noted that the vascular pattern is often absent from the distal 10 cm of the normal rectum. Sometimes, in the presence of gross microscopic disease, the rectal mucosa appears normal to the naked eye (Watts et al 1966).

Generally, in patients with gonococcal, chlamydial, herpetic and early-stage syphilitic infection, the inflammation is principally restricted to the rectum, but in amoebic and bacterial dysentery the inflammatory process is seen to exend beyond the rectosigmoid junction. Double contrast barium enema examination in patients with proctitis shows nodularity and ulceration of the mucosa (Sider et al 1982).

In patients with *chronic proctitis* symptoms are usually mild and consist of intermittent anal discharge or mucus-streaking of the stool and anorectal bleeding. The sigmoidoscopic appearance of the mucosa is usually normal (McMillan et al 1983b).

Diagnosis

The enumeration of polymorphs in a smear of rectal exudate, obtained by rolling a cotton-wool-tipped applicator stick over the mucosa, is an unreliable and unnecessary investigation when the proctoscopic and sigmoidoscopic appearance is consistent with acute proctitis. As shown in Figure 38.1, there is little correlation between the numbers of cells and the histology. Although McMillan et al (1983b), using impression

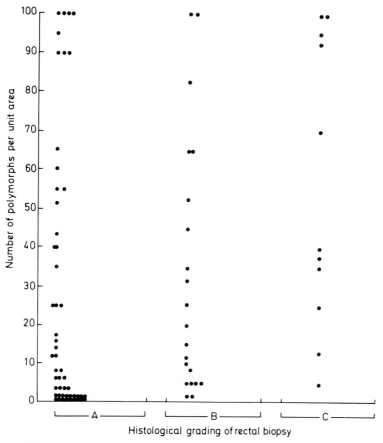

Fig. 38.1 Numbers of polymorphonuclear leucocytes per unit area of a Gram-stained smear of rectal exudate obtained by rolling a cotton-wool swab over the rectal mucosa. A = normal rectal mucosa. B = increased numbers of plasma cells and lymphocytes within the lamina propria. C = predominantly polymorphonuclear leucocyte infiltration of lamina propria. Polymorphs often seen traversing columnar epithelium.

smears, found good correlation between the cytological and histological findings in patients with acute infective proctitis, the method is inconvenient and does not lend itself to use in a busy clinic. In most cases a diagnosis can be made on the basis of the symptoms and proctoscopic findings. Cytology is of little value in the detection of chronic proctitis.

The appropriate specimens for microbiological examination should be obtained as detailed elsewhere in this chapter. When these investigations are unhelpful and the patient's symptoms persist, sigmoidoscopy with the taking of a rectal biopsy and radiological examination of the colon are indicated to exclude ulcerative proctocolitis and Crohn's disease.

Treatment

Treatment of infective proctitis is discussed in relation to the individual infecting organism. In patients with so-called non-specific proctitis every effort should be made to exclude inflammatory bowel disease and to identify any possible aetiological factor. Treatment with broad spectrum antibiotics such as tetracycline usually does not prove useful, and the use of steroids and salazopyrine has not been studied adequately to allow firm conclusions to be obtained regarding their efficacy and safety.

A. INFECTIONS ACQUIRED BY THE FAECAL-ORAL ROUTE

Eukaryotes — protozoa

The results of studies are given in Table 38.1 on the prevalence of intestinal protozoa amongst homosexual men who have attended STD specialists in developed countries or, in the series reported by Markell et al (1984), who were recruited for investigation through gay organizations. The prevalence of infection amongst heterosexuals of the western world — in countries of low incidence — is much lower, with less than 1% and

3% infected respectively with *E. histolytica* or *G. intestinalis*. As most studies have involved some form of selection, the true prevalence of enteric protozoal infections amongst homosexual men cannot readily be determined; prevalence is likely to be lower in close-coupled or asexual homosexual men than among open-coupled or functional (see Ch. 2).

Giardia intestinalis

Giardia intestinalis (lamblia) is a protozoal flagellate found in its trophozoite form in the upper small intestine (Ch. 2). Transmission occurs by ingestion of cysts, formed in the small intestine and excreted in the faeces. The microscopic features of giardia are given with those of other intestinal flagellates and ciliates in Table 38.2.

Epidemiology. Giardiasis is an infection found in both temperate and tropical countries especially where sanitation is poor. Although the protozoon is acquired mainly through the ingestion of viable cysts in faeces-contaminated water or food, person-to-person transmission of the parasite also occurs by the faecal-oral route (Kulda & Nohynkova 1978). During outbreaks of infection, many of those infected have no symptoms. The homosexual transmission of *G. intestinalis* was first recognized by Meyers and his colleagues (1977) in Seattle and later supported by Schmerin et al (1978) in New York City.

Giardia intestinalis is more likely to produce disease in patients with immunodeficiency syndromes, including selective IgA deficiency.

Pathology. In many patients with no underlying immunodeficiency, the histology of the jejunum is normal. The histological changes which have been described in association with *Giardia* infection are generally mild and include villous blunting and lymphocytic infiltration of the lamina propria. The crypt epithelium is sometimes infiltrated with neutrophils and lymphocytes (Ridley & Ridley 1976, Hartong et al 1979). More severe changes

Table 38.1 Prevalence of intestinal protozoa in homosexual men. References: 1. William et al (1978); 2. Phillips et al (1981); 3. Markell et al (1984); 4. Keystone et al (1980); 5. McMillan (1982, unpublished data); 6. McMillan (1980); 7. Chin & Gerken (1984).

Organism	Studies on prevalence (numbers examined)						
	New York City[1] (89)	New York City[2] (99)	San Francisco[3] (508)	Toronto[4] (200)	Edinburgh[5] (310)	Glasgow[6] (118)	London[7] (83)
Entamoeba histolytica	20	11	29	27	10	3	12
Entamoeba hartmanni	—	—	25	—	1	—	5
Entamoeba coli	13	—	21	—	10	—	25
Endolimax nana	11	—	38	—	5	—	22
Iodamoeba butschlii	5	—	13	—	2	1	4
Giardia intestinalis	12	4	6	13	6	2	8
Dientamoeba fragilis	1	—	1	—	0	—	—
Chilomastix mesnili	—	—	1	—	1	—	—

Table 38.2 Microscopic features of the intestinal flagellates and ciliates.

Protozoon	Shape and size	Nuclear characteristics (stained smear)	Number and position of flagella	Other features
TROPHOZOITES:				
Flagellates:				
Retortamonas intestinalis	Pear shaped 4–9 μm × 3–4 μm	Spherical nucleus anterior end of organisms.	1 anterior, 1 recurrent	Ventral cytostome extending half-way down body.
Enteromonas hominis	Pear shaped 4–10 μm × 306 μm	Anterior oval nucleus with eccentric endosome.	3 anterior, long posterior	Narrow cytostome. Prominent funis on left of cytostome extending for two-thirds of body length.
Chilomastix mesnili	Pear shaped. Rounded anteriorly, tail-like posterior projection. 6–20 μm × 4–7 μm	Round anterior nucleus with several peripheral deeply staining plaques.	3 anterior, short recurrent	Prominent cytostomal groove with long posteriorly curved right cytostomal fibre.
Giardia intestinalis	Pear shaped 10–20 μm × 5–15 μm	2 with large endosomes.	2 ventral, 2 anterolateral, 2 posterolateral, 2 caudal	
Dientamoeba fragilis	3.5 × 22 μm. Moves by extension of broad hyaline pseudopodia.	Usually 2 nuclei but not uncommonly 1 only. Large central endosome; no peripheral chromatin.	—	—
Ciliate:				
Balantidium coli	Elongated or ovoid 30–300 μm × 30–300 μm	Kidney shaped. Macronucleus enclosing micronucleus.	—	Ciliated. Peristome at anterior end. Two contractile vacuoles.
CYSTS:				
Flagellates:				
Retortamonas intestinalis	Thick-walled, oval or lemon shaped 4.5–7 μm × 3–4.5 μm	Single nucleus	—	Internal flagella and cytostomal fibres seen in stained preparations.
Enteromonas hominis	Oval. 6–8 μm × 4–6 μm	1–4 nuclei	—	—
Chilomastix mesnili	Pear or lemon shaped with hyaline anterior protuberance. 7–10 μm × 4.5 μm.	1 nucleus	—	Cytostomal fibres visible in unstained cysts.
Giardia intestinalis	Oval or round 8–20 μm	4 nuclei	—	Longitudinal fibres within cyst.
Ciliate:				
Balantidium coli	Spherical or ovoid 40–60 μm. Thick hyaline wall.	1 nucleus	—	—

are found, however, in patients with underlying immunodeficiency. Trophozoites of *G. intestinalis* appear in H&E (haematoxylin and eosin) or Giemsa-stained tissue sections as pear- or sickle-shaped organisms with two nuclei, in the lumen of the intestine or attached to the epithelial surface.

Clinical features. Many, if not most, infections with

G. intestinalis are symptomless, with the parasite being detected by chance on routine stool examination. After a prepatent period of about 10 days the onset of foul-smelling diarrhoea is sudden. Characteristically the stools tend to float on the surface of the water and the patient complains of increased flatulence, abdominal distension, cramping abdominal pain, anorexia, nausea and weight loss. Blood and pus are not present in the faeces. Untreated, symptoms usually resolve after a variable interval of up to three months. In patients with underlying immunodeficiency the illness is more prolonged with intermittent diarrhoea or steatorrhoea, increased flatulence, nausea and weight loss.

In about half of symptomatic patients, there is biochemical evidence of malabsorption (Wright et al 1977). On radiological examination after ingestion of contrast media, characteristic features, found in about 70% of cases, include thickening of the mucosal folds, particularly of the duodenum and proximal jejunum, and, as a result of excessive secretions in the gut lumen, fragmentation of the column of barium sulphate can be seen.

Diagnosis of giardiasis

1. Examination of faeces. In diarrhoeal stools, trophozoites may be seen in saline mount (Note 38.1), or in trichrome-stained preparations of fresh or preserved specimens (Note 38.2). Cysts may be found in formed stools, but, as the numbers may be too small to detect the cysts by direct microscopy, concentration by the formol-ether method (Note 38.3) is recommended. *Giardia* cannot be cultivated satisfactorily from the faeces. As cyst excretion is often intermittent, at least three stool samples, obtained on alternate days, should be examined. The ingestion of anti-diarrhoea agents, antacids, antimicrobials and barium sulphate interferes with the excretion of *Giardia* cysts, so they should be avoided while attempts at diagnosis are being made.

As the detection of *Giardia* cysts by microscopy can be difficult, immunological methods for the identification of antigen in faeces have been developed (Ungar et al 1984, Green et al 1985). Although they are not widely available at present, these methods offer considerable advantages over direct microscopy in that they are more sensitive (sensitivity is at least 92%) and do not require highly skilled technical staff.

2. Detection of Giardia trophozoites in jejunal samples. When neither trophozoites or cysts are seen in the faeces, but giardiasis is suspected clinically, jejunal intubation with aspiration of the secretions and/or biopsy may be necessary if it is important to make an organismal diagnosis. Biopsy seems to be the most sensitive for the diagnosis of *Giardia* (Kamath and Murugasu, 1974). Trophozoites may be seen by direct microscopy of the jejunal aspirate or cultured from this source in Diamond's medium (Note 38.4). Tissue impression smears, fixed in methanol and stained by Giemsa's method (Note 38.5), should also be prepared for microscopy (Kamath & Murugasu 1974). In Giemsa-stained tissue sections the trophozoites are found in the lumen of the intestine or attached to the epithelial cells of the villi or crypts.

As an alternative to duodenal or jejunal intubation and biopsy, the so-called 'string test' or Enterotest (Note 38.6) has been advocated (Beal et al 1970). The patient swallows a length of prepared thread, and after about four hours this is withdrawn and the retained secretion examined microscopically for trophozoites.

Although IgG antibodies can be detected by immunofluorescence or ELISA in the sera of the majority of patients with symptomatic giardiasis (Ridley & Ridley 1976, Smith et al 1981), serological tests are of limited value in diagnosis. Antibodies remain detectable for many months after successful treatment and their prevalence is high in currently non-infected groups.

Treatment. Mepacrine hydrochloride (Mepacrine Tablets BNF) taken orally in a dosage of 100 mg 3 times a day for 7 days (Wolfe 1975), gives a cure rate of about 95% in giardiasis (Wolfe 1975). Side effects include gastrointestinal upsets and, on very rare occasions, exfoliative dermatitis and toxic psychosis; it should not be used in patients with psychotic illness or with psoriasis.

Metronidazole (Metronidazole Tablets BNF; Flagyl Tablets, May and Baker) 200 mg 3 times a day for 7 days is less effective (cure rate of less than 70%) (Ch. 22).

Entamoeba histolytica

Amoebiasis is caused by the protozoon *Entamoeba histolytica.* After ingestion by the host, those cysts which escape the gastric juices, pass into the small intestine where they excyst to form trophozoites, which colonize the large intestine. Trophozoites may remain free-living in the intestinal lumen and in turn encyst to be excreted in the faeces; alternatively they may invade the mucous membrane of the intestinal wall, cause ulceration and sometimes produce the clinical features of amoebic dysentery. The amoebae may be carried from the intestine to the liver or, less commonly, other organs, where abscesses may develop. The microscopic features of *E. histolytica* and of the four non-pathogenic intestinal amoebae are given in Table 38.3.

Pathogenicity of *Entamoeba histolytica*. For decades, controversy has existed and still exists regarding the pathogenicity of *E. histolytica.* It is known that many symptomless individuals excrete amoebic cysts in their faeces and that comparatively few people develop serious disease as a result of the infection. Such observations prompted numerous authorities to postulate the existence of pathogenic and non-pathogenic strains of *E. histolytica.*

Although morphologically similar, virulent (that is, invasive) and avirulent (that is, non-invasive) stocks (Note 38.5) of *E. histolytica* differ in several respects. Only virulent stocks grown axenically produce hepatic

Table 38.3 Microscopic features of *Entamoeba histolytica* and of four non-pathogenic intestinal amoebae.

| Organism | Size μm | TROPHOZOOITES | | | |
| | | Nucleus | | Cytoplasm | |
		Peripheral chromatin	Endosome	Appearance	Inclusions
Entamoeba histolytica	15–50 (usually 15–20)	fine granules, beaded	small central	granular ectoplasm & endoplasm clearly differentiated	Bacteria, may have erythrocytes
Entamoeba coli	15–50 (usually 20–25)	clumped unevenly, arranged on membrane or as solid ring	large, often eccentric	granular; no differentiation into into ecto- and endoplasm	Bacteria, debris
Entamoeba hartmanni	5–12 (usually 8–10)	similar to *E. histolytica*	small, compact, often central	fine, granular	Bacteria
Endolimax nana	6–18 (usually 8–10)	absent	large, irregular, usually central	granular vacuolated	Bacteria
Iodamoeba butschlii	8–20 (usually 12–15)	absent	large, rounded; surrounded by achromatic granules	coarse granular vacuolated	Bacteria, debris

| Organism | Size μm (shape) | CYSTS | | | | |
| | | Nucleus or nuclei | | | Cytoplasm | |
		Number	Peripheral chromatin	Endosome	Chromatoidal bodies	Glycogen iodine-stained
Entamoeba histolytica	10–20 Spherical	1–4	As trophozoite	As trophozoite	Common; blunt ends	Ill-defined glycogen vacuole
Entamoeba coli	10–30 Usually spherical	1–8, seldom 2, occasionally 16	Coarse, granular, may be clumped on membrane	Large, eccentric	Infrequent; splinter-like ends	Well-defined mass lying between nuclei in binucleate cysts
Entamoeba hartmanni	5–9 Spherical	1–4, often 2	Fine granules on membrane	Small, central	Common; blunt smooth ends	Diffuse or absent
Endolimax nana	5–12 Ovoid	1–4	Absent	Large, central	Absent	Diffuse if present
Iodamoeba butschlii	6–15 Very irregular, ovoid, spherical	1, rarely 2	Absent	Large, eccentric	Absent	Large, well-defined

abscesses when inoculated into the livers of hamsters (Mattern & Keister 1977). Cultivated virulent stocks of *E. histolytica* differ in their surface properties from avirulent stocks. The virulent ingest erythrocytes at a much greater rate than the avirulent, show marked contact-dependent cytopathic effects, and agglutinate more readily when incubated with concavalin A (Martinez-Palomo 1983). Recently McGowan and colleagues (1982) isolated a heat-labile cytotoxin from highly and moderately virulent axenically-cultivated stocks of *E. histolytica*, but not from a so-called non-pathogenic stock. The partially purified cytotoxin, whose activity could be inhibited by specific immune sera and by protease inhibitors, was shown to have no enzymic activity. To render cultures of *E. histolytica*, derived from stools, free from other contaminating organisms (viz. to make axenic) is difficult, so it is not practicable to test for the elaboration of cytotoxin as a marker of pathogenicity.

Differences in the isoenzyme profiles for four enzymes (Glucose phosphate isomerase; phosphoglucomutase; L-malate: NADP$^+$ oxidoreductase; and hexokinase) have been used as the basis for classifying stocks of *E. histolytica*. Certain of these stocks, classified in this way and termed zymodemes, have been found to be associated with invasive amoebiasis (Sargeaunt et al 1982, 1984, Gathiram & Jackson 1985).

In a study of 52 stocks of *E. histolytica* obtained from the faeces of 470 homosexual men who attended STD clinics in Edinburgh and London, Sargeaunt et al (1983) found zymodemes which he recognized as 'non-pathogenic'. The non-invasive nature of *E. histolytica* in homosexual men in Edinburgh was confirmed by the clinical and histopathological study undertaken by McMillan et al (1984a). Neither trophozoites within the rectal mucosa nor significant titres of serum antibodies against the amoeba were detected. In the absence of other pathogenic organisms, however, they found a significant association between the presence of *E. histolytica* and an increased chronic inflammatory cell infiltration of the rectal lamina propria. From this study they concluded that non-invasive amoebae may induce proctitis. This finding was not, however, obtained in a study from London (Goldmeier et al 1986).

Invasive amoebiasis in homosexual men appears to be rare. Burnham et al (1980) reported acute proctitis with tissue invasion with amoebic trophozoites in a young homosexual man, and Thompson et al (1983) described a case of a hepatic amoebic abscess in a homosexual. In neither case was the zymodeme determined.

Histopathology

a. Intestinal amoebiasis. A common finding in intestinal amoebiasis is an acute inflammatory cell infiltration of varying degree of the lamina propria, with migration of polymorphs through the surface epithelium and lymphoid hyperplasia (Prathap & Gilman 1970, Pittman et al 1974), but the nature of this mucosal response is non-specific. In early invasive lesions there are foci of interglandular epithelial cell and basement membrane destruction with invasion by amoebae of the superficial lamina propria. A mild polymorph infiltration is found in the tissues adjacent to the site of amoebic infiltration. As invasion progresses, there is further necrosis with involvement of the submucosa, and the ulcer assumes the typical flask-shaped appearance.

b. Cutaneous amoebiasis The floor of the ulcer consists of necrotic tissue containing trophozoites which overlies granulation tissue. At the edge of the ulcer the epidermis shows acanthosis and papillomatosis (Purpon et al 1967).

Clinical features. In patients with amoebiasis about 90% are symptom-free; in the remainder the severity of the illness varies greatly. In symptomatic intestinal amoebiasis the patient has diarrhoea, abdominal discomfort, flatulence and blood and mucus in the stool, and may also complain of anorexia and weight loss. Sigmoidoscopy may reveal a normal rectal mucosal pattern or a mucous membrane which is red, oedematous and friable. The inflammatory reaction extends beyond the rectosigmoid junction. The appearance may, however, be identical to that of non-specific ulcerative proctocolitis (Pittman et al 1974), when there may be multiple areas of ulceration, with individual ulcers reaching up to a few millimetres in diameter with a yellow base and an erythematous margin.

The development of hepatic abscess is associated with tenderness in the right hypochondrium, fever, and weight loss. Aspiration of the abscess produces a red-brown thick fluid, in which amoebae are rarely demonstrable. Cutaneous amoebiasis may rarely produce perianal or genital ulceration. The ulcers, which are exquisitely tender, are irregularly-shaped with an undermined edge and blood-encrusted necrotic base (Purpon et al 1967). The inguinal lymph nodes are usually enlarged. Untreated, the lesions progress at a variable rate and can produce large areas of ulceration.

Diagnosis of amoebiasis. The diagnosis of intestinal amoebiasis rests on the detection of cysts and/or trophozoites of *E. histolytica* in the faeces or material obtained from rectal ulcers (Table 38.3).

Detection by microscopy of trophozoites and cysts. It is useful to examine saline mounts of faeces, rectal exudate or material scraped from a rectal ulcer for the presence of trophozoites. These are 15–25 μm in diameter and exhibit unidirectional movement with the often explosive protrusion of finger-like pseudopodia (lobopodia). The presence of erythrocytes in the cytoplasm is pathognomonic of *E. histolytica*. Differentiation of *E. histolytica* trophozoites from other non-pathogenic species of intestinal amoebae is important but, except for finding erythrocyte-containing organisms, is not possible from examination of unstained faecal preparations. Smears of faeces, rectal exudate and ulcer material, fixed in Schaudinn's fluid, and stained with modified Gomori's stain (Wheatley 1951), however, enable such differentiation but require care and experience. Microscopic features helpful in the differentiation of *E. histolytica* from other amoebae are summarized in Table 38.2.

Trophozoites are not commonly found in formed stools, which should routinely be examined for cysts of *E. histolytica* when amoebiasis is suspected. As the number of cysts in a given sample may be small, it is helpful to examine the faeces after cyst concentration by the formol-ether method — Note 38.3 (McMillan & McNeillage 1984). The characteristics which distinguish cysts of *E. histolytica* from those of the non-pathogenic amoebae are (i) size; (ii) number of nuclei; and (iii) presence in the cyst of blunt-ended chromatoidal bodies (Table 38.3). As the identification of amoebic cysts may be difficult, in cases of doubt, samples should be sent fresh or in preservative (Note 38.7) to a reference laboratory.

Detection by culture. Cultivation of intestinal amoebae is desirable from the clinical point of view. McMillan & McNeillage (1984) showed that in 11 of 48 men infection with *E. histolytica* would have been missed if culture had not been undertaken. Cultured trophozoites are required for zymodeme analysis.

Detection by immunological tests. The accurate diagnosis of *E. histolytica* trophozoites and cysts is often difficult, time-consuming and requires experience. More objective methods for the identification of amoebic infection have been described. Root et al (1978) developed an ELISA method for the detection of *E. histolytica* antigens in faeces but it did not gain general acceptance as a diagnostic test. A double antibody indirect ELISA method using a combination of monoclonal and polyclonal antibodies, however, has given encouraging results (Ungar et al 1985). Further studies are required before conclusions can be drawn regarding the value of this test in diagnosis.

Serological tests for antibodies against *E. histolytica* are of value only in the diagnosis of invasive disease (Table 38.4); in the majority of individuals with hepatic amoebic abscesses there are high titres of antibody against the protozoa. Although the indirect haemagglutination test is sensitive, the antibodies detected persist for many years even after successful treatment and for this reason the value of the test in the assessment of cure is limited. It is, however, of some value in epidemiological studies. The indirect immunofluorescent antibody test is better in determining cure of extra-intestinal disease. When treatment has been successful, the titres of antibodies detected in the test fall significantly within two months.

Treatment. In acute invasive amoebiasis immediate treatment is necessary.

Metronidazole is the drug of choice for acute invasive amoebic dysentery, for it is very effective against the trophozoites in ulcers at a dosage of 800 mg 3 times a day for 5 days. It is also effective against amoebae which may have migrated to the liver. It is given either for 10 days or for 5 days, followed by a 10-day course of diloxanide furoate 500 mg 8-hourly by mouth which is effective against the cysts of *E. histolytica*. Large hepatic abscesses may require aspiration. After completion of treatment stool samples should be examined at intervals, say monthly, for three months, for cysts and trophozoites of *E. histolytica*.

The efficacy of treatment of hepatic abscesses is assessed by clinical or radiological examination, possibly supplemented by serological testing. In most cases treated successfully titres of amoebic antibodies detected by immunofluorescence fall significantly within two months of completion of therapy.

The question of treatment of asymptomatic patients who excrete cysts is controversial. Many standard text books of tropical medicine suggest treatment for such individuals, but a recent study in India (Nanda et al 1984) has shown — surprisingly in a hyperendemic area — that spontaneous eradication of the amoebae usually occurs and the risk of the development of invasive amoebiasis is negligible. The results of similar studies amongst homosexual men are awaited.

As invasive disease is rare, in symptomatic homosexual men infected with *E. histolytica*, and in whom other causes of proctitis have been excluded, treatment with diloxanide furoate alone is necessary. It should be stressed that careful clinical examination should be undertaken before treatment is undertaken. There is always the possibility of the introduction into the homosexual community of a virulent *E. histolytica*.

Chloroquine is effective in the treatment of liver

Table 38.4 Serological tests in patients with intestinal and extra-intestinal *E. histolytica* infection.

Test	Sensitivity (%) Asymptomatic cyst carriers	Symptomatic (diarrhoea, blood, mucus)	Extra-intestinal disease	Specificity (%)
Indirect haemagglutination				
Kessel et al (1965)	66	98	100	
Juniper et al (1972)	58	61/95 (symptomatic/invasive)	83	
Complement fixation				
Kessel et al (1965)	28	33/90 (symptomatic/invasive)	100	100
Juniper et al (1972)	58	56/65 (symptomatic/invasive)	83	
Fluorescent antibody				
Jeanes (1969)	0	75	95	100
Precipitin				
Maddison et al (1965)	40	88	97	100
Agar gel diffusion				
Juniper et al (1972)	52	54/86 (symptomatic/invasive)	83	

abscess but is ineffective against other forms of amoe-biasis. It is given in a dose for adults of 600 mg (base) daily by mouth for 5 days and then reduced to 300 mg (base) daily for 14–21 days. This may be followed by a course of metronidazole. For abscesses containing more than 100 ml pus (i.e. approximately 60–100 mm in diameter) aspiration carried out in conjunction with drug therapy will greatly reduce the period of disability. A 10-day course of diloxanide furoate should be given on completion of chloroquine treatment (BNF 1987).

Cryptosporidium spp

Cryptosporidium spp are coccidian protozoal parasites of the suborder Eimeriina (Ch. 2) which are not species-specific and can infect mammals including man, reptiles and birds.

Epidemiology. On the basis of occasional case reports (Meisel et al 1976, Lasser et al 1979) human crypto-sporidiosis was recognized initially as a cause of severe protracted diarrhoea in immunodeficient patients. With the occurrence of AIDS and its frequent association with it, *Cryptosporidium* is now recognized as an important cause of morbidity in this condition. Cryp-tosporidiosis is now also being recognized, however, as an important cause of self-limiting diarrhoea in immu-nocompetent individuals in both developed and devel-oping countries (Table 38.5). All age groups can be infected, but mostly there is an increased prevalence amongst children, particularly those living in poor and unhygienic urban areas (Højlyng et al 1984). Although the coccidian can infect domestic animals and trans-mission to man from them has been described (Anderson et al 1982, Current et al 1983), human-to-human spread by the faecal- oral route is probably more important. Oocyst excretion has been found both in symptomatic and asymptomatic family contacts of patients with cryp-tosporidiosis (Casemore & Jackson 1984, Hart et al 1984). The observation by Jokipii et al (1983), that 12 of 14 patients had visited Leningrad, a city where individuals have previously acquired giardiasis (see above), suggested that the protozoon may be spread in the water supply.

The probable transmission of *Cryptosporidium* by the faecal-oral route suggests that homosexual men might be at risk. Although sporadic cases of cryptosporidiosis have been described in homosexual men who did not have AIDS (Soave et al 1984) it has not yet been found in such patients attending the Department of Genito-Urinary Medicine in Edinburgh (McMillan & McNeillage 1984).

Pathology. *Cryptosporidium* can infect the epithelial cells of the entire gastrointestinal tract, the biliary and pancreatic ducts, the gall bladder and the respiratory tract. Jejunal and ileal biopsies from infected patients show hyperplasia of the crypts, blunting and loss of villi and degenerating surface cells. There is a mild to moderate increase in the numbers of polymorphonuclear leucocytes, plasma cells and lymphocytes within the lamina propria (Meisel et al 1976). Rectal biopsies show the pattern of non-specific proctitis: there is infiltration of the lamina propria with acute and chronic inflam-matory cells, the goblet cells show some mucin de-pletion and the columnar epithelial cells may be replaced by abnormal cuboidal cells (Nime et al 1976).

In tissue sections cryptosporidia appear as small (2–3 μm) round or oval nucleate bodies on the micro-villous surface of epithelial cells. They are most numerous in the jejunum and ileum, and less common in the colon. Electronmicroscopy shows various stages in the life cycle of the parasite (Bird & Smith 1980).

Clinical features. In the *immunocompetent* cryptospori-dial infection is associated with a self-limiting diarrhoea. The diarrhoea may be intermittent or continuous and the stools are often watery and offensive but they do not contain blood or mucus. Abdominal pain before def-aecation, anorexia and vomiting are common additional features, and fever may be found in about one-fifth of patients. Unless there is concomitant infection, white blood cells are usually not detected in the faeces. The diarrhoea usually ceases in two to three weeks, but excretion of oocysts may continue for up to two weeks afterwards (Hart et al 1984).

In the *immunodeficient* the diarrhoea — which is often

Table 38.5 Prevalence of *Cryptosporidium* spp in patients with gastroenteritis.

Location of study	Number (%) of infected patients/number of patients investigated			Reference
	Number tested	Number positive	%	
Helsinki, Finland	154	14	(9.1)	Jokipii et al (1983)
Clwyd, Wales	500	7	(1.4)	Casemore & Jackson (1983)
Harbol, Liberia	278	22	(7.9)	Højlying et al (1984)
Bristol, UK	867	43	(5.0)	Hunt et al (1984)
Liverpool, UK	1967	27	(1.4)	Hart et al (1984)
Copenhagen, Denmark	800	16	(2.0)	Holten-Andersen et al (1984)

profuse, with up to 10 l of fluid stool being passed daily — is prolonged with weight loss and general debility. Many AIDS patients with cryptosporidiosis die from other opportunistic infections. In the few non-AIDS cases with cryptosporidiosis associated with immuno-suppression, discontinuation of the drug(s) has resulted in spontaneous resolution of the infection (Meisel et al 1976).

Diagnosis. The diagnosis of cryptosporidiosis relies on the detection of oocysts in the faeces or on the discovery of the various stages of its life cycle within enterocytes on histological examination of jejunal, ileal, colonic or rectal biopsies. In faecal smears stained by a modified Ziehl-Neelsen method (Henriksen & Pohlenz 1981) oocysts of *Cryptosporidium* appear as round or oval red structures, 5–6 μm in diameter, containing a single deeply-stained red 'dot' which stands out clearly against a green background (Note 38.8). With experience, the oocysts are readily distinguishable from yeasts, but for confirmation, Giemsa-stained smears (Note 38.5) should be examined also. Oocysts appear as pale blue, semi-translucent structures containing eccentrically-placed pink-staining granules.

Although a sugar flotation method for the concen-tration of oocysts is available, the HIV risks involved in its use do not justify its routine application.

Treatment. Unfortunately there is no specific treatment for cryptosporidiosis. Recently, an ornithine decarbox-ylase inhibitor — alpha-difluoromethylornithine — has proved useful in occasional patients, but more experience with the drug is required before conclusions can be drawn.

Other protozoa
With the possible exception of *Dientamoeba fragilis* (Ch. 2) the other protozoa which have been found at increased frequency in the faeces from homosexual men are not pathogenic. The increasing prevalence is prob-ably a result of sexual activity associated with faecal contamination among a promiscuous but relatively closed population.

Nematodes

Enterobius vermicularis
Enterobius vermicularis is an intestinal parasite, usually transmitted by food or fomites contaminated by ova, and is most commonly found in children. After inges-tion the ova hatch and develop within 6 weeks into adult worms, which inhabit the caecum and adjacent regions of the small and large intestines. The male worms are small, 2–5 mm in length, the females larger, 8–13 mm long. When fully mature, the females emerge from the anus and deposit eggs on the perianal skin. It is this activity which produces pruritus ani, particularly at night. Uncommonly, threadworms enter the vagina and produce vulvo-vaginitis in young girls. On rare occasions ova may be found in cervical smears.

Reports of threadworms in homosexual males (Waugh 1972), probably indicate oro-anal contact, a common practice in some homosexual men. Threadworms should therefore be excluded as a cause of pruritus ani.

Diagnosis. Adult worms may be seen in the faeces or in the anal canal or rectum, or ova may be found on the perianal skin. Alternatively, to make a diagnosis, trans-parent adhesive tape (Sellotape) sticky side down, is applied to the perianal skin, preferably in the morning before the patient has defaecated. The tape is then applied to a slide for examination by microscopy for ova. Threadworm ova are oval and flattened on one side (50–60 μ $\times$ 10–30 μ).

Treatment. Piperazine is the most widely used drug in the treatment of enterobiasis, most conveniently being given to adults and children over 6 years of age as a single sachet containing 4 g of piperazine phosphate B.P. with standardized senna (Pripsen, Reckitt and Colman) — stirred into a small glass of milk and drunk immediately. It should be repeated as a follow-up dose after 14 days. Side effects include dizziness and ataxia, but are rare. It should not be used in patients with severe bilateral renal dysfunction and its use in the first trimester of pregnancy is not advised (ABPI Data Sheet Compendium 1988–89).

Mebendazole (Vermox, Janssen Pharmaceutical Ltd.)in a single oral dose of 100 mg is satisfactory for patients of all ages. It may be given as a single tablet or as 5 ml of a 2% w/v suspension. Side effects are rare and include diarrhoea and abdominal pain. As it has been shown to be toxic in animal studies the drug is contra-indicated in pregnancy (ABPI Data Sheet Compendium 1988–89).

Strongyloides stercoralis
In the case of the nematode *Strongyloides stercoralis*, non-infective rhabitiform larvae may develop into infective filariform larvae before leaving the colon (Ch. 2). Hence, during homosexual intercourse between males, the ingestion of faeces containing these infective filari-form larvae, during oro-anal contact, will enable trans-mission to occur. Alternatively penetration of the mucosa or skin of the penis or elsewhere by infective larvae and the acquisition of *Strongyloides* infection will be possible by direct faecal contact during or following anal intercourse.

Phillips et al (1981) detected *Strongyloides* in the faeces of 2 of 51 homosexual men who attended a sexually transmitted diseases clinic (New York City), and Sorvillo et al (1983), in San Francisco, reported the probable sexual transmission of the helminth. Although the larvae most commonly infect the upper intestine, the rectum may be involved. The larvae penetrate the submucosa and induce a chronic inflammatory cell reaction with eosinophilic infiltration (Carvalho-Filho 1978).

Since overwhelming infection may occur in immunocompromised individuals, producing massive reinvasion of the ileum or colon with haemorrhage, it is very important to exclude strongyloidiasis by examination of the stool in patients to be immunosuppressed.

The diagnosis of strongyloidiasis is made by the detection of larvae in stool samples by microscopy after concentration or by culture (Garcia & Ash 1979).

Prokaryotes

Shigella spp

Most cases of bacillary dysentery occur in children of pre-school or school age, and in boys more often than girls. Generally, in adults, the sexes are affected almost equally, with a slight preponderance of cases in females. Transmission of the organism is usually by hand to mouth contact; the infected individual contaminates toilet fixtures, which are then handled and the organisms transferred to the mouth of the new host. Occasionally, infection results from contaminated water, food or fomites. In several outbreaks of the disease in the United States of America, more than two-thirds of adult cases were in young men, many of whom were homosexual; transmission occurred possibly as a result of oro-anal and oro-genital sexual contact (Dritz et al 1977). Infectivity persists throughout the acute phase of the illness, and for a variable time, usually three to four weeks thereafter. It is important to note that *Shigella* dysentery in homosexual males may be accompanied by infection with other intestinal pathogens such as *Entamoeba histolytica* or *Giardia intestinalis* and other sexually transmissible infection.

Clinical features. In the majority of cases bacillary dysentery is mild. After a prepatent period of two to seven days, the patient suffers from the frequent passage of loose stools. The following day the passage of stools becomes more frequent, but less copious, and symptoms subside after a few days; there is usually no pyrexia, and only small quantities of mucus and blood may be passed.

In some cases the disease is more severe, beginning abruptly with the frequent passage of loose stools, containing blood and mucus; there is also fever, tenesmus and abdominal tenderness. Symptoms persist for about a week and then subside, the illness occasionally passing into a chronic phase. As the disease

process is not confined to the rectum, at sigmoidoscopy the inflammatory changes in the rectum are seen to extend into the sigmoid colon.

Fulminating dysentery, with dehydration and electrolyte imbalance, is rarely seen in adults in developed countries.

Uncommon complications of bacillary dysentery include acute pyelonephritis, conjunctivitis and arthritis.

Diagnosis. Shigella can be readily cultured from stool specimens plated on to medium such as MacConkey agar, DCA (deoxycholate citrate agar). or XLD (xylose lysine decarboxylase) agar. The groups within the genus Shigella (e.g. *Sh. dysenteriae*, *Sh. flexneri*, *Sh. boydii*, *Sh. sonnei*) are identified by appropriate biochemical and serological tests.

Treatment. In management of the patient, bed rest and adequate fluid intake are necessary; careful attention to hygiene is important to prevent further transmission. Antibiotic therapy should not be given unless the illness is severe; the laboratory should confirm that the drug selected is active in vitro against the patient's isolate. In the past, antibiotic treatment has resulted in the emergence of resistant strains of the organism and clearance of the pathogen may not occur significantly earlier than when non-specific treatment has been given.

Diarrhoea may be controlled by the use of agents such as kaolin and morphine mixture, BNF, 10 ml given orally every 6 hours.

Campylobacter spp

Campylobacter jejuni is an important cause of enteritis worldwide, and *C. fetus* subspecies *intestinalis* (Ch. 2) is associated with enteritis in debilitated individuals. The organism is present in the faeces of wild or domestic animals, and contaminated water has been the source of outbreaks of disease (Mentzing 1981). Other means of acquiring the infection include the ingestion of contaminated food or milk (Robinson & Jones 1981; Blaser et al 1982) and the handling of infected animal carcasses (Jones & Robinson 1981). Person to person transfer seems to be uncommon.

Sporadic cases of infection with *C. jejuni* in homosexual men have been reported (Quinn et al 1981). The infection does not appear to be widespread, nor always a problem of homosexual males. In London, Simmons & Tabaqchali (1979) did not isolate campylobacters from the rectal material of 50 homosexual men who attended an STD clinic. McMillan et al (1984b) found a similar prevalence of serum IgG antibodies against the campylobacter in both homosexual and heterosexual men. Quinn et al (1984), nevertheless, in Seattle isolated *C. jejuni* from the faeces of 6% of 158 homosexual men with proctocolitis, and from 3% of 75 symptomless homosexuals; *C. fetus* was cultured from the faeces of 1 patient with proctitis. The Seattle group did not culture campylobacter from the faeces of 150 heterosexual men and women.

Quinn et al (1984) cultured groups of campylobacter-like organisms from rectal material from 16% of 158 homosexual men with proctocolitis and from 8% of 75 symptomless homosexuals. These organisms differed from other species of campylobacters in several respects (see Ch. 2), but their association with symptoms and signs of proctitis suggested that they were pathogenic. The occurrence of campylobacter-like organisms in a group at risk of acquiring enteric infection suggests their transmission by the faecal-oral route as a result of homosexual practices.

Clinical features. Although asymptomatic infections are known to occur, infection with campylobacters is often associated with a self-limiting diarrhoeal illness (Blaser et al 1979). After a prepatent period of up to 10 days there is sudden diarrhoea with bile-stained stools, which later become mucoid and sometimes blood-stained. There is often anorexia (but not vomiting), malaise, pyrexia, headache, cramping lower abdominal pain, myalgia, arthralgia and backache.

Reactive arthritis is a rare complication. These constitutional features are usually noted during the early stage of the illness. On sigmoidoscopy a marked proctitis is seen to extend beyond the rectosigmoid junction. Radiological examination shows a pancolitis with no distinguishing features (Lambert et al 1979). During the acute phase of the disease, rectal biopsy specimens show a non-specific acute infective proctitis pattern (see above) (Lambert et al 1979).

Untreated, the illness generally lasts for less than 10 days, the organism is eliminated within two months and radiological abnormalities resolve within six.

Diagnosis. A diagnosis based on clinical features is confirmed by culture of campylobacter on selective media, serologically by the detection of specific IgM, or by rising titres of IgG antibodies (Watson et al 1979).

Treatment. As the illness is self-limiting in mild cases,

treatment is not necessary unless the patient is a food-handler and likely to infect others. If symptoms are more severe, erythromycin in a dosage of 500 mg twice-daily by mouth for 5 days has proved useful, but resistance to this drug has been reported from Sweden (Taylor et al 1982).

Viruses

Hepatitis A virus is acquired by the faecal-oral route and can be spread amongst homosexual men during sexual activity (Ch. 30).

B. INFECTIONS SPREAD BY MUCOSAL/SKIN CONTACT DURING ANAL INTERCOURSE

Prokaryotes

Neisseria gonorrhoeae

This organism, perhaps the most common pathogen, actual or potential, acquired by anal intercourse (Table 38.6) is considered in detail in Chapters 14 and 15, and only details of rectal infection are considered here.

Clinical features. More than half of men with uncomplicated rectal gonorrhoea are symptomless; the remainder have symptoms and signs of a distal proctitis (Fluker et al 1980, McMillan et al 1983a). Perianal abscess formation and disseminated infection seem to be uncommon complications of untreated rectal gonorrhoea.

Histopathology. In about 60% of infected men the histology of the rectal mucosa is normal; in the remainder there is a generally mild proctitis with no distinguishing features (McMillan et al 1983a).

Diagnosis. Culture of the organism on selective media and identification of isolates by biochemical or immunological methods (Ch. 14) are necessary for reliable diagnosis. Although Gram-negative diplococci can be detected in stained smears of rectal exudate in only about 60% of infected patients (McMillan & Young 1978), it is useful to examine rectal smears with the aim that treatment can be commenced before the patient

Table 38.6 Prevalence of rectal gonorrhoea amongst homosexual men who attended STD clinics.

City	Rectal gonorrhoea			Reference
	Number tested	Number positive	%	
New Orleans	79	26	(32.9)	Owen & Hill (1972)
Chicago, USA	1653	153	(9.3)	Ostrow & Shaskey (1977)
Boston, USA	1533	213	(13.7)	Fiumara (1978)
London, UK	180	26	(14.4)	Munday et al (1981b)
Edinburgh, UK	176	22	(12.5)	McMillan et al (1983b)
Denver, USA	8278	1322	(16.0)	Judson (1984)

leaves the clinic. Although most rectal gonococcal infections will be detected by sampling once, about 5% of infections will not be identified unless a second sample is taken for culture some days later. There seems to be little difference in the isolation rate of gonococci from samples taken through a proctoscope or, blindly, by the passage of a swab through the anal canal (Deherogoda 1977).

Treatment. Some published reports on the treatment of rectal gonorrhoea in homosexual men are given in Table 38.7. In general, single-dose treatment with penicillin is ineffective and courses of antimicrobials are necessary. Although spectinomycin has proved useful, the emergence of resistant strains of gonococci has limited its suitability as drug of first choice in the treatment of rectal disease. Rather limited experience with the newer cephalosporins and ciprofloxacin suggests that these drugs may be of better therapeutic value. At present, we recommend ampicillin in an oral dosage of 500 mg every 6 hours for 5–7 days, or, if the patient is hypersensitive to penicillin, co-trimoxazole 2 tablets twice-daily by mouth for 5 days. Cultures should be obtained 7 and 14 days after completion of treatment to ensure that this has been successful.

Neisseria meningitidis
The significance of rectal infection with *Neisseria meningitidis* of differing serogroups is uncertain. In our experience and that of Judson et al (1978), the organism can be isolated from the rectums of about 2% of homosexual men who attend STD clinics. Janda et al (1980) did not show any correlation between the presence of the organisms and clinical features. The importance of the organism lies in its possible confusion with *N. gonorrhoeae* on culture.

Treponema pallidum
Primary syphilis of the anal margin presents often as a painful, tender, non-indurated ulcer which sometimes bleeds easily on palpation. As the clinical features, unlike those of primary genital lesions, closely resemble those of a traumatic and fissure, it is important to examine by dark-ground microscope — or by a method based on monoclonal antibody (p. 118) — material from any anal ulcer in men who have had receptive anal intercourse.

As many homosexual men with secondary syphilis give no history suggestive of a primary lesion, it is probable that the majority of rectal primary lesions do not produce symptoms. Occasionally patients with serological evidence of primary syphilis present with symptoms of proctitis and single or multiple indurated rectal masses, some of which may be ulcerated, are palpable and visible at proctoscopy (Nazemi et al 1975, Voinchet & Guivarc'h 1980). A diffuse distal proctitis may be part of the secondary stage of the disease (Akdamar et al 1977).

Biopsy specimens of these lesions show a dense infiltration of the lamina propria and submucosa with plasma cells, lymphocytes and histocytes. There is proliferation of the endothelial cells of the capillaries, and crypt abscesses may be a feature. Spirochaetes can sometimes be demonstrated in the lesions by silver staining or immunofluorescence (Quinn et al 1982).

The diagnosis of syphilitic proctitis is best made by proctoscopy backed by the results of serological testing; as profuse haemorrhage may result, biopsy of the lesions is not recommended in clinical practice.

Rectal spirochaetosis
On epithelial surfaces of the large intestine of man and other animals such as monkeys, treponemes of the genus *Brachyspira* (Hovind-Hougen 1982) and flagellated bacteria (family Spirillaceae) may be found; this situation has been referred to as intestinal spirochaetosis (Harland & Lee 1967, Takeuchi et al 1974). Although electronmicroscopy is necessary to distinguish these organisms, their presence in haematoxylin-eosin stained sections is indicated by a basophilic zone about 3 μm in width on the surface of the epithelium. As it is uncertain whether the entire mucosal surface of the intestine is occupied by these organisms, a more appropriate term may be rectal spirochaetosis. Although the condition is found in about 7% of unselected rectal biopsies (Lee et al 1971), McMillan & Lee (1981) detected rectal spirochaetosis in 36% of 100 biopsies

Table 38.7 Recommended first-line treatment schedules for rectal gonorrhoea in homosexual men.

Drug and dose	Cure rate			Reference
	Number treated	Number cured	%	
Ampicillin 250 mg by mouth q.i.d. for 5 days	103	97	(94)	John & Jefferiss (1973)
Co-trimoxazole 2 tablets by mouth twice-daily for 7 days	66	58	(88)	Waugh (1970)
Spectinomycin 2 g intramuscularly	25	25	(100)	Sands (1980)
2 g intramuscularly	56	54	(96)	
Cefuroxime 1.5 g intramuscularly	29	29	(100)	McMillan (1984* data)
Ciprofloxacin 250 mg by mouth	11	11	(100)	McMillan (1985* data)

* unpublished data

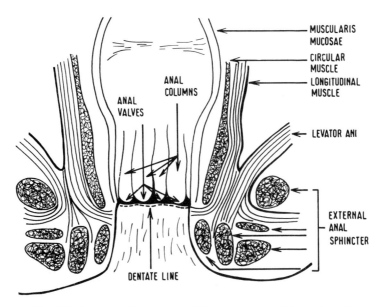

Fig. 38.2 Anatomy of ano-rectum. The mucous coat of the anal canal presents a number of permanent vertical folds known as *anal columns*. Crescentic folds which join the lower ends of the two columns are the *anal valves* and behind each are to be found the pocket-like *anal sinuses*. The pale *dentate line* is the wavy line of attachment of the *levator ani* and can be identified distal to the anal valves.

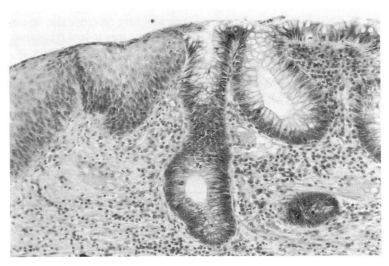

Fig. 38.3 Histology of the rectum transition zone.

defaecation, bleeding during defaecation and, as a result of the pain, he tends to become constipated. The fissure, which is usually situated at the exterior anal margin, appears as a single ulcer, almost triangular in shape. As a chancre may also be painful, it is important to exclude primary syphilis in any homosexual patients with anal fissuring or ulceration (Ch. 8). Furthermore the clinical features of primary and, less frequently, recrudescent anorectal herpes simplex virus infection

may resemble those of acute traumatic anal fissure. Features which assist the physician in reaching a correct diagnosis are summarized in Table 38.9 (McMillan & Smith 1984). In tropical countries, granuloma inguinale and tuberculous ulceration have to be considered in the differential diagnosis (Ch. 35).

Chronic anal fissure produces similar but less severe symptoms. There is usually a single elongated, somewhat indurated ulcer at the posterior anal margin and frequently a skin tag ('sentinel pile') is to be seen at the distal end of the ulcer.

Biopsy of the fissure is indicated only if there is doubt about the nature of the anal ulcer. Histologically, there is ulceration of the squamous epithelium with oedema and dense infiltration of the surrounding tissues with lymphocytes and plasma cells.

The treatment of anal fissure falls within the province of the surgeon, and methods used in management include anal dilatation and sphincterotomy. The topical application of steroid-containing ointments produces no benefit.

Lacerations of the rectal mucosa and perforation of the rectosigmoid junction may occur as a result of traumatic forms of anal intercourse, including fisting and the insertion of foreign bodies (Sohn et al 1977, Barone et al 1983). Bleeding is the cardinal symptom of mucosal lacerations, which may occur at any site within the rectum. Systemic disturbance and abdominal tenderness are not features of tears in the mucosa. However, when there is transmural laceration into the peritoneal cavity, there is usually a sudden onset of abdominal pain which may radiate to the shoulders, rectal bleeding of varying severity and pyrexia. The abdomen does not move with respiration, there is generalized tenderness with guarding and bowel sounds are absent. Radiographs of the abdomen with the patient in the erect position may show air below the diaphragm.

Pelvic cellulitis may occur as a complication of fisting (Weinstein et al 1981). The 3 patients described complained of anorectal pain, abdominal pain and fever which developed 1–7 days after the fisting episode. Although rectal tears were not visible during sigmoidoscopy there was a marked proctitis extending from 7–15 cm from the anal margin. Induration of the tissue between the rectal mucosa and pelvis was also noted in each case. The salient feature at laparotomy, undertaken in one case, was retroperitoneal oedema, particularly around the rectum. It was postulated that the cellulitis may have resulted from extraperitoneal microperforation of the rectum during fisting.

Patients with rectal tears and/or pelvic cellulitis should be treated in hospital in co-operation with surgical colleagues. If the laceration involves the rectal mucosa only, the patient does not usually require surgical treatment other than suture of the tear and blood replacement if needed. He should be observed for signs of further bleeding or intraperitoneal rupture of the rectum. Immediate laparotomy is indicated in patients with transmural laceration with signs of peritonitis. Repair of the tear, proximal colostomy and broad-spectrum antibiotics are required. In cases of pelvic cellulitis, broad spectrum antibiotics should be given, but should there be signs of continuing peritonitis, laparotomy is necessary.

SOLITARY ULCER SYNDROME OF THE RECTUM

This is a condition of young patients, with men and women being affected equally often, the aetiology of which is uncertain. The most common symptom is that of anorectal bleeding, which may be severe; perineal, sacral or iliac fissure pain, tenesmus and a feeling of incomplete defaecation are less common symptoms. At sigmoidoscopy, the characteristic sign is ulceration, which, despite the name of the syndrome, is often multiple. Rounded oval ulcers, usually about 2 cm in diameter (range 2–5 cm), are generally found within 7–10 cm of the anal margin on the anterior or anterolateral wall of the rectum (Madigan & Morson 1969). Typically, the ulcer is only slightly depressed below the surrounding mucosa and the base is covered with a whitish-grey or yellow slough. At the margin is a thin area of hyperaemia. Occasionally the base of the ulcer is granular and the surrounding mucosa is heaped up. A non-ulcerating syndrome is also well-recognized, the mucosa appearing nodular at the site of the lesion.

Histologically, the lamina propria is replaced by fibroblasts and fibrous tissue and smooth muscle fibres which emanate from a thickened muscularis mucosae and stream towards the surface of the mucosa. The mucosal surface shows goblet cell depletion and reactive hyperplasia, and the crypts sometimes show cystic dilatation. When the biopsy is taken from the centre of an ulcer, dense fibrosis of the submucosa is seen with overlying granulation tissue and necrotic cells.

The solitary ulcer syndrome is chronic and ulcers may persist unchanged for many years.

Aetiology

The aetiology of the solitary ulcer syndrome is uncertain. In some patients (Rutter 1975) there is electromyographic evidence of hyperactivity of the puborectalis muscle as is seen in the descending perineum syndrome (Parks et al 1966), and it has been suggested that during defaecation high intra-abdominal pressure forces the anterior wall of the rectum on to the contracted puborectalis. The anterior wall of the rectum may also be forced towards the anal canal with resulting ischaemia. Direct trauma to the rectal mucosa by insertion of the patient's finger into the rectum (self digitation) or the insertion of foreign bodies into the rectum has been suggested as a possible cause of the rectal ulceration (Thomson & Hill 1980). In this respect it is interesting to note that 8 of 234 homosexual men who consecutively attended a STD clinic in Edinburgh had histological changes suggestive of the syndrome viz. thickened muscularis mucosae, streaming of muscle fibres between the crypts, and fibrosis of the lamina propria. In only one of these men was there rectal ulceration.

Treatment

Treatment consists of reassurance about the benign nature of the syndrome and symptomatic therapy if severe bleeding occurs. Exclusion of STD remains a constant medical duty in the case of those at risk.

PERIANAL HAEMATOMA ('THROMBOSED EXTERNAL PILE')

A perianal haematoma is a common problem amongst homosexual men. It presents as a painful swelling of the anal margin often following, or soon after, traumatic receptive anal intercourse. On examination there is a tender dark blue-purple swelling about 2–4 cm in diameter at the anal margin. Although it has been suggested that such lesions arise from rupture of small blood vessels, it seems more likely that it results from clotting within a vein under the non-hairy anal skin (Thomson 1982).

Although the lesion will burst or regress spontaneously, rapid relief can be achieved by opening the vein through a small incision.

PROCTALGIA FUGAX

This condition, whose symptoms may be mistaken for organic disease of the ano-rectum or prostate, is characterized by episodes of sudden onset pain apparently rising deeply within the rectum and lasting a few seconds to several minutes. The pain may occur at any time, but often at night when it awakens the sufferer. There are no abnormal clinical signs and investigation of the bowel shows no evidence of organic disease.

The aetiology is unknown, but the condition may be a variant of the irritable colon syndrome (Harvey 1979).

Treatment consists of reassurance about the benign nature of the proctalgia fugax.

ANORECTAL MALIGNANCY IN HOMOSEXUAL MEN

Neoplasms may arise from: 1. the columnar epithelium of the rectum; 2. the stratified squamous epithelium of the anal canal and anal skin; and 3. from the modified stratified epithelium which lies between the columnar epithelium of the rectum and the stratified squamous epithelium of the anal canal, viz. the transitional zone, a segment of about 0.5 cm in length.

The majority (about 95%) of carcinomas of the rectum are adenocarcinomas, the others being undifferentiated anaplastic tumours and anaplastic mucus-secreting tumours ('signet-ring' cell carcinoma).

Endocrine tumours, secondry tumours, leiomyosarcomas and malignant lymphomas are less commonly found in the rectum.

Squamous cell carcinomas of the anal canal (that is those at the dentate line or above) arise from the transitional zone (cloagenic carcinoma). These carcinomas may be: 1. of the basaloid type whose morphology, but not behaviour, resembles that of basal cell carcinoma of the skin; 2. the transitional cell type; and 3. squamous cell carcinomas of the ordinary type, with considerable variation in their differentiation. Often there is an admixture of the various cell types. Mucoepidermoid carcinomas of the anal canal also arise from the transitional epithelium, but are rare. The carcinomas of the anal margin (that is those situated below the dentate line — Fig. 38.2) are almost invariably well differentiated squamous cell carcinomas. Intra-epidermal squamous cell carcinoma (Bowen's disease) of the skin of the anal region may also be found.

In a study of colonic and rectal diseases in 260 homosexual men, Sohn & Robilotti (1977) noted one case of Bowen's disease and another of squamous cell carcinoma of the anal region. Subsequently, other cases of cloagenic and squamous carcinoma of the anorectum have been reported (Cooper et al 1979, Leach & Ellis 1981, Li et al 1982).

The finding of anorectal carcinomas in homosexual men may be coincidental but it is tempting to speculate for a number of reasons that sexually transmissible agents may play a part in the aetiology. There is an association between cervical cancer and sexual intercourse at an early age and with multiple partners (Ch. 25); and furthermore there is an increased incidence of anal cancer in women with cervical squamous cell carcinomas. In addition, the transitional epithelium of the anal canal and the uterine cervix have a common origin from the embryonic cloagenic membrane. The hypothesis that sexually transmissible agents may play a part in the aetiology is supported by the study undertaken by Daling et al (1982) who showed that two correlates of homosexual behaviour (that is, having had syphilis and never having been married) were related to an increased incidence of anal carcinoma. More recently an association between certain types of human papilloma virus and malignancy of the female genital tract has been described (Ch. 30). Whether or not there is a similar association between anorectal cancer in homosexual men and certain types of HPV is as yet uncertain but anal warts are common amongst men who have had anal intercourse and malignant transformation of these warts has been described (Oriel & Whimster 1971). Recently Croxson and his colleagues (1984) reported the occurrence of intra-epithelial carcinoma in 7 homosexual men with evidence of wart virus infection of the anal region. As 4 of these patients subsequently developed AIDS, it may be that the immunological mechanisms responsible for the clearance of HPV from the body were defective, allowing persistence of infection with malignant transformation of the cells. The host defence mechanisms which operate to eliminate neoplastic cells are not fully understood, but cell-mediated immune responses are probably important. As T4 cells are necessary for the efficient mounting of such responses and as the AIDS retrovirus (Ch. 2) is T4 cell tropic, individuals with HIV infection may be at particular risk for the development of malignant disease (see Ch. 31). Clearly it is a complex subject.

Clinical features of anorectal neoplasia

Patients with anal neoplasm often complain of pain in the anal region, bleeding and anal discharge. Rectal neoplasms often produce painless bleeding, a sensation of incomplete defaecation if the lesion is in the lower part of the rectum, and alteration in bowel habit. Unless seen early, anal neoplasms may first be recognized as deeply ulcerated lesions. The appearance at sigmoidoscopy of rectal carcinomas varies considerably but in general presents as an ulcerated or polypoidal lesion. In all cases anorectal ulceration for which there is no readily-identifiable cause should be referred to a surgical colleague for biopsy.

Treatment

The treatment of anorectal neoplasm falls outside the scope of this book and interested readers are referred to textbooks of anorectal surgery (Goligher 1984).

PERIANAL ABSCESSES, ANAL FISSURES AND HAEMORRHOIDS

The prevalence of these conditions in homosexual and heterosexual men is similar. Abscesses present as painful tender perianal swellings which, unless small, require surgical drainage. Anal fistulae result from internal and external rupture of anal abscesses. Their internal orifice is often difficult to locate, but sometimes the fistulous tract can be palpated. The treatment of anal fistulae, which is often difficult, falls within the province of the surgeon. Similarly symptomatic haemorrhoids warrant surgical referral. It should be noted that the haemorrhoids may not be the cause of the patient's anorectal symptoms and that a careful rectal examination is necessary.

METAPLASTIC POLYPS

A common sigmoidoscopic finding in men and women of all ages is the presence of discoid nodules of only a few millimetres in size projecting from the mucosa. They are of the same colour as the surrounding mucosa and are seldom pedunculated. Histologically there is lengthening of the crypts which are dilated and their epithelium becomes flattened or papillary. The number of goblet cells is diminished (Morson 1978).

Using histochemical or immunohistological methods, metaplastic polyps show increased expression of carcino-embryonic antigen, reduced secretion of O-acylated sialomucin, reduced activity of cytoplasmic enzymes, and absent secretory IgA activity. As these changes are found commonly in adenomas with dysplastic changes, Jass (1983) has suggested that, although of no significance to the individual, they should be regarded as being markers of a population at high risk for the development of rectal carcinoma. This view is challenged by Rognum & Brandtzaeg (1983), who suggest that these polyps may reflect proliferative activity unrelated to oncogenesis.

Metaplastic polyps should be regarded as benign lesions which do not produce symptoms, and removal is not indicated. The management of other polyps, which may occasionally be found in homosexual men (Sohn & Robilotti 1977), falls outside the scope of the physician, and referral to a surgeon is indicated.

NOTES TO CHAPTER 38

Note 38.1: Preparation of saline mount of faeces for parasite detection

About 2 mg of faeces is collected at the end of a wooden applicator stick and emulsified in a drop (about 0.05 ml) of saline (8 g per l) at the centre of a clean microscope slide (the consistency of the resulting preparation should be such that print can be discerned through it). The drop is covered by a 22 × 22 mm cover-slip of No.1 thickness. After scanning at ×100 magnification, detailed microscopy for trophozoites, cysts, ova and larvae is undertaken at ×400 magnification.

Note 38.2: Trichrome-stained preparation of fresh or preserved specimens of faeces

The distal end of a wooden applicator stick is charged with a small quantity of faeces, which is then deposited about 2 cm from the narrow edge of a clean microscope slide. Using the middle section of the stick, the sample is spread thinly and evenly along the slide. Immediately after the preparation of the smear, the slide is fixed for 30 minutes in Schaudinn's fluid (saturated aqueous solution of mercuric chloride about 70 gl⁻ — 40 ml; absolute ethanol — 20 ml; glacial acetic acid, added just before use — 3 ml) and then stained as shown in the schedule. The fixative stain, alcohols and xylene are conveniently kept in Coplin jars.

1. Ethanol 70%   (5 min)
2. Ethanol 70% with iodine   (5 min)
3. Ethanol 70%, two changes   (5 min)
4. Stain with Trichrome stain*   (30 min)
5. 90% ethanol containing 1% v/v glacial acetic   (3 s)
   acid
6. Absolute ethanol   (3 s)
7. Absolute ethanol, two changes   (5 min)
8. Xylene (2 changes)   (3 min)
9. Mount in DPX

*Stain (Wheatley 1951)
   Chromotrope 2R   0.6 g
   Light green SF   0.3 g
   12-Tungstophosphoric acid   0.7 g
   Glacial acetic acid   1.0 ml
   Distilled water   100 ml

The acetic acid is added to the dry stains, and after 30 minutes the distilled water is added.

Note 38.3: Concentration of flagellate and amoebic cysts in faeces

A modification of the Ridley & Hagwood (1956) method is used routinely in our laboratory:

With a wooden spatula about 5 g of faeces are mixed with 10 ml of 10% (v/v) formalin.

The suspension is strained through a single-layer cotton gauze swab (Vernaid, Vernon-Carus Ltd., Preston, England, UK) into a conical centrifuge tube.

About 3 ml of diethyl ether* are added and the tube is shaken vigorously about 50 times to extract fat from the sample. After centrifugation at 600 g for 1 minute, the fatty

plug at the interface of the ether and formalin is loosened with a wooden applicator stick, and this and the liquid centres of the tube are discarded into disinfectant (Kirbyclor, Kirby, Warwick, England, UK).

With a pasteur pipette the sediment is mixed with a few drops of iodine solution (see above) and a wet-mount of the mixture is prepared.

*Diethyl ether is highly inflammable and over a period of months of storage forms explosive peroxides; ethyl acetate is a satisfactory alternative.

Note 38.4: Diamond's medium

Diamond's medium TY-5-33 (Diamond et al 1978) consists of trypticase, yeast extract, glucose, L-cysteine hydrochloride supplemented with vitamins, iron, and bovine serum.

Note 38.5: Giemsa's method for staining trophozoites of Giardia intestinalis

Smears are fixed in absolute methanol for 1 minute, air dried, and stained in Giemsa's stock stain (British Drug Houses, Poole, UK) diluted 1:20 with phosphate buffered water (pH 7.2)* for 30–45 minutes. After rinsing briefly in phosphate-buffered solution the slides are air dried.

* $NaH_2PO_4.2H_2O$ (0.2 M)   140 ml
  Na_2HPO_4 (0.2M)   360 ml
  Distilled water   to 1000 ml

Note 38.6: Enterotest in giardiasis

In in the enterotest a long thread is packed in a gelatin pharmaceutical capsule. The free end of the thread protruding from the capsule is fixed with adhesive tape to the corner of the mouth and the capsule swallowed. Within 3–4 hours much of the line is extended to the duodenum or jejunum. It is then withdrawn and the bile-stained mucus is scraped off and immediately examined microscopically (Kulda & Nohynkova 1978).

Note 38.7: Preserving faeces for later microscopy

Polyvinyl alcohol (PVA)/fixative (Brooke & Goldman 1949) is used

   Mercuric chloride saturated solution in water
   (2 pts)/95% ethanol (1 pt)   93.5 ml
   Glycerol   1.5 ml
   Glacial acetic acid   5.0 ml
   Polyvinyl alcohol (Sigma Type II low MW) 5.0 g

PVA is added with continuous stirring to the rest of the ingredients and heated slowly to about 75°C; when water-clear, 5 ml quantities are dispensed in wide-mouthed screw-capped containers. These will remain effective for about 6 months if stored at room temperatures. With an applicator stick, about 1 ml of faeces is mixed with the 5 ml of PVA/fixative in the container; this preparation will remain satisfactory for microscopy for several months. When convenient, a little of the suspension is pipetted on to a clean paper towel and, after a few minutes when most of the fluid has been absorbed, smears are made on slides using an applicator stick.

After drying the smears overnight at 37°C, they are stained as in Note 38.5.

Note 38.8: Staining schedule for *Cryptosporidium* spp

a. Carbol-fuchsin method
 1. Fix in methanol   (3 min)
 2. Fix in formaldehyde vapour (cotton-   (20 min)
    wool ball soaked in formalin staining
    dish at 37°C)
 3. Carbol-fuchsin   (5 min)
 4. Differentiate in H_2SO_4 10% v/v

 5. Rinse in tap water
 6. Counterstain in malachite green 5%   (5 min)
    w/v
 7. Rinse in tap water
 8. Blot dry
 9. Mount in DPX

b. Giemsa method
 1. Fix in methanol   (3 min)
 2. Stain in Giemsa*   (1 h)
 3. Rinse in tap water
 4. Blot dry
 5. Mount in DPX

*Giemsa stain

Giemsa stain (BDH)	1 ml
Methanol	1.25 ml
Aqueous sodium carbonate (1.4% w/v)	0.05 ml
Tap water	40 ml

REFERENCES

I. INFECTIONS

Akdamar K, Martin R J, Ichinose H 1977 Syphilitic proctitis. Digestive Diseases 22: 701–704

Anderson B C, Donndelinger T, Wilkins R M, Smith J 1982 Cryptosporidiosis in a veterinary student. Journal of the American Veterinary Medical Association 180: 408–409

Beal C B, Viens P, Grant R G L, Hughes J M 1970 A new technique for sampling duodenal contents. Demonstration of upper small-bowel pathogens. American Journal of Tropical Medicine and Hygiene 19: 349–352

Bird R G, Smith M D 1980 Cryptosporidiosis in man: parasite life cycle and fine structural pathology. Journal of Pathology 132: 217–233

Blaser M J, Berkowitz I D, LaForce F M, Cravens J, Reller L B. Wang W-L L 1979 Campylobacter enteritis: clinical and epidemiological features. Annals of Internal Medicine 91: 179–185

Blaser M J, Checko P, Bopp C, Bruce A, Hughes J M 1982 *Campylobacter* enteritis associated with.foodborne transmission. American Journal of Epidemiology 116: 886–894

Bolan R K, Sands M, Schachter J, Miner R C, Drew W L 1982 Lymphogranuloma venereum and acute ulcerative proctitis. American Journal of Medicine 72: 703–706

Bowie W R, Alexander E R, Holmes K K 1978 Etiologies of post gonococcal urethritis in homosexual and heterosexual men: roles of *Chlamydia trachomatis* and *Ureaplasma urealyticum*. Sexually Transmitted Diseases 5: 151–154

Brooke M M, Goldman M 1949 Polyvinyl alcohol-fixative as a preservative and adhesive for protozoa in dysenteric stools and other liquid materials. Journal of Laboratory and Clinical Medicine 34: 1554–1560

Burnham W R, Reeve R S, Finch R G 1980 *Entamoeba histolytica* infection in male homosexuals. Gut 21: 1097–1099

Carvalho-Filho E 1978 Strongyloidiasis. Clinics in Gastroenterology 7/1: 179–200

Casemore D P, Jackson B 1983 Sporadic cryptosporidiosis in children. Correspondence, Lancet ii: 679

Casemore D P, Jackson F B 1984 Hypothesis:

cryptosporidiosis in human beings is not primarily a zoonosis. Journal of Infection 9: 153–156

Chin A T L, Gerken A 1984 Carriage of intestinal protozoal cysts in homosexuals. British Journal of Venereal Diseases 60: 193–195

Cotton D W K, Kirkham N, Hicks D A 1984 Rectal spirochaetosis. British Journal of Venereal Diseases 60: 106–109

Current W L, Reese N C, Ernst J V, Bailey W S, Heyman M B, Weinstein W M 1983 Human cryptosporidiosis in immunocompetent and immunodeficient persons. Studies of an outbreak and experimental transmission. New England Journal of Medicine 308: 1252–1257

Curry J P, Embil J A, Williams C N. Manuel F R 1978 Proctitis associated with *Herpesvirus hominis* type 2 infection. Canadian Medical Association Journal 119: 485–486

Deherogoda P 1977 Diagnosis of rectal gonorrhoea by blind anorectal swabs compared with direct vision swabs taken via a proctoscope. British Journal of Venereal Diseases 53: 311–313

Diamond L S, Harlow D R, Cunnick C C 1978 A new medium for the axenic cultivation of *Entamoeba histolytica* and other *Entamoeba*. Transactions of the Royal Society of Tropical Medicine and Hygiene 72: 431–432

Douglas J G, Crucioli V 1981 Spirochaetosis: a remediable cause of diarrhoea and rectal bleeding. British Medical Journal 283: 1362

Dritz S K, Ainsworth T E, Garrard W F, Back A, Palmer R D, Boucher L A, River E 1977 Patterns of sexually transmitted enteric diseases in a city. Lancet ii: 3–4

Fiumara N J 1978 The treatment of gonococcal proctitis. An evaluation of 173 patients with 4g of spectinomycin. Journal of the American Medical Association 239: 735–737

Fluker J L, Deherogoda P, Platt D J, Gerken A 1980 Rectal gonorrhoea in male homosexuals: presentation and therapy. British Journal of Venereal Diseases 56: 397–399

Garcia L S, Ash L C 1979 Diagnostic Parasitology. Clinical Laboratory Manual, C V Mosby Company, St. Louis

Gathiram V, Jackson T F H G 1985 Frequency distribution

of Entamoeba histolytica zymodemes in a rural South African population. Lancet i: 719–721

Goldmeier D 1980 Proctitis and herpes simplex virus in homosexual men. British Journal of Venereal Diseases 56: 111–114

Goldmeier D, Sargeaunt P G, Price A J et al 1986 Is Entamoeba histolytica in homosexual men a pathogen? Lancet i: 641–644

Goodell S E, Quinn T C, Mkrtichian E, Schuffler M D, Holmes K K, Corey L 1983 Herpes simplex virus proctitis in homosexual men. Clinical, sigmoidoscopic and histopathologic features. New England Journal of Medicine 308: 868–871

Green E L, Miles M A, Warhurst D C 1985 Immunodiaonostic detection of Giardia antigen in faeces by a rapid visual enzyme-linked immunosorbent assay. Lancet ii: 691–693

Harland W A, Lee F D 1967 Intestinal spirochaetosis. British Medical Journal iii: 718–719, Plate between pages 708 & 709

Hart C A, Baxby D, Blundell N 1984 Gastro-enteritis due to Cryptosporidium: a prospective survey in a children's hospital. Journal of Infection 9: 264–270

Hartong W A, Gourley W K, Arvanitakis C 1979 Giardiasis: clinical spectrum and functional-structural abnormalities of the small intestinal mucosa. Gastroenterology 77: 61–69

Henriksen Sv Aa, Pohlenz J E L 1981 Staining of Cryptosporidia by a modified Ziehl-Neelsen technique. Acta Veterinaria Scandanavica 22: 594–596

Holten-Andersen W, Gerstoft J, Henriksen Sv Aa, Pedersen N S 1984 Prevalence of Cryptosporidium among patients with acute enteric infection. Journal of Infection 9: 277–282

Hovind-Hougen K, Birch-Andersen A, Henrik-Nielsen R et al 1982 Intestinal spirochaetosis: morphological characterization and cultivation of the spirochaete Brachyspira aalborgi gen. nov. sp. nov. Journal of Clinical Microbiology 16: 1127–1136

Højlying N, Mølbak K, Jepsen S, Hansson A P 1984 Cryptosporidiosis in Liberian children. Lancet i: 734

Hunt D A, Shannon R, Palmer S R, Jephcott A E 1984 Cryptosporidiosis in an urban community. British Medical Journal 289: 814–816

Janda W M, Bohnhoff M, Morello J A, Lerner S A 1980 Prevalence and site-pathogen studies of Neisseria meningitidis and N. gonorrhoeae in homosexual men. Journal of the American Medical Association 244: 2060–2064

Jeanes A L 1969 Evaluation in clinical practice of the fluorescent amoebic antibody test. Journal of Clinical Pathology 22: 427–429

John J, Jefferiss F J G 1973 Treatment of anorectal gonorrhoea with ampicillin. British Journal of Venereal Diseases 49: 362–363

Jokipii L, Pohjola S, Jokipii A M M 1983 Cryptosporidium: a frequent finding in patients with gastro-intestinal symptoms. Lancet ii: 358–361

Jones D M, Robinson D A 1981 Occupational exposure to Campylobacter jejuni infection. Correspondence, Lancet i: 440–441

Judson F N 1984 Infections with pathogenic Neisseria in homosexual men. In: Ma P, Armstrong D (eds) The acquired immune deficiency syndrome and infections of homosexual men. Yorke Medical Books, USA, p 26–39

Judson F N, Ehret J M, Eickhoff T C 1978 Anogenital infection with Neisseria meningitidis in homosexual men. Journal of Infectious Diseases 137: 458–463

Juniper K, Worrell C L, Minshew M C, Roth L S, Cypert H, Lloyd R E 1972 Serologic diagnosis of amebiasis. American Journal of Tropical Medicine and Hygiene 21: 157–168

Kamath K R, Murugasu R A 1974 A comparative study of four methods for detecting Giardia lamblia in children with diarrheal disease and malabsorption. Gastroenterology 66: 16–21

Kessel J F, Lewis W P, Pasquel C M, Turner J A 1965 Indirect hemagglutination and complement fixation tests in amebiasis. American Journal of Tropical Medicine and Hygiene 14: 540–550

Keystone J S, Keystone D L, Proctor E M 1980 Intestinal parasitic infections in homosexual men: prevalence, symptoms and factors in transmission. Canadian Medical Association Journal 123: 512–514

Kulda J, Nohynkova E 1978 Intestinal flagellates. In: Kreir J (ed) Parasitic protozoa, vol II. Academic Press, London, p 103

Kumar N B, Nostrant T T, Appelman H D 1982 The histopathologic spectrum of acute self-limited colitis (acute infectious-type colitis). American Journal of Surgical Pathology 6: 523–529

Lambert M E, Schofield P F, Ironside A G, Mandal B K 1979 Campylobacter colitis. British Medical Journal 1: 857–859

Lasser K H, Lewin K J, Ryning F W 1979 Cryptosporidial enteritis in a patient with congenital hypogammaglobulinemia. Human Pathology 10: 234–240

Lee F D, Krazewski A, Gordon J, Howie J G R, McSeveney D, Harland W A 1971 Intestinal spirochaetosis. Gut 12: 126–133

McGowan K, Deneke C F, Thorne G M, Gorbach S L 1982 Entamoeba histolytica cytotoxin: purification, characterization, strain virulence and protease activity. Journal of Infectious Diseases 146: 616–625

McMillan A, Gilmour H M, McNeillage Gillian, Scott G R 1984a Amoebiasis in homosexual men. Gut 25: 356–360

McMillan A, Sommerville R G, McKie P M K 1981 Chlamydial infection in homosexual men: frequency of isolation of Chlamydia trachomatis from the urethra, anorectum and pharynx. British Journal of Venereal Diseases 57: 47–49

McMillan A, McNeillage G J C 1984 Comparison of the sensitivity of microscopy and culture in the laboratory diagnosis of intestinal protozoal infection. Journal of Clinical Pathology 37: 809–811

McMillan A, Young H 1978 Gonorrhea in the homosexual man. Frequency of infection by culture site. Sexually Transmitted Diseases 5: 146–150

McMillan A, McNeillage G, Gilmour H, Lee F D 1983a Histology of rectal gonorrhoea in men, with a note on anorectal infection with Neisseria meningitidis. Journal of Clinical Pathology 36: 511–514

McMillan A 1980 Intestinal parasites in homosexual men. Scottish Medical Journal 25: 33–35

McMillan A, Smith I W 1984 Painful anal ulceration in homosexual men. British Journal of Surgery 71: 215–216

McMillan A, Gilmour H M, Slatford K, McNeillage G J C 1983b Proctitis in homosexual men. A diagnostic problem. British Journal of Venereal Diseases 59: 260–264

McMillan A, Lee F D 1981 Sigmoidoscopic and microscopic appearance of the rectal mucosa in homosexual men. Gut 22: 1035–1041

McMillan A, McNeillage G J C, Watson K C 1984b The prevalence of antibodies reactive with Campylobacter jejuni in the serum of homosexual men. Journal of Infection 9: 63–68

Maddison S E, Powell S J, Elsdon-Dewar R 1965 Application of serology to the epidemiology of amebiasis. American Journal of Tropical Medicine and Hygiene 14: 554–557

Mandal B K, Schofield P F, Morson B C 1982 A clinicopathological study of acute colitis: the dilemma of transient colitis syndrome. Scandinavian Journal of Gastroenterology 17: 865–869

Markell E K, Havens R F, Kuritsubo R A, Wingerd J 1984 Intestinal protozoa in homosexual men of the San Francisco Bay Area: prevalence and correlates of infection. American Journal of Tropical Medicine and Hygiene 33: 239–245

Martinez-Palomo A 1983 Parasite factors of virulence. In: The biology of Entamoeba histolytica. Research Studies Press, Chichester, Ch 6

Mattern C F T, Keister D B 1977 Experimental amebiasis. II Hepatic amebiasis in the newborn hamster. American Journal of Tropical medicine and Hygiene 26: 402–411

Meisel J L, Perera D R, Meligro C, Rubin C E 1976 Overwhelming watery diarrhea associated with a Cryptosporidium in an immunosuppressed patient. Gastroenterology 70: 1156–1160

Mentzing L-O 1981 Waterborne outbreaks of Campylobacter enteritis in Central Sweden. Lancet ii: 352–354

Meyers J D, Kuharic H A, Holmes K K 1977 Giardia lamblia infection in homosexual men. British Journal of Venereal Diseases 53: 54–55

Mindel A 1983 Lymphogranuloma venereum of the rectum in a homosexual man. British Journal of Venereal Diseases 59: 196–197

Munday P E, Thomas B J, Johnson A P, Altman D G, Taylor-Robinson D 1981a Clinical and micrcbiolcoical study of non-gonoccal urethritis with particular reference to non-chlamydial disease. British Journal of Venereal Diseases 57: 327–333

Munday P E, Dawson S G, Johnson A P et al 1981b A microbiological study of non-gonococcal proctitis in passive male homosexuals. Postgraduate Medical Journal 57: 705–711

Nanda R, Baveju U, Anand B S 1984 Entamoeba histolytica cyst passers: clinical features and outcome in untreated subjects. Lancet ii: 301–303

Nazemi M M, Musher D M, Schell R F, Milo S 1975 Syphilitic proctitis in a homosexual. Journal of the American Medical Association 231: 389

Nime F A, Burek J D, Page D L, Holscher M A, Yardley J H 1976 Acute erterocolitis in a human being infected with the protozoan Cryptosporidium. Gastroenterology 70: 592–598

Oriel J D, Reeve P, Wright J T, Owen J 1976 Chlamydial infection of the male rectum. British Journal of Venereal Diseases 52: 46–51

Ostrow D G, Shaskey D M 1977 The experience of the Howard Brown Memorial Clinic of Chicago with sexually transmitted diseases. Sexually Transmitted Diseases 4: 53–55

Owen R L, Hill J L 1972 Rectal and pharyngeal gonorrhea in homosexual men. Journal of the American Medical Association 220: 1315–1318

Phillips S C, Mildvan D, Williams D C, Gelb A M, White M C 1981 Sexual transmission of enteric protozoa and helminths in a venereal-disease-clinic population. New England Journal of Medicine 305: 603–606

Pittman F E, Hennigar G R, Charleston S C 1974

Sigmoidoscopic and colonic mucosal biopsy findings in amebic colitis. Archives of Pathology 97: 155–158

Prathap K, Gilman R 1970 The histopathology of acute intestinal amebiasis. A rectal biopsy study. American Journal of Pathology 60: 229–246

Purpon I, Jimenez D, Engelking R L 1967 Amebiasis of the penis. Journal of Urology 98: 372–374

Quinn T C, Goodell S E, Mkrtichian PA-C, Schuffler M D, Wang S-P, Stamm W E, Holmes K K 1981 Chlamydia trachomatis proctitis. New England Journal of Medicine 305: 195–200

Quinn T C, Lukehart S A, Goodell S, Mkrtichian E, Schuffler M D, Holmes K K 1982 Rectal mass caused by Treponema pallidum: confirmation by immunofluorescent staining. Gastroenterology 82: 135–139

Quinn T C, Stamm W E, Goodell S E et al 1983 The polymicrobial origin of intestinal infections in homosexual men. New England Journal of Medicine 309: 576–582

Quinn T C, Goodell S E, Fennell C et al 1984 Infections with Campylobacter jejuni or Campylobacter-like organisms in homosexual men. Annals of Internal Medicine 101: 187–192

Ridley D S, Hagwood B C 1956 The value of formol-ether concentration of faecal cysts and ova. Journal of Clinical Pathology 9: 74–76

Ridley M J, Ridley D S 1976 Serum antibodies and jejunal histology in giardiasis associated with malabsorption. Journal of Clinical Pathology 29: 30–34

Robinson D A, Jones D M 1981 Milk-borne campylobacter infection. British Medical Journal 282: 1374–1376

Root D M, Cole F X, Williamson J A 1978 The development and standardization of an Elisa method for the detection of Entamoeba histolytica antigens in fecal samples. Archivos de Investigacion Medica 9: 203–210

Sands M 1980 Treatment of anorectal gonorrhea infections in men. Journal of the American Medical Association 243: 1143–1144

Sargeaunt P G, Jackson T F H G, Simjee A 1982 Biochemical homogeneity of Entamoeba histolytica isolates especially those from liver abscess. Lancet i: 1386–1388

Sargeaunt P G, Oates J K, MacLennan I, Oriel J D, Goldmeier D 1983 Entamoeba histolytica in male homosexuals. British Journal of Venereal Diseases 59: 193–195

Sargeaunt P G, Baveja V K, Nanda R, Anand B S 1984 Influence of geographical factors in the distribution of pathogenic zymodemes of Entamoeba histolytica: identification of zymodeme XIV in India. Transactions of the Royal Society of Tropical Medicine and Hygiene 78: 96–101

Schachter J 1981 Confirmatory serodiagnosis of lymphogranuloma venereum proctitis may yield false-positive results due to other chlamydial infections of the rectum. Sexually Transmitted Diseases 8: 26–27

Schmerin M J, Jones T C, Klein H 1978 Giardiasis association with homosexuality. Annals of Internal Medicine 88: 801–803

Sider L, Mintzer R A, Mendelson E B, Rogers L F, Degesys G E 1982 Radiographic findings of infectious proctitis in homosexual men. American Journal of Roentgenology 139: 667–671

Simmons P D, Tabaqchali S 1979 Campylobacter species in male homosexuals. British Journal of Venereal Diseases 55: 66

Smith P D, Gillin F D, Brown W R, Nash T E 1981 IgG antibody to Giardia lamblia detected by enzyme-linked immunosorbent assay. Gastroenterology 80: 1476–1480

Soave P, Danner R L, Honig C L, Ma P, Hart C C, Nash T, Roberts R B 1984 Cryptosporidiosis in homosexual men. Annals of Internal Medicine 100: 504–511

Sorvilloi F, Mori K, Sewake W, Fishman L 1983 Sexual transmission of *Strongyloides stercoralis* among homosexual men. Correspondence, British Journal of Venereal Diseases 59: 342

Stamm W E 1984 Proctitis due to *Chlamydia trachomatis*. In: Ma P, Armstrong D (eds) The acquired immune deficiency syndrome and infections of homosexual men. Yorke Medical Books, USA, p 40–47

Takeuchi A, Jarvis H R, Nakazawa H, Robinson D M 1974 Spiral-shaped organisms on the surface colonic epithelium of the monkey and man. American Journal of Clinical Nutrition 27: 1287–1296

Taylor D E, DeGrandis S A, Karmali M A et al 1982 Erythromycin resistance in Campylobacter jejuni. In: Newell D G (ed) Campylobacter epidemiology pathogenesis and biochemistry. MTP Press, Baltimore, p 211–213

Thompson J E, Freischlag J, Thomas D S 1983 Amebic liver abscess in a homosexual man. Sexually Transmitted Diseases 10: 153–155

Ungar B L P, Yolken R H, Nash T E, Quinn T C 1984 Enzyme-linked immunosorbent assay for the detection of *Giardia lamblia* in fecal specimens. Journal of Infectious Diseases 149: 90–97

Ungar B L P, Yolken R H, Quinn T C 1985 Use of a monoclonal antibody in an enzyme immunoassay for the detection of *Entamoeba histolytica* in fecal specimens. American Journal of Tropical Medicine and Hygiene 34: 465–472

Voinchet O, Quivarc'h M 1980 Chancre syphilitique simulant un cancer du rectum. Gastroenterologie Clinique et Biologique 4: 134–136

Watson K C, Kerr E J C, McFadzean S M 1979 Serology of human campylobacter infections. Journal of Infection i: 151–158

Watts J McK, Thompson H, Goligher J C 1966 Sigmoidoscopy and cytology in the detection of microscopic disease of the rectal mucosa in ulcerative colitis. Gut 7: 288–294

Waugh M A 1970 Trimethoprim-sulphamethoxazole (Septrin) in the treatment of rectal gonorrhoea. British Journal of Venereal Diseases 47: 34–35

Waugh M A 1972 Threadworm infestation in homosexuals. Transactions of the St Johns' Hospital Dermatological Society 58: 224–225

Wheatley W B 1951 A rapid staining procedure for intestinal amoebae and flagellates. American Journal of Clinical Pathology 21: 990–991

William D C, Shookhoff H B, Felman Y M, DeRamos S W 1978 High rates of enteric protozoal infections in selected homosexual men attending a venereal disease clinic. Sexually Transmitted Diseases 5: 155–157

Wolfe M S 1975 Giardiasis. Journal of the American Medical Association 233: 1362–1365

Wright S G, Tomkins A M, Ridley D S 1977 Giardiasis: clinical and therapeutic aspects. Gut 18: 343–350

II. TRAUMATIC, NEOPLASTIC AND OTHER NON-INFECTIVE CONDITIONS

Barone J E, Yee J, Nealon T F 1983 Management of foreign bodies and trauma of the rectum. Surgery, Gynecology and Obstetrics 156: 453–457

Cooper H S, Patchefsky A S, Marks G 1979 Cloagenic carcinoma of the anorectum in homosexual men: an observation of four cases. Diseases of the colon and rectum 22: 557–558

Croxson T, Chabon A B, Rorat E, Barash I M 1984 Intraepithelial carcinoma of the anus in homosexual men. Diseases of the Colon and Rectum 27: 325–329

Daling J R, Weiss N S, Klopfenstein L L, Cochran L E, Chow W H, Daifuku R 1982 Correlates of homosexual behavior and the incidence of anal cancer. Journal of the American Medical Association 247: 1988–1990

Goligher J 1984 Surgery of the anus rectum and colon, 5th edn. Bailliere Tindall, London

Harvey R F 1979 Colonic motility in proctalgia fugax. Lancet ii: 713–714

Jass J R 1983 Relation between metaplastic polyp and carcinoma of the colorectum. Lancet i: 28–29

Leach R D, Ellis H 1981 Carcinoma of the rectum in male homosexuals. Journal of the Royal Society of Medicine 74: 490–491

Li F P, Osborn D, Cronin C M 1982 Anorectal squamous carcinoma in two homosexual men. Lancet ii: 391

Madigan M R, Morson B C 1969 Solitary ulcer of the rectum. Gut 10: 871–881

McMillan A, Smith I W 1984 Painful anal ulceration in homosexual men. British Journal of Surgery 71: 215–216

Morson B C 1978 The large intestine. In Symmers H S T C (ed) Systemic pathology, 2nd edn. Churchill Livingstone, Edinburgh, p 1136

Oriel J D, Whimster J W 1971 Carcinoma in situ associated with virus-containing anal warts. British Journal of Dermatology 84: 71–73

Parks A G, Porter N H, Hardcastle J 1966 The syndrome of the descending perineum. Proceedings of the Royal Society of Medicine 59: 477–482

Rognum T O, Brandtzaeg P 1983 How reliable in terms of oncogenic development are functional markers of colorectal cancer. Lancet i: 239: 37

Rutter K R P 1975 Solitary rectal ulcer syndrome. Proceedings of the Royal Society of Medicine 68: 22–26

Sohn N, Weinstein M A, Gonchar J 1977 Social injuries of the rectum. American Journal of Surgery 134: 611–612

Sohn N, Robilotti J G 1977 The gay bowel syndrome. A review of colonic and rectal conditions in 200 male homosexuals. American Journal of Gastroenterology 67: 478–484

Thomson H, Hill D 1980 Solitary rectal ulcer: always a self-induced condition? British Journal of Surgery 67: 784–785

Thomson H 1982 The real nature of 'perianal haematoma'. Lancet ii: 467–468

Weinstein M A, Sohn N, Robbins R D 1981 Syndrome of pelvic cellulitis following rectal sexual trauma. American Journal of Gastroenterology 75: 380–381

Index